POLYPLOIDY

Biological Relevance

BASIC LIFE SCIENCES
Alexander Hollaender, General Editor
Associated Universities, Inc.
Washington, D.C.

POLYPLOIDY
Biological Relevance

Edited by

Walter H. Lewis

Washington University
St. Louis, Missouri

PLENUM PRESS · NEW YORK AND LONDON

Library of Congress Cataloging in Publication Data

International Conference on Polyploidy; Biology Relevance, Washington University, 1979.
   Polyploidy, biological relevance.

   Includes index.
   1. Polyploidy—Congresses. I. Lewis, Walter Hepworth. II. Title. [DNLM: 1. Polyploidy—Congresses. QH461 1612p 1979]

QH461.I57 1979	575.2'92	80-91

ISBN 0-306-40358-7

Proceedings of the International Conference on Polyploidy: Biological Relevance,
held at Washington University, St. Louis, Missouri, May 24—27, 1979

© 1980 Plenum Press, New York
A Division of Plenum Publishing Corporation
227 West 17th Street, New York, N.Y. 10011

Printed in the United States of America

PREFACE

———

      Polyploidy as a dramatic mutational event in the process of
evolution has wide implications in nature and for the generation
of new and improved crops. The three day Conference on POLYPLOIDY:
BIOLOGICAL RELEVANCE focused on three aspects of this natural
phenomenon: the first emphasized the characteristics of polyploidy,
the second described the occurrence of polyploidy among plants
and animals, and the third considered past and future areas of
both fundamental and pragmatic research that involve polyploidy.
      New information relative to origin, cytogenetics, ecology,
physiology, biochemistry, and populational studies stress the
need to reexamine current views on the origins of polyploidy and
its significance among both plants and animals. There are major
differences in the occurrence of polyploidy between plant
groups and it is proving a much more common event among bisexual
vertebrates than heretofore considered possible. Crop development
and improvement must utilize approaches based fundamentally on
more natural systems; in fact future research should focus more
on polyploidy as a natural phenomenon that needs study at all
levels of endeavor from field-oriented populational aspects to
sophisticated molecular analyses and genome manipulations.
      This volume provides a summary of current knowledge of
polyploidy pertinent to botanists, zoologists, and agriculturists
who are interested in the evolution of natural systems and who
are concerned with the contribution that crop improvement can
make to human well-being.

                              Walter H. Lewis

St. Louis, Missouri
October, 1979

                              v

ACKNOWLEDGMENTS

The Host Committee thanks all speakers and moderators for their generous contribution to the Conference and to this volume. Their active and enthusiastic participation during the initial organizational phase and at the meeting in St. Louis, and their prompt perparation of manuscripts made the Committee's work a distinct pleasure. The Committee acknowledges the generous support from four sponsoring institutions: Monsanto Agricultural Products Company, St. Louis, National Science Foundation (DEB 7095121), Washington, D.C., University of Missouri at St. Louis, and Washington University. Their financial support was essential. The Committee also thanks those who labored throughout the Conference, particularly Dr. Memory Elvin-Lewis, Ms. Memoria Lewis, Dr. Prathibha Vinay, and Mr. Vincent Zenger.

Finally, the Editor acknowledges the dedication of staff members from the Department of Biology, Washington University, in the preparation of this volume for publication. He thanks in particular Ms. Linda Howard for her careful typing during many hours of extra time and effort.

CONTENTS

PART I

POLYPLOIDY IN PLANT EVOLUTION

ORIGINS OF POLYPLOIDS

J.M.J. deWet

Crop Evolution Laboratory, Department of Agronomy
University of Illinois
Urbana, IL 61801

Polyploidy is a conspicuous feature of chromosomal evolution
in higher plants. Stebbins (1) estimates that between 30 and 35
percent of flowering plant species have gametic chromosome numbers
in multiples of the basic number characteristic of the genus to which
they belong. Polyploidy is common in some groups and rare or absent
in others. Levin and Wilson (2) calculate that relative increase
in chromosome diversity in woody angiosperms is about 14% that of
herbaceous angiosperms. Habit, habitat and the breeding system
seem to contribute to origin and success of polyploids.

WHAT CONSTITUTES A POLYPLOID

Polyploidy is a process not an event. Polyploid evolution is
characterized by aneuploidy superimposed on waves of polyploidy.
What is recognized as a diploid at the generic level may represent
an ancient polyploid at higher levels of taxonomic categories.
Common polyploid series in the Poaceae are based on n=5, 6, 7, 8
or 9. In the tribe Andropogoneae, however, species with 2n=20 or
2n=36 regularly behave cytogenetically as diploids. Genera based
on n=5 or 9 are rare. As a general definition, polyploids combine
three or more basic genomes of the taxonomic group to which they
belong. From a practical point of view this concept is better
limited to the generic level. The basic diploid chromosome number
in the grass genus Sorghum is 2n=20, and individuals or species
with 2n=40 behave cytogenetically as tetraploids. The related
Stiposorghum, however, a genus commonly included in Sorghum, is
characterized by diploid species with 2n=10 and tetraploids with
2n=20 chromosomes.

3

KINDS OF POLYPLOIDS

Polyploids are traditionally classified, on the basis of their assumed origin, into autoploids and alloploids. These concepts date back to the classic paper of Kihara and Ono (3) in which they state: "Unter Polyploidie mussen wir heute zwei verschiedene Erscheinungen unterscheiden, nämlich die Autoploidie und die Allopolyploidie. Unter Autopolyploidie versteht man die Verdoppelung desselben Chromosomensätzes; unter Allopolyploidy die durch das Zusammenkommen verschiedener Chromosomensätze auf dem Weg der Bastardierung erfolgte Chromosomenvermehrung." These concepts, describing autoploidy as a doubling of the diploid genome, and alloploidy as hybridization followed by doubling of two different haploid genomes, were useful five decades ago, but have become misleading rather than informative. First, as will be discussed later, polyploidy involves sexual functioning of cytologically non-reduced gametes rather than somatic chromosome doubling. Second, most natural polyploids fall somewhere in between the typical auto-ploid and typical alloploid recognized by Kihara and Ono (3). Poly-ploidy involves a single self-fertilizing individual, different individuals within an interbreeding population, differently adapted populations within a species, different species with a genus, or even species of different genera. The most successful natural poly-ploid is tetraploid, and probably combines the genomes of two differently adapted, but cytogenetically closely allied taxa.

MODES OF ORIGIN

Genetic and evolutionary implications of polyploidy are fre-quently discussed (1,4-9). Modes of origin are less well understood. Chromosome doubling (3) implies a somatic event, either in the zygote to produce a polyploid individual, or in some apical meristem to produce a polyploid chimera. These have generally been accepted as the common modes of origin of polyploids. Polyploids also arise through formation and sexual functioning of cytologically non-reduced female and male gametes (10-14).

Zygotic Chromosome Doubling

Diploid parents occasionally produce tetraploid offspring. These polyploids may result from chromosome doubling in the zygote, or from cytologically non-reduced male and female gametes that com-bine to produce functional tetraploid zygotes. Both pathways to polyploidy are extremely rare, and which one of them operates in the origin of a particular polyploid is almost impossible to deter-mine.

Zygotic chromosome doubling was first proposed by Winge (15). It was his impression that chromosomes of the female gamete pair with those of the male gamete in the zygote, and that when gametes were

sufficiently different, chromosomes fail to pair and the zygote
perishes. Should the chromosomes in a hybrid zygote split long-
itudinally, however, each chromosome has a homologous mate, homologues pair, and an embryo with double the parental number of
chromosomes develops. The spontaneous appearance of tetraploid
Oenothera lamarckiana Ser. (16), and the amphidiploid hybrids produced in Nicotiana (17) are commonly accepted as proof of polyploidy
through zygotic chromosome doubling. Clausen and Goodspeed (17)
crossed tetraploid Nicotiana tabacum L. (2n=48) with diploid N.
glutinosa L. (2n=24) and obtained two hybrid seedlings, the one
sterile and the other fertile. When the fertile F_1 hybrid was
selfed, it produced 220 morphologically more or less uniform offspring. Individuals studied cytologically were amphidiploid (2n=72),
suggesting that their hybrid parent was similarly polyploid. Chromosome doubling, however, did not necessarily occur in the zygote.
Polyploidy may have resulted from coming together of cytologically
non-reduced male and female gametes to produce a zygote with 2n=72
chromosomes. Moreover, the hybrid may have been triploid (2n=36)
and produced functionally cytologically non-reduced gametes. Hybrids
between tetraploid N. rustica L. (2n=48) and diploid N. paniculata
L. (2n=24) are partially fertile although they are characterized
by 12 chromosome pairs and 12 single chromosomes during meiotic
prophase of sporogenesis (18). Among 37 F_2 offspring of such a
triploid hybrid, 30 were hexaploid (2n=72), and the chromosome numbers
of the remaining seven ranged between 2n=38 and 2n=58. Critical
supporting evidence of polyploidy through somatic chromosome doubling
in the zygote is lacking, and a great deal of evidence is available
that contradicts this concept.

Meristematic Chromosome Doubling

        Chromosomes are readily doubled in developing seedlings to pro-
duce polyploid plants, or in active apical meristematic tissues to
produce polyploid chimeras by the application of chemicals such as
colchicine. Spontaneous somatic chromosome doubling, however, is
a rare event (19). The only well documented case is the origin of
Primula kewensis Watson. A hybrid seedling with P. verticillata
Forssk. (2n=18) as the pollen parent appeared among offspring of
P. floribunda Wall. (2n=18) at the Royal Botanic garden in Kew
during 1899. This hybrid was highly sterile sexually, although
chromosome pairing was essentially normal during meiotic prophase
and sporogenesis proceeded regularly to produce cytologically
balanced gametes (20). This sterile hybrid was vegetatively propagated and widely distributed as an ornamental. Twenty-six years
after the hybrid first appeared, fertile shoots appeared on a
sterile plant that was being maintained at the John Innes Institute.
These shoots turned out to be tetraploid, and produced an abundance
of tetraploid offspring (21). This clearly is a case of somatic
chromosome doubling. Earlier, in 1904, fertile tetraploid offspring

were obtained by pollinating a pin-eyed flower on one hybrid
plant with pollen from a thrum-eyed flower from another hybrid
plant of the same original hybrid stock. These tetraploids
probably originated from fertilization of a cytologically non-
reduced female gamete with a similar male gamete, rather than
from parthenogenetic development after chromosome doubling in the
megagametophyte. Attempts to cross P. floribunda with P. verticillata resulted in two fertile hybrids, both of which were tetraploid
(21). They could have resulted from zygotic chromosome doubling.
But, they more probably originated as a result of fertilization
of a diploid female gamete of one species by a diploid male
gamete of the other species.

Gametic Chromosome Non-Reduction

        Sporogenesis is a complex process and occasional failure of
chromosome reduction during meiosis has been observed in many
species. Chromosome reduction either fails to take place during
the first meiotic division, or cytokinesis fails during the
second meiotic division. The result is a gametophyte with the
same chromosome number as the sporophyte. Franke (13) lists 31
plant families in which functional cytologically non-reduced
gametes were reported. DenNijs and Peloquin (22) demostrate that
cytologically non-reduced gametes are commonly produced in species
of Solanum and hybridization among diploids frequently results
in polyploidy. Cytologically non-reduced gametes are probably
produced in most individuals, and Löve (23) suggests that polyploid
individuals occur in most large, sexually reproducing diploid
populations. Most such polyploids, however, do not compete
successfully with their parents and are soon eliminated from the
population.
        Polyploids derived through sexual functioning of cytologically
non-reduced gametes are more commonly triploid (2n+n) than tetraploid (2n+2n). Diploid male and female gametes may be produced
at equal frequencies. However, the probability is small that a
rare diploid female gamete is going to be fertilized by an equally
rare diploid male gamete. Moreover, diploid pollen compete
poorly with haploid pollen on diploid stigmas. Diploid maize
pollinated by a mixture of pollen from diploid and tetraploid
races, rarely produces triploid offspring. Union of a diploid
female gamete with a normal haploid male gametes is far more
common than diploid-diploid union. Triploid embryos, recognized
by their poorly differentiated endosperm, are encountered in
ears of maize. This occurs at a relatively high frequency in
some inbreds. Tetraploid embryos, on the other hand, are extremely
rare.
        Genotype as well as phenotype determine the frequency with
which diploid gametes are produced. Grant (24) found that adverse
growing conditions increase the number of cytologically non-

reduced gametes produced in populations of <u>Gilia</u>. This is probably
true in many species. The genotype of the individual also plays
a major role. Alexander and Beckett (25) demonstrate that among
selected inbreds of <u>Zea mays</u> L. frequency of diploid eggs varied
from 0 to 3.5% when they are grown under identical conditions.
Furthermore, it is known that the gene 'elongate' on chromosome
three of maize increases the number of diploid eggs produced. It
delays cell division and upsets meiosis, and is used to produce
tetraploid maize breeding lines (26,27).
    Hybridity also promotes the formation of cytologically non-
reduced gametes. Diploid gametes are often the only functional
ones in inter-specific hybrids. Numerous spontaneous polyploids
obtained experimentally originated in this way. Harlan and deWet
(14) list 68 genera in which functional cytologically non-
reduced gametes were produced in F_1 hybrids that resulted from
fertilization of a normal haploid female gamete by a normal haploid
male gamete. Hybrids between <u>Tripsacum dactyloides</u> (L.) L. (2n=36)
and <u>Zea mays</u> L. (2n=20), as an example, are male sterile but
female fertile (28, 29). Functional eggs are cytologically non-
reduced, and the hybrid can be backcrossed with either parent as
the pollen donor (30).
    Chromosome increase through sexual functioning of cytologi-
cally non-reduced gametes may give rise to first generation
hybrid polyploids, or diploid hybrids may produce polyploid
offspring. Polyploidy occurs at diploid levels, as well as at
polyploid levels. Polyploidy buffers the shock of absorbing
foreign genomes, and diploid species that are otherwise reproductively isolated often cross when cytologically non-reduced female
gametes function sexually. Similarly, species that are genetically isolated at the diploid level may cross at the autotetraploid
level to produce amphidiploids.

                        SUCCESS OF POLYPLOIDS

    Polyploidy is a rare event, but occurs at a sufficiently
high frequency for polyploid individuals to occur in large populations of many sexually reproducing diploid species. Few of these
polyploids survive beyond one generation. They are eliminated
in competition with their parents for available habitats. They
must compete for the parental habitat or invade new habitats, and
are often lower in fertility than their parents.

<u>Colonizing Ability</u>

    Polyploids are successful only if they are able to compete
successfully with their parents and other taxa for available
habitats. Competition for the habitat has two principal components,
ability of newly formed polyploid seedlings to become established,

and the ability of these seedlings to produce adaptive offspring.
Such competition tends to favor perennials. Once established,
the polyploid perennial has several generations in which time
desirable gene combinations capable of competing successfully for
available habitats can be sorted out. All polyploids, however,
are not perennial. Numerous annual polyploids are equally successful.

A primary requirement for success is colonizing ability.
The South African Oxalis pescapre L. is characterized by a sexually
fertile tetraploid (2n=28) and a sexually sterile pentaploid
(2n=35) race. Both races seem equally successful in their native
habitat. They were widely introduced into Europe, Asia, and
North America as cultigens, and both races escaped from cultivation. However, it is the sexually sterile pentaploid that
produces by means of tubers, rather than the seed producing
tetraploid that has become a weed. It is now widely distributed
in Australia and parts of California (13).

Successful polyploids are commonly allopatric with their
closest relatives. When sympatric, polyploids differ from their
diploid parents in habitat preference. The widely distributed
Themeda triandra Forssk. is a principal component of the grass
flora of subtropical Africa. In southern Africa it is characterized by sympatric diploid and polyploid races, but frequencies of
ploidy levels differ from one vegetation zone to another (32).
Diploids dominate in tropical forests, with triploids (3%) and
tetraploids (13%) occurring together in some diploid populations.
Polyploids fare better in other veld types. In the arid karroo
and semi-arid bushveld diploids represent about 50% of Themeda
populations. In these veld types, triploids (21%), and higher
polyploids (8%) occur with, and are as widely distributed as,
diploids. Polyploids dominate in the grass veld. Triploids
(19%), tetraploids (37%), pentaploids, and hexaploids (25%) are
widely distributed, with diploids (19%) present as relatively
rare individuals in most populations. Diploids and polyploids of
Themeda have equally wide distributions in South Africa, but
differ in efficiency to exploit different habitats. Only in the
grass veld do polyploids have a significant selective advantage
over diploids in habitat adaptation. Yet, polyploids are continuously being produced, and do compete successfully also in other
veld types. Frequencies of chromosome races, however, remain
essentially stable in all veld types from year to year.

Polyploids do not show consistent differences in patterns of
distribution when compared with their diploid relatives. Successful polyploids compete with their parents for the same habitat,
or they colonize new habitats. The reed Phragmites australis
(Cav.) Trin. ex Steud. is characterized by races with 2n=36, 48,
72, 84 or 96 chromosomes that occur in mixed populations across
the range of the species in Europe (33). On the other hand, in
the genus Epilobium species and races are adapted to different
habitats (34,35).

Frequency of polyploids among flowering plants commonly increases in the northern hemisphere with an increase in latitude. A similar increase is often also noticeable from lower to higher altitudes. This seems to suggest that polyploids are better capable of withstanding severe climates than are their diploid relatives. However, it is equally likely that the arctic environment selects for characters associated with polyploidy, rather than in favor of the polyploid condition itself (36). Löve and Löve (37,38) propose that polyploids of northern floras originated in areas with more equitable climates and were later forced into more severe climates. It was shown by Johnson and Packer (39) that frequency of polyploids in Alaskan flora is associated with local habitat rather than the overall arctic environment. The high frequency of polyploids among northern floras is probably due to the superior ability of herbaceous perennials to colonize habitats made available by retreating glaciers (1). Among modern genera, the highest frequency of polyploids occurs among herbaceous perennials in all environments, the lowest among annuals, with wood perennials intermediate in polyploid frequency between these two extremes (2).

Polyploidy and Fertility

Newly produced polyploids are less fecund than their diploid parents. Autoploids are characterized by meiotic chromosomal irregularities and cytologically unbalanced gametes are produced. These gametes either do not function, or they produce cytologically unbalanced offspring. Amphidiploids are characterized by regular meiotic behavior, and cytologically balanced gametes are produced. However, gametes that combine two well differentiated haploid genomes do not always function successfully.

Fertility is improved in polyploids through cytological diploidization of the genome, or through a change to asexual reproduction. Gillie and Randolph (40) note a statistically significant reduction of quadrivalent frequency in tetraploid maize after ten generations of sexual reproduction. Selection for increased fertility coupled with selection for overall agronomic fitness also significantly increases yield of tetraploid maize. Dudley and Alexander (41) improved seedset from around 50% to as much as 73% within ten cycles of intense selection pressure. Cytological studies in the Crop Evolution Laboratory reveal that increased fertility is correlated with an increase in percentage cytologically balanced gametes produced. Tetravalent frequency at early diakinesis remained essentially the same for all ten selection cycles, but in populations with the highest percentage seedset, tetravalents fall apart at late diakinesis and the chromosomes reach the metaphase plate as bivalents. Later meiotic chromosome movements are regular, and cytologically balanced gametes are produced. Eventually the genomes of even autoploids

may be diploidized. Most natural polyploids behave cytologically
as diploids. An alternative method to overcome partial sexual
sterility is asexual reproduction.

Gametophytic Apomixis and Polyploidy

Numerous polyploids reproduce asexually by means of gametophytic apomixis (42). The more successful ones are facultatively
sexual. Functional cytologically reduced and non-reduced female
gametophytes are produced, and either gametophyte may develop
parthenogenetically or function sexually to produce viable seed
(43).
Gametophytic apomixis is closely associated with polyploidy.
All polyploids are not apomicts, but nearly all gametophytic
apomicts are polyploid. Polyploids commonly originate as a
result of the formation, and sexual functioning of cytologically
non-reduced female gametophytes. Formation of cytologically non-
reduced female gametophytes is also a required first step in
shifting from sexual reproduction to gametophytic apomixis. The
only further requirement is for this gametophyte to develop
parthenogenetically into a seed. Selection pressures for increase
in fertility may lead to apomictic seed production as well as
genomic diploidization. Gametophytic apomixis provides a convenient
method to bypass meiosis in autoploids, and thus prevent the
formation of cytologically unbalanced offspring. Gametophytic
apomicts are not all autoploid in origin. Alloploids may also
reproduce asexually. These commonly originate as hybrids between
autotetraploid gametophytic apomicts. They may also combine
diploid genomes that are so alien that the amphidiploid is sexually
sterile.
Apomicts, as do polyploids, do not show consistent patterns
of distribution when compared with their diploid relatives. They
may compete successfully with their diploid parents for similar
habitats or occupy completely different habitats. Apomixis
stabilizes selected genotypes and often allows for rapid colonization of pioneer habitats. Polyploid agamospecies are successful
despite their asexual mode of reproduction, not necessarily
because they reproduce apomictically.

REVERSIBLE TETRAPLOIDY

Haploids are characterized by the gametic chromosome number
of their parents. They arise through parthenogenetic development
of unfertilized eggs. Offspring of gametophytic apomicts commonly
include haploids (43). Haploids also appear occasionally among
offspring of sexually reproducing species (44). Haploids derived
from naturally occurring tetraploids are often vigorous and
sometimes fertile. The question thus arises whether reversible

tetraploidy played any part in plant evolution and speciation
(45-47).

Monoploids are derived from diploid species and have a
single haploid genome. Although sometimes surprisingly vigorous,
they are sterile. The probability that monoploids played a significant role in speciation can be ruled out. Dihaploids derived
from tetraploids are diploid in chromosome number. Those derived
from amphidiploids are cytologically similar to diploid hybrids
between the original parents. Reversible tetraploidy among
autoploids reconstitutes the parental diploid.

Reversible tetraploidy is commonly regarded as playing at
most a minor role in population evolution in higher plants (1).
This is not necessarily true. Haploids derived from amphidiploids
are highly sterile. This is not surprising. But they resemble
interspecific hybrids in genome constitution, and polyploidy
superimposed on hybridization is an accepted mode of speciation.
Dihaploids often produce functional cytologically non-reduced
gametes and the parental amphidiploid can be recovered. New
amphidiploids can also be produced when dihaploids are backcrossed
in succession to the original parental diploids. This allows for
introgression between the established amphidiploid and its close
diploid relatives. Successive backcrosses with the same diploid
can result in autotetraploids with introgression from the amphidiploid. Whether such introgression actually occurs in nature is
difficult to determine with certainty. Phenotypically the same
effects can be achieved through hybridization and polyploidy.
Diploid (AA) crosses with diploid (BB) will give rise to a hybrid
(AB) that resembles dihaploid (AB). Backcrosses of hybrid or
diphaploid with the parental diploids may result in either establishing an amphidiploid (AB-x-BB gives ABB-x-AA gives AABB), or
an autoploid (AB-x-AA gives AA*B*-x-AA gives AAA*B*-x-AA gives
AAA*A*) with two haploid genomes contaminated by genetic material
of the non-backcross diploid parent. Introgression of this
nature has been achieved in hybrids between Zea mays and Tripsacum
dactyloides (30,48). Phylogenetically significant is the subtle
genetic differences between diploid hybrids and dihaploids derived
from amphidiploids or established autotetraploids.

Haploids derived from newly formed autoploids are cytologically
diploid. Randolph and Fischer (49) obtained fully fertile diploids
from autotetraploid maize, and we have obtained normal diploids
from tetraploid maize after fifteen successful selection cycles
for increase in percentage seedset. Natural autotetraploids are
characterized by various degrees of genome differentiation.
Dihaploids derived from tetraploid species of the section Tuberosum
of Solanum are often fertile (50). Dihaploids obtained from
tetraploid populations of Tripsacum dactyloides range from fully
fertile to completely sterile. These dihaploids differ phenotypically from diploids. This is not surprising. The genomes of
established tetraploids are variously diploidized. The presence
of fertile dihaploids may therefore significantly change gene

frequencies of diploid populations. Dihaploids may also establish
diploids in areas where parental diploids do not exist. An
apparent dihaploid of recent origin is out competing the parental
tetraploid Dichanthium caricosum (L.) A. Camus as a weed near
Pretoria in South Africa (46).

It is difficult to determine how successful and widespread
reversible tetraploidy is in nature. Numerous species are characterized by diploid and tetraploid races, and many of these have
diploid biotypes that resemble tetraploids in phenotype and
habitat preference. Anderson (51) suspects that diploid Flaveria
campestris Johns. is of haploid origin. Dihaploids certainly are
playing significant roles in maintaining variability among some
apomictic tetraploids. Tripsacum dactyloides is characterized by
a narrow-leaved diploid (2n=36) and broad-leaved tetraploid race
in its northern range (52). Some tetraploid populations, however,
are characterized by phenotypically similar diploids. The diploids
cross with the differently adapted narrow-leaved diploids where
they are sympatric. Hybrids give rise to polyploids through
sexual functioning of cytologically non-reduced gametes, and they
act as a bridge for gene transfer between diploid and tetraploid
races. In Dichanthium annulatum (Forssk.) Stapf diploids occur
as rare individuals among apomictic tetraploids (53,54). These
diploids are of haploid origin and are sexually fertile. They
produce sexual tetraploids when pollinated by apomictic tetraploids,
and provide a means by which the population maintains contact
with sexuality. Successful dihaploids are rare in nature, but
haploidy plays a role in maintaining and increasing variability
within diploid as well as tetraploid populations of numerous
species.

SUMMARY

1.   Polyploidy is a conspicuous feature of chromosomal
evolution in higher plants. It is common in many genera, and
numerous species are characterized by diploid and polyploid
races.
2.   Polyploid evolution is a process not an event.
3.   Polyploidy may involve somatic chromosome doubling or
sexual functioning of cytologically non-reduced gametes.
4.   Spontaneous chromosome doubling, either in the zygote to
produce a polyploid plant or in apical meristem to produce a
polyploid chimera, is a rare event.
5.   The common mode of polyploidy is through the formation
and sexual functioning of cytologically non-reduced gametes.
Increase in chromosome number can occur in the first or later
hybrid generations.
6.   Polyploidy via cytologically non-reduced gametes is
commonly a two step process. A diploid (2n) female gamete is
fertilized by a haploid (n) male gamete to produce a triploid

(3x), which in turn produces cytologically non-reduced triploid (3n) female gametes that are fertilized by haploid (n) gametes of the diploid parents and result in tetraploid (4x) offspring.

    7. Fertilization of a rare diploid (2n) female gamete by an equally rare diploid (2n) male gamete to directly produce a tetraploid (4x) is extremely rare but does occur.

    8. Polyploidy is successful only if the new polyploids are able to compete with their parents. Success depends on availability of suitable habitats, as well as the ability to produce successful offspring.

    9. The most successful polyploids combine the diploid genomes of cytogenetically allied, but differently adapted taxa.

    10. Fertility is restored in polyploids through cytological diploidization of the genomes or through gametophytic apomixis.

    11. Reversible tetraploidy is part of polyploid evolution.

LITERATURE CITED

1. Stebbins, G.L., 1971, "Chromosomal Evolution in Higher Plants," Addison-Wesley Publ. Co., Reading, Mass. 216 p.

2. Levin, D.A., Wilson, A.C., 1976, Rates of evolution in seed plants. Net increase in diversity of chromosome numbers and species number through time. Proc. Nat. Acad. Sci. USA 73: 2086-2090.

3. Kihara, H., Ono, T., 1926, Chromosomenzahlen und systematische gruppierung der Rumex arten. Zeitschr. Zellf. Mikrosk. Anat. 4: 475-481.

4. Ehrendorfer, F., Krendl, F., Habeler, E., Sauer, W., 1968, Chromosome numbers and evolution in primitive angiosperms. Taxon 17: 337-468.

5. Jones, K., 1970, Chromosome changes in plant evolution. Taxon 19: 172-179.

6. deWet, J.M.J., 1971, Polyploidy and evolution in plants. Taxon 20: 29-36.

7. Jackson, R.C., 1976, Evolution and systematic significance of polyploidy. Ann. Rev. Ecol. Syst. 7: 209-234.

8. Raicu, P., 1976, Les complexes polyploides chez les vegetaux. Bull. Soc. Bot. France 123: 249-260.

9. Gottschalk, W., 1976, "Die Bedeutung der Polyploidie für die Evolution der Pflanzen," Gustav-Fischer, Stuttgart. 501 p.

10. Buxton, B.H., Darlington, C.D., 1931, Hybrids of Digitalis ambigua and Digitalis purpurea, their fertility and cytology. J. Genetics 19: 269-279.

11. Müntzing, A., 1932, Cytogenetic investigations on synthetic Galeopsis tetrahit. Hereditas 16: 105-154.

12. Clausen, J., Keck, D.D., Hiesey, W.M., 1945, Experimental studies on the nature of species. II. Plant evolution through amphiploidy and autoploidy with examples from the Madiinae. Carnegie Inst. Wash. Publ. 564: 1-174.

13. Franke, R., 1975, Über das auftreten von unreduzierten Gamenten bei angiospermen. Arch. Züchtungsforsch. Berlin 5: 201-208.

14. Harlan, J.R., deWet, J.M.J., 1975, On Ö. Winge and a prayer: the origins of polyploidy. Bot. Rev. 41: 361-390.

15. Winge, Ö., 1917, The chromosomes. Their numbers and general importance. Compt. Rend. Trav. Lab. Carlsberg 13: 131-175.

16. Gates, R.R., 1924, Polyploidy. Brit. J. Exp. Biol. 1: 153-182.

17. Clausen, R.E., Goodspeed, T.H., 1925, Interspecific hybridization in Nicotiana. II. A tetraploid glutinosa-tabacum hybrid, an experimental verification of Winge's hypothesis. Genetics 10: 279-284.

18. Lammerts, W., 1931, Interspecific hybridization in Nicotiana. XII. The amphidiploid rustica-paniculata hybrid: its origin and cytogenetic behaviour. Genetics 16: 191-211.

19. Jahr, W., Skiebe, V., Stein, M., 1965, Die herstellung von Neuen Allopolyploiden für die Züchtung. Züchter 34: 7-14.

20. Digby, L., 1912, The cytology of Primula kewensis and of other related Primula hybrids. Ann. Bot. 26: 357-388.

21. Newton, W.C.F., Pellew, C., 1929, Primula kewensis and its derivatives. J. Genetics 20: 405-467.

22. DenNijs, T.P.M., Peloquin, S.J., 1977, 2n gametes in potato species and their function in sexual polyploidization. Euphytica 26: 585-600.

23. Löve, A., 1964, The biological species concepts and its evolutionary structure. Taxon 13: 33-45.

24. Grant, V., 1952, Cytogenetics of the hybrid Gilia mellefoliata x achilleaefolia. I. Variations in meiosis and polyploidy rate as affected by nutritional and genetic conditions. Chromosoma 5: 372-390.

25. Alexander, D.E., Beckett, J.B., 1963, Spontaneous triploidy and tetraploidy in maize. J. Heredity 54: 103-106.

26. Rhoades, M.M., 1956, Genetic control of chromosome behaviour. Maize Genet. Coop. Newsletter 30: 38-42.

27. Alexander, D.E., 1957, The genetic induction of autotetraploidy: a proposal for its use in corn breeding. Agron. J. 49: 40-43.

28. Mangelsdorf, P.C., Reeves, R.G., 1939, The origin of Indian corn and its relatives. Texas Agric. Exp. Sta. Bull. 374: 1-315.

29. Newell, C.A., deWet, J.M.J., 1973, A cytological survey of Zea-Tripsacum hybrids. Canad. J. Genet. Cytol. 15: 763-778.

30. deWet, J.M.J., Harlan, J.R., 1974, Tripsacum-maiz interaction: a novel cytogenetic system. Genetics 78: 493-502.

31. Baker, H.G., 1965, Characteristics and modes of origin of weeds. in "The Genetics of Colonizing Species," Baker, H.G., Stebbins, G.L. (eds.), Academic Press, New York.

32. deWet, J.M.J., 1960, Cytogeography of Themeda triandra in South Africa. Phyton (Argentina) 15: 37-42.

33. Gorenflot, R., 1976, Le complexe polyploide du Pharagmites australis (Cav.) Trin. ex Steud. (P. communis Trin.). Bull.

Soc. Bot. France 123: 261-267.

34. Mosquin, T., 1967, Evidence for autopolyploidy in _Epilobium_
     angustifolium (Onagraceae). Evolution 21: 713-719.
35. Small, E., 1968, The systematics of autoploidy in _Epilobium_
     latifolium (Onagraceae). Brittonia 20: 169-181.
36. Johnson, A.W., Packer, J.G., Reese, G., 1965, Polyploidy,
     distribution and environment, _in_ "Quaternary of the United
     States, "Wright, H.E., Frey, D.G.(eds.), Inter. Assoc. Quatern.
     Res. Publication.
37. Löve, A., Löve, D., 1971, Polyploidie et goebotanique. Nat.
     Canad. 98: 469-494.
38. Löve, A., Löve, D., 1975, Cryophytes, polyploidy and continen-
     tal drift. Phytocoenologia 2: 54-65.
39. Johnson, A.W., Packer, J.G., 1965, Polyploidy and the environ-
     ment in arctic Alaska. Science 148: 237-239.
40. Gillie, L., 1912, The cytology of _Primula_ _kewensis_ and of
     other related _Primula_ hybrids. Ann. Bot. 26: 357-388.
41. Dudley, J.W., Alexander, D.E., 1969, Performance of advanced
     generations of autotetraploid maize (_Zea_ _mays_ L.) synthetics.
     Crop Sci. 9: 613-615.
42. Nygren, A., 1967, Apomixis in the angiosperms. Handb. Pflan-
     zenphysiol. 18: 551-596.
43. deWet, J.M.J., Stalker, H.T., 1974, Gametophytic apomixis and
     evolution in plants. Taxon 26: 689-697.
44. Kimber, G., Riley, R., 1963, Haploid angiosperms. Bot. Rev.
     29: 480-531.
45. Ornduff, R., 1969, Reproductive biology in relation to system-
     atics. Taxon 18: 121-144.
46. deWet, J.M.J., 1971, Reversible tetraploidy as an evolutionary
     mechanism. Evolution 25: 545-548.
47. Raven, P.H., Thomas, H.J., 1964, Haploidy and angiosperm
     evolution. Amer. Nat. 98: 251-252.
48. Newell, C.A., deWet, J.M.J., 1973, A cytological survey of
     Zea-Tripsacum hybrids. Canad. J. Genet. Cytol. 15: 763-778.
49. Randolph, L.F., Fischer, H.E., 1939, The occurrence of parthe-
     nogenetic diploids in tetraploid maize. Proc. Nat. Acad.
     Sci. USA 25: 161-164.
50. Hougas, R.W., Peloquin, S.I., Ros, R.W., 1958, Haploids of
     the common potato. J. Heredity 49: 103-106.
51. Anderson, L.C., 1972, _Flaveria_ _campestris_ (Asteraceae): a
     case of polyhaploidy or relict ancestral diploidy. Evolution
     26: 671-673.
52. Newell, C.A., deWet, J.M.J., 1974, Morphological and cytologi-
     cal variability in _Tripsacum_ _dactyloides_ (Gramineae). Amer.
     J. Bot. 61: 652-664.
53. deWet, J.M.J., Harlan, J.R., 1970, Apomixis, polyploidy and
     speciation in _Dichanthium_. Evolution 24: 270-277.
54. deWet, J.M.J., 1968, Diploid-tetraploid-haploid cycles and
     the origin of variability in _Dichanthium_ agomospecies.
     Evolution 22: 394-397.

CYTOGENETICS OF POLYPLOIDS

R. C. Jackson and Jane Casey

Department of Biological Sciences
Texas Tech University
Lubbock, TX   79409

Following Winge's classic paper on polyploidy (1), there have been a large number of publications dealing with various aspects of the subject. However, this symposium is probably the first to bring together at one place and at one time so many different viewpoints and disciplines dealing with this subject.

Many earlier papers dealt with the general cytology of polyploids, but very few utilized the requisite cytogenetic principles and methodologies in arriving at conclusions concerning the kind of polyploidy involved. Stebbins put many of the problems in perspective in his first classification of polyploids, and most cytogeneticists and plant systematists have since followed his system but often without adequate data. It is clear from a perusal of a small part of the vast literature that basic cytogenetic information is lacking or ignored in many studies of both synthetic and natural polyploids. Detailed and meaningful quantitative comparisons therefore are impossible in most cases, but we believe that such problems can be overcome if better methods are used and the data reported in a uniform manner.

Polyploidy is but one category of heteroploidy. The latter may be defined as any deviation from the normal chromosome number in a cell, tissue, or whole organism (2,3). The categories of heteroploidy are monoploidy (haploidy), diploidy, polyploidy, polyhaploidy, and aneuploidy. Polyploids have three or more genomes and have been classified in various ways. However, the classification by Stebbins (4-6), who broadened and refined that offered by Clausen, Keck, and Heisey (7), is the one generally accepted and referred to in the literature. This classification utilizes the terms autopolyploidy, segmental allopolyploidy, allopolyploidy, and autoalloploidy. Stebbins recognized and emphasized that while these categories are not always sharply defined, they are nevertheless useful in discussing the evolution of different types. He further emphasized that interpretations of polyploid origin must take into consideration information from all sources. We agree completely with this viewpoint, but we also consider those factors that affect chromosome pairing to be of major importance in classifying and understanding the evolution of polyploids.

In this discussion we have tried to emphasize some of the fundamental cytogenetic factors relating to analyses of polyploids. We have not attempted to cover parthenogenetic systems, polyhaploidy, nor factors promoting the formation and maintenance of polyploids. Some of these topics were treated in an earlier review (3).

FACTORS AFFECTING MEIOTIC CHROMOSOME PAIRING

The process of meiosis depends upon the action and synchrony of many genes (8), and the process is being dissected by the study of mutations in many organisms suitable for genetic analysis. The normal function of genes affecting meiosis also may be responsible for mitotic functions so that both soma and germ lines may reflect the effects of a single mutation but in different ways. The action and synchrony of these genes may be greatly influenced by environmental factors such as high or low temperature, chemicals, radiation, and nutrition. It has become clear that these environmental factors as well as certain other genes can exert their effects on the germ line in premeiotic cells.

Premeiotic Effects on Chromosome Pairing

The early work of Okamoto (9), Riley and Chapman (10), and Sears and Okamoto (11) initiated a series of elegant experiments that have led to a better understanding of chromosome pairing in hexaploid wheat, Triticum aestivum (AABBDD). Later work demonstrated that pairing between the different genomes, homoeologous pairing, is suppressed by a dominant gene, termed Ph for pairing homoeologous (3,12). The gene was localized to the long arm of chromosome 5B.

The most probable mode of action of Ph was first suggested by Feldman (13) who found homoeologous pairing in wheat plants containing six $5B^L$ arms (tri-isosomic $5B^L$) instead of the normal two. The extra strength of Ph was demonstrated by also suppressing homologous pairing. He suggested that Ph exerted its effect by its action on premeiotic chromosomes.

It was supposed (13) that with the normal Ph dose (two 5B chromosomes) the homologues within each genome set are in closer proximity than to homoeologues of another genome. With six Ph genes present, the effect might be to disrupt even the close association of homologues such that with the onset of zygotene

there would be a possibility of some homoeologues close enough
together so that intergenomal pairing would occur. Using telocentrics, it was found (14) that non-homologous telocentrics in
homozygous Ph plants were positioned at random in root tip cells
while homologues were significantly closer together.

These findings (14) have not always been verified; the
suitability of the model has been questioned and alternative
statistical methods suggested (3,12). Nevertheless, the original
hypothesis has strong experimental backing. In one study (15)
colchicine was applied to developing florets of hexaploid wheat
after the completion of the last premeiotic mitosis. Multivalents
caused by homoeologous pairing were quite frequent, and their
mean frequency was only slightly lower than Feldman (13) had
obtained with six doses of the Ph gene. The conclusion was that
colchicine applied before meiosis inhibits association of homologues in premeiotic nuclei. This was corroborated and extended
by additional experiments (3,12,16-19) which also tested the
effects of temperature and other chemicals on premeiotic chromosome
positioning.

Dover and Riley (19) treated immature florets of _Triticum_
aestivum, _T. aestivum_ X _Aegilops_ _mutica_, and _T. aestivum_ X
Secale _cereale_ hybrids with 0.5% colchicine. When the treatment
occurred at the time of the last premeiotic mitosis in the anthers,
asynapsis was induced at metaphase I irrespective of whether the
potential pairing partners were homologous or homoeologous.
Treatment of _T. aestivum_ nullosomic for chromosome 5B showed
homoeologous pairing was absent and homologous pairing was reduced,
indicating that homoeologous pairing was first affected. Use of
dilute colchicine (0.01%) during the last mitosis prior to meiosis
induced multipolar spindles and microsporocytes with varying
chromosome numbers in the species and hybrids. In _T. aestivum_ X
S. cereale (2n=28) meiocytes had 22 to 28 chromosomes. Chloral
hydrate had no effect on pairing. This presumably was due to the
fact that, while it prevents the polymerization of the tubulin
subunits of the continuous spindle fibers, it does not interfere
with reinitiation of centromeric microtubule formation. This
means that chromosome movement could still be possible so that
normal premeiotic association would occur.

One study is particularly instructive concerning the effects
of premeiotic events on meiotic ones. Driscoll and Darvey (20)
treated _Triticum_ _aestivum_ monoisosomic for 5D^L with 0.03% colchicine at the premeiotic state and compared chiasma frequencies
with untreated plants of the same chromosomal constitution. In
the untreated material, the mean chiasma formed per pair of
chromosome arms was 0.96 while in the isochromosome arms it was
0.97. In colchicine treated material, the normal chromosomes
formed an average of 0.44 chiasma per arm pair, and in the
isochromosome arms it was 0.96. This demonstrates two separable
events in meiosis. The first is a close spatial arrangement of
homologues that can be disrupted by colchicine. The second event

results in synapsis and crossing over (20). Colchicine did not
disturb pairing and crossing over in the isochromosome 5D^L
because the two homologous arms were attached to the same centromere and were always in close proximity while the spatially
separated normal chromosomes were often too far apart for normal
synapsis. Whether all organisms have the system demonstrated for
wheat remains moot. However, this system is very plausible and
offers one explanation for asynaptic mutants in diploids, namely,
that premeiotic factors responsible for moving homologues into
close proximity are ineffective. Avivi (16,17) has suggested
that somatic association genes may act in the diploid state in
such a way that pairing behavior in artificially doubled plants
may be predicted. However, the somatic association found in
wheat and other species (12) may not characterize all species.
For example, no somatic association has been found in Nicotiana
otophora and Lilium longiflorum. It is possible though that in
some species the premeiotic association may be found only in
meiocytes immediately after their formation and before leptotene.

Somatic association, presumably related to premeiotic
alignment, has been reported for diverse groups of organisms, but
these findings usually have concerned other than premeiotic
cells. It is perhaps most extreme and best known in the Diptera
but has been found in other taxa (3,21).

The cause of somatic association is unknown, but it may be
brought about by anaphase movement in which the chromosomes are
moved into proximity as they near the end of the spindle (21,19).
An alternative explanation is some controlled arrangement of the
centromeric microtubules or chromosome parts on the reconstituted
nuclear membrane (3,12,16,17). Under normal circumstances the
association may be to a specific part of the nuclear membrane
perhaps governed in part by nuclear pore complexes transmitted
through the gametes. The nucleoplasmic part and the central
pore of the complex are reported to contain DNA and are considered
(22) to be a detachable chromosome element. Disruption of the
centromeric spindle elements could cause a malorientation on the
new nuclear membrane via the pore complexes, and new connections
with their homologous chromosomes may place homoeologues in close
proximity.

All data on the subject point toward the centromere, centric
heterochromatin, or other special sites as being responsive to
Ph or Ph-like gene action and this action being modified by
chemicals that will precipitate tubulin or tubulin-like protein.
Whether the action of Ph-like genes is effective at the last
mitotic anaphase before synapsis or in the premeiotic sporocyte
is still moot. The effect, however, is proven.

Ph-like suppression has been reported or suggested for other
species (3,12). As information on this type of gene has spread,
unsophisticated comments have been made over the years to the
effect that cytogenetic analysis is of minor importance in determining relationships, and that chromosome pairing may be

controlled by a single gene. This is akin to saying that the
metabolism of an organism is controlled by a single gene because
one homozygous, non-functional locus can cause death. Certainly
the Ph gene is important in controlling homoeologous pairing in
wheat, but there are other genes in common wheat and its relatives
that likewise affect pairing, as recently reviewed by Sears(12).

Meiotic Chromosome Pairing

Early requisites to a normal meiosis are a precise synapsis
of homologous chromosomes by formation of a synaptonemal complex
and by exchanges between non-sister chromatids. The function of
the synaptonemal complex is to provide a stabilized area in the
nucleus which allows for specific molecular matching of homologous
DNA segments that are preselected for crossing over (23). As
detailed in the previous section, certain premeiotic events are
necessary preliminaries in some species.

Enough detailed ultrastructural studies of widely divergent
taxa now have accumulated to allow some generalizations (24,25,
26,23). In the meiocytes, a lateral component (LC) of the synaptonemal complex (SC) is formed on the chromosome prior to or
during synapsis, and the end of the LC is attached to a limited
area of the nuclear membrane. Homologous chromosomes move to
200-300 nm apart, and the SC is completed by addition of a central
component between the LC's. The central component (CC) is
initiated from points near the LC attachment sites on the nuclear
membrane or from various sites along the bivalents. Putative,
non-homologous SC's have been reported. However, it is not clear
whether this is truly non-homologous pairing or whether it is
pairing initially begun in response to duplications. The appearance
of the SC is different in euchromatic and heterochromatic regions
at pachytene and is correlated with crossover and non-crossover
positions (26). The chromosomes at pachytene are synapsed with
precision and are generally detached from the nuclear membrane at
this stage. Various length measurements have demonstrated that
only a small part of the total bivalent DNA can be bound in the
SC. In _Neurospora_, _Zea_ _mays_, and _Lilium_ _longiflorum_ the SC bound
DNA is 0.3, 0.014-.017, and 0.0006%, respectively, of total DNA
length, while it is about 0.2 in _Drosophila_ and 0.12% in _Bombyx_
mori females (25). The small fraction of the total DNA involved
with the SC in any one chromosome of a particular cell may help
explain why relatively small segments of non-homologous regions
show up as buckles in some meiocytes and are absent in others.
Since there is little or no change in SC length during pachytene,
light microscopic observations on length changes from early to
late stages may be due to squashing, cell to cell variation, or
the removal of part of the complex as pachytene proceeds.
Perhaps early diplotene may be confused with late pachytene under
the lower resolution light optics.

The synaptonemal complex is usually shed beginning with early diplotene. However, in achiasmate species it may persist until metaphase or anaphase I as a substitute for chiasmata until the bivalents are properly aligned at metaphase I to insure orderly disjunction.

Control of Chiasmata. Chiasmata are necessary for a normal meiosis in those organism that are chiasmate. Factors that affect chiasmata formation are all of the premeiotic and pairing components discussed previously plus those of the environment. Natural environmental factors with known effects are those of temperature and nutrition.

Temperature effects have been documented in numerous taxa (27,28), but the precise cell cycle stage in which effects were initiated usually was unknown in earlier work. In certain fungi, heat treatments have both premeiotic and meiotic effects on crossing over while cold treatment primarily affects the pachytene stage.

The work by Grant (29) on chiasma frequency among F_1 hybrid siblings of Gilia is very instructive for those who rely only on information from natural populations. Hybrids grown in sand had a very low chiasma frequency compared to siblings grown in rich soil. A pot-bound allotetraploid showed a significant increase in chiasmata after it was watered with mineral solution. In barley and rye a higher chiasma frequency was caused by increasing the concentration of phosphate. Increased chiasma frequency in Lolium has been produced by a high concentration of potassium at $30°C$ while no effect was evident at $20°C$. Even the small number of environmental effects cited point out the necessity of a controlled environment when chiasma frequency and the kind of pairing configurations in polyploids are to be determined (3).

Genetic control of chiasmata may occur at several levels. General effects on all of the chromosomes may be demonstrated and are probably quantitatively controlled. In addition, chiasma frequency in a specific segment of a bivalent may be controlled by additively acting genes, maternal factors, epistasis, and dominance (30). Structural heterozygosity and its concomitant effect on reducing chiasma frequency in one bivalent may result in increased crossover frequencies in others (31). Position of chiasmata, terminally or at random, can be controlled by a single gene. Moreover, chromosome specific control is known for three genera of Compositae: Crepis (32), Haplopappus (Jackson and Casey, unpublished), and Hypochoeris (33). There is recent evidence for separate genetic control and chiasmata maintenance in maize (34).

Pairing, Chiasmata, and Multivalents. Unless otherwise qualified, our following discussion deals with sets of completely homologous chromosomes. Furthermore, the basic chromosome number is x=1.

If we consider an autotetraploid with 2n=4x=4, there are
four identical chromosomes. Each chromosome has an equal probability of pairing with any one of the other three. The model
suggested for this situation (35,36) assumes that the arm of any
particular chromosome pairs independently of the other arm. This
can be better envisioned by referring to Fig. 1. The homologous
centromeres are labeled 1 to 4 for convenience. The upper arms
are all termed a while the lower ones are b. Thus, 1 refers to
chromosome arm 1a or 1b.

During pachytene, it is assumed that each arm is paired with
another whole arm throughout its length. All arms are paired and
each pair of arms forms one distal chiasma. Taking the four a
arms two by two (Fig. 1), we have three different ways they may
pair: (1a-2a, 3a-4a), (1a-3a, 2a-4a), (1a-4a, 2a-3a). The same
possibilities exist for the four b arms. Now one can construct a
simple matrix and determine the frequency with which arm a and
arm b of the same chromosome are paired with both arm a and arm b
of another chromosome. We will consider two examples. The first
pairing arrangement of a arms on the left side of the matrix in
Fig. 1 may occur with any one of the four b arm arrangements at
the top. Taking the b arm arrangement, the paired chromosome arm
combinations 1a-2a, 3a-4a may occur with 1b-2b, 3b-4b. This
yields two bivalents. The same a arm combinations may occur also
with the second b arm combinations of 1b-3b, 2b-4b. This yields
a quadrivalent. When all possibilities of the a arm combinations
are combined with the b arm combinations two by two, the expected
probable arrangements of the independently paired a and b arms
are two-thirds quadrivalents and one-third bivalents at pachytene.
Although the number of bivalents and quadrivalents is the same,
the number of chromosomes in quadrivalents is twice that in
bivalents.

In a triploid 2n=3x=3, the a arm pairing combinations two by
two are three, as are the b arms. The possible random pairing of
a arms inter se and of b arms likewise yields two-thirds of the
time a possibility of a trivalent and one-third of the time a
bivalent and a univalent. However, the number of trivalents is
twice that of bivalents, and the number of chromosomes in trivalents is 1.5 times that in bivalents. Univalents are one-sixth
the total chromosomes in trivalents.

In pentaploids and higher levels, the possible arm pairing
arrangements become more complex. With the basic number of x=1,
the possible types of a arm arrangements of triploids through
octoploids are given in Table 1. The b arm arrangements would
occur in the same frequency. The matrix derived from the possible
combinations becomes increasingly complex as the ploidy level
increases, but the univalent, bivalent, and multivalent frequency
can be determined by using only the first arrangement of b arms
combined with each of the a arm pairing combinations.

One formula for determining the number of pairing arm
combinations, two by two, with even ploidy levels and x=1 is

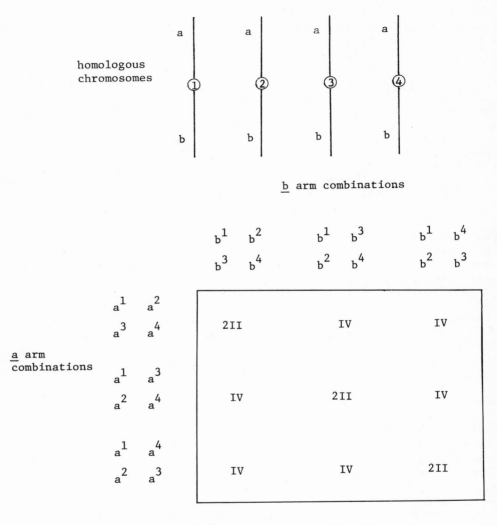

Fig.1. Top. Four homologous chromosomes. Arms a may pair at random, two by two as may arms b. a and b arms pair independently. Bottom. Random combinations of a and b arms pair to give 2 bivalents or 1 quadrivalent.

$$\frac{N!}{(N-C)!\,2^{C}}$$

where N equals the ploidy level and C equals N divided by 2. The expected fraction of bivalents is 1 over the above formula, and the fraction for maximum number of chromosomes in a multivalent should be $(C-1)!\,2^{C-1}$ over the formula.

These formulas are not applicable to odd-numbered ploidy levels, but in each case the odd-numbered polyploid will have the same number of end arrangements as the next highest even number. The different configurations and their frequencies expected under the assumptions of the model in Fig. 1 and derived from the combinations in Table 1 are given in Table 2 for 3x to 8x ploidy levels. Note that the number of bivalents does not equal the number of quadrivalents except with the tetraploids mentioned earlier. Since the formulas given above apply to only one chromosome and its homologues, suitable probability methods need to be used for numbers greater than this.

It should be emphasized that the configurations and frequencies listed in Table 2 are those expected under the strict limitations of the model of pairing and chiasma function given earlier (Fig. 1). Pairing configurations at pachytene may conform to expectations, but lack of a suitable number of chiasmata may give a misleading impression of this if the cells are scored at metaphase I. On the other hand, if the chiasma frequency per bivalent is greater than two, quadrivalent frequency will be greater than two-thirds (35).

Table 1. Numbers of different pairing end combinations for different ploidy levels at pachytene when x=1.

Ploidy level	Number of two-by-two pairing arm combinations.
3x	3
4x	3
5x	15
6x	15
7x	105
8x	105
9x	945
10x	945

Table 2. Ploidy levels and theoretical chromosomal configurations and their frequencies. Based on x=1, random pairing of
chromosome ends, and two distal chiasmata per bivalent (see Fig.
1).

Ploidy level	Chromosomal configurations and frequencies
3x	3III (.666); II, I (.3333)
4x	IV (.6666); 2II (.3333)
5x	V (.5333); IV, I (.1333); III, II (.2666); 2II, I (.0666)
6x	VI (.5333); IV, II (.4000); 3II (.0666)
7x	VII (.4571); VI, I (.0762); V, II (.2286); IV, III (.1143); IV, II, I (.0571); III, 2II (.0571); 3II, I (.0095)
8x	VIII (.4571); VI, II (.3048); 2IV (.1143); IV, 2II (.1143); 4II (.0095)

As pointed out elsewhere (3), most cytological studies of
meiosis in polyploids utilize diakinesis or metaphase I for
analyses of pairing configuration. This may lead to a misinterpretation of actual pachytene pairing and an underestimation
of homology. For example, in tetraploids of _Allium_ _porrum_ the
metacentric chromosomes have proximally localized chiasmata,
usually on each side of the centromere. Most meiocytes had
quadrivalents at pachytene, but mostly bivalents were observed at
metaphase I; only 2.6% of the cells had quadrivalents.
Tetraploids of other _Allium_ species with more randomly distributed
chiasmata had 1-5 quadrivalents in each cell (37). This
emphasizes the necessity of pachytene studies in making judgements
concerning the classifications of polyploids.
    Several mathematical techniques and models have been employed
for pairing analysis (3,35,36). Probably the most detailed
examination of the issue was by John and Henderson (35) who
conducted studies on polyploid meiocytes in otherwise diploid
insects. The advantages in their kind of analysis were recognizable chromosomes, ease of chiasmata determination at diplotene, and
comparison of chiasmata frequency in diploid and tetraploid
cells of precisely the same genotype because the newly arisen
tetraploid cells had not undergone selection. There was a slightly
higher frequency of chiasmata in the tetraploid than in the
diploid cells. Chiasma frequency in autotetraploids may be more
than or less than the diploids. In insects it appears that

quadrivalent formation is a function of chromosome length and
chiasma number. In the tetraploid plants that have been analyzed,
namely, cereal grasses (38), the chromosomes conform well to the
model of Fig. 1 in which chiasmata usually occur in each effective
pairing region at or near the chromosome ends.
     The effects of differing chiasma frequencies in a theoretical
tetraploid of 2n=4x=8 are shown in Table 3. It is apparent from
Table 3 that, following random pairing, the number and placement
of chiasmata determine the late prophase and metaphase I configurations. Note that with the capability of only one chiasma per
bivalent fewer quadrivalents are expected. These data show the
need for as much information as possible about natural polyploids
and their presumed diploid ancestors. It is apparent that one can
determine whether or not an organism has autoploid or some type of
alloploid behavior by analyzing meiotic metaphase I configurations
in the polyploid. As done in some examples in Table 3, one can
determine theoretically the possible frequencies of the different
types of multivalents and bivalents. For example, for an autotetraploid with x=7 that fits the model in Fig. 1, there are only two
classes of configurations, quadrivalents and bivalents. One can
then use the binomial $(p+q)^7$. In the expanded binomial, the frequency of cells with various numbers of quadrivalents (p) and
bivalents (q) is as follows:

$$p^7 + 7\ p^6\ q^1 + 21\ p^5q^2 + 35\ p^4q^3 + 35\ p^3q^4 + 21\ p^2q^5 + 7\ p^1q^6 + q^7$$

However, because p and q are unequal (Fig. 1), the coefficients
must be recalculated with p = 2/3 and q = 1/3. The corrected
coefficients for the now skewed binomial are given in Table 5 and
should be considered as frequencies of the different configurations
expected among cell distributions. Other than dealing with
unequal frequencies of p and q the method is straightforward.
The normal coefficients can be obtained from tables and the new
values recalculated easily. Predicted and observed values of the
frequencies of quadrivalents and bivalents and their distribution
among the meiocyte population can be tested statistically. However, when chiasma frequencies are not those used in the model
of Fig.1, the solution is more difficult. A recent solution to
this problem has been obtained in the article cited under Table 3.
This method employs a series of constants derived from different
chiasma frequency probabilities so that mean chiasma frequency per
cell is all that is needed to determine expected numbers of multivalents, bivalents and univalents. Thus the expected distributions
for autoploids still can be calculated, and if the observed data
for a natural polyploid do not fit the expected, then it is the
investigator's responsibility to explain the deviation if he
describes the organism as an autoploid.

     Preferential Pairing. Preferential pairing or differential
affinity refers to a situation wherein three or more chromosomes

Table 3[a]. Theoretical metaphase I configuration frequencies, mean chiasma, and c values per cell for autotetraploids (2n=4x=8) derived from races of a diploid species with different chiasma frequencies.

Mean No. chiasma per cell	c value	O IV	C IV	III	O II	C II	I
8.0	1.0	1.33	----	----	1.33	----	----
7.2	0.9	0.88	0.39	0.06	1.09	0.27	0.08
6.4	0.8	0.55	0.55	0.18	0.87	0.51	0.37
4.0	0.5	0.08	0.33	0.43	0.36	1.10	2.14

[a]The method for calculating configuration frequencies is that of Driscoll, C.J., Bielig, L. M., and Darvey, N.L., 1979. Genetics 91: 755-767. The letters O and C before the II and IV indicate circle bivalent and quadrivalent and chain bivalent and quadrivalent. The c value is obtained by considering that all bivalents in a cell have two chiasmata. This number is divided into the mean number of chiasmata per cell observed.

of different degrees of homology may form bivalents according to which two are the most homologous. For example, Rhoades (39) has shown that preferential pairing occurs in corn plants that are trisomic for normal chromosome 10 (k10) and a morphologically distinct form of this chromosome called K10, found in a number of races from Latin America. K10 differs from the normal type by a large, mostly heterochromatic segment added to the long arm and in the chromomeric structure of the distal one-fifth of the long arm. Preferential pairing at pachytene occurs in trisomic K10 k10 k10 or K10 K10 k10. If pairing is random, in plants with K10 K10 k10 there should be a ratio of 2:1 K10 to k10 univalents. However, in a sample of 216 microsporocytes with K10 K10 k10, a K10 chromosome was the univalent in only 69 of the meiocytes (31.9%), whereas if pairing and crossing over had been random, about 144 cells (66.6%) should have had K10 as a univalent. The normal k10 was univalent in 147 cells (68%) whereas it was expected to occur in only about 72 cells (33.3%). In k10 k10 K10 plants, a total of 166 cells had k10 univalents in only 28 cells (16.6%); they should have occurred in about 111 cells (66.6%). The K10 chromosome was univalent in 138 cells (83.1%) and was expected randomly to occur in only about 55 (33.3%).

The work on preferential pairing in maize trisomics has been expanded to preferential pairing in autoploids. Using tetraploids duplex for the chromosome inversion 3A, Doyle (40,41) was able to demonstrate both genetically and cytologically that preferential pairing occurred between the homomorphic inverted chromosomes. Shaver (42) used duplex 3A inversions in a tetraploid with two corn and two teosente genomes and also demonstrated preferential pairing. Using the K10 chromosome discussed above, Snope (43) produced a tetraploid maize duplex for K10. The expected frequency of K10 K10 and k10 k10 homomorphic bivalents is 33.3%, but homomorphic bivalents were found in 82% of the microsporocytes.

Two genetically controlled factors thus have been shown to affect pairing: premeiotic chromosome orientation and structural differences. But what causes the complete lack of pairing as might be expected in a strict alloploid? The possibility that enough structural change has occurred to preclude pairing is not very feasible, especially when the literature on multiple translocations and inversions in hybrids is examined. The explanation for lack of pairing may lie in control of premeiotic chromosome orientation such that homoeologues in the F_1 are situated so that normal meiotic synaptic forces cannot act. Other possibilities are genetically determined differences between lateral elements, defects in the central element of the synaptonemal complex, and differential contraction of the homoeologues.

Factors Affecting Later Meiotic Stages and Fertility

Metaphase I Configurations. Most meiotic analyses of pairing configurations in polyploids utilize late prophase or metaphase I. Possible interpretational errors due to analysis at this time were pointed out earlier. Various models and statistical treatments for M_I analyses have been proposed (44,3,35,36,45), but none can compensate completely for the study of the pachytene stage.

In order to obtain maximum information from M_I analyses, it is best if data are presented according to distribution of various chromosomal configurations in numbers of cells. Chiasma frequency data should be given, and, if the chromosomes can be identified, chiasma frequency and placement should be scored according to the sets of identifiable homologues. This will allow for comparisons with known or putative parental diploids and analysis of expected versus observed configurations. Further, it gives information that can be quantified and used for comparison with other examples.

Through the kindness of Dr. Douglas Dewey, we have access to some of his data on the Hordeum violaceum complex of Iran (46). The basic chromosome number is x=7. The diploid race in his excellent Fig. 1 (46) shows seven circle bivalents, indicating two distal chiasmata per bivalent. For purpose of illustration, we will assume that each bivalent of the diploid regularly has this configuration and that chiasma frequency is not reduced in the tetraploid. The model presented earlier then can be used in analysis of the data to determine whether or not the tetraploid H. violaceum fits the expectation for an autoploid. His data, with modifications for redistribution of univalents, trivalents, and a hexavalent, are given in Table 4.

The data in Table 4 have been compared with expected frequencies of bivalents and quadrivalents according to their binomial distribution among cells in Table 5. Because the expected frequency of quadrivalents (p) is two-thirds and of bivalents (q) is one-third, the binomial distribution is skewed. Considering first the original bivalent frequency, it is apparent that the total number of bivalents does not equal the number of quadrivalents as expected in the model. The total number of chromosomes in bivalents should be 1858 (33.3%) but 5116 (65.7%) were observed. Total chromosomes in quadrivalents should have been 5171 (66.6%), but only 2484 (32%) were observed. The average number of quadrivalents per cell should have been about 4.6, but 2.2 were observed (46). This is true also for the rearranged data. The distribution of configurations among cells (Table 5) also departs significantly from expectation.

There are several possible explanations for the nonagreement of the cytological data and those required for an autoploid according to requirements of the model of Fig. 1.

The first possibility is that the tetraploid H. violaceum is in fact a segmental alloploid derived from genetically different

Table 4. Metaphase I chromosome configuration in 2n=4x=28
Hordeum violaceum Boiss. & Huet.

Configurations and number of chromosomes in each

I[a]	II	III	IV	VI[b]	No. Cells
	14	1			10
2	13				8
4	12				3
6	11				1
1	12	1	0(1)		3
2	10	2	0(2)		1
	12		1		64
2	11		1		8
4	10		1		1
1	10	1	1(2)		4
5	8	1	1(2)		1
	10		2		61
2	9		2		4
4	8		2		1
1	8	1	2(3)		2
3	7	1	2(3)		3
	8		3		45
2	7		3		3
1	6	1	3(4)		2
	6		4		25
	4		5		13
	2		6		10
	0		7		3
	1(2)		5(6)	1	1
Σ 99	2558	17	621	1	277
c 99	5116	51	2484	6	7756

[a] Where appropriate, the correct number of univalents has been
added to the trivalents to increase the number of quadrivalents.
The correct quadrivalents number is then indicated in parentheses
in that column.
[b] The hexavalent was partitioned to a quadrivalent and a
bivalent since it probably resulted from translocation heterozygosity.
[c] Total number of chromosomes.

Table 5. Binomial distribution of quadrivalents (p) and bivalents (q) (p=2/3; q=1/3) of 2n=4x=28 with expected frequencies and observed and expected numbers of cells having different combinations of the configurations.

$(p+q)^7 =$	p^7	$+$ p^6q^1	$+$ p^5q^2	$+$ p^4q^3	$+$ p^3q^4	$+$ p^2q^5	$+$ p^1q^6	$+$ q^7
Configurations	7IV	6IV,2II	5IV,4II	4IV,6II	3IV,8II	2IV,10II	IV,12II	14II
Expected frequencies of cells	.0585	.2048	.3073	.2561	.1280	.0384	.0064	.0004
Observed number of cells[a]	3	10(11)	14(13)	25(27)	50(55)	71(72)	78(76)	10
Expected number of cells	16.2	56.7	85.1	70.9	35.5	10.6	1.8	0.1

a Number in parentheses are recalculated values from Table 4 only where trivalents have been converted to quadrivalents by adding a univalent or by converting a hexavalent to a quadrivalent and a bivalent. Observed data are from Hordeum violaceum.

populations. The higher than expected frequency of bivalents
might be explained by preferential pairing within the partially
differentiated genomes. Homoeologous pairing without sufficient
chiasmata could account for the univalents.

The second possibility is that the chiasma frequency in the
parental diploid was not the two per bivalent required by the
model. This could lead to increased bivalent frequency at the
expense of quadrivalents (Table 3). However, even if all trivalents and univalents are allocated to the quadrivalent class,
the ratio of quadrivalents is still too low. Furthermore, a
decrease in quadrivalents should result in an appreciable increase
of trivalents over that observed.

The third possible explanation for an excess of bivalents is
that chromosome associations prior to pachytene may have been
positioned in such a way that synapsis most frequently involved
only two chromosomes. Evidence for such a mechanism is well known
in the segmental allohexaploid Triticum aestivum. However, there
is now evidence for the same or a similar mechanism in diploids
and their autoploids.

Timmis and Rees (47) studied four autoploids from four
inbred lines of Secale cereale (2n=2x=14). Rye has most of the
requirements for the model of autoploids being used. Microsporocytes that were selected for analysis contained not more
than one rod bivalent. The remaining bivalents were rings, and
any univalents were allocated to trivalents. These were the only
considerations for sample selection; presence or absence of
quadrivalents was ignored. This was to assure that a deficiency
of chiasmata caused by asynapsis or ineffective synapsis was not
a limiting factor in the analysis. In a selected sample of
meiocytes, 94% of the multivalents were quadrivalents; the 6%
trivalents were attributed to the lack of at least three chiasmata
in a pachytene quadrivalent. However, a significant excess of
bivalents over the expected 50% was found in each of the autotetraploids from the four inbred lines. The cytological evidence
from meiosis indicated that in these lines the chromosomes were
associated to a significant degree in groups of two prior to
synapsis so that pachytene configurations were inferred to have a
higher frequency of bivalents than expected from random pairing
of four homologues. The reasoning concerning synapsis was that
in rye it follows the model used earlier for the occurrence and
placement of chiasmata and that effective chiasmata sites occur
only distally where synapsis begins. Nevertheless, because
pachytene stages were not analyzed, multivalents formed by inter-
stitial pairing may have occurred but were ineffective in chiasma
formation. But even if this were true, still unknown is the
mechanism responsible for the bivalent associations at the pairing
sites.

An explanation for the excess bivalents in both Secale and
Hordeum may be found in the results from Avivi's (16,17) work
with Triticium longissimum (2n=2x=14). This is a wild diploid

species of wheat with intermediate and low pairing lines. When
crossed with hexaploid T. aestivum, the intermediate pairing line
either promotes homoeologous pairing or does not suppress it, but
the low pairing line neither promotes nor suppresses homoeologous
pairing. The intermediate and low pairing lines do not differ in
their chiasma frequency at the diploid level. Autotetraploids
produced from each line also do not differ in chiasma frequency.
However, the two lines do differ significantly in quadrivalent
frequency at metaphase I. The 4x intermediate pairing line had a
mean of 4.35 ± 0.11 quadrivalents per cell while the low pairing
line had a quadrivalent frequency of 3.40 ± 0.20. The combination
of low quadrivalent and high bivalent frequency in the low pairing
line indicates that there was probably a positioning of the
chromosomes in groups of two when synapsis began. The effect of
the low pairing gene(s) was to maintain an arrangement of this
type in the autoploid while the high pairing line gene(s) did
not.

     Colchicine treatment of premeiotic cells in the anthers of
the intermediate pairing line of T. longissimum and of the high
pairing line of T. speltoides produced phenocopies of the low
pairing line of T. longissimum. There was an insignificant
difference in chiasma frequency, and tetraploid cells showed
complete pairing in the intermediate pairing line of T. longissimum.
In contrast with the induced tetraploid of this line with a mean
quadrivalent frequency per cell of 4.53, the meiocytes that had
mild colchicine premeiotic treatment had a mean quadrivalent
frequency of only 0.15 per cell. Essentially the same results
were found for T. speltoides. In both species there was a distinct
switch toward a higher frequency of bivalents without disrupting
normal chiasma frequency. Clearly there was a phenocopying
effect by the colchicine of the low pairing gene(s). This suggests
that the mild colchicine treatments of the premeiotic cells
disrupts the normal position of homologue attachment on the
nuclear membrane (16,17,18,48,49). When colchicine induces
tetraploidy, bivalent formation occurs mostly between the newly
replicated sister chromosomes because of their close proximity.

     The work by Avivi (16,17) thus suggests that the four auto-
tetraploids of inbred rye lines may have carried genes equivalent
to the low pairing gene(s) of Triticum longissimum. Timmis and
Rees discuss the effect of selection for improved fertility in
rye autoploids. In at least some lines, increased fertility was
correlated with increased quadrivalent frequency for reasons that
were not entirely clear. One might suppose that selection had
included an intermediate pairing gene as in T. longissimum in
combination with another factor influencing fertility.

     In regard to Hordeum violaceum, the tetraploid described may
be either a segmental allotetraploid or an autoploid. The higher
than expected frequency of bivalents may be due in part to low
pairing genes in the species. In both Hordeum and Secale, it is
important to inquire whether or not premeiotic positioning occurs.

The colchicine test used by Avivi and others could provide an answer.

Metaphase I Orientation and Disjunction. The final orientation of chromosomes at metaphase I normally will determine the anaphase I disjunction patterns. Various disjunctional configurations are possible, depending upon premeiotic positioning, differential affinity, ploidy level, and chiasma frequency and position. Multivalents in polyploids may behave variously, but their metaphase orientation and disjunctional patterns are not so closely tied to fertility as in translocation heterozygotes which produce multivalents. For example, in a whole arm translocation heterozygote involving two non-homologous metacentrics, a maximum configuration with distal chiasmata in all arms would be a circle of four chromosomes at metaphase I. The only two-by-two disjunctional patterns that are genetically balanced come from alternate chromosomes in the circle. In contrast, any two adjacent or alternate chromosomes from a circle in an autotetraploid will be genetically balanced. In polyploids, problems of genetic balance in the gametes is usually encountered to a greater extent in those with odd numbers of genomes. These will be discussed separately from even number types.

Even numbers of genomes with chiasma position and number discussed in the earlier model (Fig. 1) should be reasonably fertile if chromosomal balance is the limiting factor. For example, diploid, tetraploid, and hexaploid Hordeum violaceum do not appear to have significantly different pollen fertilities. Stebbins (5) has discussed several examples, however, in which chromosomal behavior and fertility are not correlated.

There are three types of disjunctional orientations of quadrivalents that form a circle of four. Two are concordant and one is discordant (50). Only the latter should produce chromosomally unbalanced gametes because there is a tendency for the central chromosomes to lag at anaphase I and not be included in daughter nuclei. If only three chiasmata are formed in the pachytene quadrivalent, a chain of four chromosomes occurs at metaphase I. The orientation on the metaphase plane may be convergent, parallel, indifferent or linear. The two latter types frequently may lag at anaphase and lead to sterility as with similar chromosomes from the discordant type.

The behavior of univalents has been documented in many species. Unless univalents initially have some special disjunctional mechanism or are otherwise preadapted for this state, certain predictions can be made about their behavior (51,52,50). They may frequently lag behind the disjoining bivalents and be left out of the regular nuclei at telophase I. They also may undergo centric misdivision by a break through the centromere, thus producing in some cases stable telocentric chromosomes. Repair of the DNA in the centric region by joining the double helix of the two sister chromatids may yield isochromosomes with

identical arms. Additionally, sister chromatids may separate at
anaphase I, but this frequently causes lagging, and both separated
chromatids may be left out of daughter nuclei. However, some
chromatids do manage to reach the poles and be included in the
normal nuclei. At the second anaphase they may undergo misdivision
or lagging or both. Chromosomes not included in normal nuclei
will usually form micronuclei. In further development each may
ultimately become a very small non-functional pollen grain. In
estimating fertility, counting of these small pollen grains may
give greater sterility than theoretically possible (53).

Much of the sterility in tetraploids is due to disjunction
of trivalents and univalents. Different types of trivalent
arrangements are convergent, linear, and indifferent (50). The
two latter types may leave the middle chromosomes behind at
anaphase I. The univalents may behave as those described.

With premeiotic association as in wheat or with preferential
pairing and at least one chiasma per bivalent, metaphase orientation and anaphase disjunction should be normal for even-numbered
polyploidy levels.

Odd numbers of genomes may result in several types of orientations at metaphase I; one or more genomes completely unpaired,
unpaired chromosomes with some special disjunctional mechanism,
or a mixture of multivalents, bivalents, and univalents.

If three genomes are present and two are paired as bivalents,
the third genome univalents may behave in several ways. Theoretically, they should move individually and at random to either pole.
Their distributions in telophase I nuclei can then be calculated
by expanding the binomial $(p + q)^n$, where n equals the number of
univalents chromosomes and p and q represent the two spindle poles.
It is clear that with increasing n the probability of getting
chromosomally balanced gametes decreases. In actual practice some
univalents may lag for various reasons so that cells with all
theoretical expectations may not be found. If the chromosomes can
be identified individually at later stages, one can test for
individual differences in lagging and loss frequency (51).

An odd number of genomes may not appreciably decrease fertility in cases with preferential disjunction of univalents. The
classical example is Rosa canina (2n=5x=35). In megasporocytes
there are seven bivalents and twenty-one univalents. At anaphase
I, the univalents all move to the micropylar end, while the seven
bivalents disjoin normally. The second meiotic division is
equational for the univalents so that meiosis yields two megaspores
with twenty-eight chromosomes and two with seven. In microsporocytes, seven bivalents and twenty-one univalents are found
at metaphase I. The seven bivalents disjoin normally, but the
univalents behave so that very few are included in the microspores. Pollen grains with seven chromosomes predominate and
are selected for during pollen tube growth. Since one of the
28 chromosome megaspores produces the nuclei of the embryo sac, a

28 chromosome egg and a seven chromosome sperm reconstitute the pentaploid condition in this species.

To some extent directed disjunction of univalents occurs in the meiocytes of Leucopogon juniperinum (2n=3x=12). At metaphase I there are four bivalents and four univalents. The bivalents disjoin normally, but the four univalent chromosomes do not follow a binomial distribution. Instead, they occur in the two telophase nuclei in a higher than expected frequency. Non-random disjunction was observed in the microsporocytes where the cytological analysis was made. Here 41.2% of the cells showed univalent distribution of 0↔4 (54).

Autotriploids are usually characterized by mixtures of trivalents, bivalents, and univalents. Because there are no special mechanisms to insure balanced disjunction of univalents and trivalents, they are usually rather sterile and produce large numbers of aneuploid gametes.

ANEUPLOIDY AND POLYPLOIDY

Aneuploidy is an increase or decrease by less than a complete genome in a cell, tissue, or whole organism. It may develop as a result of either meiotic or mitotic irregularities. In somatic tissue of polyploids, multiple spindles may cause decreases in number and tissue mosaics (55-59). In some species there is a regular decrease by euploidy to a basic number (58), and the decrease may continue until few chromosomes are found in the cell. Chromosomal elimination has been reported for numerous species (55). In hybrids of Hordeum bulbosum (2x or 4x) with other species, there may be complete elimination of H. bulbosum chromosomes through a series of cell divisions in the embryo.

The term aneuploidy if used alone can result in illogical ideas of genetic balance, so modifying terms have been proposed (2). These are holaneuploidy and meroaneuploidy. Holaneuploidy involves an increase or a decrease in chromosome number by entire chromosomes and their gene systems as they normally occur. This type of aneuploidy therefore involves additions such as primary trisomics and tetrasomics or losses to give monosomics or nullosomics. Nullosomics are expected only in polyploids, and usually autosomal monosomics are found more frequently in polyploids. Supernumerary chromosomes in their normal state may be classified as a kind of holaneuploid situation. This is because even though their origin in some groups is postulated as a derivative of regular chromsomes, it remains uncertain in most species.

Meroaneuploidy involves increases or decreases by parts of the original parental chromosomes. Centric fusion (Robertsonian translocation) decreases actual numbers of chromosomes as separate linkage groups, but the requisite genetic material of the chromosome is not lost, only the centromere and adjacent centric heterochromatin. In some cases the break may be such that some parts of two centromeres are involved in the rejoining (2,60). With

telocentric or subtelocentric chromosomes and centric heterochromatin, the chromosome number may be reduced by half if whole
arm translocations are involved. This same result may be obtained
with smaller translocations, but the process is more complicated.
There are numerous examples of meroaneuploid reduction in diploids
(2). The process has been suggested for a number of chromosomally
variable plant groups suspected of polyploidy, but adequate
cytogenetic verification is usually lacking. However, in a long
series of studies in the Commelinaceae, the elegant analyses of
Jones (61,62) have done much to solve some of the problems of
polyploidy and aneuploidy in the family. Representatives of the
genera Gibasis and Cymbispatha can serve as examples of chromosomal
changes in the family.

Gibasis schiediana has two cytotypes, 2n=10 and 2n=16. The
former is a self-sterile diploid and the latter a self-fertile
tetraploid. The haploid karyotype of the diploid has two metacentric chromosomes (M) and three acrocentrics (A). A basic (X)
karyotype of the tetraploid has three M and two A chromosomes.
Size relationships and meiotic analyses show that the extra M
chromosome came from centric fusion of two acrocentrics similar
to two of those in the diploid.

The F_1 hybrid has 13 chromosomes, eight M and five A. Four
M and two A from the tetraploid are structural homologues of two
M and one A of the diploid. These are expected to form trivalents,
bivalents, and univalents in the usual way, and their numbers did
not differ significantly from expected when chiasma frequencies
were used in the calculations.

Four chromosomes remain. The two metacentrics from the
tetraploid each have, for example, an a arm and a b arm. Of the
two acrocentrics from the diploid, one has an a arm and the other
a b arm. If pairing is random among these four chromosomes, and
if a single crossover occurs in each arm, four configurations in
various frequencies are possible. These are $1M_{II}$, $2A_I$ (1/9); 1
M-M-A$_{III}$, $1A_I$, (4/9); 2 M-A$_{II}$ (2/9); 1 A-M-A$_{III}$, M_I (2/9). These
were recognized and scored separately, and the frequency of the
M_{II} bivalent was far in excess of expected (62). This nonrandom
pairing may be taken as an indication that the chromosomes have
undergone differentiation, possibly in the polyploid.

In addition to the difference in breeding system and the
centric fusion in the tetraploid, there appear to be differences
in rhizome production (62). Thus the karyotype may be paralleling
morphological differentiation, and further study may indicate the
two cytotypes should be separate taxa. F_1's are highly pollen
sterile but have some female fertility. For all practical
purposes, however, they are mostly reproductively isolated.

The second example from the Commelinaceae is the genus
Cymbispatha with chromosome numbers of 2n=12,14,16,22,28, and 30
(62). Only the two species with 2n=14 will be discussed here
(C. geniculata and one chromosomal race of C. commelinoides).
All species and cytotypes have the fundamental arm number in

double or in multiples of seven. C. geniculata has 14 acrocentric
chromosomes (A) wile C. commelinoides has 14 metacentrics. This
suggests that the latter is a tetraploid that has undergone centric
fusions beginning with a tetraploid karyotype (2n=4x=28) based on
one similar to C. geniculata. That this is true is indicated by
meiotic pairing in 2n=14 C. commelinoides which forms up to three
quadrivalents per cell in unimodal frequencies. However, centric
fusion of whole arms can account for only 12 of the 14 chromosomes.
The remaining metacentric pair must have resulted from a fusion
between homologous acrocentric chromosomes to yield a pseudoiso-
chromosome. Duplication of the fusion isochromosome could then
yield the 2n=14 M karyotype of the polyploid. Evidence for the
fusion of homologous arms was found in one plant which had one or
two circle univalents in some cells. Isochromosomes have been
detected in three other genera of Commelinaceae, and Jones (62)
has discussed their evolutionary implication.
    Centric fusion, while being recognized as a major factor in
chromosomal evolution of many animals and some plants, must now
be considered as proved for some aneuploid modification in polyploids.

STRUCTURAL CHANGES IN POLYPLOIDS

    There is no reason why there should be a lack of structural
chromosome changes in polyploids. In terms of frequency, they
might be expected to be found more often in polyploids than in
diploids. This is because various deletions may be compensated
for by a normal genome in tetraploids and higher ploidy levels.
Also, there may be certain selective advantage when structural
changes become homozygous because this could lead to preferential
pairing and a more regular meiosis.
    Translocation systems may not be detected in polyploids
during meiosis if the interchange is among members of a homologous
set, but they are evident when the number of chromosomes in a
multivalent is greater than expected for a particular ploidy
level. There are few detailed studies of translocations in
natural polyploids. The analysis among populations of Haworthia
reinwardtii var. chalumnensis by Brandham (63), however, is of
interest because he found an interchange frequency of over 99% in
tetraploids and of 34% in triploids. This is all the more remarkable because the determinations were based on recognizable unequal
interchanges in somatic cells. An equally large number of equal
interchanges also might be expected. Because there was a low
frequency of homozygotes, there appears to be selection for
interchange heterozygotes, possible because they are more vigorous
than homozygotes.
    Both paracentric and pericentric inversions in polyploids
have been studied in detail in Brandham's (64,65) excellent
analyses. The major importance of these structural changes,

other than their possible effect on preferential pairing, is to change chromosome morphology and gene balance.

Paracentric inversion heterozygotes may transmit terminal deletions to progeny (64). Also, because dicentric bridges may be included in microspore or megaspore nuclei, there is a chance for continued breakage in embryos or later somatic tissue.

Pericentric inversion heterozygotes may produce chromosomes with both deletions and duplications. Because of compensation by an additional genome, these may be transmitted to progeny. The two ends of the duplication-deficiency chromosome are homologous so internal pairing may produce isochromosome behavior (64). If such chromosomes become homozygous, mostly external pairing could occur. The isochromosome-like behavior might not become apparent then until outcrossed hybrids were analyzed.

CONCLUDING STATEMENT

We have stressed many of the fundamental factors that should be considered in cytogenetic analyses of polyploids. To be of maximum use for comparative work, certain data items from controlled environments need to be part of any study. These may be enumerated as follows. For Parental or suspected parental taxa: (1) karyotype; (2) mean chiasma frequency per bivalent; (3) male and female fertility. For F_1 hybrids: same data as for parental taxa plus pachytene analysis. For Polyploids: same data as for parental or suspected parental taxa and F_1 hybrids. In addition, the multivalent, bivalent, and univalent numbers per cell or chromosome set should be listed so that they can be compared with expected distributions based on information derived from the parental taxa and F_1 hybrids. Tests for premeiotic association also should be carried out.

There are many non-cytogenetic items of information that are necessary. Some of these are comparative morphology, distribution, ecology, biochemistry, frequency of natural hybrids, and evidence of gene flow at the diploid and polyploid levels.

LITERATURE CITED

1.   Winge, Ö., 1917, The chromosomes. Their number and general importance. Carlsberg Lab., Copenhagen C.R. Trav. 13: 131-275.
2.   Jackson, R.C., 1971, The karyotype in systematics. Ann. Rev. Ecol. Syst. 2: 327-368.
3.   Jackson, R.C., 1976, Evolution and systematic significance of polyploidy. Ann. Rev. Ecol. Syst. 7: 209-234.
4.   Stebbins, G.L., 1947, Types of polyploids: Their classification and significance. Adv. Genet. 1: 403-429.

5.   Stebbins, G.L., 1950, "Variation and Evolution in Plants,"
     Columbia Univ. Press, New York.
6.   Stebbins, G.L., 1971, "Chromosomal Evolution in Higher
     Plants," Addison-Wesley, Reading, MA.
7.   Clausen, J., Keck, D.D., Hiesey, W.M., 1945, Experimental
     studies on the nature of species. II. Plant evolution
     through amphiploidy and autoploidy with examples from the
     Madiinae. Carn. Inst. Wash. Publ. 564: 174 pp.
8.   Baker, B.S., Carpenter, A.T.C., Esposito, M.S., Esposito,
     R.E., Sandler, L., 1976, The genetic control of meiosis.
     Ann. Rev. Genet. 10: 53-134.
9.   Okamoto, M., 1957, Asynaptic effect of chromosome V. Wheat
     Inf. Serv. 5: 6.
10. Riley, R., Chapman, V., 1958, Genetic control of the cytologi-
     cally diploid behaviour of hexaploid wheat. Nature 182:
     713-715.
11. Sears, E.R., Okamoto, M., 1958, Intergenomic chromosome
     relationships in hexaploid wheat. Proc. X Inter. Congr.
     Genet. 2: 259-269.
12. Sears, E.R., 1976, Genetic control of chromosome pairing in
     wheat. Ann. Rev. Genetics 10: 31-51.
13. Feldman, M., 1966, The effect of chromosome 5B, 5D, and 5A
     on chromosome pairing in Triticum aestivum. Proc. Nat. Acad.
     Sci. USA 55: 1477-1453.
14. Feldman, M., Mello-Sampayo, T., Sears, E.R., 1966, Somatic
     association in Triticum aestivum. Proc. Nat. Acad. Sci. USA
     56: 1192-1199.
15. Driscoll, C.J., Darvey, M.L., Barber, H.N., 1967, Effect of
     colchicine on meiosis of hexaploid wheat. Nature 216:
     687-688.
16. Avivi, L., 1976, The effect of genes controlling different
     degrees of homoeologous pairing on quadrivalent frequency in
     induced autotetraploid lines of Triticum longissimum.
     Canad. J. Genet. Cytol. 18: 357-364.
17. Avivi, L., 1976, Colchicine induced bivalent pairing of
     tetraploid microsporocytes in Triticum longissimum. Canad.
     J. Genet. Cytol. 18: 731-738.
18. Bennet, M.D., Stern, H., Woodward, M., 1974, Chromatin
     attachment to nuclear membrane of wheat pollen mother
     cells. Nature 252: 395-396.
19. Dover, G.A., Riley, R., 1973, The effect of spindle inhibitors
     applied before meiosis on meiotic chromosome pairing. J.
     Cell Sci. 12: 143-161.
20. Driscoll, C.J., Darvey, N.L., 1970, Chromosome pairing:
     Effect of colchicine on an isochromosome. Science 169:
     290-291.
21. Brown, W.V., Stack, S.M., 1968, Somatic pairing as a regular
     preliminary to meiosis. Bull. Torrey Bot. Club 95: 369-378.

22.   Engelhardt, P., Pusa, K., 1972, Nuclear pore complexes:
      "press-stud" elements of chromosomes in pairing control.
      Nature New Biol. 240: 163-166.
23.   Stern, H., Westagaard, M., von Wettstein, D., 1975, Presy-
      naptic events in meiocytes of Lilium longiflorum and their
      relation to crossing over: A preselection hypothesis.
      Proc. Nat. Acad. Sci. USA 72: 961-965.
24.   Gillies, C.B., 1975, Synaptonemal complex and chromosome
      structure. Ann. Rev. Genetics 9: 91-110.
25.   Holm, P.B., 1977, Three-dimension reconstruction of chromosome
      pairing during the zygotene stage of meiosis in Lilium
      longiflorum (Thonb.). Carlsberg Res. Commn. 42: 103-151.
26.   Moens, P.B., 1978, Ultrastructural studies of chiasma
      distribution. Ann. Rev. Genetics 12: 433-450.
27.   Lu, B.C., 1974, Genetic recombination in Coprinus. IV. A
      kinetic study of the temperature effect on recombination
      frequency. Genetics 78: 661-677.
28.   Wilson, J.Y., 1959, Chiasma frequency in relation to tempera-
      ture. Genetica 29: 290-303.
29.   Grant, V., 1952, Cytogenetics of the hybrid Gilia millefoliata
      X achilleaefolia. I. Variation in meiosis and polyploidy rate
      as affected by nutritional and genetic conditions. Chromosoma
      5: 372-390.
30.   Landner, L., Ryman, N., 1974, Genetic control of recombination
      in Neurospora crassa II. Polygenic and maternal control in
      two proximal chromosome regions - a quantitative analysis.
      Hereditas 78: 169-184.
31.   Valentin, J., 1972, Interchromosomal effects of autosomal
      inversions in Drosophila melanogaster. Hereditas 72:
      243-254.
32.   Tease, C., Jones, G.H., 1976, Chromosome-specific control of
      chiasma formation in Crepis capillaris. Chromosoma 57:
      33-49.
33.   Parker, J.S., 1975, Chromosome-specific control of chiasma
      formation. Chromosoma 49: 391-406.
34.   Maguire, M.P., 1978, Evidence for separate genetic control
      of crossing over and chiasma maintenance in maize. Chromo-
      soma 65: 173-183.
35.   John, B., Henderson, S.A.,1962, Asynapsis and polyploidy in
      Schistocerca paranensis. Chromosoma 13: 111-147.
36.   Sved, J.A., 1966, Telomere attachment of chromosomes. Some
      genetical and cytological consequences. Genetics 53:
      747-756.
37.   Levan, A., 1940, Meiosis of Allium porrum, a tetraploid
      species with chiasma localization. Hereditas 26: 454-462.
38.   Morrison, J.W., Rajhathy, T., 1960, Chromosome behaviour in
      autotetraploid cereals and grasses. Chromosoma 11: 297-309.
39.   Rhoades, M.M., 1952, Preferential segregation in maize, pp.
      66-80, in "Heterosis," Iowa State College, Ames.

40. Doyle, G.G., 1963, Preferential pairing in structural
     heterozygotes of Zea mays. Genetics 48: 1011-1027.
41. Doyle, G.C., 1969, Preferential pairing in trisomics of Zea
     mays. Chromosomes Today 2: 12-20.
42. Shaver, D.L., 1963, The effect of structural heterozygosity
     on the degree of preferential pairing in allotetraploids of
     Zea. Genetics 48: 515-524.
43. Snope, A.J., 1967, Meiotic behaviour in autotetraploid maize
     with abnormal chromosome 10. J. Heredity 58: 173-177.
44. Elci, S., Sybenga, J., 1976, Incomplete preferential pairing
     in a tetraploid Secale hybrid carrying translocations:
     Multivalent configuration frequencies and marker segregation.
     Genetica 46: 177-182.
45. Sybenga, J., 1975, The quantitative analysis of chromosome
     pairing and chiasma formation based on the relative frequen-
     cies of MI configurations. VII. Autotetraploids. Chromosoma
     50: 211-222.
46. Dewey, D.R., 1979, The Hordeum violaceum complex of Iran.
     Amer. J. Bot. 66: 166-172.
47. Timmis, J.N., Rees, H., 1971, A pairing restriction at
     pachytene upon multivalent formation in autotetraploids. J.
     Heredity 26: 269-275.
48. Hotta, Y., Shepard, J., 1973, Biochemical aspects of colchi-
     cine action on meiotic cells. Mol. Gen. Genet. 122: 243-260.
49. Rimpau, J., Lelley, T., 1972, Zur anheftung der meiotis
     chromosomen an die kernmembran. Z. Pflanzenzuechtg. 67:
     167-201.
50. Lewis, K.R., John, B., 1963, "Chromosome Marker," Little,
     Brown and Co., Boston.
51. Giraldey, R., Lacadena, J.R., 1976, Univalent behavior at
     anaphase I in desynaptic rye. Chromosoma 59: 63-72.
52. Khush, G.S., 1973, "Cytogenetics of Aneuploids," Academic
     Press, New York.
53. Jackson, R.C., 1973, Chromosomal evolution in Haplopappus
     gracilis: a centric transposition race. Evolution 27:
     243-256.
54. Smith-White, S., 1948, Polarised segregation in the pollen
     mother cells of a stable triploid. Heredity 2: 119-130.
55. Kasha, K.J., 1974, Haploids from somatic cells, pp. 67-90,
     in "Haploids in Higher Plants," University of Guelph,
     Guelph, Ont.
56. Ladizinsky, G., Fainstein, R., 1978, A case of genome
     partition in polyploid oats. Theor. App. Genet. 51: 159-160.
57. Snoad, B., 1955, Somatic instability of chromosome numbers
     in Hymenocallis calathenum. Heredity 9: 219-234.
58. Storey, W.B., 1968, Mitotic phenomena in the spider plant.
     J. Heredity 59: 23-27.
59. Tan, G-Y, Dunn, G.M., 1977, Mitotic instabilities in tetra-
     ploid, hexaploid, octoploid Bromus inermis. Canad. J.
     Genet. Cytol. 19: 531-536.

60.   John, B., Freeman, M., 1975, Causes and consequences of
      Robertsonian exchange.   Chromosoma 52: 132-136.
61.   Jones, K., 1969, Telocentric chromosomes in plants.   Chromo-
      somes Today 2: 218-222.
62.   Jones, K., 1979, Aspects of chromosome evolution in higher
      plants.   Adv. Bot. Res. 6: 159-194.
63.   Brandham, P.E., 1974, Interchange heterozygosity among
      populations of Haworthia reinwardtii var. chalumnensis.
      Chromosoma 47: 85-108.
64.   Brandham, P.E., 1977, The meiotic behaviour in polyploid
      Aloinae.   I.   Paracentric inversions. Chromosoma 62: 69-84.
65.   Brandham, P.E., 1977, The meiotic behaviour of inversions in
      polyploid Aloinae.   II.   Pericentric inversions.   Chromosoma
      62: 85-91.

POLYPLOIDY AND DISTRIBUTION

Friedrich Ehrendorfer

University of Vienna
Vienna, Austria A-1030

Since polyploidy has been recognized as a widespread and common phenomenon among eukaryotes, particularly higher plants, biologists have been interested in possible causal connections between polyploidy and distribution, and have tried to present relevant generalizations and "rules." A quick historical survey of this topic takes us back to the first relevant studies on angiosperms during the thirties: Hagerup (1) and Tischler (2) demonstrated a frequency increase of polyploids from southern to northern latitudes and interpreted it as the result of greater hardiness of polyploids under extreme ecological conditions. Manton (3), on the basis of her studies on Biscutella in glaciated and unglaciated areas in Europe, was the first to stress the better colonizing potential of polyploids. The further elaboration of this question in the forties and fifties can be exemplified by contributions from A. and D. Löve (4,5), Stebbins (6,7), and many others. During the same time studies concerned with polyploidy and distribution were extended to some animal and other plant groups (cf. contributions in this Conference), foremost to the pteridophytes, again by Manton (8). Her finding of very high chromosome base numbers in many fern plants paved the way to our understanding of paleopolyploidy, a phenomenon to which publications by Favarger (9) and S. and G. Mangenot (10) have further contributed during the sixties. First steps to elucidate the role of polyploids in different plant communities, succession lines, and ecosystems can be linked with papers by Knapp (11), Ehrendorfer (12,13), and Pignatti (14).

No dramatically new aspects have been proposed in regard to problems of polyploidy and distribution during the last decade, but a steady increase in well-documented detailed information

offers us a much broader basis for comparisons and critical
surveys of the problem today.

Since the thirties two approaches have offered themselves to
tackle the problems of polyploidy and distribution: Inquiries a)
into the relationships of diploid and polyploid taxa within
species, genera, or families, and b) into the relative frequency
of diploid and polyploid taxa among local floras or plant communities. One could illustrate these two approaches and our present
position in regard to polyploidy and distribution by giving a
rather general survey of the extensive literature, but such
surveys and literature compilations are available in very adequate
form (15-19, see Lewis p. 103). As an alternative, I propose to
present a number of cases of sexual polyploid complexes from the
angiosperms and of polyploid spectra from Austrian plant communities with which our Vienna research group has worked during the
past years. From these case studies it should become apparent
that some trends can be recognized in regard to the role of
polyploidy in distribution; but on the whole, a much more critical
attitude towards relevant generalizations still in vogue is to be
recommended.

NEOPOLYPLOIDY IN XEROPHYTES FROM THE
MEDITERRANEAN AND NEAR EAST

Two polyploid complexes from the Rubiaceae-Rubieae, both
consisting of outbreeding perennial herbs, have been chosen to
illustrate some basic aspects of polyploidy and distribution.
The first example concerns two very closely related species of
the genus Cruciata (20-21 for details and distribution maps):
Cruciata laevipes (=Galium cruciata) is diploid throughout and
rather uniform. As a mesophyte of the temperate deciduous forest
vegetation of Europe, it ranges from Portugal to n. Persia (with
a disjunct occurrence in the w. Himalaya), and from s. Greece to
Scotland. In contrast, C. taurica s.l. (= C. coronata) represents
an intricate polyploid complex with various 2x, 4x, 6x, and 8x
cytotypes, and very considerable morphological polymorphism.
Basically xerophytic, this complex occupies a remarkable variety
of open habitats from the colline to the alpine zone, radiating
from c. Anatolia to the w. Aegean, Crimea, and w. and n. Persia,
and adjacent Turkmenia. The apparent racial chaos of C. taurica
s.l. can be elucidated considering the distribution of the various
cytotypes: The diploids, morphologically uniform and well separated, are limited to local areas and to open habitats outside the
forest since ancient times, e.g., rock fissures within the n.
Anatolian forest belt (near Trabzon), montane talus slopes and
alpine rock steppes above timberline in the mountains of s.w.
Antolia, and extremely xeric primary steppes near the salt lake
Tuz Göll in c. Antolia. The tetraploids are linked in several

ways with the diploids and have radiated into considerably larger
areas with races concentrated in the Crimea, the mountain areas
from w. and n. Anatolia through Transcaucasia to w. and n. Persia,
and the steppe regions of c. and s.w. Anatolia, and of w. Iraq
through Syria to n. Israel. The hexaploids and octoploids,
finally, display a bewildering array of character combinations.
They obviously have been derived from hybridization between the
various diploids, tetraploids, and their locally interspersed
autopolyploids. These polyploids of hybrid origin have occupied
a variety of more recent open forest steppe habitats, have filled
the distribution gaps between the tetraploid races, and have
further extended the area of the C. taurica complex.

The polyploids within C. taurica s.l. obviously are neopolyploids (9), i.e., they are very similar and closely related to
extant diploids (or lower polyploids), so that they can be placed
into the same species (comparium, species aggregate, or closely
knit series). These neopolyploids are clearly less adapted to
extreme environments (drought, cold, etc.) than their diploid
relatives (and possible ancestors), but they obviously have been
superior in colonizing more recently opened up dry habitats in
the Near East: the areas occupied by 4x, 6x, and 8x members of
C. taurica s.l. are much more extensive than those held today by
the diploids. All this is well in line with our understanding of
the Pleistocene and Postglacial history of the Near East which
has suffered dramatic climatic and vegetational changes up to the
present, particularly in regard to the expansion of non-forested
areas from small initials. The explosive evolution of the C.
taurica polyploid complex obviously has been stimulated by these
events and the lability of the Near East environments.

In contrast, the mesic forest environment of the closely
related Cruciata laevipes has been rather stable and has allowed
the survival of this certainly ancient and uniform taxon on the
diploid level. During the postglacial expansion of deciduous
climax forests in Europe, this diploid C. laevipes even has been
able to occupy an area about three times as extensive as all the
diploids and polyploids of C. taurica s.l. put together. The
case of Cruciata, therefore, clearly illustrates that we can
understand the problems of polyploidy and distribution only if we
include historical and environmental aspects into our considerations.

The next example refers to a more advanced species aggregate,
i.e., the Galium incurvum agg. According to the latest survey
(Ehrendorfer and Ancev, in preparation) this complex includes
eight diploid and six tetraploid species, and ranges from s.w.
Romania, e. Yugoslavia and Bulgaria through Greece, the Aegean
Islands, and Anatolia to Transcaucasia and Lebanon. Habitats are
always dry and open, and range from woodland to rock fissures,
and from sea level to the alpine zone. The tetraploid members of
G. incurvum agg. are mostly intermediate in morphology, ecology,
and distribution between diploids, and apparently have originated

from them. Apart from diploids of the G. incurvum agg., two more diploids from the closely related G. mollugo agg. (e.g., G. heldreichii) seem to have contributed genomes to these tetraploids. A comparison of diploids and tetraploids in regard to local versus extensive distribution, or relatively ancient versus more recent habitats reveals no obvious regularities: in woodland habitats there are wide diploids, e.g., G. heldreichii (throughout the Aegean), and wide tetraploids, e.g., G. subuliferum s.l. (including G. flavescens p.p. and G. scabrifolium p.p.; throughout Bulgaria, n. and c. Anatolia). On the other hand, very local endemics from rocky habitats are again found, both among the diploids, e.g., G. bornmuelleri (in n. Anatolia) and the tetra-ploids, e.g., G. velenovskyi (in the Bulgarian Rhodope Mts.). Diploids and tetraploids within G. incurvum agg. often have widely overlapping geographical ranges. In such instances species integrity is maintained by a tendency to occupy somewhat different ecological niches and by the different ploidy level acting as a crossing barrier.

An interpretation of the evolution in the G. incurvum agg. has to consider it as part of the eastern (sub)mediterranean flora, an old, strongly differentiated, rich, and "saturated" flora which has evolved and radiated in an ecologically and geographically very diverse environment. In such rather stabilized floras polyploidy often underlies the origin of intermediate "fill-in" taxa and isolates them from their ancestors with which they often coexist in a parapatric fashion. In this way, poly-ploidy contributes to a more intensive partitioning of habitats into narrower and more specific ecological niches and a progressive "saturation" of established floras.

NEO-AND MESOPOLYPLOIDY IN PLANT GROUPS
OF THE GLACIATED EUROPEAN MOUNTAINS

The two following cases concern polyploid complexes from the European mountains, particularly the Alps, and illustrate the role of polyploids during and after glaciation periods from the beginning of the Pleistocene to the present. Again the examples are sympetalous Angiosperms and perennial herbaceous outbreeders.

Within the Dipsacaceae members of Knautia sect. Trichera radiated into a variety of mesic to dry habitats of the sub-mediterranean and temperate zone of Europe, ranging from the lowlands to above timberline. This differentiation has primarily taken place on the diploid level and by gene mutations. Few changes in chromosome structure have been involved, and due to incomplete crossing barriers, hybridization and the origin of hybrid polyploids were of importance in subsequent phases of evolution (13,22, and unpublished). Looking at the present distribution of the basic diploids (and some closely related tetraploids) of the Knautia drymeia and K. longifolia aggregates,

one can recognize widely disjunct areas which coincide with well
known ice age refugia while the distributional gaps are clearly
related to glaciation centres. The members of K. drymeia agg.
inhabit the warmer forest zones and extend from the w. Balkans to
Bohemia, the eastern and southern foothills of the Alps, the
French Plateau Central and the Pyrenees. In contrast, the rather
distinct species within K. longifolia agg. mainly occupy subalpine to
lower alpine meadows in isolated areas of the Balkan and e.
Karpathian Mts., the s.e. and w. Alps, the French Plateau Central,
and the e. Pyrenees. From extensive character analyses and
crossing experiments we know that members of these two ancient
and well-differentiated aggregates have been the main ancestors
of a polymorphic neopolyploid complex with tetraploids and hexaploids, the K. dipsacifolia agg. (=K. sylvatica agg.). This
complex takes an intermediate position in regard to morphology,
ecology, and distribution between K. drymeia agg. and K. longifolia
agg. Preferred habitats are montane to subalpine tall herb
communities. Two successive evolutionary phases are apparent:
the 4x members of K. disacifolia agg. occur in the mountains of
the Karpathians, c. Germany, and w. France, less affected by the
glaciation periods, while the most recent 6x cytotypes have
occupied their area in the c. and n. Alps only after the last
glaciation. Still, the size of the 6x area is inferior to that
held by the 4x cytotypes and the ancestral aggregates.

The K. dipsacifolia agg. is thus another good example of the
well-established generalization that neopolyploids which combine
genomes from different diploids (or lower polyploids) often
surpass their ancestors in variation, adaptability, and invasion
potential in new habitats and virgin areas, e.g., those which
have become available after the retreat of the extensive Pleistocene ice sheets.

As a contrast to the still very closely knit neopolyploid
Knautia groups, I shall now turn to the alpine members of Artemisia
group "Leucophorae" (Asteraceae/Anthemideae,23). This exemplifies
a much more mature and already somewhat "fragmented" polyploid
complex which is made up of mesopolyploid taxa. This term (9)
can be applied to polyploids which have clearly diverged from
extant diploids (or lower polyploids) at the species level, but
which are still close enough to them or related polyploids that
they can be placed into the same series, section, or small genus.

On the basis of detailed analysis of morphological, anatom-
ical, and karyological characters (including Giemsa-banded karyotypes), it has been possible to reveal the most likely phylogenetic
relationships among the group "Leucophorae" (Figs. 1 and 2). The
diploid basis of the group first consists of a pair of taxa with
n=9 (chromosome base number in Artemisia) and karyotype E with
very few heterochromatic bands; it includes the primitive and
strongly disjunct A. eriantha with alpine populations in the
Balkan and Karpathian Mts., the c. Appennin, the w. Alps and the
Pyrenees, and the advanced nival A. genipi which has successful

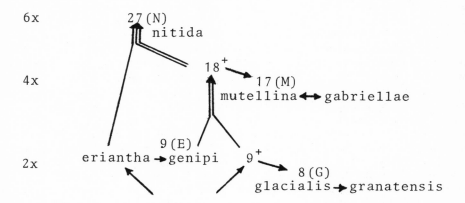

Fig. 1. Scheme of postulated phylogenetic relationships
between alpine members of Artemisia group "Leucophorae" with
references to ploidy levels (2x-4x-6x), haploid chromosome numbers,
hypothetical extinct types (+), and karyotypes (letters). Data
partly from Gutermann (23).

expanded throughout the high Alps. Another diploid branch,
probably of separate immigration, has the derived chromosome
number n=8 and karyotype G with many heterochromatic bands: it is
represented by two very distinct species of highest altitudes,
i.e., A. glacialis in the w. Alps and A. granatensis in the
Sierra Nevada of s. Spain. On a subtetraploid level with n=17
and karyotype M, we encounter two closely related alpine taxa, A.
mutellina which has expanded from an extensive area in the Alps
to the n. Appennin, the Pyrenees, and the Sierra Nevada, and A.
gabriellae, an endemic of the e. Pyrenees. These two subtetra-
ploids certainly had one common ancestor (probably in the Alps)
and combine characters from both the A. eriantha and the A.
glacialis subgroup. But their karyotypes definitely exclude the
possibility of a direct origin (suggested by the karyotype formula
E+G=M) and suggest participation of an extinct G-precursor, still
with n=9, and on the tetraploid level a reduction from an eutetra-
ploid M-precursor, also extinct: n=18→17. This interpretation
is supported by the fact that the group "Leucophorae" contains an
euhexaploid member, A. nitida, with n=27 and karyotype N which
shares some characters with the A. mutellina subgroup and with A.
eriantha. On behalf of its karyotype, relict habitat: (sub)-
alpine limestone rock fissures, and disjunct area in the s. Alps
and Alpe Apuane, A. nitida must be a very ancient member of the
group "Leucophorae" with its ancestors doubtful (A. eriantha ?)
or vanished.

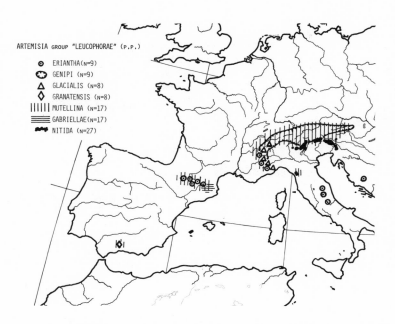

Fig. 2. Distribution map of alpine members of <u>Artemisia</u>
group "<u>Leucophorae</u>". Data from Gutermann (23).

The study of the relationships of diploids and mesopolyploids
within the group "<u>Leucophorae</u>" of <u>Artemisia</u> by Gutermann (23)
indicates the difficulties inherent in reconstructing the history
of older polyploid complexes. Furthermore, here is another clear
warning against uncritical generalizations in regard to our
topic: there are, side by side, at the diploid level ancient and
extremely localized relics like <u>A</u>. <u>granatensis</u> and evidently much
younger, successful nival migrants like <u>A</u>. <u>genipi</u>; and at the
polyploid levels we encounter a similar situation, comparing <u>A</u>.
<u>nitida</u> and <u>A</u>. <u>mutellina</u>. Circumstances like this certainly
should make us skeptical in assuming any direct role of polyploidy
in expansion and distribution.

PALEOPOLYPLOIDY IN TROPICAL WOODY FAMILIES

Our survey of polyploidy and distribution would be incomplete
without reference to woody angiosperms from (sub)tropical environments and comments on the phenomenon of paleopolyploidy. For an
illustration, I propose to discuss the Dilleniaceae (Dilleniales)
and the vesselless Winteraceae (Magnoliales).

DILLENIACEAE

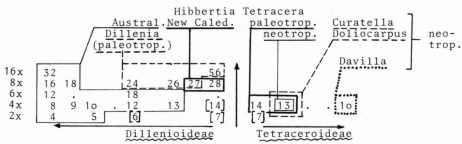

Fig. 3. Scheme of postulated relationships between haploid chromosome numbers within the Dilleniaceae with Dillenioideae and Tetraceroideae. Horizontal arrows signal dysploid lineages, the vertical arrow stands for polyploid lineages. Different lines surround coherent chromosome numbers and link them with generic names and areas.

On the basis of detailed morphological, phytochemical, and geographical analyses (24-27), together with karyological informa- tion (chromosome numbers, structure of interphase nuclei, etc., Ehrendorfer unpublished), our present knowledge about relationships, polyploidy and dysploidy, and distribution of the Dilleniaceae has been condensed into Fig. 3 and 4. A basic chromosome number of x=7 is postulated. Diploids with n=7 apparently are extinct, but polyploids on that base number have been found in paleotropical members of both subfamilies, the Tetraceroideae (on 4x) and the Dillenioideae (on 8x,16x). From this, the center of diversity and the concentration of primitive characters, a paleotropical origin of the ancient family with Dillenioideae-like ancestors can be assumed. In the neotropics evolution of the morphologically more advanced Tetraceoideae has proceeded at the 4x chromosome level and by descending dysploidy to n=13 and n=10. In the paleotropics the Dillenioideae are represented by the morphologi- cally quite primitive genus Dillenia. Its species are trees of humid rain forests for which only high polyploidy (8x, with some dysploidy, and 16x) has been recorded so far. This contrasts with the enormous karyological diversity in the related, but phylogenetically more progressive, genus Hibbertia which has radiated extensively from mesophytic trees to xerophytic pygmy shrubs, particularly in Australia (27). It is most remarkable in this context that the morphologically most primitive members of Hibbertia in the relict flora of New Caledonia are polyploids on the ancient chromosome base number x=7 (with n=28 and 27, Ehren- dorfer unpublished). The more advanced Australian species have

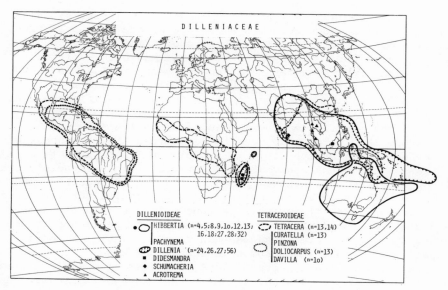

Fig. 4. Distribution map of Dilleniaceae, with references
to haploid chromosome numbers within genera. Data partly from
Kubitzki (25,26).

followed a line of descending dysploidy, with n=6 missing, but with
the very progressive diploid base numbers n=5 and n=4 still
preserved; on these, further polyploid lines with 4x, 6x, 8x and
16x taxa have originated.

The Dilleniaceae thus clearly illustrate various phases in
the evolution of polyploid complexes: Australian species of
Hibbertia are still in a relatively juvenile stage; their
progressive differentiation is reflected by dysploidy on the
diploid level, subsequent polyploid lines are still complete and
they correspond to the neo- and mesopolyploid pattern. In contrast, the New Caledonian species of Hibbertia, and particularly
members of Dillenia, represent much more mature and senescent
stages of polyploid complexes; as paleopolyploids (9) they have
become isolated because all of their diploid and lower polyploid
ancestors are now extinct or have diverged beyond recognition.
Such paleopolyploids are relict types, often preserve primitive
morphological features, adhere to original and stable habitats,
and occupy local or disjunct refugial areas as remnants of a
formerly more extensive distribution. What a contrast to the
neopolyploids which we have discussed, e.g., in Cruciata taurica
or in Knautia dipsacifolia! It is obvious that we shall fail in
generalization about polyploidy and distribution if we do not
differentiate between neo-, meso- and paleopolyploids, and recognize their dramatic differences.

Let us conclude this chapter on woody (sub)tropical paleopolyploids with short comments about one of the most primitive
families of angiosperms, the Winteraceae. From recent studies
(see 28, also for further references), it has been verified that
this predominantly Southern Hemisphere family includes a bulk of
morphologically most primitive hermaphroditic genera with a
remarkably disjunct distribution: in the s.w. Pacific there are
Bubbia (New Guinea to n.e. Australia, New Caledonia, and Lord
Howe Island), Belliolum (New Caledonia and Solomon Islands),
Exospermum (New Caledonia), and Pseudowintera (New Zealand), and
in the New World Drimys s.s. In my opinion Takhtajania from
Madagascar is not as aberrant as described (single carpels!) and
also belongs to this central group of the Winteraceae for which
(with the exception of Exospermum and Takhtajania, not yet studied
karyologically) the remarkable paleopolyploid chromosome number
n=43 has been documented. On New Caledonia there is a further
genus, Zygogynum, more advanced than the others by its fused
carpels, with n=86; its chromosome number has been doubled once
more, but its habitats, nevertheless, often are extremely ancient
and stable communities with Araucaria and other relict taxa. An
aberrant and morphologically more advanced element of the Winteraceae is the dioecious genus Tasmannia, formerly often included
under Drimys. It ranges from New Guinea south to Tasmania and
north to the Philippine Islands, and has n=13, a chromosome
number which apparently represents a tetraploid level in comparison
with the bulk of the family with n=43, to be interpreted as
dodecaploid (12x) (20); this would make the New Caledonian endemic
Zygogynum 24-ploid.

It is apparent that the data on the Winteraceae support our
skepticism in regard to rash generalizations about polyploidy,
habitat, and distribution and enforce a consideration of the
great variety of different polyploid types.

NEW APPROACHES TO POLYPLOID SPECTRA

If polyploidy has a direct or indirect effect on the ecology
and distribution of plants it should be possible to trace it by
comparing relative frequencies of diploid and polyploid taxa from
different habitats and different floras. Classical examples for
this approach are the polyploid spectra (18,30) from the n.
Sahara through Europe to n. Greenland which indicate an increase
from 37.8% to 85.9%. Originally this trend has been taken as an
indication of greater hardiness of the polyploids (1,2), and
later as the result of more recent establishment of the northern
floras (30,31). Favarger (16) and Stebbins (17), among others,
have pointed to the many fallacies of such global calculations
and generalized conclusions: foremost, the frequency of polyploidy
differs among different growth forms (e.g., more polyploids among
perennial herbs as compared with woody plants or annuals). As

floras vary greatly in their growth form spectra, polyploid
spectra, too, are greatly affected. Significant comparisons
therefore are only possible between floras of comparable structure.
Furthermore, the relative frequency of polyploids tends to increase
within groups, but also within floras, as a result of evolutionary
age; thus, there is a gradual accumulation of polyploids through
a shift from basic diploids to neopolyploids and on to meso-and
paleopolyploids. Consequently, ancient tropical floras have a
considerably greater proportion of polyploids (often paleopolyploids) than juvenile temperate floras. We can expect reasonable results from such spectra only when we differentiate between
different polyploid types. Finally, calculations of diploid/poly-
ploid frequencies should be based on local karyological research
and not on the often misleading literature data (cf. the common
occurrence of infraspecific polyploidy, etc.).

On the basis of the guiding principles outlined above, data
on four plant communities from near Vöslau, south of Vienna,
Lower Austria, have been assembled in the upper half of Table 1.
Two of these communities are situated on dolomite and more or
less shallow rendzina soils. They are permanent, extra-
successional communities: succession is compensated by erosion.
The Black Pine forest (Pinetum nigrae) is a relict community
which has persisted in the area at least throughout the last
glaciation. The adjacent rock steppe (Fumaneto-Stipetum) on
steeper slopes is rich both in dealpine relict species and in
early postglacial (sub)mediterranean-illyric immigrants. The
other two communities grow on limestone and brown forest soils of
later postglacial origin. First, there is a deciduous oak-
hornbeam forest (Querco-Carpinetum), established as a climax
community in the area approximately 6,000 years ago, and an
adjacent man-made meadow, a Mesobrometum, maintained by mowing
(and some grazing), and not older than that type of management,
i.e., several hundred years. These two communities can be regarded
as successional, as the meadow reverts to the deciduous forest
within a few decades without human interference. The growth form
spectra of all four communities are not so different as to distort
the following calculation.

The underlying classification of taxa into diploid/poly-
ploid types has been refined beyond customary procedures in Table
1: there is a first separation of uniformly diploid or polyploid
groups as stable from those with an internal diploid/polyploid
differentiation as labile. "Groups" are understood here in a
relative sense, i.e., as medium-sized genera, as sections of
larger genera, or as groups of small and closely related genera.
Conclusions about the relative age of floras and taxa are significant only when they are based on labile groups and on closely
related diploids and polyploids within groups. Stable groups
which lack current polyploidization indicate a rather steady
course of evolution in less disturbed environments. Polyploidization in labile groups points to hybridization and saltatory

Table 1. Proportions of diploids and polyploids in plant communities of Lower Austria and the Ivory Coast (values as percents).

Community	Number of species	Stable		Labile			
		diploids	polyploids	basic diploids	neo-polyploids	meso-polyploids	paleo-polyploids
I. Temperate Flora: Europe, Lower Austria, Vöslau (Ehrendorfer et al., unpublished)							
Deciduous forest (climax) (Querco-Carpinetum)	72	43.1	16.7	13.9	11.1	12.5	2.8
Pine forest (permanent) Pinetum nigrae	85	40.0	10.6	24.7	10.6	12.9	2.2
Rock Steppe (permanent) (Fumaneto-Stipetum)	40	27.5	12.5	37.5	12.5	10.0	--
Meadow (anthropogenous) (Mesobrometum)	104	38.5	8.7	14.4	27.9	10.6	--
II. Tropical Flora: Africa, Ivory Coast (data from 10)							
Rainforests	510	45.5	19.2	12.9	2.0	5.7	14.7
Savannas	45	51.1	15.7	8.9	6.7	11.1	6.7

evolution under more strongly fluctuating conditions. A high
frequency of basic diploids from such groups suggests a mature
parental flora which has engaged in the origin of juvenile daughter
floras where neo-(and meso-) polyploids are more prominent.
Paleopolyploids, on the other hand, indicate a senescent flora
whose origin lies in the distant past and which has survived to
the present under equable conditions.

A comparison of the figures for these diploid/polyploid
types in Table 1 reveals remarkable differences between the four
plant communities studied in Lower Austria: the two forest
communities have more stable diploids and polyploids (59.8% and
50.6%) than the rock steppe (40.0%) and the meadow (47.2%). The
forests also have a few paleopolyploids (2.8% and 2.2%) which are
altogether lacking in the open communities. There are more basic
diploids which have participated in the origin of polyploids in
the relict pine forest (24.7%) as compared with the postglacial
deciduous forest (13.9%). Basic diploids are most prominent in
the permanent rock steppe (37.5%), indicating the leading role
the species of this older community have played in the origin of
more recent neopolyploids of temperate central European open
habitats. Such neopolyploids, correspondingly, abound in the
most recent, man-made meadows (27.9%).

As a contrast to the temperate European diploid/polyploid
spectra, data from the rainforests and savannas of tropical West
Africa, Ivory Coast, have been incorporated into the lower half
of Table 1. The breakdown of the original chromosome reports by
S. and G. Mangenot (10) into the various types recognized is my
own and necessarily provisional. Nevertheless, the higher proportion of stable diploids and polyploids and of paleopolyploids in
comparison with the temperate communities is very obvious and
attests to the greater age and more steady evolution of the
tropical communities under more equable environments. But in
addition to that, there are apparently significant differences
between the rainforest and the savanna data, for the greater
frequency of stable polyploids (19.2%) and of paleopolyploids
(14.7%) in the rainforest flora suggests an unrivalled prominence
of ancient "senescent" and stasigenetic groups, while the good
proportion of basic diploids (12.9%) indicates certain potentials
for evolutionary radiation. The top values for stable diploids
(51.1%) and the somewhat higher figures for neo- and meospolyploids
(6.7% and 11.1%) in the savannas signal a more recently evolved
flora with numerous ana- and kladogenetic groups.

These results from improved and more discriminative diploid/
polyploid spectra correspond with a general scheme (12,13) proposed
for the different "compartments" of ecosystems, with differentiation, hybridization, and polyploidization prevailing in the more
labile, successional communities, with expansion promoted in the
climax, and conservation in the more stable permanent and extra-
successional communities.

CONCLUSIONS

With selected examples of sexual polyploid complexes from the angiosperms and of diploid/polyploid spectra from plant communities, I have tried to illustrate some aspects of polyploidy and distribution. From this it is evident that there are no direct and general causal connections between polyploidy on the one hand and ecology, habitat, or distribution of Angiosperms on the other. Still, a number of more general conclusions appear to be warranted.

1) Successful neopolyploid races tend to originate under more or less unstable environmental conditions and in areas of contact and hybridization between diploid (and lower polyploid) ancestors; this often involves local autopolyploid derivatives of the ancestral types.

2) The chances for the origin, establishment, and expansion of neopolyploids are best in widespread successional to subclimax communities and in areas which are being settled by invasion floras. Under such conditions the faster and more efficient mobilization of hybrid variability and the better genetic adaptability of neopolyploids often make them superior to their immediate diploid (lower polyploid or autopolyploid) ancestors.

3) Under more stable enviromental conditions, in the permanent communities of edaphically restricted and geographically localized habitats, and in well balanced climax communities, stable diploids and older polyploids prevail and limit the origin and expansion of neopolyploids. If neopolyploids are established under such conditions, their habitats and areas often are quite narrow in comparison with their ancestors. This results in a finer partitioning of ecological niches and an increasing "saturation" of mature floras.

4) Older polyploids, particularly meso- and paleopolyploids, often have suffered profound shifts and reductions of their habitats and distributions areas. Genetic divergence in such meso- and paleopolyploids often is slowed down considerably. Therefore, they often conserve primitive morphological, ecological, and distributional features, while related diploids (or lower polyploids) have greatly changed in this respect. Original relationships, therefore, often are blurred beyond recognition.

We should continue to be critical about these and similar generalizations. We should check and recheck them by further careful and many-sided analyses of polyploid complexes and by thoroughly documented and discriminative karyological surveys of diverse floras and vegetation types. Only in this way will we gain a deeper understanding of the role polyploidy and other cytogenetic mechanisms play in the extremely complex and dynamic evolution of our biosphere.

LITERATURE CITED

1. Hagerup, O., 1932, Über Polyploidie in Beziehung zu Klima, Ökologie und Phylogenie. Hereditas 16: 19-40.
2. Tischler, G., 1934, Die Bedeutung der Polyploidie für die Verbreitung der Angiospermen, erläutert an den Arten Schleswig-Holsteins, mit Ausblicken auf andere Florengebiete. Bot. Jahrb. 67: 1-36.
3. Manton, I., 1934, The problem of Biscutella laevigata L. Zeitschr. Indukt. Abst.-u. Vererbungsl. 67: 41-57.
4. Löve, A., Löve D., 1943, The significance of differences in the distribution of diploids and polyploids. Hereditas 29: 145-163.
5. Löve, A, Löve, D., 1949, The geobotanical significance of polyploidy. I. Polyploidy and latitude. Portug. Acta Biol. (A) special. vol. (R.B. Goldschmidt): 273-352.
6. Stebbins, G.L., 1942, Polyploid complexes in relation to ecology and the history of floras. Am. Nat. 76: 36-45.
7. Stebbins, G.L., 1950, "Variation and Evolution in Plants," Columbia Univ. Press, New York.
8. Manton, I., 1950, "Problems of Cytology and Evolution in Pteridophyta," Cambridge Univ. Press, London.
9. Favarger, C., 1961, Sur l'emploi des nombres de chromosomes en géographie botanique historique. Ber. Geobot. Inst. Rübel 32: 119-146.
10. Mangenot, S., Mangenot, G., 1962, Enquête sur les nombres chromosomiques dans une collection d'espèces tropicales. Rev. Syt. Biol. Vég. 25: 411-447.
11. Knapp, R., 1953, Über Zusammenhänge zwischen Polyploidie, Verbreitung, systematischer und soziologischer Stellung von Pflanzenarten in Mitteleuropa. Zeitschr. Indukt. Abst.-u. Vererbungsl. 85: 163-179.
12. Ehrendorfer, F., 1959, Differentiation-hybridization cycles and polyploidy in Achillea. Cold Spring Harbor Symp. Quant. Biol. 24: 141-152.
13. Ehrendorfer, F., 1962, Cytotaxonomische Beiträge zur Genese der mitteleuropäischen Flora und Vegetation. Ber. Deutsche Bot. Ges. 75: 137-152.
14. Pignatti, S., 1960, Il significato delle specie poliploidi nelle associazioni vegetali. Atti Ist. Venet Sc. Lett. Arti 118: 75-98.
15. Tischler, G., Wulff, H.D., 1953-1963, Allgemeine Pflanzen-karyologie, Angewandte Pflanzenkaryologie, in K. Linsbauer et al. (eds.), "Handbuch der Pflanzenanatomie," 2, Ergänzungs-band, Bornträger, Berlin.
16. Favarger, C., 1967, Cytologie et distribution des plantes. Biol. Rev. 42: 163-206.
17. Stebbins, G.L., 1971, "Chromosomal Evolution in Higher Plants," E. Arnold, London.

18. Gottschalk, W., 1976, "Die Bedeutung der Polyploidie für
     die Evolution der Pflanzen," G. Fischer, Stuttgart.
19. Jackson, R.C., 1976, Evolution and systematic significance
     of polyploidy. Ann. Rev. Ecol. Syst. 7: 209-234.
20. Ehrendorfer, F., 1970, Mediterran-mitteleuropäische Floren-
     beziehungen im Lichte cytotaxonomischer Befunde. Feddes
     Rep. 81: 3-32.
21. Ehrendorfer, F., 1971, Evolution and eco-geographical
     differentiation in some South-West Asiatic Rubiaceae, in
     P.H. Davis et al. (eds.), "Plant Life of South-West Asia,"
     Botanical Society of Edinburgh.
22. Ehrendorfer, F., 1962, Beiträge zur Phylogenie der Gattung
     Knautia (Dipsacaceae), I. Cytogenetische Grundlagen und
     allgemeine Hinweise. Österr. Bot. Zeitschr. 109: 276-343.
23. Gutermann, W., 1979, Systematik und Evolution einer alten,
     dysploid-polyploiden Oreophyten-Gruppe: Artemisia mutellina
     und ihre Verwandten (Asteraceae: Anthemideae). Diss.
     Formal-und Naturw. Fak., Univ. of Wien.
24. Kubitzki, K., 1969, Flavonoide und Systematik der Dilleni-
     aceae. Ber. Deutsche Bot. Ges. 81: 238-251.
25. Kubitzki, K., 1971, Doliocarpus, Davilla und verwandte
     Gattungen (Dilleniaceae). Mitt. Bot. Staatssamml. München
     9: 1-106.
26. Kubitzki, K., 1975, Relationships between distribution and
     evolution in some heterobathmic tropical groups. Bot.
     Jahrb. Syst. 96: 212-230.
27. Stebbins, G.L., R.D. Hoogland, 1976, Species diversity,
     ecology, and evolution in a primitive angiosperm genus:
     Hibbertia (Dilleniaceae). Plant Syst. Evol. 125: 139-154.
28. Ehrendorfer, F., Silberbauer-Gottsberger, I., Gottsberger,
     G., 1979, Variation on the population, racial, and species
     level in the primitive relic angiosperm genus Drimys (Winter-
     aceae) in South America. Plant Syst. Evol. 132: 53-83.
29. Ehrendorfer, F., Krendl, F., Habeler, E., Sauer, W., 1968,
     Chromosome numbers and evolution in primitive angiosperms.
     Taxon 17: 337-353.
30. Reese, G., 1958, Polyploidie und Verbreiung. Zeitschr. Bot.
     46: 339-354.
31. Reese, G., 1966, Apropos: Alter einer Flora. Ber. Deutsche
     Bot. Ges. 79: 177-181.

PHYSIOLOGY OF POLYPLOIDS

Moshe Tal[1]

Department of Biology
Ben Gurion University of the Negev,
Beer Sheva, Israel

A number of facts suggest that the multiplication of the genome has played an important role in the evolution of all major phylogenetic groups (1-4). Multiplication might be achieved either by an increase of the DNA/chromosome ratio (cryptic polyploidy) or by the doubling of the entire chromosome complement (conventional polyploidy), the latter being widespread in higher plants. Polyploidy has been found in at least 30% of the genera of flowering plants. Moreover, it has been suggested that most genera of flowering plants with a basic gametic chromosome number of 12 or more are the product of an ancient polyploidy (4).

Polyploidy raises questions of "why" which are concerned with the evolutionary reasons for the phenomenon and of "how" which deal with genetic and physiological mechanisms.

It has been suggested that polyploid plants tend to be more successful than diploid plants as invaders of relatively disturbed habitats, such as those vacated by pleistocene glaciers (4). Such habitats may, according to Pojar (5), also include sand dunes, salt marshes and subalpine meadows, all of which are characterized by frequent, drastic, irregularly recurring distur- bances and which are therefore nearly always available for colonization. Dobzhansky et al. (6) suggested that successful polyploid invaders, including those which cytologically behave as autopolyploids, are of hybrid origin. It has also been suggested that a high capacity for invading new habitats is related to intensive hybridization in plants (4). However, while hybridiza-

---

[1]I thank Miss Dorot Imber and Dr. Alan Witztum for their advice.

tion on the diploid level is accompanied by sterility and/or excessive segregation, chromosome doubling following hybridization might eliminate the sterility and reduce the amount of genetic recombination that characterizes diploid hybrids (16). This mechanism will be referred to as "balanced hybridity". Dobzhansky et al. (6) concluded that "contrary to earlier opinions, polyploids are not usually more successful than their diploid ancestors in regions having climates characterized by severe cold or drought; in many instances, they occur in regions that are more mesic and favorable than some or all of their diploid ancestors".

In addition to the advantage of balanced hybridity, genome multiplication per se may also contribute to the success of polyploids. Since natural polyploids may differ from their diploid counterparts in the various genetic changes accumulated during evolution, the effect of genome multiplication per se can be studied independently of other effects only in autopolyploids newly derived from ancestral strains.

The specific contribution of genome multiplication is not necessarily related to a specific structure or process, but is most likely a result of the integrated functioning of all components of the organism. However, since the research on this subject is very scanty, the data are still scarce and fragmentary. The existing fragmentary knowledge on the physiological aspects of genome multiplication will be reviewed according to the level of organization or function.

GENE ACTION

DNA which Codes for rRNA

By the use of DNA-rRNA hybridization, Cullis and Davis (7) found that in newly produced polyploids of Datura, the rDNA/total DNA ratio is the same at different ploidy levels. In Vicia (8), which is largely a diploid genus, and Nicotiana (9), which contains diploid and polyploid species, the genomic fraction of rDNA decreases as the DNA content increases. Cullis and Davies (7) suggested that contrary to the situation in the newly derived polyploids of Datura, mechanisms controlling the number of cistrons were envolved during the evolution of Vicia and Nicotiana. Mahr and Fox (8) suggested that with the increase of DNA content in Vicia, fewer of its genes are transcribed, and therefore less rRNA is necessary to meet the requirements of translation.

Modification of Enzyme Activity

Albuzio et al. (10) compared the activity of various enzymes in a diploid cultivated tomato variety and in an autotetraploid derived from it. The comparison included enzymes involved in the carbon pathway of photosynthesis, electron-transport chain of respiration and nitrogen assimilation. The lower capacity for CO_2 assimilation in the polyploids was explained by the reduced activity of ribulose diphosphate carboxylase in these plants, which was not compensated by the decrease in the activity of the enzymes involved in photorespiration. The study also included six enzymes associated with carbohydrate metabolism. The change in the activity of these enzymes was not necessarily related to the change of gene dosage; the activity of three enzymes increased, in one it remained unchanged and in the other two it decreased in the polyploid as compared with the diploid plants. Albuzio et al. (10) interpreted this enzyme behavior in the polyploid plants as "ambiguous" and suggested that this ambiguity is the cause for disturbed metabolic regulation and consequently the abnormality of development and reproduction processes in the polyploid plants.

The study of peroxidase activity in polyploid series of gametophytes and sporophytes in the fern Todea barbata is interesting as it reflects biochemical changes accompanying gene duplication (11). DeMaggio and Lambrukos (11) found that while total peroxidase activity increased at the higher somatic ploidy levels, the activities of individual isozymes varied, as did the enzymes of carbohydrate metabolism in tomato (10) - some were lower, some were the same and others were higher in the polyploid than in the diploid plants. Carlson (12) studied a number of enzymes in primary and secondary trisomics of Datura and found a marked gene-dosage effect on enzyme activity. He suggested that the rate of transcription of each structural gene is constant and independent of its number, and consequently the increase in the amount of gene product and enzyme activity is related to the increase in the number of that gene. DeMaggio and Lambrukos (11) suggested that in the fern the absence of a direct relationship between gene dosage and enzyme activity indicates that some form of regulation mechanism, in addition to transcription rate, controls isozyme activity in the polyploid plants.

Total RNA and protein

Tal (13) studied the concentration of RNA, which is probably mostly rRNA, and protein in an artificial autotetraploid of tomato. He found that the RNA and protein contents per haploid genome of the polyploid plants were about 85% of those of the diploid plants. The lower RNase activity found in the polyploid plants suggests that the reduced RNA content results from a lower rate of RNA synthesis in this plant. The decrease in RNA synthesis in the polyploid plant may result from the repression of the rDNA cistrons. The decrease in protein synthesis in the autopolyploid tomato was indicated by the somewhat lower percentage of incorporation of labeled leucine into protein in these plants (13).

Similar findings were reported by Albuzio et al. (10) in the
tomato. They found that although the activity of the enzymes
associated with nitrate assimilation was increased, the rate of
protein synthesis was greatly reduced in the autotetraploid
tomato. They postulated that the activity of enzymes concerned
with the transcriptional and translational processes is regulated
independently of that of the enzymes associated with intermediary
metabolism. Albuzio et al. (10) suggested this phenomenon as
another example of the unfavorable balance in the polyploid
tomato plants.

DNA CONTENT, CELL CYCLE, AND CELL DIMENSIONS

According to Stebbins (4), the most common primary effect of
polyploidy is the increase of cell size, with the consequent
decrease in the cell surface/volume ratio. Similar changes in
cell dimensions were found in the autotetraploid tomato as measured
in naked protoplasts isolated from leaves of diploid and polyploid
plants (Tal, unpublished). Dermen (14) speculated that some of
the physiological effects attributed to polyploids may be related
to changes in the relationship between volume and surface in
chromosomes, nuclei and other cell constituents. Price (15), who
carried out an extensive study on a number of different plant
species, concluded that there is a direct relation between the
amount of DNA per cell, nuclear volume and cell volume in plants.
Van't Hof (16) found in roots of germinating seedlings of distantly
related plants a direct relationship between the duration of the
cell cycle and both the S period and the amount of DNA per cell.
Evans (17) also found that the duration of the mitotic cycle in
comparable tissues of different plant species is closely correlated
with the amount of nuclear DNA. In agreement, reduced number of
cell divisions during development is characteristic of polyploidy
(4). In contrast to Van't Hof (16), Troy (18) found in diploid-
autotetraploid comparisons performed in several higher plants
that the duration of the S period is relatively constant and does
not depend on the DNA content. Similar findings have been reported
in ferns (19). It was proposed, therefore that the increase of
gene number in the cell is accompanied by a proportional increase
in the activity of the enzymes involved in DNA synthesis (18).

According to the nucleotypic theory of Bennett (20), certain
physical parameters of the plant, including mitotic cycle time,
duration of mitosis, chromosome size and nuclear and cell volumes,
are determined by the amount of DNA per nucleus regardless of the
information content of the DNA. He suggested, therefore, that
nuclear DNA content and devlopmental rates are inversely related,
i.e., the lower the DNA content the faster the developmental
rate. Price and Bachman (21) found that the change in DNA content
influences cell volume to a larger extent than it does the duration
of the mitotic cycle. They concluded, therefore, that plants

with a high DNA content apparently have the potential to differentiate more mass in a given period of time than low-DNA forms,
but they do this in fewer and larger cells. They suggested that
different strategies can be employed for rapid developmental
rates either through a selection for low DNA content and small
cell and plant size or a selection of high DNA content and con-
comitantly greater cell size.

GROWTH SUBSTANCES

The balance of growth substances may have a regulatory
influence on most functions of the plant. Very little is known,
however, on this balance in autopolyploid plants. Gustafsson
(22) found a lower content of a growth substance, probably an
auxin, in autotetraploid Lycopersicon pimpinellifolium as compared
with the diploid plants. An indirect indication of higher
activity of auxin in autotetraploid tomato derived from a cultivated diploid variety was obtained from the response of callus
growth to auxin supplied externally (Tal, unpublished). Tal
found that the growth of callus tissue derived from the polyploid
tomato was suppressed to a greater extent than that of the diploid
species by increasing the concentration of α-naphthalene acetic
acid in the medium from 0.2 to 2.0 mg/L. In addition, symptoms
characteristic of excess of ethylene and/or auxin (25) appeared
in the autopolyploid tomato during its development (Tal, unpublished). These symptoms included pronounced leaf epinasty and
stem swelling. A high activity of auxin, even at a low concentration, might result from a low concentration of an auxin antagonist. Tal (38) also found that the content of abscisic acid was
lower in the polyploid than in the diploid plant. Whether the
latter hormone plays the role of an auxin antagonist in the
tetraploid plant is not known. Since the data are very fragmentary
and since hormones usually interact with one another, a better
understanding of the role of hormone balance in the polyploid
plants requires simultaneous analyses of all the major hormones
in the plant.

WATER BALANCE

A higher water content and, consequently, a lower osmotic
pressure, has been found in an autotetraploid cultivated tomato
as compared with the diploid species (24,25,26). Györffy (27)
found that under low humidity, in contrast to high humidity, the
polyploid plants developed a higher osmotic pressure than the
diploid plants. In agreement with previous results, Tal and
Gardi (28) found that autotetraploid cultivated tomato plants had
a higher water content, as expressed by succulence, and a higher
relative water content than in the diploid plants. They suggested

that the higher relative water content in the polyploid plants
might result from the lower transpiration and possibly, to some
extent, from the higher root pressure. Lower transpiration in
polyploid plants than in diploid plants was also observed by Chen
and Tong (29) in barley.

Two of the major resistances to water flow which govern
water status in the plant are the resistance to water absorption
in the root and the resistance to water loss in the leaf, which
is controlled mainly by the stomata (30). Although the circumference and area of the aperture of the individual stomata in
the polyploid plant was greater than that in the diploid plant,
the total circumference and area of all apertures per unit leaf
area is smaller in the polyploid. This fact can explain the
lower transpiration in the polyploid plant.

Higher root pressure in the polyploid tomato was indicated
by the greater guttation of polyploid leaves at night as well as
by the larger amount of root exudate in these plants (28). The
higher root pressure in the polyploid may contribute to their
growth. During the night, when transpiration is low, root pressure
may have a significant effect on plant turgor and consequently on
cell and plant growth (28). It is well known, however, that cell
size and the ability of the plant to survive drought are inversely
related (31). Steudle et al. (32) found that smaller cells
require much lower changes of turgor pressure to reach a certain
degree of cell well extension, i.e., growth may be slowed as cells
increase in volumn. Cutler et al. (33) found that the decrease
of cell size permits the development of lower osmotic potentials
in the cell, and consequently the ability of the cell to preserve
the turgor required for growth increases. The disadvantage
conferred by the greater cell size of the polyploid plant on its
turgor pressure may be compensated by the lower transpiration and
probably also by the higher root pressure in these plants.

ION BALANCE

Cacco et al. (34) studied the uptake of SO_4^{-2} and K^+ by
roots of diploid and polyploid wheat, sugar beet, and tomato.
They found that at increasing ploidy, wheat and sugar beet showed
higher efficiency and tomato lower efficiency for the uptake of
these ions. Natural selection may improve the uptake of nutrients
existing in limited amounts by either one or both strategies: a.
velocity strategy, i.e., increasing V_{max}, b. affinity or efficiency
strategy, i.e., decreasing K_m (35). While in wheat and sugar beet
the higher ploidy was characterized by high V_{max} and unchanged or
decreased K_m, in tomato it was reflected by a small decrease in
K_m and a greater decrease in V_{max}. Cacco et al. (34) thus concluded
that, in spite of the small decrease of K_m, the decreased efficiency in the tomato results from the decrease of V_{max} (velocity
strategy).

Albuzio et al. (10) distinguish between metabolic and transport activities which are responsible, respectively, for transformation and supply of nutrients. They suggest that nutrient
supply has a priority in the general regulation of plant metabolism, since the rate of transformation of a metabolite cannot be
greater than its rate of uptake. The lower efficiency of the
transport system in the roots of the polyploid tomato may,
according to their opinion, be the major expression of the
unbalanced gene regulation in this plant. Most recently, Tal and
Morton (unpublished) found in a preliminary experiment that the
activity of $(K^+ + Na^+)$-activated adenosine triphosphatase (ATPase)
was not lower in the root of the autotetraploid cultivated tomato
as expected from the results of Cacco et al. (34). If the suggestion (36) that ATPase is involved in the active uptake of K^+
in the plant root is correct, and if our preliminary result is
correct, then the lack of direct relation between the efficiency
of K^+ uptake and ATPase activity in the tetraploid tomato raises
a big question.

DEVELOPMENT, PHENOTYPIC STABILITY, AND FERTILITY

The influence of polyploidy on the phenotype of the plant is
characterized by its gigas effect and the change it causes in the
shape and texture of organs. The leaves, for example, are usually
thicker, broader, and shorter than those of the diploid ancestors
(4). However, the increase of cell size, which generally characterizes polyploids, does not necessarily lead to increased size
of the plant as a whole or even of its individual organs because
of the reduction in the number of cell divisions in these plants
(4). These generalizations also seem to be correct for the
autotetraploid tomato – compared with its diploid progenitor –
which was found to have shorter, wider, and thicker cotyledons and
leaves, and a slower growth rate, at least during the early phase
of development (28).
Another important aspect of plant performance is the
stability of its phenotypic expression, especially for traits
important for survival. Faberge (37) found that autotetraploid
tomato plants were less variable than the diploid ancestor in
respect to weight of the whole plant and the fruits. Tal (unpublished) found that the variability of the leaf width/length ratio
as well as of the cell size was about the same in the autotetraploid tomato and the diploid plant. Whether or not the
stability of these characteristics is important for survival of
the plant is still an open question. The results indicate,
however, that the multiplication of the genome does not decrease
the stability of the phenotypic expression of certain characters,
but on the opposite, it might even increase it in certain cases.
Lowered fertility is a common effect of autopolyploidy (4).
The lower fertility may result from either cytological or phys-

iological causes or from both of them. Tal and Gardi (28) found, in agreement, that autopolyploid tomato plants were less fertile than their diploid progenitor. Since meiosis in the polyploid plants was found to be regular, i.e., the chromosomes were equally distributed during anaphase I, it can be concluded that the lower fertility of these plants resulted from physiological disturbances.

The decreased fertility and retarded growth rate, characteristic of newly derived autopolyploids, contribute to their adaptive inferiority, as found in autopolyploid-diploid comparisons in many genera (4). According to Stebbins (4), during evolution this adaptive disadvantage of genome multiplication might have been compensated by genetic-evolutionary processes, e.g., 1) gradual genetic modification through mutation, genetic recombination and selection, 2) modification through hybridization, either preceding or following the doubling of chromosomes, and selection of adaptive segregants.

RESPONSES OF POLYPLOIDS TO STRESS

Salinity

Tal and Gardi (28) and Tal (13) compared the responses to salinity stress of diploid and autotetraploid plants of the cultivated tomato. They (28) found that under salinity, dry weight of the whole plant and relative water content decreased to a smaller extent in the polyploid plants than in the diploids and suggested that the better growth of the former under salinity stress results, in part, from the better water balance in these plants. It was suggested, therefore, that certain constituents and functions which are known to be influenced by water stress would be less affected by salinity in the polyploid plant. Contrary to expectation, the polyploid plants resembled the diploids in their metabolic adaptation to salt stress. Salinity affected diploid and polyploid plants similarly with respect to the content of DNA, protein, ABA, RNase activity, and leucine incorporation.

Irradiation and Mutagenesis

Sparrow and Miksche (38) found that polyploid plants are more tolerant to irradiation than diploid plants. Baetcke et al., (39) suggested that radiosensitivity is directly related to the chromosome size and the volume occupied by the DNA.

Sparrow et al. (40) suggested that the greater radiation resistance found in some polyploids as compared with related diploids, is more likely to be due to their reduced chromosome volume rather than to the radioprotective effect of gene redundancy. Swaminathan et al. (41), however, claimed that the

resistance to mutagenesis by ethyl methane sulphonate in induced
tetraploid barley resulted from the increased genetic redundancy.

Herbicides

Tomkins and Grant (42) studied the response of various weeds
to different herbicides. They found that of all the different
plant characteristics studied, e.g., organization, life-form, and
various physiological and cytological factors, only the level of
ploidy was significantly related to herbicide resistance. Polyploid plants were more resistant than diploid plants. They
suggested that two mechanisms are responsible for the higher
resistance in the weed species, i.e., increased heterozygozity in
the allopolyploids and increased genetic redundancy in the autopolyploids.

DISCUSSION AND CONCLUSIONS

The success of polyploid plants is, as suggested above, due
to balanced hybridity and possibly also to the effect of genome
multiplication per se. The effect of the latter can be studied
independently of the effect of other genetic changes only in
autopolyploids newly derived from single ancestral strains.
However, compared with their diploid progenitors these autopolyploids usually exhibit adaptive inferiority which might be compensated by other genetic processes only during evolution (4).
During the process of adaptation, the positive contributions of
genome multiplication to the physiology of the plant may be
manifested.
When studying the physiological changes associated with the
multiplication of the genome, we attempt to differentiate between
those changes that might contribute to the inferiority of the
autopolyploid plant and those that might contribute to the success
of natural polyploids.
Albuzio et al. (10) interpreted the lack of a consistant
relationship between the changes in the activities of certain
enzymes and the change of gene dosage, found in the autotetraploid
tomato, to be among the causes for the upsetting of metabolic
regulation and consequently the developmental abnormalities of
this plant. Their interpretation is correct if the rate of
transcription of each structural gene is constant and independent
of its number and consequently the increase in the amount of gene
product and enzyme activity is related to the increase in the
amount of that gene. It is possible, however, that the absence
of a direct relationship between gene dosage and enzyme activity
results from another form of regulation mechanism. It is,
therefore, impossible at the present stage to decide unequivocally
whether one pattern of enzymatic response to the multiplication

of the genome is more favorable than another to the plant. More
objective assessment of the contribution of specific changes to
the performance of the plant as a whole may be obtained only on
the basis of an integrated study of all major changes caused by
genome multiplication and their effect on the performance of the
whole plant and preferable under a variety of conditions.

Although the available information is fragmentary and based
on a very narrow spectrum of plant types, some tendencies are
indicated (Table 1):

1) The amounts of RNA and protein per cell were not doubled
following the doubling of the whole genome. The change of RNA
and protein levels seem to be related to the change of cell
surface, which represents the cytoplasm, and not to the change of
volume which represents mainly the vacuole. The possible direct
relation between the levels of RNA and protein and the space
occupied by the cytoplasm, suggests that the concentration of
these macromolecules in the cytoplasm was unchanged with the
increase of ploidy level. It seems, therefore, as if the total
activity of the genes involved in the production of RNA and
protein is related to the volume occupied by the cytoplasm and is
controlled by the concentration of these macromolecules. The
validity of this hypothesis, however, should be confirmed by
additional experiments.

2) Various activities including RNA and protein synthesis,
CO_2 assimilation, transpiration and ion uptake, as well as the
level of auxin and abscisic acid were found to decrease in the
polyploid plant as compared with the diploid one.

3) The autotetraploid tomato plant has a better water balance.

4) The stability of the expression of certain phenotypic
characters is similar or even greater in the autotetraploid
tomato as compared with the diploid plant.

These facts and the better performance of the autotetraploid
tomato plants under salinity stress (28) and of other autopolyploid
plants exposed to herbicides (43), might represent positive
contributions of genome multiplication. However, since the
available information is fragmentary and based mainly on only one
plant type, e.g., the tomato, any generalization on the effect of
genome multiplication must wait for more data derived from
additional experimantal systems.

Representative experimental systems may include diploid-
autopolyploid comparisons in cultivated vs. wild plants or in
genetically homozygous vs. heterozygous plants. Following this
line, our study in the physiology of polyploids that dealt with
the cultivated tomato, is, therefore, being extended to the wild
tomato species Lycopersicon peruvianum. This species, which is
more tolerant to salinity (44) and probably also to drought than
the cultivated species, is self-incompatible and consequently
highly heterozygous (45).

An additional approach recommended in the study of the
physiology of polyploid plants is the comparison of diploids and

Table 1. Quantitative changes in the cultivated tomato (4x/2x).

Cell volume	1.90	Transpiration	0.84
Cell surface	1.60	Stomata	
DNA/Cell[a]	2.00	Size	1.76
		Aperture area/ unit of leaf area	0.81
RNA/Cell	1.70	Circumference/ unit leaf area	0.90
Protein/Cell	1.60	Root pressure	>1
Dry matter/Cell	1.85	Water content	>1
		Relative Water content	>1
RNA Synthesis	<1		
Protein Synthesis	<1	Uptake efficiency[d]	
		K^+	0.79
Auxin Level[b]	0.63	SO_4^{2-}	0.72
Auxin Activity	>1(?)		
Abscisic acid level	0.73	Activity of (K^++Na^+)-ATPase	1(?)
CO_2 assimilation[c]	<1	Stability of pheno- typic expression[e]	≩1

[a] A calculated value.

[b] From Gustafsson (22). Auxin level was determined in Lycopersicon pimpinellifolium.

[c] From Albuzio et al. (10).

[d] From Cacco et al. (34).

[e] From Faberge (37) and Tal (unpublished).

All other values are from Tal (13), Tal and Gardi (28), Tal, and Tal and Morton (unpublished). Question marks signify results based only on preliminary experiments.

polyploids on different organizational levels. The study of
isolated tissues and cells, for example, may help to answer the
question whether the specific behavior of the polyploid, as
compared with the diploid, is related to a cellular characteristic
or to the organization of the cells in the tissues in the whole
plant.

SUMMARY

Polyploidy, a multiplication of the whole chromosomal complement, is a very widespread phenomenon in higher plants. Natural
polyploids have been suggested to be more successful than their
diploid progenitors under certain conditions. This success may
be due to "balance hybridity," i.e., the combination of the
advantage of hybridity together with the balancing of excessive
segregation and sterility by chromosome doubling, and possibly
also to the effect of genome multiplication per se. The latter
effect can be studied independently of the effect of other genetic
changes only in autopolyploid newly derived from single ancestral
strains. The existing knowledge on the effect of genome multiplication on the physiology of the plant is fragmentary and based
on too narrow a representation of plant types; much of the information available on the effect of genome multiplication pertains
to the tomato. Various aspects of polyploidy are discussed
according to levels of function and organization: gene action,
cell characteristics, growth substances, water balance, ion
balance, stability of phenotypic expression and the response of
polyploid plants to stress.
Future work on the physiology of autopolyploid plants should
be directed towards: (1) the investigation of more representative
experimantal systems that should include genetically homogeneous
and heterogeneous species of both wild and cultivated plants; and
(2) diploid-polyploid comparisons on the level of isolated tissues
and cells, in addition to the whole plant.

LITERATURE CITED

1. Riley, M., Anilionis, A., 1978, Evolution of the bacterial
    genome. Ann. Rev. Microbiol. 32: 519-560.
2. Sparrow, A.H., Nauman, A.F., 1976, Evolution of genome size
    by DNA doubling. Science 192: 524-529.
3. Stebbins, G.L., 1950, "Variation and Evolution in Plants,"
    Columbia University Press, New York.
4. Stebbins, G.L., 1971, "Chromosomal Evolution in Higher
    Plants," E. Arnold, London.
5. Pojar, J., 1973, Levels of polyploidy in four vegetation types
    of southwestern British Columbia. Canad. J. Bot. 51: 621-628.

6. Dobzhansky, T., Ayala, F.J., Stebbins, G.L., Valentine, J.W., 1977, "Evolution," W.H. Freeman, San Francisco.

7. Cullis, C., Davies, D.R., 1974, Ribosomal RNA cistron number in a polyploid series of plants. Chromosoma 46: 23-28.

8. Mahr, E.P., Fox, D.P., 1973, Relationship between nuclear DNA content and rRNA gene number in Vicia faba. Nature New Biol. 245: 170-171.

9. Siegel, A., Lightfoot, D., Ward, O.G., Keener, S., 1973, DNA complementary to ribosomal RNA: Relation between genomic proportion and ploidy. Science 179: 682-683.

10. Albuzio, A., Spettoli, P., Cacco, G., 1978, Changes in gene expression from diploid to autotetraploid status of Lycopersicon esculentum. Physiol. Pl. 44: 77-80.

11. DeMaggio, A.E., Lambrukos, J., 1974, Polyploidy and gene dosage effects on peroxidase activity in ferns. Biochem. Genet. 12: 429-440.

12. Carlson, P.W., 1972, Locating gene loci with aneuploids. Mol. Gen. Genet. 114: 273-280.

13. Tal, M., 1977, Physiology of polyploids plants: DNA, RNA, protein, and abscisic acid in autotetraploid and diploid tomato under low and high salinity. Bot. Gaz. 138: 119-122.

14. Dermen, H., 1940, Colchicine polyploidy and technique. Bot. Rev. 6: 599-635.

15. Price, H.J., Sparrow, A.H., Nauman, A.F., 1973, Correlations between nuclear volume, cell volume and DNA content in meristematic cells of herbaceous angiosperms. Experientia 29: 1028-1029.

16. Van't Hof, J., 1965, Relationships between mitotic cycle duration, S period duration and the average rate of DNA synthesis in the root meristem cells of several plants. Exp. Cell. Res. 39: 48-58.

17. Evans, G.M., Rees, H., 1971, Mitotic cycles in dicotylendons and monocotyledons. Nature 233: 350-351.

18. Troy, M.R., Wimber, D.E., 1968, Evidence for a constancy of the DNA synthetic period between diploid-polyploid groups of plants. Exp. Cell Res. 53: 145-154.

19. Hannaford, J.E., DeMaggio, A.E., 1970, Cell cycle kinetics and cytophotometric analysis in polyploid fern prothalli. Amer. J. Bot. 57: 741.

20. Bennett, M.D., 1972, Nuclear DNA content and minimum generation time in herbaceous plants. Proc. Roy. Soc. London (B) 181: 109-135.

21. Price, H.J., Bachman, K., 1976, Mitotic cycle time and DNA content in annual and perennial Microseridinae (Compositae, Cichoriaceae). Pl. Syst. Evol. 126: 323-330.

22. Gustafsson, F.G., 1944, Growth hormone studies of some diploid and autotetraploid plants. J. Heredity 35: 269-272.

23. Abeles, F.B., 1973, "Ethylene in Plant Biology," Academic Press, New York.

24. Faberge, A.C., 1936, The physiological consequences of polyploidy. I. Growth and size in the tomato. J. Genetics 33: 365-382.

25. Kostoff, D., Axamitnaya, I.A., 1935, Studies on polyploid plants. Comp. Rend. Doklady 2: 295-297.

26. Schlosser, L.A., 1936, Befruchtugs schwierigkeitenbei autopoly- ploiden und ihre uberwindung. Der Züchter 8: 295-301.

27. Györffy, B., 1941, Untersuchungen uber der osmotichen poly- ploiden pflanzen. Planta 32: 15-37.

28. Tal, M., Gardi, I., 1976, Physiology of polyploid plants: water balance in autotetraploid and diploid tomato under low and high salinity. Physiol. Pl. 38: 257-261.

29. Chen, Shao-Lin, Tong, P.S., 1945, Studies on colchicine induced autotetraploid barley, Amer. J. Bot. 32: 177-181.

30. Tal, M., Imber, D., 1971, Abnormal stomatal behavior and hormonal imbalance in flacca, a wilty mutant of tomato. III. Hormonal effects on the water status in the plant. Pl. Physiol. 47: 849-850.

31. Iljin, W.S., 1957, Drought resistance in plants and physio- logical processes. Ann. Rev. Pl. Physiol. 8: 257-274.

32. Steudle, E., Zimmermann, U., Luttge, U., 1977, Effect of turgor pressure and cell size on the wall elasticity of plant cells. Pl. Physiol. 59: 285-289.

33. Cutler, J.M., Rains, D.W., Loomis, R.S., 1977, The importance of cell size in the water relations of plants. Pl. Physiol. 40: 255-260.

34. Cacco, G., Ferrari, G., Lucci, G.C., 1976, Uptake efficiency of roots in plants at different ploidy levels. J. Agric. Sci. Camb. 87: 585-589.

35. Crowley, P.H., 1975, Natural selection and the michaelis constant. J. Theor. Biol. 50: 461-475.

36. Kylin, A., Kähr, M., 1973, The effect of magnesium and calcium ions on adenosine triphosphatase from wheat and oat roots. Physiol. Pl. 28: 452-457.

37. Faberge, A.C., 1936, The physiological consequences of polyploidy. II. The effect of polyploidy on the variability in the tomato. J. Genetics 33: 383-397.

38. Sparrow, A.H., Miksche, J.P., 1961, Correlation of number, volume and DNA content with higher plant tolerance to chronic radiation. Science 134: 282-283.

39. Baetcke, K.P., Sparrow, A.H., Nauman, C.H., Schwemmer, S.S., 1967, The relationship of DNA content to nuclear and chromo- some volumes and to radiosensitivity (LD_{50}). Proc. Nat. Acad. Sci. USA 58: 533-540.

40. Sparrow, A.H., Sparrow, R.C., Schairer, L.A., Pond, V., 1965, Evidence that genetic redundancy does not have a radioprotective effect in polyploids of higher plants. Rad. Res. 25: 243-244.

41. Swaminathan, M.S., Chopra, V.L., Bhaskaran, S., 1962, Chromo-
     some aberrations and the frequency and spectrum of mutations
     induced by ethyl methane sulphonate in barley and wheat.
     Indian J. Genet. Pl. Breed. 22: 199-207.

42. Tomkins, D.J., Grant, W.F., 1978, Morphological and genetic
     factors influencing the response of weed species to herbi-
     cides. Canad. J. Bot. 56: 1466-1471.

43. Tal, M. Imber, D., Erez, A., Epstein, E., 1979, Abnormal
     stomatal behavior and hormonal inbalance in flacca, a wilty
     nutant of tomato. V. Effect of abscisic acid on indoleacetric
     acid metabolism and ethylene evolution. Pl. Physiol. 63:
     1044-1048.

44. Tal, M., Heikin, H., Dehan, K., 1978, Salt tolerance in the
     wild relatives of the cultivated tomato: Responses of callus
     tissue of Lycopersicon esculentum, L. peruvianum and Solanum
     pennellii to high salinity. Z. Pflanzenphysiol. 86:
     231-240.

45. Rick, C.M., 1963, Barriers to interbreeding in Lycopersicon
     peruvianum. Evolution 17: 216-232.

CHEMISTRY OF POLYPLOIDS:

A SUMMARY WITH COMMENTS ON PARTHENIUM (ASTERACEAE-AMBROSIINAE)

James A. Mears

Herbarium and Phytochemistry Laboratory
Academy of Natural Sciences of Philadelphia
Philadelphia, PA 19103

The chemistry of polyploids will be considered in terms of three major subjects: the chemical nature of hybrid complementation, chemical changes that occur during chromosome doubling, and chemical changes that occur as the result of evolution of polyploid genotypes. Several questions that seem particularly relevant to the evolutionary potential of polyploids are addressed by the chemical evidence presented: Is there chemical evidence of natural autoploid species? Are there chemical differences related to polyploidization itself? How do natural polyploid species differ from colchicine-induced polyploids? Is there evidence of unique adaptive capacities related to the chemistry of induced or natural polyploids? What are the chemical characteristics of different levels of polyploidy? Is there chemical evidence of diploidization of the genome of induced and natural polyploids?

Although it is probably impossible to demonstrate that any natural polyploid arose from the doubling of a genome which did not arise from interecotypic hybridization of some type (1), it is useful to consider two groups of polyploids: one (here called alloploids) in which the chemistry or the morphology suggests a combination of characteristics from two or more chemical or morphological types, and one (here called autoploids) in which the chemistry and morphology suggest an origin from only a single chemical and morphological type. Certainly nearly all natural polyploids (perhaps all) are intermediates to the categories of strict alloploids and strict autoploids (2). Nearly all the useful chemical information available about polyploids involves studies of phenolics, probably because phenolic patterns of parental species are often inherited as co-dominants in hybrids (3,4) and because phenolics have so often been useful in characterizing species.

77

CHEMICAL STUDIES OF ALLOPLOIDS

Chemical studies of alloploids originated as attempts to determine the parentage of natural polyploids. About 30-35% of all species of flowering plants have chromosome numbers which are multiples of some chromosome numbers within their own genera (1). Since alloploids have been regarded as much less likely than autoploids to overlap in characteristics with their diploid parents (1,5), natural polyploids have often been assumed to be alloploids. The realization that hybrids often produce phenolic profiles which are combinations of the phenolic profiles of the parental types (4) suggested a means of determining the parentage of polyploids distinct from the means employed in morphological studies and employing more readily quantifiable units (6). The additional discovery that hybrids sometimes produce non-parental phenolics (7), with structures produced by combinations of parental biosynthetic capacities (8,9), increased the incentive for chemical studies of presumed alloploids.

When phenolic profiles (sometimes, more specifically, fla-vonoid profiles) in presumed natural hybrids and alloploids have been near complements of the apparent parental profiles, parentage has been considered demonstrated; non-complementary profiles often have been rejected, neglected, and not reported (10,11). The determination of parentage of alloploids has been least complicated when parental profiles include many species-specific compounds, but it has been possible to determine two and even three parental phenolic genotypes of some alloploid species when there were few parent-specific compounds (12,13,14). The absence of hybrid-specific compounds has not been a significant deterrent to determining parentage when complementation of parental profiles occurred predominantly (6,15,16,14). The production of hybrid compounds has been explained as the modification of products of one parental genome by the genome of the other parent (17,18,19), probably representing the overcoming of blockages in one parent by the genome of the other parent since the hybrid-specific compounds are often found in other species of the genus. (The biosynthetic steps most often involved in the production of hybrid compounds from parental compounds are O-glycosylation, methylation and hydroxylation, all processes widespread in plants but differing in the identity of the specific substrates modified in different species (20).)

The general correspondence of induced and natural tetraploids of recent origin (probably less than a century) was demonstrated in a study of three introduced diploid _Tragopogon_ species, their reciprocal hybrids, allotetraploids induced from the reciprocal hybrids and two natural allotetraploid species derived from the diploids (21-24). Complementation was observed generally but some hybrid- (and some allotetraploid-) specific compounds occurred; some parental compounds were missing from F_1's and some, from both induced and natural allotetraploids. Some parental compounds missing from the diploid F_1's were detected in F_2's and in both induced and natural allotetraploids. In general, the natural and induced alloploids were similar.

Levin and Levy have studied flavonoid inheritance in several natural allotetraploid species of Phlox derived from three very distinct diploid species, which do not share specific phenolic constituents. Artificial F_1's produced chromatographic profiles which are complements of the parental profiles, but each natural allotetraploid produced a profile consisting of part of one parental profile plus many allotetraploid-specific compounds (11). (One allotetraploid did produce some parts of both parental profiles.) Levy and Levin (19) used the term "stabilized inter-genomic segregates" to characterize the groups of compounds from one parental genome carried to a greater degree of biosynthetic modification by the genome of the other parent.

However, not all hybrid or allotetraploid-specific compounds are more modified than the compounds of either parent. Some are simpler compounds, apparently precursors in one parent concentrated in the hybrid or alloploid (11,18,25).

Missing compounds have proven a greater problem with most studies of hybrids and alloploids. While hybrid compounds could be readily accepted as reflecting combinations of parental capacities, missing compounds could not be so readily explained. Belzer and Ownbey (23), looking at cytological and chemical data, suggested that deviations from complementation, particularly missing compounds, could be related to the high degree of sterility of the F_1's which apparently resulted from chromosomal trans-locations and inversions in the diploid parental genomes. When several strains of tetraploid and hexaploid wheat were crossed with diploid rye to produce allohexaploid and allooctoploid X Triticale, an average of 94% of the wheat phenolics were produced in the X Triticale strains, while an average of 78% of the rye phenolics were produced (12). There were certain compounds from rye which tended to be missing from X Triticale when any wheat strain was used to produce the alloploids.

Eliminated parental compounds are apparently those which are further modified by the hybrid genome (perhaps into hybrid compounds) or those which are not produced because an earlier bio-synthetic step is blocked in the hybrid genome (18,11). The recovery of missing compounds in later generations of hybrids and allotetraploids is apparently related to intergenomic segregation (19).

Fig. 1 shows a model of flavonoid production designed to illustrate the origins of various kinds of hybrid-specific compounds and the occurrence of parental compounds which are missing in hybrids and alloploids. This model is based on many concepts but owes much to the Phlox studies of Levin and Levy; however, the steps and structures do not refer to any specific organisms.

It is convenient to regard the flavonoids detected as indications of points of product release from biosynthetic pathways.

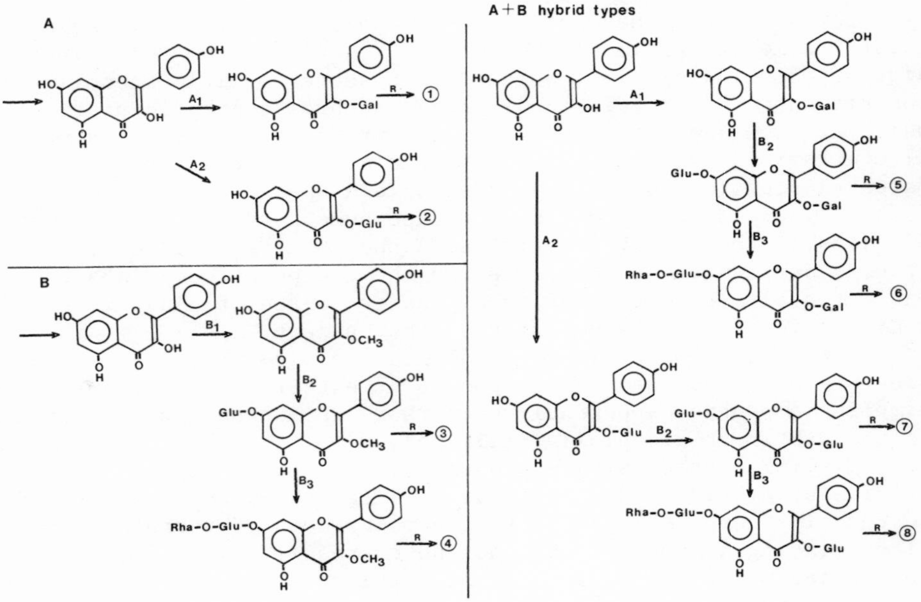

Fig. 1.   A model of flavonoid expression in a hybrid genome
(A X B).

If every biosynthetic process observed in an individual occurred
with all available precursors, one would not observe the concentration of structural intermediates. Yet intermediate structures
are often detected. Therefore, there must be many multiple
complexes of biosynthetic steps (enzymes), some fundamentally
different in the nature of the enzymes involved and in the nature
of the modifications produced, others differing in the points at
which products are released from a biosynthetic pathway. Biosynthetic complexes which release products which are structurally
intermediate to other products of the same genome may consist of
some mutant, ineffective enzymes. In Fig. 1, the model indicates
that in genome A some biosynthetic complexes carry the kaempferol
precursor through process A_1 to the 3-0-galactoside (compound 1)
while some biosynthetic complexes carry the kaempferol precursor
through process A_2 to the 3-0-glucoside (compound 2). Genome A
does not modify kaempferol at C_7 (see Fig. 3) and does not produce
a build-up of kaempferol. Parental genome B carries the precursor
kaempferol through three processes: B_1, methylation of the 3-
hydroxyl; B_2, 0-glucosylation at C_7; and B_3, 0-rhamnosylation of

the glucose at C_7. Neither kaempferol nor 3-methyl kaempferol is released by genome B, but some biosynthetic complexes release the 7-0-glucoside of 3-methyl kaempferol (compound 3) and some release only the most modified product of genome B, 7-0-rhamnoglucoside of 3-methyl kaempferol (compound 4). In the model R designates release.

In the F_1 hybrid and allotetraploid of the A and B genomes, all the biosynthetic complexes could be organized exactly as in the parental genomes; the parental flavonoids would occur - compounds 1,2,3,4. But combinations of parental biosynthetic steps could occur in some biosynthetic complexes, as indicated in Fig. 1. Compounds 5,6,7 and 8 represent hybrid compounds, which could not be produced by either parent.

If all biosynthetic steps acted independently in hybrids and alloploids only hybrid compounds would be produced. When complementation plus hybrid compounds are observed in hybrids and alloploids, it is probable that there are some biosynthetic complexes still composed exactly as in the parental types while other biosynthetic complexes combine some biosynthetic steps derived from each parent.

Compounds present in parents but missing in hybrids or alloploids are accounted for in the following ways: If all the biosynthetic complexes include step A_1 and step B_2 together so that step B_2 modifies all the product of A_1, compound 1 should be missing in the hybrid genome because it is all modified to compound 5 or 6 (Fig. 2a); the presence of biosynthetic step B_2 (attachment of glucose at C_7) might block or prevent the function of step A_2 (the attachment of glucose C_3), then parental compound 2 should be missing in the hybrid and hybrid compounds 7 and 8 should not occur (Fig 2b).

A precursor compound could appear as product in the hybrid genome if, as the result of combination of parental biosynthetic steps, some biosynthetic complexes contain ineffective associations leading to the release of structural intermediates. For example, 3-methyl kaempferol might be released if step A_2 (glucosylation at C_3) blocked or prevented step B_2 (glucosylation at C_7) (Fig. 2c).

In later generations of hybrids and allotetraploids, there should be a breakdown of simple complementation as specific biosynthetic steps are lost or as specific combinations of all the available biosynthetic steps become stabilized. In such advanced generations there should be more compounds reflecting the integration of parental biosynthetic capacities and fewer parental compounds.

This model should apply as well to C-glycosylated flavonoids as to non-C-glycosylated flavonoids. Studies of plants which produce C-glycosides-Tragopogon (21,23), Phlox (11), grasses (12-14)- have produced such clear results apparently because C-glycosylation is not a terminal process biosynthetically (26). Flavonoids with unsubstituted phenolic hydroxyls are rarely

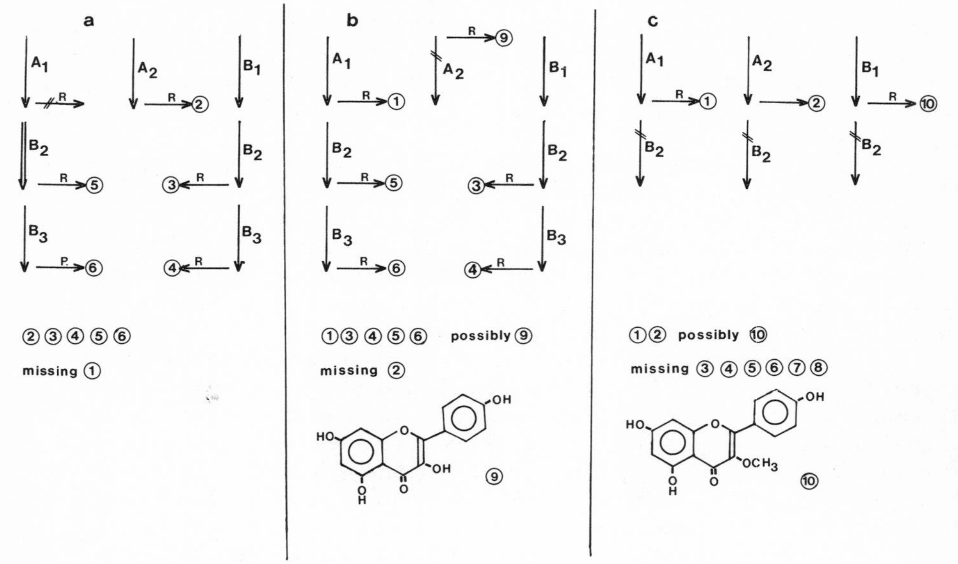

Fig. 2. A model for missing parental flavonoids and for the expression of parental precursors in hybrids and alloploids. See tex for symbols.

detected in living tissues (27) and are presumably toxic to plant metabolism. A major exception, however, is the class of compounds with glycosides attached at C_6 or C_8 through a carbon-carbon bond (Fig. 3). The biosynthetic steps which modify the phenolic hydroxyls of flavonoids (methylations and O-glycosylation) are regarded as terminal steps, probably occurring after the basic three ring structure of flavonoids is produced (27). C-Glycosylation, however, apparently occurs before the closure of the central ring (26). Therefore studies of species with produce C-glycosides can involve such distinct processes as presence and absence of terminal steps (such as O-glycosylation and hydroxylation), while studies of species which produce only non-C-glycosides involve differences in specific sugars at various hydroxyl positions.

Studies of isozymes have also documented parental complementation in F_1's and in induced alloploids, as well as the presence of hybrid- and alloploid-specific isozymes. Bhatia et al. (28,29) produced allotetraploids of barley, rye, wheat and X Triticale with increased numbers of isozyme bands and with alloploid-specific isozyme bands in several enzyme systems. Barber et al. (30,31) detected a new esterase isozyme in octoploid X Triticale derived from hexaploid wheat and diploid rye; he noted that

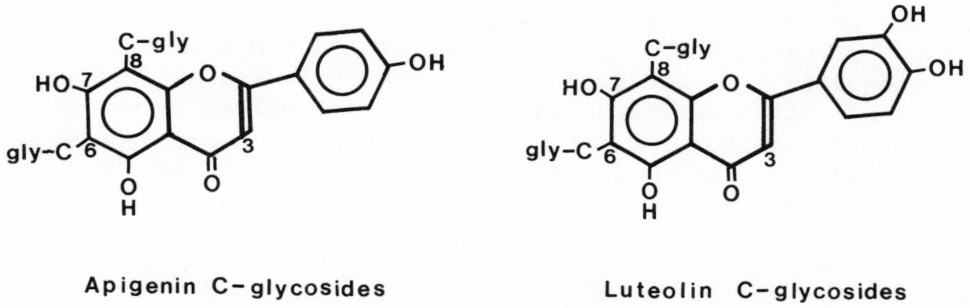

Apigenin C-glycosides   Luteolin C-glycosides

Fig. 3.   The C-glycosyl flavonoid types of Briza media L.

Schwartz and Laughner (32) found a higher range of enzyme activity
with such hybrid isozymes.

Sing and Brewer (33) determined in a study of eight enzyme
systems in allotetraploid and allohexaploid wheat that only
phosphoglucomutase isozymes showed hybrid complementation. While
most of the hybrid isozyme patterns were more complex than in the
parents, alkaline phosphatase patterns were simpler in the
alloploids than in the parents. A study of 13 isozyme systems in
natural Tragopogon alloploids of recent origin (24) demonstrated
that the alloploids have a fixed heterozygosity of 33 to 43% of
genes involved while the diploids were not detectably heterozygous.

The evidence available from chemical studies of diploid F_1's
and in induced and natural alloploids indicates

1) there often is recognizable complementation of parental
phenolic and isozyme profiles in diploid F_1's and in induced and
natural alloploids;

2) there often are phenolics and isozymes present in F_1's and
induced and natural alloploids which result from interactions of
parental genotypes, i.e., nonparental (hybrid) compounds and
isozymes;

3) often there are a few parental phenolics of isozymes which
are not observed in F_1's or in alloploids;

4) natural alloploids generally reflect a greater degree of
integration of parental genomes and "stabilized intergenomic
segregates" (19) than do F_1's and induced alloploids;

5) induced and natural alloploids generally express a richer
phenolic and isozyme diversity than either parent, representing
distinct chemical types available for natural selection.

CHEMICAL STUDIES OF AUTOPLOIDS

Haskell (34) compared the phenolics of colchicine-induced tetraploids of two diploid strains of raspberry to the phenolics of two spontaneous autotetraploids that arose apparently from root cuttings. The spontaneous autotetraploids differed more from the diploids studied than did the colchicine-induced autoploids. Moreover, the spontaneous autoploids produced slightly fewer phenolics than the diploids. Although it was not stated by Haskell that the spontaneous autoploids were derived from the diploid cultivars used to produced the experimental autoploids, and although the degree of variation of phenolics in raspberry cultivars was not noted; the important points of his study are probably justified: some colchicine-induced autoploids are different chemically from some spontaneous autoploids derived from chromosome doubling in vegetative tissue, and diploids and induced autoploids may differ in phenolic constituents.

In some studies of induced autotetraploids, qualitative differences in phenolics and isozymes of diploids and autoploids have not been detected (11,28,29). However, Levy (35) found qualitative differences in the glycoflavone profiles of 14 of 15 autotetraploids induced from cultivars of Phlox drummondii Hook., including 14 instances of flavonoids not detected in a diploid cultivar but detected in its autoploid and eight instances of flavonoids detected in a diploid cultivar but not detected in its autoploid derivative. Many changes in tissue specificity were detected. The 15 cultivars studied produced glycoflavonoid profiles which were subsets of the range of glycoflavonoids identified from wild types of the species. All the flavonoids which were detected not in a diploid cultivar but in its tetraploid derivative were identified in some specimens of P. drummondii. There were no new compounds for the species produced in the autotetraploids. The autotetraploid induced from a wild diploid, P. drummondii ssp. mcallisteri (Whitehouse) Wherry, produced no autoploid-specific compounds. However, five compounds detected in diploid ssp. mcallisteri were not detected in its autotetraploid.

Levy (35) has interpreted the Phlox drummondii glycoflavone data as best explained as disturbance of the mechanisms which regulate the biosynthesis of individual compounds. Because the wild species, in its several forms, does produce all the glycoflavones detected in the autotetraploids induced from the several diploid cultivars, the loss of diploid compounds is explained as functional repression of existing structural genes. Gain of compounds in the autoploids is explained as functional derepression of previously silent structural genes. The implication is that structural genes which occur in some wild P. drummondii became silent during the development of the studied cultivars and were, in some cases, derepressed by colchicine-induced chromosome doubling.

While most studies of flavonoid profiles of diploids and induced and natural autotetraploids indicate qualitative similarity of the profiles, there is an example which demonstrates that doubling the chromosome number can change the chemical type of the flavonoids expressed. Briza media L. consists of diploid and tetraploid forms with different geographical distributions in Europe (36,37). The diploids produce C-glycosyl derivatives of apigenin while the natural tetraploids produce C-glycosyl derivatives of luteolin (Fig. 2). Colchicine-induced autotetraploids of the C-glycosyl apigenin-producing diploids produce the C-glycosyl luteolin types found in the wild tetraploids. Triploid hybrids of the natural diploids and tetraploids all produce luteolin type flavonoids. Such a change in flavonoid structural type should be related to a change in hydroxylase activity, but attempts to isolate the relevant enzyme failed. Instead, it was determined that the induced autotetraploid has a flavonoid isomerase profile which is substantially different from that of the diploid: there is a flavonoid isomerase in the autotetraploid which has a greater range of heat stability than those of the diploid.

DeMaggio and Lambrukos (38) studied soluble protein and peroxidase isozymes in an induced series (1x,2x,4x) of gametophytes and an induced series (2x,4x) of sporophytes of Todea barbara (L.) Moore. Some bands of the total soluble protein of gametophytes of different ploidy levels varied in intensity of staining. In the gametophyte series, total peroxidase activity per cell increased to about 3.5 times the haploid activity with a change from 1x to 4x. Similar isozymes of peroxidase were detected in the 1x and 4x gametophytes but major differences in specific isozyme contribution to total peroxidase activity were reported. Of the 18 peroxidase isozyme bands studied, there were three bands about three times more active in the 4x than in the 1x, while four bands were much less active in the 4x than in the 1x. In the sporophyte material two peroxidase bands detected in the 4x material were not detected in the 2x material and apparently represent novel autoploid isozymes in the sporophyte. Many differences, quantitative and qualitative, were noted in the 4x gametophyte and the 4x sporophyte. It was concluded that some form of regulation of genes, in addition to transcription rate, controls peroxidase isozyme activity in Todea barbara, resulting in different isozyme characteristics at different ploidy levels (38).

Levin et al. (39) have also studied enzyme (alcohol dehydrogenase) activity in diploids, induced autotetraploids of six Phlox drummondii cultivars, and wild type P. drummondii ssp. mcallisteri. About twice as much alcohol dehydrogenase specific activity was detected in the autotetraploids as in the diploid cultivars. There was considerable variability and the consistent increase was "cultivar-dependent." In the wild type, there was no similar increase in alcohol dehydrogenase specific activity with chromosome doubling; indeed, there was a slight decrease in specific activity. Nakai (40) found increased esterase activity in 17 of 29 induced autotetraploids compared to the diploids.

These examples demonstrate that colchicine-induced chromosome doubling can produce increased enzyme activity per cell and per mg. protein, changes in the balance of isozyme activities, some isozyme activities and stabilities not detected in the relevant diploids, and major and minor changes in flavonoid profiles. If colchicine has not caused structural mutations which result in these changes, there should be few if any differences in the structural genes in the studied systems. Therefore these differences are explained in terms of disruption of the regulation of gene expression, using Britten and Davidson (41) as a model.

How much of the differences in diploid and induced and natural autotetraploids is due to colchicine itself? Although colchicine-induced mutants have been detected (42), colchicine is probably not responsible for most of the differences noted here. While there may be differences in autotetraploids produced from different tissues, particularly in those which are produced from vegetative cells versus those produced from reproductive cells (34,38), the chemical correspondence of the colchicine-induced autotetraploids with the natural tetraploids of Briza media is certainly related primarily to chromosome doubling.

If colchicine-induced genome doubling is correlated with disruptions of regulatory mechanisms, perhaps it is the colchicine which causes the regulatory disruptions and the regulatory disruptions which cause the genome doubling and the chemical differences. Is it possible that the regulatory disruptions which coincide with genome doubling are also the sources of a tendency to apomixis in some diploids and polyploids? Perhaps both apomixis and genome doubling occur through specific or general disruptions in gene regulation, particularly frequently in the presence of relatively distinct genomes. What is the chemical environment of the genome immediately before circumvention of meiotic reduction? None of the chemical data seems to relate to these questions directly.

Do true autopolyploids exist outside laboratories, greenhouses, and cultivated fields? Although it is probably impossible to distinguish a natural, true autoploid from a segmental alloploid in which all the observed characteristics were identical in the parental ecotypes, it apparently is not necessary to postulate more than one parental type to explain the flavonoid chemistry of the tetraploid Briza media.

GENE REGULATION, GENE DOSAGE COMPENSATION AND DIPLOIDIZATION

Conspicuous physiological differences of isogenic cells at different stages of development have supported the concept of a mechanism regulating the sequence of activation of isoalleles

(43). Britten and Davidson (41) have suggested that at higher
levels of organization (than that in procaryotic organisms),
evolution may be considered chiefly as changes in the regulatory
system. Nair et al. (44) point out the inactivation during
metamorphosis of an allele in Drosophila ochrobasis while the
same allele remains active in both larval and adult stages in D.
setosimentum, a near sibling species.

DeMaggio and Lambrukos (38) found major differences in the
isozyme profiles of genetically identical tetraploid gametophytes
and tetraploid sporophytes of Todea barbara; tetraploids derived
from fused gametes were quite different in isozyme profile from
tetraploids derived from redoubled somatic genomes. Ross et al.
(45) found that a shift from monokaryon to dikaryon stages mediated
a major change in the nature, quantity or distribution of the
proteins of a bipolar Coprinus. The many changes in flavonoid
tissue specificity which occurred during induction of autotetraploids from diploid cultivars of Phlox drummondii (35) are
evidence of changes in regulatory mechanisms as the result of
doubling the genome.

Apparently regulation of genetic activity is disrupted by
doubling the genome. While the differences observed in alloploids
may not demonstrate the point because there are two relatively
dissimilar genomes interacting in unpredictable ways, the data
from induced autoploids is clear: a considerable amount of chemical
change of a more or less unpredictable type occurs when autoploids
are produced from diploids. It is probable that changes in the
regulatory mechanism account for some of the differences in
hybrids and alloploids characterized by Levy and Levin (19) as
stabilized intergenomic segregates.

Noggle (46), in a review of the literature on the physiology
of polyploids, indicated that the amounts of some chemical constituents could be altered by increasing chromosome numbers. Yet
there is evidence from gene dosage studies that nonadditive
effects occur in some polyploids. While Carlson (47) found that
the presence of an additional gene increased the overall rate of
transcription and resulted in an increase in enzyme activity in
Solanum, DeMaggio and Lambrukos (38) found a direct correlation
between gene dosage and peroxidase activity in gametophytes of
Todea barbara but no significant difference in different ploidy
levels of sporophytes. Kostoff and Axamitnaja (48) found not
much difference in the phenolics content in some Nicotiana F_1's
and amphidiploids. Wolf et al. (49) found that the expression of
"regulatory genes of phosphodiesterase" is dosage dependent in
wheat, while Nakai (40) found esterase activity related to gene
dosage in 17 of 29 diploid/autoploid pairs. Nakai reported
dosage compensation in four pairs of Aegilops and two pairs of
Triticum. A comparison of diploid and tetraploid Datura stramonium
L. showed complete dosage compensation for peroxidase (50). In
Phlox drummondii (39) alcohol dehydrogenase activity was gene
dosage related in four cases (specific activity in the autote-

traploids of 1.79 to 2.18 times the diploid level), slightly less
in two cases and entirely compensated in the autotetraploid of
the wild type ssp. mcallisteri.

The kinds of changes that may occur in a tetraploid which
will eventually result in some approach to disomic inheritance
may be initiated during polyploidization by disruption of the
regulatory mechanism, but should eventually involve chromosomal
translocations and inversions. Del Pero de M. and Swain (51)
have studied a species, Gibasis schiedeana (Kunth) Hunt, in which
polyploidization is correlated with a Robertsonian fusion. The
diploid number is 2n=10, with two metacentric and three acrocentric
chromosomes; and the tetraploid is 2n=16, with three metacentric
and one acrocentric chromosomes. There are three flavonoid
chemical types in the diploids (a,b,c) and four types in the
tetraploids (b,c,a + trace of b,b + trace of a).

It appears that Robertsonian fusion has disturbed a part of
the genome which controls the production of some part of the
flavonoid patterns. The tetraploids producing either pattern b
or c may be autoploids, but the tetraploids producing pattern a +
trace of b or pattern b + trace of a appear to be alloploids with
the basic information to make both patterns a and b. Del Pero de
M. and Swain suggested that those which produce pattern a +
trace of b have chromosomes in which the information to make
pattern b has been disturbed through the process of Robertsonian
fusion. Indeed, pattern b + trace of a is produced by those
tetraploids which have B chromosomes. The information necessary to
produce pattern b is apparently involved with the B chromosomes
in such tetraploids. More evidence for that interpretation is
provided by a single individual without B chromosomes from a
population with B chromosomes normally producing pattern a +
trace of b; the individual without the B chromosomes produced
pattern b + trace of a (51).

It is not clear whether Robertsonian fusion was followed by
genome doubling or whether genome doubling was followed by several
similar Robertsonian fusions. Some tetraploids appear to be
autoploids; some, alloploids. In either case it appears that the
Robertsonian fusion, rather than the genome doubling per se has
been responsible for the nonparental chemical types in Gibasis
schiedeana.

In Thelesperma simplicifolium Gray (n=8,9,10,11,12,22), the
exceptional differences in major phenolic constituents in a
diploid (n=10) and a "tetraploid" (n=22) could not be sorted into
the effects of introgression, polyploidy, and aneuploidy (52).
Although Lotus corniculatus L. was once thought to be of autoploid
origin from L. tenuis Waldst and Kit. (9), the phenolic profiles
of the two species are distinct in hydroxylation patterns. It
has been suggested that L. corniculatus is therefore of alloploid
origin from two cryptic species within the L. tenuis group (1,9,53).

In a study of a polyploid series of Potentilla pensylvanica
L., Kohli and Denford (54) detected most of the kaempferol and

apigenin glycosides in the diploids, tetraploids and octoploids
(2n=14,28,56), but kaempferol-3-0-diglucoside was not detected
in the octoploid while kaempferol-3-0-diglucosyl-7-0-glucoside
was found in the tetraploid only. Apigenin-7-galactoside was
found in the octoploid only. While these differences are concerned
entirely with terminal glycosylation and might be expected to be
the kind of changes observed in different levels of natural
autoploids the existence of chemical discontinuity in the different ploidy levels can support arguments of separate origins of
the tetraploid and the octoploid.

The demonstrated disruption of regulatory mechanisms during
polyploidization and the gene dosage compensation observed in
some autoploids provides evidence that the genome of some if not
all new polyploids behaves in some ways like a diploid. Diploidization of the tetraploid genome need not depend entirely on
chromosomal structural changes (55,56).

PROBLEMS IN DETERMINING PARENTAGE OF NATURAL POLYPLOID SPECIES

Since deviations from complementation of parental phenolic
and isozyme profiles can be expected in allopolyploids and autopolyploids, less correspondence of the chemical characteristics
of natural polyploids with those of their diploid sources is
anticipated. If the diploid species which once produced an
allopolyploid exist at the time of the search for parental types,
evolution may have occurred in both the diploid and polyploid
lines to the extent that the parallel genomes may no longer be
entirely homologous (33,57). Subsequent hybridization may have
occurred at the polyploid or diploid levels. In Aegilops there
is evidence that some allotetraploid species hybridize naturally,
so that attempting to determine parentage in terms of interactions
of diploid species is unrealistic (58,59). Kaltsikes and Dedio
(14) have found it difficult to assign parentage to genomes in
hexaploid Aegilops, since there is hybridization in the tetraploid
species and since all tetraploid and hexaploid genomes are very
similar to genomes of one group of diploid species. Similar
examples of hybridization at both diploid and tetraploid levels
occur in Phlox (19) and Coreopsis (60). In a study of Saccharum
spontaneum L. (2n=40,48,50,54,56,60,64,80,96,112) problems related
to the identification of material and hybridization with other
species at the several ploidy levels were noted (61,62).

Allopolyploids derived from closely related parental types
should produce chemical profiles which are an integral part of
the variability of the taxonomic group of the parental types.
Parthenium tetraneuris Barneby is a tetraploid (2n=72) differing
from the diploid (2n=36) P. alpinum (Nuttall) T. & G. in very few
characteristics (63-66). While P. alpinum occurs on a variety of
soils associated with gypsum and limestone in central and eastern
Wyoming, P. tetraneuris occurs on gypsum nodules in southcentral
Colorado. The flavonoids (66) and the sesquiterpene lactones

(67,68) of both species have been studied (Fig. 4). The concentrations of both kinds of constituents are greater in P.
tetraneuris, where more flavonoids and more sesquiterpene lactones
have been detected; the constituents of P. alpinum are also the
major constituents of P. tetraneuris. All the flavonoids and
sesquiterpene lactones of P. tetraneuris may indeed occur in P.
alpinum, but flavonoid glycosides have not yet been detected in
P. alpinum. While it is possible that P. tetraneuris is an
autotetraploid derivative of P. alpinum or of some similar,
extinct common ancestor, it is equally probable that P. tetraneuris
is an allotetraploid which originated from hybridization of an
ecotype morphologically and chemically very similar to P. alpinum
with some unknown (probably extinct) close relative of P. alpinum
with similar morphological characteristics and with a chemistry
which included flavonoid glycosides.

In studies of Pityrogramma triangularis (70,71), Artemisia
(72), and Ambrosia (73,74), analysis of the distribution of
certain chemical types provides data which correlates with distribution of chromosomal and morphological characteristics while
analysis of other chemical studies provides data which does not
correlate with chromosomal and morphological data.

In Parthenium section Partheniastrum there are a number of
morphologically distinct ecotypes recognized as a total of two
species and five varieties (75). The flavonoid constituents of
section Partheniastrum have been determined (Mears, unpublished).
A study of chromosome numbers and pollen characteristics
has shown that pollen size is indicative of ploidy level in all
the sections of Parthenium, exluding the apomictic series (Mears,
unpublished). Therefore, it has been possible to correlate the
flavonoid patterns of specimens traditionally identified as P.
integrifolium L. var. integrifolium (diploid and tetraploid),
var. hispidum (Raf.) Mears (all tetraploid) and var. hispidum
f. repens (Eggert) Mears (all tetraploid) where they overlap and
interact (in Missouri, Arkansas, and surrounding states), with
ploidy levels; moreover, it has been possible to characterize the
distribution of ploidy levels in specimens examined in a numerical
taxonomic, principal component study of morphological characters.
In Fig. 5 specimens from the region of overlap and interaction of
var. hispidum and var. integrifolium are graphed according to the
two major complex morphological components. In that figure the
polyploids are represented by solid squares while the diploids
are hollow circles. The specimens which possess the set of
characteristics identified with var. hispidum, and those
which also possess the few special characteristics of f. repens,
are circumscribed and are seen to be all polyploids. The few
specimens which group with the type of var. integrifolium (in an
analysis of specimens from the total range of the species, not
shown here) are also indicated. The majority of specimens
examined are morphologically intermediate to the var. integrifolium
group and the var. hispidum group. While the few specimens which

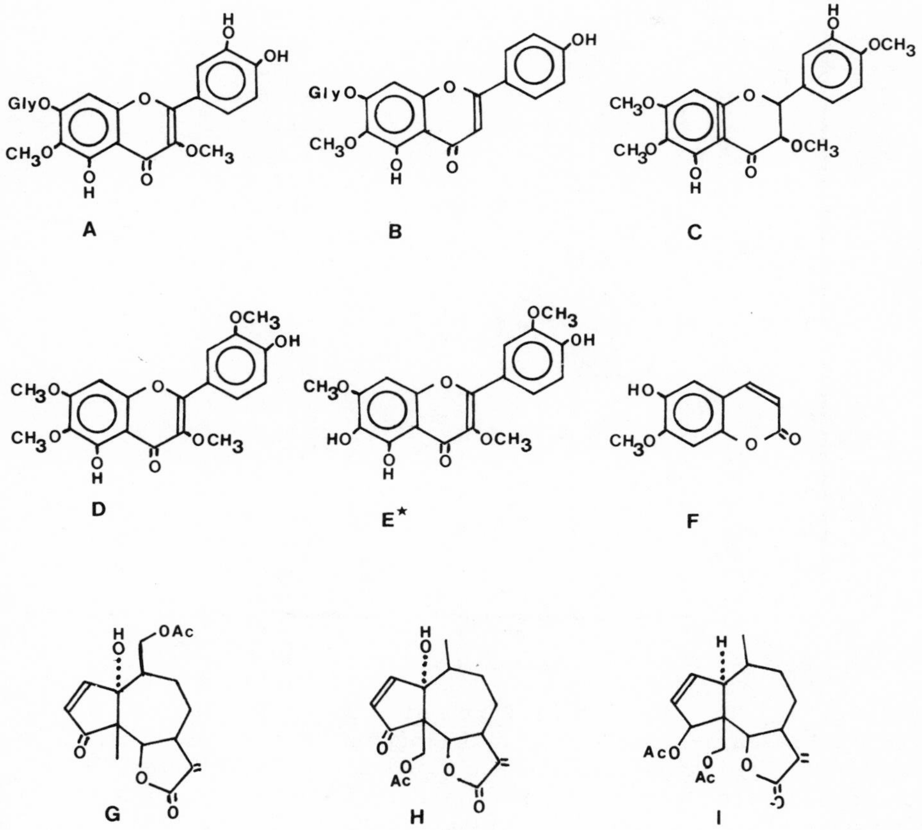

	A	B	C	D	E*	F	G	H	I
Tet	+	+	+	+	+	+	+	+	+
Alp	—	—	+	+	+	+	—	+	—

Fig. 4. Flavonoid (A,B,C,D,E), coumarin (F) and sesquiterpene lactone constituents of Parthenium alpinum (Alp) and P. tetraneuris (Tet). From Rodriquez et al. (68) and Mears (66).

*Compound E was not earlier identified (66) but matches chromatographically a constituent recently identified (69) from another Parthenium species.

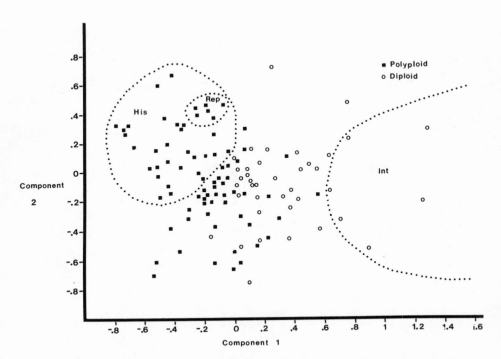

Fig. 5. Distribution of Parthenium integrifolium specimens
from the Missouri-Arkansas-Illinois region in two dimensions
representing principal components 1 and 2 of a multidimensional
scaling analysis of selected morphological characteristics.
Polyploids are indicated as solid squares; diploids, hollow circles.
Int - var. integrifolium; His - var. hispidum; Rep - var. hispidum
f. repens.

group with var. integrifolium in this study are diploids (there
are sporadic polyploids in the eastern part of the range), the
morphological intermediates are a mixture of diploids and polyploids, with the polyploids more closely associated morphologically
with var. hispidum.
     Of the 39 phenolics included in a study of Parthenium (Mears,
in preparation), 20 are found in P. integrifolium var. integrifolium and var. hispidum (including f. repens). They are
glycosides and aglycones of variously methylated derivatives of
quercetin, quercetagetin, kaempferol, and 6-hydroxykaempferol,
as well as coumarins and phenolic acids. Their distribution

Table 1. Distribution and frequency of twenty phenolics in Parthenium intergrifolium var. integrifolium, var. hispidum, and var. hispidum f. repens.

Biological groups[a]	Flavonoid Aglycones								Flavonoid Glycosides							Phenolic Acids			Coumarins		Number of specimens examined
	6	7	12	15	14	13	18	19	20	21	22	23	24	25	28	35	36	37	38	39	
Int																					
2xE	0.0	0.1	0.0	1.0	0.8	0.5	0.4	1.0	0.0	0.5	1.0	0.0	0.0	0.5	0.0	0.4	1.0	1.0	1.0	1.0	38
2xW	0.0	0.0	0.0	0.3	0.0	0.3	0.3	0.9	0.5	0.4	0.9	0.1	0.1	0.4	0.0	0.5	1.0	0.6	0.8	0.8	43
4xW	0.2	0.0	0.0	0.5	0.2	0.2	0.0	1.0	0.2	0.3	1.0	0.0	0.3	0.7	0.2	0.5	1.0	0.8	0.8	0.8	28
His	0.2	0.0	0.0	0.2	0.3	0.0	0.3	0.8	0.2	0.2	0.9	0.4	0.2	0.1	0.2	0.4	0.8	0.9	1.0	0.4	57
Rep	0.0	0.0	0.0	0.6	0.0	0.0	0.0	1.0	0.0	0.0	1.0	0.0	0.0	0.0	0.0	0.4	1.0	1.0	0.0	0.9	19

aThe compounds are represented by numbers which refer to the 39 phenolics included in a study of Parthenium (Mears, in preparation). The biological group symbols are Int_{2xE} - diploid var. intergrifolium from east of the Appalachians, Int_{2xW} - diploid var. integrifolium from west of the Appalachians, Int_{4xW} - polyploid var. integrifolium from west of the Appalachians, His - polyploid var. hispidum (f. hispidum) from west of the Appalachians, and Rep - polyploid var. hispidum f. repens from west of the Appalachians.

and frequency of detection in var. integrifolium and var. hispidum
are shown in Table 1.

What is the origin of the tetraploids? What is the nature
of the interaction which produces so many morphological intermediates? There are certain morphological characteristics of
some tetraploids (very large capitula, non-tuberous rhizomes)
which are strongly correlated with limestone habitats (dolomitic
limestone glades, for example): such tetraploids are recognized
as var. hispidum. Only two compounds have been found in var.
hispidum but not in diploids of var. integrifolium (flavonoid 6,
which is 3,7,3'-trimethylquercetagetin, and flavonoid 28, which
is 3-methylkaempferol-7-glycoside). The presence of both in
the polyploid var. integrifolium suggests some interaction of
var. hispidum and var. integrifolium at the tetraploid level.
Forma repens expresses much less phenolic diversity than either
var. hispidum (as a whole) or var. integrifolium, producing only
compounds commonly found in both varieties.

The biochemical distances (16) calculated on the basis of
the phenolic frequencies indicate that the western diploids of
var. integrifolium are most similar to the tetraploids of var.
integrifolium, but are also very similar to var. hispidum. The
tetraploids of var. integrifolium are more similar to the tetraploids of var. hispidum than they are to the eastern diploids of
var. integrifolium. Forma repens is somewhat more similar to the
western diploids of var. integrifolium than to var. hispidum in
general. Fig. 6 shows a plausible representation of the origin
of the western forms, based on the primary biochemical distances.

It is probable that western diploids of P. integrifolium
var. integrifolium gave rise to tetraploids which became isolated
on limestone glades, eventually resulting in some ancestral form
of var. hispidum. A renewed contact of var. integrifolium and
some ancestral form of var. hispidum occurred, possibly after
considerable isolation of the eastern and western diploids of var.
integrifolium. The presence of probably segmental alloploid var.
integrifolium in the region of geographic overlap facilitated
infraspecific hybridization and movement of genes into var.
hispidum and into tetraploid var. integrifolium. Variety hispidum
has now been modified considerably by its interaction with var.
integrifolium (possibly diploids as well as tetraploids, although
no evidence of triploids has been found), with forma repens
perhaps representing some of the characteristics of the ancestral
type.

The flavonoid chemistry does not specify all the detail,
neither does the morphology. In a complex of species and varieties
where genome doubling occurs sporadically in partially isolated
groups, where morphological isolates are primarily segregates of
characteristics found in the most widespread and variable variety,
one should not expect to resolve the origins and relationships
with chemical or morphological studies alone.

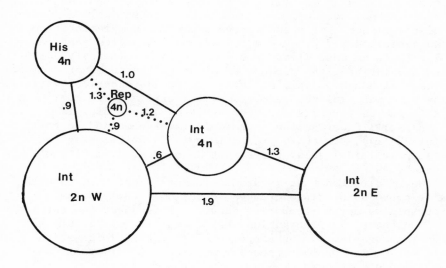

Fig. 6. Relationship of diploid and tetraploid groups of Parthenium integrifolium from the Missouri-Arkansas-Illinois region as indicated by biochemical distances calculated from Table 1.

CHEMICAL EVIDENCE OF THE EVOLUTIONARY SIGNIFICANCE OF POLYPLOIDS

An examination of the chemistry of natural polyploid species and induced polyploids supports the argument that polyploids, including autoploids, can be sufficiently different from their diploid ancestors to encounter selection in unique ways. The production of an esterase isozyme in allooctoploid X Triticale not present in either parent has been called (31,32) an example of the chemical basis of heterosis.

Alloploids possess a richness of phenolic diversity compared to diploid parental types; they also tend to produce novel compounds. Should diversity of phenolic types be important to chemical defenses in certain environments, alloploids may have a considerable advantage over their parents. Kaltsikes and Dedio (13,14) found that resistance to rusts in certain Aegilops alloploids was correlated with the shared presence or the shared absence of phenolics.

Feeny (76) has developed a concept of two basic groups of chemical defenses: (1) unusual compounds in concentrations sufficient to prevent a predator from continuing its attack, and (2) a pool of compounds possessing general negative action on the digestive system of the predator. It is quite possible that diversity of structural types in the general negative action pool is important in environments which present a variety of predators. Therefore, polyploids may exist with an advantage from the beginning if they are derived from parents sufficiently different to confer a richness of phenolic types through complementation.

An autoploid may produce a nonparental phenolics profile (36,37). Such an unpredictable variation in a relatively homogeneous population might produce an advantage in terms of chemical defenses. Although polyploids have been found to be less variable in flavonoid patterns than diploids (Perideridia, 77; Aegilops, 14), this may be a result of "few biotypes at the diploid level and still fewer at the tetraploid level combined to form hexaploids" (14). In those groups in which hybridization can occur at polyploid levels, there must be a great diversity of chemical types (61,62).

deWet (78) noted that in apomictic tetraploid species with sexually reproducing diploid races, occasional fully sexual autotetraploids may be temporary genetic bridges between apomictic types. Moreover, in Dichanthium, haploidization may insure a bridge with sexuality. Therefore, cycles of polyploidization and haploidization may promote phenolic and isozymic diversity in some polyploid complexes.

Alloploids derived from parental species which share few chemical characteristics are likely to be more chemically diverse than alloploids derived from chemically similar ecotypes. Alloploids derived from very distinct parental species are probably the only biological type which is likely to preserve much of the recombined genome of such diverse genotypes. It is clear that alloploidy represents a means of interaction and possibly recombination of those diverse genotypes which can produce hybrids.

In Parthenium, the development of guayule as a desert latex crop may involve hybridization of P. argentatum with various other species of Parthenium. Will it be with the other shrubby species of section Parthenichaeta, with which Rollins (79) produced viable hybrids? Will it be with the tuberous and rhizomatous perennial herbs of section Partheniastrum, some of which also produce latex? Will it be with the somewhat shrubby or herbaceous, perennial or annual species of section Argyrochaeta? All of these are possible. (Rollins got a hybrid of P. argentatum and P. hysterophorus L.) If they are possible in the garden they may be possible in populations in Mexico in which three to five Parthenium species coexist.

Alloploidy provides a mechanism for the association of diverse genotypes in a single organism, and provides a unique combination of characters upon which selection may occur.

Much of the chemical information about polyploids indicates the possibility that polyploids, alloploids, and autoploids may express unique subsets of the chemical constituents found throughout a genus. None of the evidence suggests that chemical characteristics new for the genus have originated within a functionally polyploid species. Yet, if a totally new enzyme or chemical defense should originate in one diploid species of a genus, it might occur in the future in combinations with morphological and chemical characteristics of other species than that in which is originated, through the intermediacy of polyploids.

ACKNOWLEDGMENTS

The Parthenium research was accomplished while several grants and a traineeship were in effect: NSF grants GB-26276 and GB-37666 and NIH traineeship 5-TOI-M-00789. Some of the ideas included in this paper originated or were developed as the result of conversation with Thomas Uzzell. Helen R. Mears has assisted much in laboratory and field work with Parthenium and has prepared the figures in this paper.

LITERATURE CITED

1. Stebbins, G.L., 1971, "Chromosomal Evolution in Higher Plants," Addison-Wesley, Reading, MA.

2. Stebbins, G.L., 1947, Types of polyploids; Their classification and significance. Adv. Genetics 1: 403-439.

3. Alston, R.E., Turner, B.L., 1959, Application of paper chromatography to systematics: Recombination of parental biochemical components in a Baptisia hybrid population. Nature 194: 285-286.

4. Alston, R.E., Turner, B.L., 1962, "Biochemical Systematics," Prentice-Hall, Inglewood Cliffs, N. J.

5. Stebbins, G.L., 1950, "Variation and Evolution in Plants," Columbia University Press, New York.

6. Stebbins, G.L., Harvey, B.L., Cox, E.L., Rutger, J.N., Jelencovic, G., Yagil, E., 1963, Identification of the ancestry of an amphidiploid Viola with the aid of paper chromatography. Amer. J. Bot. 50: 829-839.

7. Garber, E.D., 1958, The genus Collinsia. VI. Distribution of pigments in the flowers. Bot. Gaz. 119: 240-243.

8. Turner, B.L., Alston, R.E., 1959, Segregation and recombination of chemical constituents in a hybrid swarm of Baptisia laevicaulis X B. viridis and their taxonomic implications. Amer. J. Bot. 46: 678-686.

9. Harney, P.M., Grant, W.F., 1964, The cytogenetics of Lotus (Leguminosae). VII. Segregation and recombination of chemical constituents in interspecific hybrids between species closely related to L. corniculatus L. Canad. J. Genet. Cytol. 6: 140-146.

10. Stromnaes, O., Garber, E.D., 1963, The genus Collinsia. XXI. A paper chromatographic study of root extracts from fifteen species and six interspecific hybrids. Bot. Gaz. 124: 363-367.

11. Levin, D.A., 1968, The genome constitutions of eastern North American *Phlox* amphidiploids. Evolution 22: 612-632.

12. Dedio, W., Kaltsikes, P.J., Larter, E.N., 1969, A thin-layer chromatographic study of the phenolics of *Triticale* and its parental species. Canad. J. Bot. 47: 1589-1593.

13. Kaltsikes, P.J., Dedio, W., 1970, A thin-layer chromatographic study of the phenolics of the genus *Aegilops*. I. Numerical chemotaxonomy of the diploid species. Canad. J. Bot. 48: 1775-1780.

14. Kaltsikes, P.J., Dedio, W., 1970, A thin-layer chromatographic study of the phenolics of the genus *Aegilops*. II. Numerical chemotaxonomy of the polyploid species. Canad. J. Bot. 48: 1781-1786.

15. Smith, D.M., Levin, D.A., 1963, A chromatographic study of reticulate evolution in the Appalachian *Asplenium* complex. Amer. J. Bot. 50: 952-958.

16. Olsson, U., 1967, Chemotaxonomic analysis of some cytotypes in the *Mentha* X *verticillata* complex (Labiatae). Bot. Not. 120: 249-261.

17. Alston, R.E., Rösler, H., Naifeh, K., Mabry, T.J., 1965, Hybrid compounds in natural interspecific hybrids. Proc. Nat. Acad. Sci. USA 54: 1458-1465.

18. Fahselt, D., Ownbey, M., 1968, Chromatographic comparison of *Dicentra* species and hybrids. Amer. J. Bot 55: 334-345.

19. Levy, M., Levin, D.A., 1975, The novel flavonoid chemistry and phylogenetic origin of *Phlox floridana*. Evolution 29: 487-499.

20. Harborne, J.B., Mabry, T.J., Mabry, H., 1975, "The Flavonoids," 2 vols, Academic Press, London.

21. Brehm, B.G., Ownbey, M., 1965, Variation in chromatographic patterns in the *Tragopogon* *dubius-pratensis-porrifolius* complex (Compositae). Amer. J. Bot. 52: 811-818.

22. Kroschewsky, J.R., Mabry, T.J., Markham, K.R., Alston, R.E., 1969, Flavonoids from the genus *Tragopogon*. Phytochem. 8: 1495-1498.

23. Belzer, N.F., Ownbey, M., 1971, Chromatographic comparison of *Tragopogon* species and hybrids. Amer. J. Bot. 58: 791-802.

24. Roose, M.L., Gottlieb, L.D., 1976, Genetic and biochemical consequences of polyploidy in *Tragopogon*. Evolution 30: 818-830.

25. Levy, M., Levin, D.A., 1971, The origin of novel flavonoids in *Phlox* allotetraploids. Proc. Nat. Acad. Sci. USA 68: 1627-1630.

26. Wallace, J.W., Mabry, T.J., Alston, R.E., 1969, On the biogenesis of flavone-O-glycosides and C-glycosides in the Lemnaceae. Phytochem. 8: 93-99.

27. Harborne, J.B., 1967, "Comparative Biochemistry of the Flavonoids," Academic Press, London.

28. Bhatia, C.R., Mitra, R.K., Jaganath, D.R., 1968, Polyploidy and isoenzymes. Genetics 60: 162 (Abstr.).

29. Mitra, R., Bhatia, C.R., 1971, Isoenzymes and polyploidy. I. Qualitative and quantitative isozyme studies in the Triticinae. Genet. Res. 18: 57-69.

30. Barber, H.N., Driscoll, C.J., Long, P.M., Vickery, R.S., 1968, Protein genetics of wheat and homoeologous relationships of chromosomes. Nature 218: 450-452.

31. Barber, H.N., 1970, Hybridization and the evolution of plants. Taxon 19: 154-160.

32. Schwartz, D., Laughner, W., 1969, A molecular basis for heterosis. Science 166: 626-627.

33. Sing, C.F., Brewer, G.W., 1969, Isozymes of a polyploid series of wheat. Evolution 61: 391-398.

34. Haskell, G., 1968, Biochemical differences between spontaneous and colchicine-induced autotetraploids. Heredity 23: 139-141.

35. Levy, M., 1976, Altered glycoflavone expression in induced autotetraploids of Phlox drummondii. Biochem. Syst. Ecol. 4: 249-259.

36. Murray, B.G., Williams, C.A., 1973, Polyploidy and flavonoid synthesis in Briza media L. Nature 243: 87-88.

37. Murray, B.G., Williams, C.A., 1976, Chromosome number and flavonoid biosynthesis in Briza L. (Gramineae). Biochem. Genet. 14: 897-904.

38. Demaggio, A.E., Lambrukos, J., 1974, Polyploidy and gene dosage effects on peroxidase activity in ferns. Biochem. Genet. 12: 429-439.

39. Levin, D.A., Torres, A.M., Levy, M., 1979, Alcohol dehydrogenase activity in diploid and autotetraploid Phlox. Biochem. Genet. 17: 35-43.

40. Nakai, Y., 1977, Variation of esterase isozymes and some soluble proteins in diploids and their induced autotetraploids in plants. Jap. J. Genet. 52: 171-179.

41. Britten, R.J., Davidson, E.H., 1969, Gene regulation for higher cells: a theory. Science 165: 349-357.

42. Foster, A.E., Ross, J.G., Franzke, C.J., 1955, Genetic analysis of F_2 populations from crosses involving colchicine-induced mutants in Sorghum. Proc. S. Dak. Acad. Sci. 34: 21-22.

43. Ohno, S., 1970, "Evolution by Gene Duplication," Springer, New York.

44. Nair, P.S., Carson, H.L., Sene, F.M., 1977, Isozyme polymorphism due to the regulatory influence. Amer. Nat. 111: 789-791.

45. Ross, I.K., Martini, E.M., Thoman, M., 1973, Changes in patterns between monokaryons and dikaryons of a bipolar Coprinus. J. Bacter. 114: 1083-1089.

46. Noggle, G.R., 1946, The physiology of polyploidy in plants. I. Review of the literature. Lloydia 9: 153-173.

47. Carlson, P.S. 1972, Locating genetic loci with aneuploids. Mol. Gen. Genet. 114: 273.

48. Kostoff, D ., Axamitnaja, I., 1935, Studies on polyploid plants. VII. Chemical analysis of F_1 hybrids and their amphidiploids. Compt. Rend. Acad. Sci. URSS (Doklady) n.s. 1: 325-329.

49. Wolf, G., Rimpan, J., Lelley, T., 1977, Localization of structural and regulatory genes for phosphodiesterase in wheat (Triticum aestivum). Genetics 86: 597.

50. Smith, H.H., Conklin, M.E., 1975, Effects of gene dosage on peroxidase isozymes in Datura stramonium trisomics. in Markert, C.L. (ed.), "Isozymes," vol. 3, Academic Press, New York.

51. del Pero de Martinez, M., Swain, T., 1977, Variation in flavonoid patterns in relation to chromosome changes in Gibasis schiedeana. Biochem. Syst. Ecol. 5: 37-43.

52. Melchert, T.E., 1966, Chemo-demes of diploid and tetraploid Thelesperma simplicifolius (Heliantheae, Coreopsidineae). Amer. J. Bot. 53: 1015-1020.

53. Harney, P.M., Grant, W.F., 1964, A chromatographic study of phenolics of species of Lotus closely related to L. corniculatus and their taxonomic significance. Amer. J. Bot 51: 621-627.

54. Kohli, B.L., Denford, K.E., 1977, A study of the flavonoids of the Potentilla pensylvanica complex in North America. Canad. J. Bot. 55: 476-479.

55. Ferris, S.D., Whitt, G.S., 1977, Duplicate gene expressions in diploid and tetraploid loaches (Cypriniformes, Cobitidae). Biochem. Genet. 15: 1097-1112.

56. Ferris, S.D., Whitt, G.S. 1977, Loss of gene expression after polyploidization. Nature 265: 258-260.

57. Riley, R., 1965, Cytogenetics and the evolution of wheat, in Hutchinson, J. (ed.), "Crop and Plant Evolution," Cambridge University Press, London.

58. Zohary, D., Feldman, M., 1962, Hybridization between amphidiploids and the evolution of polyploids in the wheat (Aegilops-Triticum) group. Evolution 16: 44-61.

59. Feldman, M., 1965, Further evidence for natural hybridization between tetraploid species of Aegilops section Pleionathera. Evolution 19: 162-172.

60. Crawford, D.J., 1970, Systematic studies on Mexican Coreopsis (Compositae). Coreopsis mutica: flavonoid chemistry, chromosome numbers, morphology and hybridization. Brittonia 22: 92-111.

61. Smith, R.M., Smith-Martin, M., 1978, Hydrocarbons in leaf waxes of Saccharum and related genera. Phytochem. 17: 1293-1296.

62. Smith, R.M., Smith-Martin, M., 1978, Triterpene methyl ethers of Saccharum and related genera. Phytochem. 17: 1307-1312.

63. Rollins, R.C., 1950, The guayule rubber plant and its relatives. Contr. Gray Herb. Harvard Univ. 172: 1-72.

64. Mears, J.A., 1970, The systematics of Parthenium section
     Bolophytum: Biochemical, morphological and ecological.
     Ph.D. Dissertation, University of Texas at Austin.
65. Mears, J.A., 1973, Systematics of Parthenium section Bolophytum:
     A correlation of morphological, biochemical and habitat
     data. Proc. Acad. Nat. Sci. (Philadelphia) 125: 121-135.
66. Mears, J.A., 1973, Flavonols of Parthenium section Bolphytum.
     Phytochem. 12: 2265-2268.
67. Rüesch, H., Mabry, T.J., 1969, The isolation and structure
     of tetraneurin-A, a new pseudoguaianolide from Parthenium
     alphinum var. tetraneuris (Compositae). Tetrahedron 25: 805-811.
68. Rodriguez, E., Yoshioka, H., Mabry, T.J., 1971, The ses-
     quiterpene lactone chemistry of the genus Parthenium
     (Compositae). Phytochem. 10: 1145-1154.
69. Rodriguez, E., 1977, Ecogeographic distribution of secondary
     constituents in Parthenium (Compositae). Biochem. Syst.
     Ecol. 5: 207-218.
70. Star, A.E., Seigler, D.S., Mabry, T.J., Smith, D.M., 1975,
     Internal flavonoid patterns of diploids and tetraploids of
     two exudate chemotypes of Pityrogramma triangularis (Kaulf.)
     Maxon. Biochem. Syst. Ecol. 2: 109-112.
71. Seigler, D.S., Smith, D.M., Mabry, T.J., 1975, n-Alkanes
     from diploid, triploid and tetraploid plants of Pityrogramma
     triangularis flavonoid chemotypes. Biochem. Syst. Ecol. 3:
     5-6.
72. Kelsey, R.G., Thomas, J.W., Watson, T.J., Shafizadeh, F.,
     1975, Population studies in Artemisia tridentata ssp. vaseyana:
     Chromosome numbers and sesquiterpene lactone races. Biochem.
     Syst. Ecol. 3: 209-213.
73. Seaman, F.C., Mabry, T.J., 1979, Sesquiterpene lactones of
     diploid and tetraploid Ambrosia camphorata. Biochem. Syst.
     Ecol. 7: 3-6.
74. Seaman, F.C., Mabry, T.J., 1979, Sesquiterpene lactone
     patterns in diploid and polyploid Ambrosia dumosa. Biochem.
     Syst. Ecol. 7: 7-12.
75. Mears, J.A., 1975, The taxonomy of Parthenium section
     Partheniastrum DC. (Asteraceae-Ambrosiinae). Phytologia
     31: 463-482.
76. Feeny, P.P., 1975, Biochemical coevolution between plants
     and their insect herbivores, in Gilbert, L.E., Raven, P.H.
     (eds.), "Coevolution of Plants and Animals," University of
     Texas Press, Austin.
77. Giannasi, D.E., Chuang, T.I., 1976, Flavonoid systematics of
     the genus Perideridia (Umbelliferae). Brittonia 28: 177-194.
78. deWet, J.M.J., 1968, Diploid-tetraploid-haploid cycles and
     the origin of variability in Dichanthium agamospecies.
     Evolution 22: 394-397.
79. Rollins, R.C., 1946, Interspecific hybridization in Parthenium.
     II. Crosses involving P. argentatum, P. incanum, P. stramonium,
     P. tomentosum and P. hysterophorus. Amer. J. Bot. 33: 21-30.

POLYPLOIDY IN SPECIES POPULATIONS

Walter H. Lewis

Department of Biology
Washington University
St. Louis, MO   63130

Polyploidy in populations of well-differentiated plant species
is now widely recognized (1,2). Most reports, however, are limited
to a few individuals from one or several populations and thereby
illustrate only a fraction of the extant genomic diversity in most
species. They rarely purport populational dynamics involving polyploidy as an evolutionary process. Nevertheless, there are recent
notable exceptions and these will be utilized freely in this review
of polyploidy within species populations.

TERMINOLOGY

In order to avoid ambiguity it is imperative to define a
number of terms. Polyploidy may be infraspecific (intraspecific)
or interspecific, i.e., it may be formed from one basic genome
of one unit we call species, or from two or more genomes representing two or more species. Even though the judgement of what
circumscribes a species varies according to the botanist and to the
data available (3,4), that judgement particularly from a specialist
is the best approximation we have of the unit to which populational
studies must relate and may modify. Terms such as ecotype and
population are valid and useful, but their circumscription and
limits can be equally as difficult as those of species as anyone
accustomed to field-oriented populational studies can attest.
The terms autoploidy and alloploidy parallel infraspecific
and interspecific polyploidy, respectively. As I am considering
polyploidy as a mutational event that is a part of the evolutionary
process involving polyploidy within species populations, multiplication of genomes "applies to cases ranging from the homozygous
individual...at one extreme, to the polyploid derivates of a
hybrid between subspecies or ecotypes of a species at the other."

This quote defining autoploidy from Clausen, Keck, and Heisey (5)
"appears to be both logical and in close agreement with the
original concept of the term" (5) as defined by Kihara and Ono
(6). It contrasts with polyploid amphiploidy and alloploidy
whereby there is the addition of all chromosomes from distinct
species. This distinction is sometimes difficult and arbitrary,
yet the terms are usefully applied to the majority of situations
where polyploidy is understood within or between species. In
addition, species complexes beyond the tetraploid level may
involve both phenomena; these autoalloploids may be widespread
among plant groups where polyploidy is an important aspect of
their evolutionary process.

Infraspecific polyploidy is divisable into: homozygous
autoploidy involving genomes from only one individual, as among
many chemically-induced polyploids, and heterozygous autoploidy
including genomes from two or more genotypes. The least heterozygous polyploids will be those formed between individuals of the
same population and gene pool, while the most heterozygous may
occur between individuals of more distant populations with
distinct gene pools and ecological adaptations, although pollen
dispersal is obviously limiting to distant cross-fertilizations (4).

In the broad sense of some geneticists, hybridization is a
term used to describe fertilization between any two individuals
with the resulting progeny known as hybrids. This extreme use
essentially equating interindividual sexual reproduction with
hybridization is not a common practice among holistic biologists;
rather, they generally restrict the use of hybridization to
crossing of individuals belonging to two unlike populations, and
rarely use the term to designate crossing between biotypes of
like populations or to call the progeny of such matings or crossing
hybrids. As the majority of sexual reproduction in nature is
between individuals of one population and those of adjacent
populations, most of which would tend to be similar, then most
sexual reproduction is not by definition hybridization, but is
simply cross-fertilization. In this review I consider that
individuals of distinct species populations may hybridize to
produce hybrids, while individuals more closely related genetically,
i.e., within species, may fertilize to give progeny. This simplistic and by no means dogmatic approach is useful, for it
equates interspecific polyploidy-alloploidy-hybridization on the
one hand and infraspecific polyploidy-autoploidy-fertilization on
the other.

ORIGIN AND FREQUENCY OF POLYPLOIDY IN SPECIES POPULATIONS

Homozygous Autoploidy

Somatic polyploidy, unreduced gametes when selfed, and
zygotic doubling of selfed gametes are all immediate sources of
new polyploids that involve only the multiplication of one genome.

Most polyploidy induced by chemicals or wounding is of this type, but spontaneous development of polyploids in nature is also known to occur. For example, the origin of triploids from diploids via unreduced gametes following self-fertilization (2n+n) is known under natural conditions in Zea mays and rice; additionally, homozygous autoploids occur at the tetraploid level in Zea mays from triploids by further development of unreduced gametes (3n+n) (1). Another example of spontaneous polyploidy was reported by Hedberg (7) among selfed diploids of Anthoxanthum odoratum in which one individual proved to be triploid and it produced eventually one tetraploid, both steps presumably by unreduced gametes. Undoubtedly similar events occur in nature among self-fertilizing individuals, but they are not often found and their survival as dynamic evolving elements of populations may be infrequent or rare.

Development of polyploids directly by the fusion of two unreduced gametes (2n+2n) is undoubtedly very infrequent. A more probable genesis of polyploidy is the formation of diploid gametes from tetraploid cells in somatic tissues provided that the plant is self-fertile. D'Amato (8,9), for example, described the formation of adventitious polyploid buds in stems of several plants following decapitation and/or growth substance treatment, the origins of which trace back to mitotic stimulation of a single endopolyploid cell. Growth and development of this bud would give rise to polyploid sporocytes and reduced but doubled gametes. Indeed the frequency of endopolyploidy in the somatic tissue of higher plants, even though not always leading directly to the germ line and even though some endopolyploid nuclei divide only once, is astounding and surely represents a reservoir of potentially valuable cells for polyploid development under particular circumstances. A few examples of endopolyploidy among angiosperms with levels of ploidy are given in Table 1 (10,11); less dramatic, but significant nevertheless, are the increases of sporocyte chromosomes (aneuploid and/or polyploid) compared to somatic ones from the same individual in Claytonia (12), Haplo-pappus (13), Poa (14), Sorghum (15), and Xanthisma (16) to note but a few. These infraindividual multiple genomes in the germ line may be important sources of diversity among gametes of both homozygous or heterozygous autoploids depending on the mechanism of fertilization.

Heterozygous Autoploidy

Infraspecific polyploids may arise from different individuals having unreduced gametes following fertilization between diploid or polyploid gametes and haploid gametes, or rarely between two diploid gametes (1,17). In this way the diversity of the species at the diploid level may be incorporated into the polyploids by bringing together adapative genotypes from similar and/or different ecotypes of two or more individuals among allogamous species.

Table 1. Maximum endopolyploidy levels in representative angiosperms (10,11).

Family	Species	Cells/tissues	Endopoly-ploidy x=genome
Araceae	Arum maculatum	endosperm austoria	24,576x
Cucurbitaceae	Cucumis sativus	nucellus	16x
Fabaceae	Lupinus regalis	tapetum	8x
	Phaseolus coccineus	suspensor	4,096x
	P. vulgaris	endosperm	96x
	Vicia faba	stem epidermis	61x
Geraniaceae	Geranium phaeum	integument	512x
Rosaceae	Prunus sp.	fruit	32x
Crassulaceae	Crassula arborescens	mesophyll	16x

Fertilization between individuals of a single population or
of different populations both near and more rarely afar allows
the union of genetically diverse genomes. Polyploidy is then
superimposed on this system via unreduced gametes in one individual (1,17). The new triploid formed (perhaps AAA_1 or AA_1A_1)
will be by and large sterile; it may survive in the population
only if perennial with some means of vegetative reproduction.
Modest success under these circumstances may depend in large
measure on the heterozygosity of certain alleles brought together
by these unique events and thus provide the basis for a fitness
within the evolving population complex. A probable example was
the recent discovery of a triploid cytotype of Thalictrum alpinum
with different ecophysiological properties from the diploid (18)
as discussed more fully on p.130.
    The second stage in this evolutionary process that will
obviously be more common among perennials than annuals is an
increase to tetraploidy following fertilization of unreduced
gametes from the same, similar, or different individuals.
Assuming cross-fertilization, which would in fact be in the
majority, a second opportunity exists for incorporating a third
set of different chromosomes into the genome of a new polyploid
and thereby increase substantially the heterozygosity at some if
not many loci. This reinformed diversity may be an important
factor in adaptability of tetraploids and higher polyploids.
Tetraploids (e.g., 3n+n) with such complements as AAA_1A_2 and
$AA_1A_1A_2$ are not homozygous; in fact, by the tetraploid level
among outcrossing individuals they have accumulated and in part

duplicated the allelic diversity of three individuals from one or
several populations.

Subsequent production of polyploid gametes could give rise
to a pentaploid (4n+n or 3n+2n) and ultimately to a $\pm$ stable
hexaploid (5n+n, 4n+2n, 3n+3n) either by step-by-step increase
via unreduced gametes (e.g., $AAA_1A_2A_3A_4$, $AA_1A_2A_3A_4$), by somatic
polyploidy of triploids (e.g., $AAAAA_1A_1$, $AAA_1A_1A_2A_3A_4$) to form a
second type of hexaploid without nearly the amount of heterozygosity as the first example, or by several other ways, all with
potentially variable genomic combinations resulting in different
autoploid potentialities. Nevertheless it is a consequence of
their genetic richness and expression that many are able to
survive and compete successfully in or near population sites
already occupied by diploids having genomes from only two individuals.

Are unreduced gametes found in species populations and is
the phenomenon common enough to be of significance in this model?
Harlan and deWet [1] list 68 genera for which polyploid individuals
are known or suspected of having formed from unreduced gametes,
and in his survey Franke [19] included plants from 31 families.
Both compilations include diverse organisms spanning the angiosperms and a few gynmosperms; undoubtedly polyploid gametes will
be found more frequently in nature as sporocytes are examined for
meiotic behavior from multiple individuals of different populations. Recently several such studies illustrate the general
occurrence of spontaneous unreduced gametes:

(1) Achillea millefolium, n=9 [20]: 8 populations from BC,
OR, and WA examined of which 19.2-43% of tetraploids produced 4n
spores; 4x, 5x, and 6x plants were indistinguishable morphologically.

(2) Claytonia virginica, n=6,7,8 [21,22]: 1 population from
MO examined of which 9% of triploids had some unreduced 6n microsporocytes (2x,3x, and 4x plants were morphologically similar); a
second population from MO was found with 9.5% of tetraploids with
some 8n microsporocytes (only 4x plants sampled).

(3) Perityle rupestris, n=17 [23]: 1 population from TX in
which five diploids were found with 0.83-5.8% 4n microsporocytes;
2x and 4x plants were morphologically indistinguishable.

Determinants exist that govern the formation of diploid
gametes (see p. 6). Adverse growing conditions, for example,
result in an increased frequency of unreduced gametes in Gilia,
and a gene in Zea mays greatly increases the number of diploid
eggs produced. These and other environmental causes as well as
gene regulation that lead to meiotic failure and the production
of restitution nuclei with a somatic number may be frequent.

Most angiosperm families of any size for which chromosomal
data are available have members illustrating infraspecific polyploidy. As chromosome counts accumulate for populations so
indeed does the reality of this statement that even a very few

years ago would have been scorned. Lewis (this volume, p.103)
lists frequencies for dicotyledons by superorders. Why autoploidy
should be so common among species of some predominantly herbaceous
families and genera and much less frequent among those that are
woody is unknown. Perhaps in part it is a sampling bias, for
woody plants are not as readily studied as herbaceous ones, but
perhaps it is a real difference governed by genes that, for
example, regulate unreduced gamete production and thus set the
stage for polyploid formation among certain herbaceous groups or
taxa in different life forms. A discussion particularly of the
rates of evolution involving chromosome increase between herbaceous
and woody plants is currently available (24).

Autoalloploidy (or Alloautoploidy)

Speciation for many plants has progressed by hybridization
between distinct species forming allodiploids (interspecific
hybrids) that are partially or wholly sterile. Hybrids may have
formed from distantly related species and be totally sterile, or
from sibling species that by homoeologous pairing of chromosomes
may have meiotic behavior sufficiently regular to produce some
viable gametes. Often diploid hybrids will produce unreduced
gametes and give rise to allotriploids and ultimately allotetraploids (amphiploids), or occasionally to allotetraploids in
one step, that are completely fertile and capable of evolving a
successful independent future.
Although alloploids are not considered by definition a part
of infraspecific polyploidy, it is sometimes difficult, even
after a study of morphology, chemistry, meiotic behavior, etc.,
to determine whether or not alien genomes are present and so be
able to characterize the type of polyploidy in the continuum from
homozygous autoploidy to well-defined alloploidy. This is particularly acute among polyploid complexes at or beyond the tetraploid
level involving sibling species. Many polyploid complexes of
species involving both alloploidy and autoploidy are known and
they contribute markedly to the adaptive potential and evolution
of higher plants (e.g., 25-29).

In conclusion, allogamy of unreduced gametes is one of the
most, if not the most important, mechanism whereby polyploid
individuals arise in sexually reproducing species populations.
In Table 2 are listed 20 examples that underscore the significance
of autoploid evolution among related individuals from allied
species populations; additional examples are found in Gottschalk
(30).

Table 2. Polyploidy (probably heterozygous autoploidy) in species
populations.

Plant and chromosome number	Ploidy	Author remarks/ summary (reference)
Achlys triphylla n=6	2x,4x	2x appear superior in sexual reproduction, the 4x superior in asexual reproduction, autotetraploidy indicated; also few 3x (31).
Allium caeruleum n=8	2x,3x	Giemsa C-band somatic karyotypes show perfect replication of 3x from 2x and trivalent formation indicates autotriploidy (32).
Agropyron cristatum n=7	2x,4x,6x	Two additional species with autotetraploid races known, A. spicatum and A. stipifolium (33).
Anthoxanthum odoratum n=5	2x,4x	Autoploidy has played an important role in the origin of the 4x race; 4x karyotype I replicates 2x (34).
Arctostaphylos uva-ursi ssp. uva-ursi n=13	2x,4x	Cytotypes cannot be distinguished morphologically or chemically, evidence suggests autoploidy (35).
Artemisia douglasiana (et al.) n=9	2x,4x,6x	Reasonable doubt now caste on the putative amphiploid origin of the 6x race via hybridization (36).
Dactylis sp. ssp. mairei n=7	2x,4x	Relict diploid race coexisting with its autoploid derivative in a specialized habitat (37).

(Table 2 continued)

Erigeron potosinus (et al.) n=9	2x,4x	Strong circumstantial evidence that auto-ploids are being formed; 6 of 22 species with two or more cytotypes (38).
Galax aphylla n=6	2x,3x,4x	Unreduced pollen in 2x race, morphologica similarity of races, and 4x with multi-valents all suggest autoploidy (39,40).
Galium palustre n=12	2x,4x	4x race of ± auto-ploid origin (41).
Hordeum violaceum n=7	2x,4x,6x	4x and 6x races be-have cytologically as autoploids and have gigas charac-teristics (42).
Larrea divaricata ssp. tridentata n=13	2x,4x,6x	No major difference in morphology and in phenolic and protein patterns among 2x,4x, and 6x races; auto-ploidy is involved in the origin of the 4x and 6x popu-lations (43).
Lesquerella engelmannii (et al.) n=6	2x,4x, 6x,8x	In all cases of popu-lation polyploidy, no instance where interspecific hybri-dization is involved; 12 of 45 species known with two or more cytotypes (44, 45).
Melanpodium cinereum var. cinereum M. leucanthum var. leucanthum n=10	2x,4x	Morphology, meiosis, and chemical pro-files (nearly iden-tical chromatographic patterns of phenolic compounds) confirm that these cytotypes are of autoploid origin (46).

(Table 2 continued)

Nerisyrenia camporum (et al.) n=9	2x,4x aneuploids	Polyploid populations may be of auto- ploid origin; 5 of 10 species with two or more cytotypes (47,48).
Pancratium triflorum n=11	2x,3x	Spontaneous 3x race in 2x population, autoploid origin because somatic karyotype of 3x a replication of 2x including satel- lites and secondary constrictions (49).
Panicum amarium n=18	4x,6x	Virtually identical phenolic compounds, and similar habitats and morphology, all suggest that 6x race arose by autoploidy via unreduced gametes (50).
Rumex paucifolium n=7	2x,4x	4x race is sub- stantially autoploid in origin; the species is distinct from any other (51).
Sedum wrightii n=12	2x,4x, 6x,8x	On the basis of evi- dence from chromo- some pairing, auto- polyploidy appears to be common in Mexican Crassulaceae (52).
Sowerbaea alliacea n=4	2x,4x	Tetraploids are structural auto- ploids, probably arising within established biotypes (53).
Tradescantia micrantha n=6	4x	Concluded that the species is an auto- tetraploid (54).

CHARACTERISTICS OF POLYPLOIDS IN SPECIES POPULATIONS

Morphology and Cell Size

The most widespread effect of polyploidy is an increase in cell size. This does not always increase plant size, for a common result of polyploidy is a reduced number of cell divisions during growth and development. Gigas effects of polyploidy are commonly found, however, particularly in organs that have a determinate growth pattern, such as flowers and seeds. In many instances, polyploidy causes changes in shape and texture of organs: leaves and petals are often thicker and firmer than those of their diploid progenitors, leaves and other organs are usually shorter and broader, the amount of branching may be reduced (55), and slower growth generally brings about later flowering and fruiting (22). The latter feature of temporal divergence may prove significant in reducing or preventing gene flow between the earlier flowering diploids and the latter flowering polyploids or, occasionally, vice versa.

Typically, cell size throughout the plant increases with increased ploidy level (56,57). Pollen and epidermal cells, particularly guard cells, have been the classic means by which diploid and polyploid cytotypes and allied species are distinguished (29). In fact the distinction between diploidy and tetraploidy is usually so clear that a tentative determination of ploidy level is possible from plant material where chromosome counts cannot be made. Pollen of polyploid origin, moreover, may also be altered sufficiently in other features, such as aperture number (Table 3) and sexine thickness.

Even the best indicators, however, have their exceptions. Pollen of Bigelowia nudata from diploid (20.6–29.4μm) and tetraploid (26.1–26.8μm) races overlap in size, although the hexaploid pollen is larger (34.2–35.6μm) (59), and neither pollen nor stoma showed consistent size differences between diploid and tetraploid

Table 3. Pollen size and aperture number of 2x and 4x cytotypes of Oldenlandia corymbosa (58).

	2x[a]	4x[a]
Diameters (means averaged, μm)	21.9 x 20.3	28.7 x 24.8
Apertures 3	98.8%	63.1%
Apertures 4	1.2%	36.9%

[a]Based on 9 and 10 collections, respectively.

races of <u>Saxifraga</u> <u>ferruginea</u> (60). Environmental influences may affect cell size, but genetic control is also a factor at least among pollen. Even though pollen of <u>Hedyotis</u> <u>caerulea</u> is dimorphic, that of diploids and tetraploids is similar in size. However, differences exist between pollen of the two floral types of this heterostylous species as illustrated in Table 4: pollen from short-styled flowers is larger than pollen from long-styled flowers irrespective of ploidy level. This is in marked contrast to homostylous rubiaceous genera (58,62).

Ecogeography

Once formed from diploid progenitors, what chance does a new polyploid have to survive? According to the minority exclusion model proposed by Levin (63), the substitution of diploids by tetraploids following the appearance of one or a few of the latter will occur only if the tetraploids are far superior to the diploids. The results of several experiments that can test this model or answer this fundamental question have been ambivalent, for when diploids and autoploids were grown together the raw, artificially-induced autotetraploids of barley were competitively inferior to the diploids (64), but when seedlings from naturally-occurring populations of <u>Sedum</u> <u>pulchellum</u> were compared, the hexaploids had the best survival rate in all experiments, the tetraploids were intermediate, and the diploids had the poorest competitive ability (65). The divergence results probably relate more to the differences in the starting material, viz., more homozygous autoploids in the first instance and more heterozygous autoploids in the second example, than to the species themselves or to the experimental methods used. Clearly the perennial <u>Sedum</u> polyploids obtained from wild populations had the opportunity to sort out desirable gene combinations and to have these polyploids selected for a unique role within or near the diploid population long before the experiment began. These well-adapted polyploids with increased heterozygosity compared to the diploids would be superior to the diploids if the minority exclusion model were valid (63). In constrast, the chemically-induced tetraploids of barley are homozygous autoploids with no greater heterozygosity

Table 4. Pollen size of 2x and 4x cytotypes of heterostylous <u>Hedyotis</u> <u>caerulea</u> (values are means averaged, μm) (61).

	Short-styled	Long-styled
2x	28.2 x 26.6	24.1 x 23.9
4x	29.7 x 31.1	23.9 x 21.9

than the diploids and with little time to sort out desirable gene combinations. They would not be expected to have a competitive edge over the diploids and, according to the model, would not survive. In retrospect these disparate results are not ambivalent; rather they can be anticipated for the majority of polyploid events.

There is, however, an important exception to this simplistic dichotomy, for sometimes the multiplication of genomes per se is sufficient to endow the new polyploid with unique characteristics that may be adaptive (see further discussions under Physiology and Chemistry). In an experiment designed by Stebbins (66,67) three decades ago, seeds of diploids and artifically-induced autotetraploids of a number of plants were grown. As expected the majority of the tetraploids failed to become established and perished, yet there was one important exception: the perennial grass Ehrharta erecta did not succumb and in fact spread from an original site on the University of California campus at Berkeley to a new habitat. In brief the events relevant to this discussion were as follows. (1) Both diploids and tetraploids multiplied by natural reseeding. (2) In a hilly area where the topography is steep, where soil drainage is particularly good, and where shade is relatively deep, the tetraploids became dominant even to the exclusion of the diploids. It was an area newly colonized by the tetraploids; the diploids apparently could not successfully colonize and/or compete. (3) Elsewhere, presumably at sites where diploids had a competitive advantage, only diploids or diploids plus a few scattered tetraploids were found. The important aspects of this experiment are, first, that newly produced tetraploids survived for 30 years in competition with the diploids, and secondly, that the ones that did had an adaptive advantage without much opportunity for preadaptation and without new genic material except for a few mutations that may have accumulated during the 30-year period. In other words, the mutational event of polyploidy involving gene multiplication alone was sufficient to allow the tetraploids to adapt and become established in a unique habitat. Even man-made tetraploids can fashion an independent role in nature under particular circumstances.

The newly formed autoploids in nature must have the ability to colonize by seeds dispersed to sites suitable for the diploids to occupy but by chance are not inhabited by them, or they must possess ecological requirements different from their progenitors (50). Should ecological differences exist then new polyploid populations could be established within the range of the diploids as well as marginally. In the absence of such differences, the opportunities for expansion of the tetraploid within the range of the diploid would be limited because a proportion of suitable habitats would be occupied. If the tetraploid populations were established toward the species boundary, concomitant with species expansion in that direction, the opportunity for polyploid colonization would be enhanced, and an area of ecologically comparable

populations of diploid and polyploid plants could develop. This
would correlate with the occasional reports of coexisting cytotypes
that apparently lack subniche differentiation (2). Additionally,
successful new polyploids tend to originate when environmental
conditions are more or less unstable, as in pioneer and subclimax
communities, while in stable climax areas polyploids have greater
difficulty becoming established and if they do their habitats and
areas of distribution are quite narrow compared to the diploids
(68,69).

Based on the frequency of reports, the spontaneous occurrence
of polyploids in nature and their successful establishment in
populations are high among angiosperms and ferns. A sample of 40
species having polyploid and/or diploids with differing ecogeographic preferences has been brought together in Table 5.   The
list includes only angiosperms, but similar examples could be
added from among the cryptogams. The table has been divided into
six, somewhat arbitrary, parts based broadly on the type of
colonization known among infraspecific polyploids, viz., distinct
geographic areas, different latitudinal distributions, different
altitudinal distributions, specific areas and habitats, different
moisture regimes, and different soil types.

Distinct geographic areas. Both diploids and tetraploids
may range widely, although the diploid cytotype is usually more
limited as in relictual distributions. Polyploid populations
often radiate from the diploids, or they may be sporadic in
occurrence throughout the range of the species, particularly the
higher polyploids and the triploids. The wide distribution of
many polyploids suggests adaptations to many ecotypes, some
undoubtedly distinct from diploid progenitors.

Differing latitudinal distributions. Depending on the
species, diploids may be distributed toward higher latitudes
(polar areas) and polyploids toward lower latitudes (equatorial
areas), or conversely. Often this is a generic or familial
tendency. Diploid cytotypes of Galium verum and Hedyotis caerulea
in the Rubiaceae, for example, both have more southerly ranges in
Europe and North America, respectively, while the tetraploid
cytotypes have more northerly ranges. In contrast diploid cytotypes of members of the Campanulaceae, Ericaceae, Portulacaceae,
and others are more boreal and the tetraploids are distributed
more toward the lower latitudes (Table 5). These polyploid range
extensions presumably representing more extreme environmental
conditions require an important qualification: what is adverse
or extreme for one plant group may be quite different for another
and polyploid distributions may vary accordingly.

Differing altitudinal distributions. In this sample infraspecific diploids colonize predominantly the high elevations, and
the tetraploids primarily the lowland habitats. However, higher
polyploids (6x,8x) often occur in the upper alpine sites while
their ancestral tetraploids inhabit lower elevations. Seemingly,
therefore, a parallel situation exists between latitude and

Table 5. Ecogeography of naturally-occurring diploids and their
infraspecific polyploids or of polyploids alone.

_____

Polyploids colonizing distinct often large geographic areas

Crocus cancellatus (70) n=4	e. Mediter- ranean area	2x 4x	Middle East to s.c. Turkey s.w Turkey and Greece (aneuploids between these areas and to the east)
Cuthbertia graminea (71) n=6	s.e. U.S. (Fig. 1)	2x 4x 6x	Confined to NC sandhills (with 3x) Widespread, coloniz ing large areas of s.e. available afte sea retreated (with 6x) Sporadic, extreme s. range
Diospyros virginiana (72) n=15	s.e. U.S. (Fig. 2)	4x 6x	c. and s.e., limite range Peripheral and larg range
Eupatorium (7 spp.) (73) n=10	e. U.S.	2x 4x	Limited ranges Widespread, mostly radiating from 2x
Heteropogon contortus (74) n=20	Australia	4x 4x-10x	Tropical latitudes only Subtropical lati- tudes
Nymphoides indica (75) n=9	pantropics	2x 4x	Old World New World
Oldenlandia corymbosa (58) n=9	pantropics	2x 4x 6x	Old World (discontinuous), New World Old World Coastal West Africa
Phacelia ranunculacea (76) n=6,7	e. U.S.	2x 4x	Midwest lowlands Atlantic Coastal Plain; bicentric distribution
Sedum ternatum (77) n=8	e. U.S. (Fig. 3)	2x 4x 3x,6x	c. Appalachian Mts. a central limited range Widespread, radiat- ing from 2x Sporadic

(Table 5 continued)

Polyploids distributed in higher or lower latitudes.

Allium grayi (78)	Japan	2x,3x	Rare, almost extinct
		4x,5x,6x	Tendency for higher polyploids to grow in the north, 6x most northern
Campanula rotundifolia (79)	Greenland	2x	Arctic
		4x	Subarctic
Claytonia virginica (80) n=6,7,8	e. North America (Fig. 5)	2x	More northern, s. Canada and n. U.S. to the Ozarks
		4x	More southern and western, n. U.S. to Kansas and Texas
		3x	Intermediate in range
Empetrum nigrum (81) n=13	Europe	2x	Lower elevations in temperate zone; dioecious
		4x	Higher elevations in temperate zone, also subarctic and arctic; bisexual
Epilobium angustifolium (82) n=18	N. Hemisphere	2x	Coldest climate (most northern)
		4x	Warmer climate
		6x	Warmest climate (most southern)
Epilobium latifolium (83) n=18	N. Hemisphere	2x	Colder regions of Arctic and alpine (with 3x)
		4x	Milder regions of Iceland, Greenland, s.e. Canada; in E. Hemisphere occupies more southerly area than 2x
Fraxinus americana (84) n=23	e. North America	2x	Diploids widespread, but north of 40°N

(Table 5 continued)

		4x,6x	Polyploids south of 40°n (DNA in root tip cells: 2x 3.22, 4x 5.96, 6x 8.51 pg)
Galium verum (85) n=11	Europe	2x	s.e. range (with few 4x)
		4x	n. range and Atlantic Coast (no 2x)
Hedyotis caerulea (86) n=8	e. U.S. (Fig. 4)	2x	More southern range, predominantly s. of the Pleistocene glaciation
		4x	More northern and including glaciated areas
Suaeda maritima (87) n=9	Old World	2x	Tropical (halophytic) areas
		4x	Temperate (cooler) areas
Vaccinium uliginosum (88) n=12	circumpolar	2x	Markedly arctic distribution
		4x	Subarctic, the northern distribution near s. limit of 2x

Polyploids colonizing upland or lowland areas

Achlys triphylla (31) n=6	Pacific Coast, BC–CA	2x	High elevations usually mountainous slopes, well-lighted habitats (also 3x)
		4x	Flat, lowland habitats, usually in deep shade
Anthoxanthum odoratum (89,90) n=5	Europe, Iceland	2x	Alpine and subalpine
		4x	Lower areas along mountain transect, lowlands

(Table 5 continued)

Calamagrostis canadensis (91) n=14	Alaska	4x	Disturbed areas and herblands at lower elevations
		6x,8x	Restricted to higher, alpine sites
Claytonia cordifolia (2) n=5	Washington	2x	Higher mountain slopes 1400-1600m
		4x	Lower mountain slopes, 1200m
Dactylis sp. n=7 (37) ssp. juncinella	Spain	2x	Above 2500m, micaceous soil in cliffs between boulders
ssp. hispanica		4x	Below 2500m, usually clay
Goodyera maximowicziana (92) n=14	Japan	2x	Higher elevations
		4x	Lower elevations
Panicum virgatum (93)	Oklahoma	4x	Lowland
		8x	Upland (with aneuploids)

Polyploids colonizing specific areas and habitats

Biscutella laevigata (94) n=9	Europe	2x	Unglaciated river valleys
		4x	Vigorous post-glacial immigrants occupying nearly whole area covered by Alpine Ice Sheet
Claytonia perfoliata (95) n=6	w. North America	2x,4x	Woodland, chaparral, coastal strand, and occasionally ruderal
		6x,8x,10x	largely ruderal

(Table 5 continued)

Dactylis glomerata (96) n=7	Middle East	2x	Small, higher enclaves in 4x territory, typical Mediterranean dwarf shrub, no less than 55cm rainfall annually, confined to calcareous soil
		4x	Lower, warmer foothills; similiar to 2x plus semi-steppe and desert (never more than 30cm rainfall annually), red sandy loam, sandstone and basal soils.
		3x	In mixed 2x-4x narrow belts
Galium anisophyllum (97) n=11	Europe	2x	Refugia only, not recolonizing
		4x-10x	Active alpine colonizers
Grindelia camporum (98) n=6	California	2x	Relatively undisturbed native associates (climax)
		4x	Consistently colonizing habitats disturbed by man (pioneer)
Parnassia palustris (99) n=9	Holland	2x	Unglaciated areas
		4x	Glaciated areas
Ptilotus obovatus (100) n=27	Australia	2x	Local, isolated relicts
		4x	Recolonizers of arid areas following Recent arid maxima
Saxifraga ferruginea (60) n=10	n.w. North America	2x	Unglaciated areas to south, few sites inside margin
		4x	Glaciated areas, disturbed terrain

(Table 5 continued)
_____

Polyploids adapted to different moisture regimes

Cardamine
    pratensis (101)   Sweden   4x   Water table not
    n=8   Denmark   too high, ground
                                                    flooded only in
                                                    early spring;
                                                    pastures
                                             8x   Wet habitats in or
                                                    near bogs and by
                                                    rivers; pastures
                                            10x   Extremely wet
                                                    habitats; bare
                                                    moist soil along
                                                    lake margins

Eragrostis
    cambessediana (102)   W. Africa   2x   Wet habitats, silty
    n=10   edge of small
                                                    lakes, dies an-
                                                    nually when water
                                                    floods area
                                             4x   Base of near-by
                                                    dunes in narrow
                                                    zone above silt
                                                    habitat; perennial
                                             8x   Very dry dunes,
                                                    sand temperature
                                                    may reach 80C;
                                                    perennial

Galax aphylla (39,40)   e. U.S.   2x   More xeric habi-
    n=6   tats
                                             4x   More mesic habi-
                                                    tats
                                             3x   Intermediate
                                                    habitats, or in
                                                    close proximity
                                                    to other cytotypes

Koeleria cristata (103)   w. North   2x   mountains and
    n=7   America   plains
                                             4x   sagebrush grass-
                                                    lands including
                                                    driest sites
                                                    samples

(Table 5 continued)

| Valeriana officinalis (104) n=7 | Britain | 4x | Xeric, limited to ± dry habitats in hilly regions |
| | | 8x | Mesic habitats, higher acidity, and lower elevations when sympatric with 4x |

Polyploids adapted to different soil types

| Aster pilosus (105) n=16 | Ontario | 4x | Fine textured silt plains and limestone outcroppings |
| | | 6x | Glacial sand till soils and coarse gravel fill |

altitude i.e., higher and lower ploidy levels may occur at higher or lower elevations depending on what the extreme or marginal habitat for a particular species or taxon is.

   Specific areas and habitats. Tetraploids of species populations consistently colonize glaciated, including alpine, areas (e.g., Biscutella laevigata, Parnassia palustris, Saxifraga ferruginea), while their diploid progenitors remain largely in unglaciated areas often limited to refugia or relictual areas. Diploids also remain in relatively undisturbed, climax areas; polyploids in contrast often colonize more ruderal, pioneer, and disturbed habitats. Two examples (Ptilotus obovata, Dactylis glomerata) illustrate tetraploid adaptations to more arid conditions than diploids (Table 5).

   Different moisture regimes. Adaptation is toward both extremes, for diploids and polyploids may be dominant in either xeric or mesic (and alkaline or acidic) conditions according to the group. The diploid of Eragrostis cambessediana inhabits wet flood plains, whereas its derived tetraploid and hexaploid races occupy progressively drier and hotter sand dunes, yet Galax

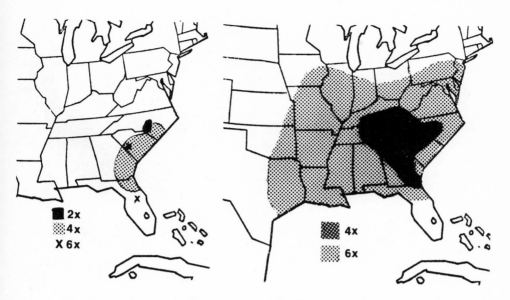

Fig. 1 (left). Distribution of <u>Cuthbertia</u> <u>graminea</u> cytotypes in the southeastern U.S. (from 71). Fig. 2 (right) Distribution of <u>Diospyros</u> <u>virginiana</u> cytotypes in the southeastern U.S.
(from 72).

<u>aphylla</u> diploids grow in more xeric habitats than their derived
tetraploids (Table 5).

<u>Different soil types</u>. Different plants of the same species
may grow in a wide range of soils, yet infraspecific diploids and
tetraploids do sometimes adapt to distinct soil conditions as
found for <u>Aster</u> (Table 5). Allied species differing in ploidy
level may also respond antithetically to a soil type: diploid
species of <u>Dianthus</u>, for example, grow poorly on calcareous soils
and prefer granitic soils, while tetraploid species thrive on
calcareous soils (106).

Certain adaptations, therefore, appear unidirectional for
ploidy levels of particular species. For latitude and altitude,
and thus broadly to climate, adaptations are sometimes opposite
for different species. The reason for this difference is unknown,
though it may represent genotypic responses predicated by the
ancestral or floristic origin of the taxon. An illustration of
this possibility is found in the research of Johnson and Packer
(107) on a modern portion of the Arcto-Tertiary geoflora of
northwestern Alaska that survived in refugia. According to my
hypothesis, polyploids arising and colonizing in this region
should adapt in general in one direction in response to most

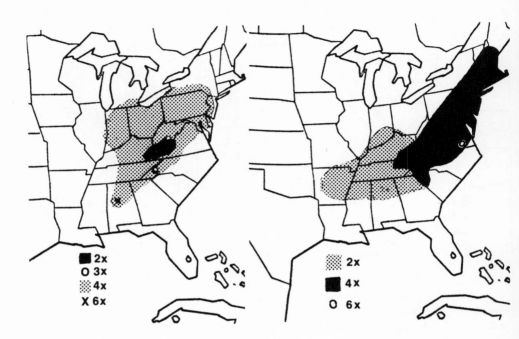

Fig. 3 (left). Distribution of Sedum ternatum cytotypes in the eastern U.S. (from 77). Fig. 4 (right). Distribution of Hedyotis caerulea cytotypes in the eastern U.S. (from 86).

climatic and edaphic conditons, and apparently they do, for there is a strong correlation between habitat and ploidy level. Polyploids were found in highest frequency in the colder wet lowlands and lowest on the well-drained warmer slopes and uplands, while the reverse was true for diploids. Even though these data were not directed toward infraspecific polyploidy per se, they do lend support to the idea that by and large elements of the same ancestral flora respond to certain major environmental parameters similarly.

The research in Alaska and also that in the Canadian Arctic Archipelago (108) support the conclusion of Löve and Löve (109,110) that polyploids are genetically by differentiation and fixed heterozygosity better adapted for survival under adverse, more extreme climatic and edaphic conditions than their diploid progenitors. (Remember, however, that extreme conditions for one species or group may not be the same for another element of the

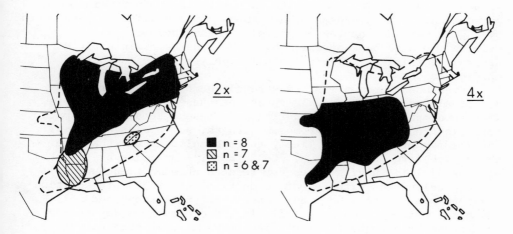

Fig. 5. Distribution of diploid and tetraploid cytotypes of
Claytonia virginica in eastern North America (modified from 80, 3x
omitted).

modern flora.) Finally, the report by Hancock and Bringhurst
(111) illustrates the importance of ecological differentiation in
determining ecogeographic adaptations among polyploid complexes
themselves.

Reproduction

    A commonly used feature distinguishing infra- and inter-
specific polyploids is the frequency by which chromosomes associate
at meiosis into quadrivalents and trivalents instead of bivalents
(55). This is a useful guide to chromosomal homology or lack of
it and hence plant origin, but it is only a guide. There are a
number of reasons for exceptional meiotic behavior as recently
reviewed in detail by Jackson (112) and Golubovskaya (113).
    Events in premeiotic cells can drastically affect meiotic
pairing. For example, chromosomes may carry genes that suppress
pairing among different genomes so that intergenomal (homoeologous)
pairing does not occur. Until this discovery it had been assumed
that the three diploid species whose genomes made up hexaploid

wheat were strongly differentiated, for how else could one explain
the near absence of meiotic pairing in haploids of the hexaploid
species? This model of an alloploid series became suspect when
it was shown that corresponding chromosomes of the three different
genomes were genetically very closely related. That the homoeologues had so little tendency to pair with each other remained a
paradox until the discovery that homoeologous pairing is suppressed
by a gene or genes on the long arm of chromosome 5B (114).
Pairing may also be suppressed by B chromosomes as in diploid
species of Triticum. The effects are very similar to that of
chromosome 5B.

Even when chromosomes are strongly homologous, tetraploids
do not always form quadrivalents at metaphase I as, for example,
when chiasmata fail to form during pachytene. Because chiasmata
formation can depend on chromosome length, polyploids with small
chromosomes are much less likely to form multivalents than are
those with large chromosomes. Genic control may also be involved
so that diploids having genes for reduced chiasma frequency will
produce polyploids with few or no multivalents (55). In addition
environmental factors such as temperature, nutrition, and soil
may alter chiasma frequency (115,116), and even from day to day
on the same plant quadrivalent frequency may vary significantly
(117).

Autotetraploid races sometimes deviate from anticipated
quadrivalent formation by having a reduced number of multivalents
(112). This suggests some genetically-controlled mechanism
operating to restrict quadrivalent formation and to form an
excess of bivalents, as reported for induced autotetraploids of
rye (118,119). Autotetraploids in nature with almost complete
bivalent formation and male fertility found among such disparate
genera as Arctostaphylos (35), Claytonia (2,22,80,91), Hedyotis
(86), Nerisyrenia (47), and Oxalis (120), suggest that such a
mechanism is widespread in angiosperms. Diploidization occurs
rapidly in raw autoploids of Zea mays (121) and rye (122) indicating, in addition, that selection can alter the frequencies of
quadrivalents and bivalents with concomitant increases in seed
set (123). Similar selections in nature would assist significantly
the otherwise disadvantaged autoploids as they become established
in populations adjacent to meiotically regular and usually highly
fertile diploid parents. However, even raw induced tetraploids
of Ehrharta erecta (C_2 generation) with viable seeds formed in
60-80% of florets were only "slightly lower than that of diploids"
growing together under natural conditions (66).

Many other factors affect the reproductive capacity and
survival of infraspecific polyploids. Apomixis, for instance,
may accompany the development of polyploidy and can be important,
at least initially, for the survival and dispersal of polyploids
(124). Greater self-compatibility may also be an outcome of
polyploidy and is important in sympatric speciation (125), and
the phenomenon of asymmetric genomic reduction (126) that could

lead to polyhaploidy and thereby reverse a normally unidirectional evolutionary trend are all features of infraspecific polyploidy that may relate to the process of polyploid evolution.

Pairing may also be supressed by B chromosomes as in diploid species of Triticum. The effects are very similar to that of chromosome 5B (96).

Physiology

Populations growing in different environments are subject to different selections and hence may be genetically as well as physiologically distinct. Comparative studies of the physiological ecology of these populations provide data on the selective significance of particular components of the environmental complex. In addition, these studies may illustrate by what specific physiological mechanisms similar biotypes have been altered to meet dissimilar environmental stresses (18).

As a background to current physiological studies on populations involving polyploids, the review 30 years ago by Noggle (127) provides an important synthesis of their physiological/chemical characteristics in relation to diploid progenitors.

(1) Polyploids grow and develop slower than their diploid ancestors. This decreased rate may correlate directly with reduced amounts of growth hormones present in polyploid tissues, as reported for Lycopersicon, Tagetes, and Sedum (65,128), and with their lowered rates of respiration (129). It can lead to later flowering of the polyploids (130) and thereby to temporal divergence with a degree of inter- or infrapopulational isolation (Table 6, showing initial diploid flowering followed by triploids and ultimately tetraploids.) Among polyploid cytotypes, from tetraploidy to nonoploidy, phenology can be important in climatic adaptation, for in Heteropogon contortus earlier flowering and polyploidy have been selected as higher polyploids were able to migrate into subtropical from tropical latitudes (74).

(2) Tetraploids show a higher moisture content and this correlates with an increase in cell size and a consequent decrease in osmotic pressure. Seedlings of tetraploids transpire less water than do diploid seedlings (131), and tetraploid seeds generally possess a higher imbibition capacity than seeds from diploid plants (127).

(3) Organic compositions of diploids and infraspecific tetraploids vary. Diploids contain a higher percentage of nitrogen than tetraploids, although this difference is not universal. Polyploids possess a greater percentage of total sugar, non-reducing sugar, reducing sugar, and starch than diploids, but diploids contain greater precentages of structural constituents such as cellulose, hemicellulose, and crude fiber. Nicotine, organic acids, crude fat extracts, and vitamin C are in greater concentration among polyploids than diploids. Leaves of tetraploids contain less chlorophyll than diploids; however, per unit area,

Table 6. Temporal divergence of coexisting diploids (n=8) and
polyploids (n=12, $\pm$ 16) in two flowering populations of Claytonia
virginica from the vicinity of St. Louis, MO (21,22).

	2x		3x		4x	
	N	%	N	%	N	%
Population 1: 1975						
March 1-15	24	51.0	23	49.0	0	–
March 16-31	0	–	92	79.3	24[a]	20.7
April 1-15	0	–	0	–	6	100
Population 2: 1976						
February 15-29	4	8.3	27	56.3	17	35.4
March 1-15	0	–	4	7.5	49	92.5
March 16-31	0	–	0	–	25	100
April 1-15	0	–	0	–	47	100

[a]Includes one 5x plant.

tetraploids are richer in chlorophyll and in general have higher
pigment contents than their diploid progenitors. Among the
enzymes, catalase activity of seeds is greater among tetrapoids
than diploids, diastatic activity of tetraploid malt extract is
higher as well, but dehydrogenase activity of leaf extracts is
similar (127).
        (4) Of the inorganic components, soluble ash content of the
tetraploids is in all cases higher than that of the diploids,
metallic elements are also higher than that of the diploids, but
the acid elements are lower.
        The same year that Noggle's review was published the results
of a detailed account comparing morphological and physiological
characteristics of a diploid-polyploid complex involving diploids,
tetraploids, and hexaploids of the self-fertile annual Sedum
pulchellum also appeared (65). All cytotypes originated from
populations found in the species range in east-central U.S.
Meiosis of the diploid was regular, while that of the tetraploids
and hexaploids exhibited some multivalent association (132). The
origin of the complex was postulated by hybridization between S.
nevii and the distinct S. nuttallianum forming the allodiploid S.
pulchellum (n=11) that by doubling formed the autoallotetraploid
S. pulchellum (n=22) and on further duplication the hexaploid
(n=33). Evidence is scanty for this origin and needs experimental
studies, particularly to explain the regular meiotic behavior and

fertility of the F_1 between two disparate species. Recently
Clausen (133) has proposed an alternative explantation: the
species is a specialized derivative of S. nevii that evolved by
autoploidy and subsequent loss of chromosomes. This appears the
more plausible origin based on cytological as well as morphological
evidence, but final disposition must wait experimentation.
Nevertheless, the cytotypes are widely accepted as S. pulchellum
and a comparison of the three levels of ploidy when grown together
in a common garden at the University of Michigan can be most
instructive (65). Only ecophysiological responses are summarized.

(1) Effects of excess and deficient water. Diploids were
most sensitive to both an excess and a deficiency of water, for
they wilted first and most severely. Soil saturation was more
injurious than drought to both diploids and tetraploids, whereas
the hexaploids appeared to withstand soil saturation slightly
better than drought. Hexaploids were best able to withstand both
an excess and a shortage of water, diploids were the least able
to withstand these extreme conditions of soil moisture, and the
tetraploids were intermediate.

(2) Soils. Acid soil (pH4.5) was tolerated best by the
diploids, least by the hexaploids, and the tetraploids were
intermediate. Alkaline soil (pH8) was tolerated best by hexaploids
and they possessed the healthiest appearing roots, while alkalinity
was tolerated least by the diploids and their roots were the
least healthy in this soil. The tetraploids were again intermediate in their response.

(3) Competition. Seedlings from each cytotype were grown
for various periods of time in plots having particular mixed
arrangements. The results of three experiments were as follows:
(a) 120 plants, the survivors after 184 days were 2x 25%, 4x
32.5%, and 6x 52.5%; (b) 224 plants, the survivors after 108 days
were 2x 39.3%, 4x 55.7%, and, after 176 days, 6x 66.6%; (c) 81
plants surviving after an unknown time were 2x 40.7%, 4x 63.0%,
and 6x 74.1%. In all experiments the hexaploids had the best
survival rates in competitive plots, the diploids had the poorest
survival rate, and the tetraploids were intermediate.

(4) Root development of cuttings. After 11 days, the
tetraploids had significantly longer roots than the average
lengths of the longest roots of either the diploids or the hexaploids. The experiment was designed to provide an indication of
ability to propagate asexually.

(5) Growth hormone content. Measured as relative amounts
of growth hormone by curvature of Avena coleoptiles, the diploids
had the greatest amount of hormone, the hexaploids the least
amount, and the tetraploids were intermediate.

(6) Time of flowering. Diploids flowered about 12 days
earlier than the tetraploids that in turn flowered about 4 days
earlier than the hexaploids. Retardation of maturity in relation
to ploidy was striking.

(7) <u>Dry weight and water content</u>. Tetraploids had significantly greater dry weight; that of the other races was about
equal. There was no significant difference in water content
among the races.

The diversity of physiological response of S. pulchellum to a
wide variety of experimental conditions may exemplify the many
species known to have infraspecific chromosomal races. Smith's
data, for example, show that the ecotypes of the diploid cytotypes
are better adapted to acidic soils than those of the polyploid
cytotypes, that they develop rapidly, and that they would favor
conditions leading to rapid flowering and maturity. On the other
hand, the polyploid ecotypes are adapted to dissimilar niches
favoring a slower growth rate and later maturity, more alkaline
soils, and extremes of water excess and deprivation. Moreover,
the competitive experiments emphasize that should the three
cytological races be in direct competition at this stage of their
evolution the polyploids would eventually eliminate the diploids.

The S. pulchellum diploid-polyploid complex is one of considerable antiquity. The report by Mooney and Johnson (18) of diploid
(2n=14) and triploid (2n=21) races of the Alaskan <u>Thalictrum
alpinum</u> in nearby populations is an example of adaptation by a
neoautoploid. Origin of the autotriploid by hybridization
(sensu lato) was ruled out by the authors; it probably arose by
cross-fertilization of reduced and unreduced gametes. The triploid
inhabits the moist, shaded walls of a creek tributary, a habitat
not ordinarily occupied by the diploid race and thus demonstrates
its ability to exist in nature even though sterile. Its unique
physiological attributes (Table 7) though not necessarily superior
to those of the nearby diploids, are sufficiently different to
favor the adaptation and persistance of the triploid in a new
niche. As a perennial, persumably with some means of vegetative
reproduction, it may possess a limited independent future, but
more importantly it may ultimately give rise to a more independent
tetraploid population by continuing the process of cross-
fertilization of unreduced and reduced gametes. In summary, the

Table 7. Distinct physiological properties of 2x and 3x cytotypes
of <u>Thalictrum</u> <u>alpinum</u> (18).

Characteristics	2x	3x
Optimum photosynthetic rate	less	greater
Photosynthetic light efficiency	less	greater
Vigor	less	greater
Leaf reflectance in the visible	greater	less

autotriploid of T. alpinum possesses a number of unique physiological properties sufficient to allow it to colonize a distinct
niche, it presents a reservoir of genetic variability that by
backcrossing could contribute to the evolutionary potential of
the diploid populations, and it may serve as the intermediate
step in the evolutionary process leading to the formation of a
stable tetraploid population.

     Another set of physiological responses are exemplified by
Larrea divaricata that grows in the very different environment of
the southwestern deserts. Yang and Lowe (134) describe two major
ecocytotypes for this species: an eastern (Chihuahuan Desert)
one with 2n=2x=26, and a western (Sonoran Desert) population with
2n=4x=52, and subsequently Yang (135) discovered a third with
2n=6x=78. The differences in geography (Fig. 6), ecophysiology
(Table 8), and morphology apparently reflect the diverse climatic
and edaphic conditions to which the populations have adapted, the
diploid to a climate of greater preciptiation and relatively low
winter temperature, the tetraploid to a dissimilar macroclimate
of reduced precipitation and higher winter temperature, and the
hexaploid intermediate between them and variable. Larrea
divaricata presents an example of the successful adaptation of
three cytologically distinct ecotypes of which marked reduction
in precipitation represents the extreme environmental condition
tolerated by the tetraploid ecocytotype.

     Adaptation of cytological races under natural conditions may
not possess apparent physiological bases. For example, the
sympatric and morphologically similar cytotypes of Viola adunca
(2x,4x,6x) indigenous to Alberta do not differ with respect to:
the effect of light on net CO_2 assimilation, the effect of
temperature of net CO_2 assimilation and dark respiration from 0
to 45C, water potential and its component potentials, minimum and
maximum leaf resistance, and the effects of moisture stress on

Table 8. Distinct physiological properties of 2x and 4x ecocytotypes of Larrea divaricata (134).[a]

Characteristics	2x	4x
Seed germination	faster	slower
Seedling growth rate	faster	slower
Tolerance for low temperature	greater	less
Tolerance for low moisture	less	greater

[a]A hexaploid ecocytotype is known but poorly understood.

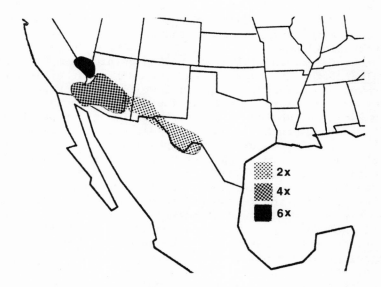

Fig. 6 Distribution of <u>Larrea</u> <u>divaricata</u> ssp. <u>tridentata</u>
cytotypes in southwestern North America (from 133,134).

leaf resistance and net CO_2 assimilation (136). Polyploids of
this species do not respond more favorably to extremes of temperature and water potential than diploids, and therefore ploidy
per se does not affect the response of <u>V</u>. <u>adunca</u> to its environment in this instance. It would be interesting to test for
physiological responses of cytotypes from different populations
to learn whether or not adaptation to dissimilar environmental
stresses occurs.

A comparison of physiological responses between diploids and
their induced polyploids is an important experimental tool, for
the data not only apply to manipulated products, but by inference
they also extend to the evolutionary processes occurring in
nature. As shown by Tal and Gardi (137) and Tal (138,139) for
tomatoes, colchicine-induced tetraploids may be physiologically
distinct in many ways from their immediate diploid progenitors.
Doubling of the genome alone resulted in 12 dissimilar and
important, though not necessarily advantageous, responses relative
to plant function (Table 9). Hall (140) also reported distinct
responses of autotetraploid rye seedlings that required 40-50%
higher oxygen concentrations at their root surface for normal
respiration to occur compared to diploids. This infers that

Table 9. Distinct properties and physiological responses of 2x
and colchicine-induced 4x cytotypes of tomato (137,138).

Characteristics/conditions	2x	4x
RNA content	greater	less
Protein content	greater	less
Saline conditions:		
protein level/unit DNA	less	greater
RNase activity	greater	less
Abscisic acid content	greater	less
Uptake and incorporation of		
labeled leucine	greater	less
Hormone ABC content	greater	less
Water content	less	greater
Water loss under salinity	greater	less
Dry weight under salinity	greater	less
Water loss during stomatal closure	greater	less
Root pressure	less	greater

tetraploid rye is less tolerant of high soil temperatures and it
may hinder the development of rye polyploids in warmer climates.
If such major changes can be promulgated by genomic doubling,
then gene duplication and heterozygosity both play significant
roles in the evolutionary process that involves polyploidy.

Chemistry

At this Conference Mears (141) has shown that the most
pertinent information on the chemistry of infraspecific polyploids
to date involves the study of phenolics, probably because phenolic
patterns are often inherited as co-dominants in hybrids and
because phenolics have so often been useful in characterizing
species. An intriguing aspect of his survey is the number of
recent reports indicating both qualitative and quantitative
chemical changes that occur following the development of new
polyploidy races within species. Some autoploids, induced or
natural, may exhibit qualitative similarities with their diploid
progenitors and show only quantitative chemical differences or
none that is discernible while other polyploids may express
novel "nonparental" compounds such as a distinct flavonoid
isomerase profile (Briza media) or two apparently new isozymes
(4x sporophyte of Todea barbara). These and a number of other
chemical differences of autoploids are summarized in Table 10.
The remarkable phenomenon may be explained by the repression of
genes among the diploid parents that on doubling are derepressed

Table 10. Quantitative and qualitative chemical attributable to
induced genomic doubling (141).

Plant (Reference)	Diploid to autotetraploid
Briza media (142,143)	Produce C-glycosyl derivates of luteolin from C-glycosyl apigenin-producing diploids (paralleling 2x and 4x wild cytotypes). Develop novel flavonoid isomerase profile.
Phlox drummondii (144)	Loss of certain glycoflavones and gain of others (but known in diploid cultivars).
Phlox drummondii (145)	About twice as much alcohol dehydrogenase activity (but variable).
Todea barbara (146) gametophyte	Peroxidase activity increased about 3.5 times per cell. Of 18 peroxidase isozyme bands studied, 3 were 3 times more active, 4 bands were much less active.
sporophyte	Two apparently novel isozymes.

and thereby allowed distinct chemical expressions. If different
profiles can arise during autoploidy by gene derepression, extreme
caution must be exercised in assuming that novel hydroxylation
patterns and phenolic profiles among polyploids represent interspecific parentage and are products of hybridization, or even
that they are expressions of crosses between different eocotypes
of one species. Allotetraploids of Tragopogon also express novel
heteromeric enzymes not produced in either one of their parents
(142). Chemical data alone may in fact be quite misleading and,
like other characteristics of the organism, must be considered a
part of the whole before categorical, far-reaching conclusions
are reached.

Other compounds may be altered markedly by polyploidy (see
also under Physiology above). Colchicine-induced tetraploids of
Datura stramonium were reported (148,149) as having about double
the amount of tropane alkaloids (L-hyoscyamine, atropine, and
scopolamine) as their diploid parents in aerial parts. In roots
of similarly produced tetraploids, the same alkaloids were
increased up to threefold over the corresponding diploid controls
(150). Moreover, a maximum increase in alkaloids of 153.6% was

recorded for tetraploids of the allied <u>Atropa</u> <u>belladonna</u> compared
to their diploids (149).

Significant diversity in secondary metabolites need not be
confined to man-manipulated ploidy complexes or to alkaloids.
Naturally-occurring <u>Achillea</u> <u>millefolium</u> triploids form azuleno-
genic substances over a complete growing season, yet phenotypically
identical hexaploids show no azulenes during a similar period in
any plant organ (151). This difference is important, for azulenes
may inhibit plant growth and they may also be cytotoxic to
animals; presence or absence of these sesquiterpenoids in similar
races of the same ssp. <u>millefolium</u> is fundamental to an understanding of its growth and development as well as of its toxicity
in relation to human and grazing animal health.

Short-term evolution of many plants is dominated by both
auto- and alloploidy, for the process may increase biochemical
diversity at the primary enzyme level and in other ways. It
allows the immediate expression of derepressed enzymes with
different properties from the diploids that may extend the range
of environments and habitats in which normal and successful
development can occur (142,143,147,152). Is this one of the
primary reasons for the success of polyploids among angiosperms
and ferns?

NAMING OF POLYPLOIDS IN SPECIES POPULATIONS

How to differentiate infraspecific polyploids from diploids
and distinct polyploid cytotypes from one another is not a simple
task. Speciation may have proceeded sufficiently in some instances
to designate confidently populations of sibling species with
appropriate Latin binomials, but in others no significant and
readily detectable morphological, physiological, or ecological
changes may yet accompany polyploidy. In these cases there is
little justification for insisting that taxonomy reflect the
polyploid genome (44). Anyone planning wholesale naming of
thousands of cytotypes with specific epithets ought to reconsider
this approach before flooding the taxonomic literature with
impractical names simply to satisfy man's interpretation of a
biological species concept. A better way might be to tag cytotypes
with a ploidy level (2x,4x, etc.) following a legitimate binomial
(2).

SUMMARY

1. Genome multiplication within species populations (autoploidy) is a common mutational event among angiosperms. It
contributes markedly to the evolutionary process leading to
speciation, particularly among herbaceous perennials where the
greatest frequency of infraspecific polyploidy is found.

2. Autoploids may be homozygous or heterozygous, i.e., the
first arising by chromosomal duplication via somatic polyploidy,

unreduced gametes, and zygotic doubling without genic material
from another individual and the second forming by similar
mutational events with the benefit of cross-fertilization. The
latter is undoubtedly more common in nature, the former by induced
polyploids using chemicals and other techniques. Heterozygosity
will be less in individuals formed from genetically identical or
similar genomes and greater when formed from genetically
dissimilar genomes within the species. By maximizing allelic
diversity it is believed that neopolyploids may compete successfully in populations dominated by their diploid progenitors.

     3. Most polyploids have probably arisen by unreduced gametes
(nonreduction of sporocytes during meiosis or reduction of polyploid premeiotic cells that appear unreduced) followed by fertilization with reduced gametes giving, step-by-step, triploids,
tetraploids, and high polyploids. These steps involve cross-
fertilizations within and between individuals of species populations and they do not involve hybridizations between distinct
species.

     4. Examples of diploid and infraspecific polyploid adap-
tations are given to illustrate distinct geographic areas, different
latitudinal and altitudinal distributions, specific areas and
habitats, different moisture regimes, and different soil types.
For latitude and altitude in particular, and therefore broadly
for climate, adaptations are sometimes opposite for different
species. Differences may be predicated by the ancestral or
floristic origin of the taxon. Nevertheless, neopolyploids
characterized by genetic divergence and heterozygosity are
better adapted for survival under adverse, extreme conditions
than are their diploid progenitors.

     5. Although neoautoploids often possess high frequencies of
abnormal meiotic behavior and reduced fertility as a consequence,
the meiotic process can be controlled by genes that either suppress
multivalent formation or elevate pairing and allow diploidization
of homologous and homoeologous chromosomes.

     6. A wide range of different physiological properties can
exemplify neopolyploids, including those of homozygous and heterozygous origins. It appears that genic duplication may trigger in
some polyploids sufficiently advantageous processes that multiplication of genetic material per se may play a significant role
in the evolutionary process.

     7. Neoautoploids may increase biochemical diversity at the
primary enzyme level and in other ways by immediate derepression
of repressed genic expressions of the diploid. This may extend
the range of environments and habitats in which successful development of polyploids occurs.

LITERATURE CITED

1.   Harlan, G.R., deWet, J.M.J., 1975, On Ö. Winge and a prayer:
      the origins of polyploidy. Bot. Rev. 41: 361-390.

2.   Lewis, W.H., 1967, Cytocatalytic evolution in plants. Bot.
     Rev. 33: 105-115; This volume, p. 103.
3.   Cronquist, A., 1978, Once again, what is a species?, pp.
     3-20, in "Biosystematics in Agriculture," Beltsville Symp.
     Agr. Res. 2, Allanheld, Osmun and Co., Montclair, NJ.
4.   Levin, D.A., 1979, The nature of plant species. Science
     204: 381-384.
5.   Clausen, J., Keck, D.D., Hiesey, W.M., 1945, Experimental
     studies on the nature of species. II. Plant evolution through
     amphiploidy and autoploidy, with examples from the Madiinae.
     Carnegie Inst. Wash. Publ. 564, 1-174.
6.   Kihara, H., Ono, T., 1926, Chromosomenzahlen und Systematische
     Gruppierung der Rumex-arten. Zeitschr. Zellforsch. 4:
     475-481.
7.   Hedberg, I., 1967, Cytotaxonomic studies on Anthoxanthum
     odoratum L. s. lat. II. Investigations of some Swedish and
     of a few Swiss population samples. Symb. Bot. Upsal. 18(5):
     1-86.
8.   D'Amato, F., 1952, Polyploidy in the differentiation and
     function of tissues and cells in plants. A critical exami-
     nation of the literature. Caryologia 4: 311-358.
9.   D'Amato, F., 1964, Endopolyploidy as a factor in plant
     tissue development. Caryologia 17: 41-52.
10. Nagl, W., 1976, Nuclear organization. Ann. Rev. Pl. Physiol.
     27: 39-69.
11. Nagl, W., 1978, "Endopolyploidy and Polyteny in Differen-
     tiation and Evolution," North-Holland, Amsterdam. 283 p.
12. Lewis, W.H., Oliver, R.L., Luikart, T.J., 1971, Multiple
     genotypes in individuals of Claytonia virginica. Science
     172: 564-565.
13. Östergren, G., Fröst, S., 1962, Elimination of accessory
     chromosomes from the roots of Haplopappus gracilis. Hereditas
     48: 363-366.
14. Müntzing, A., 1946, Different chromosome numbers in root
     tips and pollen mother cells in a sexual strain of Poa
     alpina. Hereditas 32: 127-129.
15. Darlington, C.D., Thomas, P.T., 1941, Morbid mitosis and the
     activity of inert chromosomes in Sorghum. Proc. Roy. Soc.
     London 130: 127-150.
16. Berger, C.A., Witkus, E.R., 1954, The cytology of Xanthisma
     texanum DC. I. Difference in the chromosome number of root
     and shoot. Bull. Torrey Bot. Club 81: 489-491.
17. deWet, J.M.J., 1980, Origins of polyploids. This volume, p.3
18. Mooney, H.A., Johnson, A.W., 1965, Comparative physiological
     ecology of an arctic and alpine population of Thalictrum
     alpinum L. Ecology 46: 721-727.
19. Franke, R., 1975, Über das Auftreten von unreduzierten
     Gameten bei Angiospermen. Arch. Züchtungsforsch. Berlin 5:
     201-208.

20. Tyrl, R.J., 1975, Origin and distribution of polyploid Achillea (Compositae) in western North America. Brittonia 27: 187-196.
21. Lewis, W.H., Suda, Y., 1976, Diploids and polyploids from a single species populations: temporal adaptations. J. Heredity 67: 391-393.
22. Lewis, W.H., 1977, Temporal adaptation correlated with ploidy in Claytonia virginica. Syst. Bot. 1: 340-347.
23. Powell, A.M., Sikes, S.W., 1975, On the origin of polyploidy in Perityle rupestris (Asteraceae). Sci. Biol. J. 1: 132-137.
24. Levin, D.A., Wilson, A.C., 1976, Rates of evolution in seed plants: net increase in diversity of chromosome numbers and species numbers through time. Proc. Nat. Acad. Sci. USA 73: 2086-2090.
25. Babcock, E.B., Stebbins, G.L., Jr., 1938, The American species of Crepis. Carnegie Inst. Wash. 504, 1-199.
26. Heckard, L.R., 1960, Taxonomic studies in the Phacelia magellanica polyploidy complex. Univ. Calif. Publ. Bot. 32: 1-126.
27. Uhl, C.H., 1970, Heteroploidy in Sedum glaucophyllum. Rhodora 72: 460-479.
28. Morton, J.K., 1979, Observations on Houghton's goldenrod (Solidago houghtonii). Mich. Bot. 18: 31-35.
29. Stebbins, G.L., 1950, "Variation and Evolution in Plants," Columbia Univ. Press, New York. 643 p.
30. Gottschalk, W., 1976, "Die Bedeutung der Polyploidie für die Evolution der Pflanzen," Gustav-Fischer, Stuttgart. (particularly Tables 5-8).
31. Fukuda, I., 1967, The biosystematic of Achlys. Taxon 16: 308-316.
32. Al-Sheikh Hussain, L.A., Elkington, T.T., 1978, Giemsa C-band karyotypes of diploid and triploid Allium caeruleum and their genomic relationship. Cytologia 43: 405-410.
33. Dewey, D.R., 1975, Genome relations of diploid Agropyron libanoticum with diploid and autotetraploid Agropyron stipifolium. Bot. Gaz. 136: 116-121; Dewey, D.R., Asay, K.H., 1975, The crested wheatgrasses of Iran. Crop Sci. 15: 844-849.
34. Hedberg, I., 1970, Cytotaxonomic studies on Anthoxanthum odoratum L. s. lat. IV. Karyotypes, meiosis and the origin of tetraploid A. odoratum. Hereditas 64: 153-176.
35. Packer, J.G., Denford, K.E., 1974, A contribution to the taxonomy of Arctosytaphylos uva-ursi. Canad. J. Bot. 52: 743-753.
36. Estes, J.R., 1969, Evidence for autoploid evolution in the Artemisia ludoviciana complex of the Pacific Northwest. Brittonia 21: 29-43.
37. Borrill, M., Lindner, R., 1971, Diploid-tetraploid sympatry in Dactylis (Gramineae). New Phytol. 70: 1111-1124.

38. Nesom, G.L., 1978, Chromosome numbers in Erigeron and Conyza (Compositae). Sida 7: 375-381.
39. Baldwin, J.T.,Jr., 1941, Galax: the genus and its chromosomes. J. Heredity 32: 249-254.
40. Nesom, G.L., 1979, Personal communication.
41. Teppner, H., Ehrendorfer, F., Tuff, C., 1976, Karyosystematic notes on the Galium palustre-group (Rubiaceae). Taxon 25: 95-97.
42. Dewey, D.R., 1979, The Hordeum violaceum complex in Iran. Amer. J. Bot. 66: 166-172.
43. Hunziker, J.H., Palacios, R.A., de Valesi, A.G., Poggio, L., 1972, Species disjunctions in Larrea: evidence from mor-phology, cytogenetics, phenolic compounds, and seed albumins. Ann. Missouri Bot. Gard. 59: 224-233.
44. Rollins, R.C., Shaw, E.A., 1973, "The Genus Lesquerella (Cruciferae) in North America," Harvard University Press, Cambridge. 288 p.
45. Clark, C., 1975, Ecogeographic races of Lesquerella engel-mannii (Cruciferae): distribution, chromosome numbers, and taxonomy. Brittonia 27: 263-278.
46. Stuessy, T.F., 1971, Systematic relationships in the white-rayed species of Melampodium (Compositae). Brittonia 23: 177-190.
47. Bacon, J.D., 1978, Taxonomy of Nerisyrenia (Cruciferae). Rhodora 80: 159-227.
48. Rollins, R.C., Rüdenberg, L., 1979, Chromosome numbers of Cruciferae IV. Bussey Inst. Harvard University, pp. 79-92.
49. Ponnamma, M.G., 1978, Studies on bulbous ornamentals. I. Karyomorphology of diploid and triploid taxa of Pancratium triflorum Rosb. Cytologia 43: 717-725.
50. Palmer, P.G., 1975, A biosystematic study of the Panicum amarum-P. amarulum complex (Gramineae). Brittonia 27: 142-150.
51. Smith, B.W., 1968, Cytogeography and cytotaxonomic relation-ships of Rumex paucifolius. Amer. J. Bot. 55: 673-683.
52. Uhl, C.H., 1972, Intraspecific variation in chromosomes of Sedum in the southwestern United States. Rhodora 74: 301-320.
53. Stewart, D.A., Barlow, B.A., 1976, Genomic differentiation and polyploidy in Sowerbaea (Liliaceae). Austral. J. Bot. 24: 349-367.
54. Jones, K., Colden, C., 1968, The telocentric complement of Tradescantia micrantha. Chromosoma 24: 135-157.
55. Stebbins, G.L., 1971, "Chromosomal Evolution in Higher Plants," Addison-Wesley, Reading, MA. 216 p.
56. Gates, R.R., 1924, Polyploidy. Brit. J. Exp. Biol. 1: 153-182.
57. Torrey, J.G., 1965, Physiological bases of organization and development in the root. Encycl. Pl. Physiol. 15(1): 1256-1327.

58. Lewis, W.H., 1964, Oldenlandia corymbosa (Rubiaceae). Grana
    Palynolog. 5: 330-341.
59. Anderson, L.C., 1977, Studies on Bigelowia (Asteraceae).
    Syst. Bot. 2: 209-218.
60. Randhawa, A.S., Beamish, K.I., 1970, Observations on the
    morphology, anatomy, classification, and reproductive cycle
    of Saxifraga ferruginea. Canad. J. Bot. 48: 299-312.
61. Lewis, W.H., 1976, Pollen size of Hedyotis caerulea (Rubia-
    ceae) in relation to chromosome number and heterostyly.
    Rhodora 78: 60-64.
62. Bremekamp, C.E.B., 1963, On pollen dimorphism in heterostylous
    Psychotrieae, especially in the genus Mapouria Aubl. Grana
    Palynolog. 4: 53-63.
63. Levin, D.A., 1975, Minority cytotype exclusion in local
    plant populations. Taxon 24: 35-43.
64. Sakai, K., Suzuki, Y., 1955, Studies on competition in
    plants. VII. Competition between diploid and autotetraploid
    plants of barley. J. Genetics 53: 11-20.
65. Smith, H.E., 1946, Sedum pulchellum: a physiological and
    morphological comparision of diploid, tetraploid, and hexa-
    ploid races. Bull. Torrey Bot. Club 73: 495-541.
66. Stebbins, G.L., 1949, The evolutionary significance of
    natural and artificial polyploids in the family Gramineae.
    Proc. 8th Inter. Cong. Genetics, Hereditas suppl. 461-485.
67. Stebbins, G.L., 1972, Research on the evolution of higher
    plants: problems and prospects. Canad. J. Genet. Cytol.
    14: 453-462.
68. Ehrendorfer, F., 1980, Polyploidy and distribution. This
    volume, p.45.
69. Stebbins, G.L., 1980, Polyploidy in plants: unsolved problems
    and prospects. This volume, p.495.
70. Brighton, C.A., 1976, Cytological problems in the genus
    Crocus (Iridaceae): II. Crocus cancellatus aggregate. Kew
    Bull. 32: 33-45.
71. Giles, N.H., Jr., 1942, Autopolyploidy and geographical
    distribution in Cuthbertia graminea Small. Amer. J. Bot.
    29: 637-645.
72. Baldwin, J.T., Jr., Culp, R., 1941, Polyploidy in Diospyros
    virginiana L. Amer. J. Bot. 28: 942-944.
73. Sullivan, V.I., 1976, Diploidy, polyploidy, and agamospermy
    among species of Eupatorium (Compositae). Canad. J. Bot.
    54: 2907-2917.
74. Tothill, J.C., Hacker, J.B., 1976, Polyploidy, flowering
    phenology and climatic adaptation in Heteropogon contortus
    (Gramineae). Austral. J. Ecol. 1: 213-222.
75. Ornduff, R., 1970, Cytogeography of Nymphoides (Menyanthaceae).
    Taxon 19: 715-719.
76. Chuang, T.I., Constance, L., 1977, Cytogeography of Phacelia
    ranunculacea (Hydrophyllaceae). Rhodora 79: 115-122.

77. Baldwin, J.T.,Jr., 1942, Polyploidy in Sedum ternatum Michx. II. Cytogeography. Amer. J. Bot. 29: 283-286.
78. Kurita, M., Kuroki, Y., 1964, Polyploidy and distribution of Allium gray[i]. Mem. Ehime Univ. Sect 2, Ser. B 5: 37-45.
79. Böcher, T.W., 1936, Cytological studies on Campanula rotundifolia. Hereditas 22: 269-277.
80. Lewis, W.H., Semple, J.C., 1977, Geography of Claytonia virginica cytotypes. Amer. J. Bot. 64: 1078-1082.
81. Hagerup, O., 1927, Empetrum hermaphroditum (Lge.) Hagerup. A new tetraploid, bisexual species. Dansk Bot. Arkiv. 5: 1-17.
82. Mosquin, T., 1967, Evidence for autopolyploidy in Epilobium angustifolium (Onagraceae). Evolution 21: 713-719.
83. Small, E., 1968, The systematics of autopolyploidy in Epilobium latifolium (Onagraceae). Brittonia 20: 169-181.
84. Schaefer, V.G., Miksche, J.P., 1977, Mikrospectrophotometric determination of DNA per cell and polyploidy in Fraxinus americana L. Silvae Genetica 26: 184-192.
85. Fagerlind, F., 1937, Embryologische, zytologische, und bestäubungs-experimentelle Studien in der Familie Rubiaceae nebst Bemerkungen über einige Polyploiditäts-probleme. Acta Horti Berg. 11: 195-470.
86. Lewis, W.H., Terrell, E.E., 1962, Chromosomal races in eastern North American species of Hedyotis (Houstonia). Rhodora 64: 313-323.
87. Sharma, A.K., Dey, D., 1967, A comprehensive cytotaxonomic study on the family Chenopodiaceae. J. Cytol. Genet. 2: 114-127.
88. Hagerup, O., 1933, Studies on polyploid ecotypes in Vaccinium uliginosum L. Hereditas 18: 122-128.
89. Östergren, G., 1942, Chromosome numbers in Anthoxanthum. Hereditas 28: 242-243.
90. Hedberg, I., 1969, Cytotaxonomic studies on Anthoxanthum odoratum L. s. lat. III. Investigations of Swiss and Austrian population samples. Sv. Bot. Tidskr. 63: 233-250.
91. Mitchell, W.W., 1968, Taxonomy, variation, and chorology of three chromosome races of the Calamagrostis canadensis complex in Alaska. Madroño 19: 235-246.
92. Tanaka, R., 1965, Intraspecific polyploidy in Goodyera maximowicziana Makino. La Kromosoma 60: 1945-1950.
93. Brunken, J.N., Estes, J.R., 1975, Cytological and morphological variation in Panicum virgatum L. Southwest. Nat. 19: 379-385.
94. Manton, I., 1937, The problem of Biscutella laevigata L. II: The evidence from meiosis. Ann. Bot. (n.s.) 1: 439-462.
95. Miller, J.M., 1976, Variation in populations of Claytonia perfoliata (Portulacaceae). Syst. Bot. 1: 20-34.
96. Nur, U., Zohary, D., 1959, Distribution patterns of diploid and tetraploid forms of Dactylis glomerata L. in Israel. Bull. Res. Council Israel, sect. D, Botany, 7D: 13-22.

97. Ehrendorfer, F., 1965, Dispersal mechanisms, genetic systems, and colonizing abilities in some flowering plant families, pp. 331-352, in Baker, H.G., Stebbins, G.L. (eds.), "The Genetics of Colonizing Species," Academic Press, New York.

98. Stebbins, G.L., 1965, Colonizing species of native California flora, pp. 173-195, in Baker, H.G., Stebbins, G.L. (eds.), "The Genetics of Colonizing Species," Academic Press, New York.

99. Gadella, W.J., Kliphuis, E., 1968, *Parnassia palustris* in the Netherlands. Acta Bot. Neerl. 17: 165-172.

100. Stewart, D.A., Barlow, B.A., 1976, Infraspecific polyploidy and gynodioecism in *Ptilotus obovatus* (Amaranthaceae). Austral. J. Bot. 24: 237-248.

101. Lövkvist, B., 1956, The *Cardamine pratensis* complex: outlines of its cytogenetics and taxonomy. Symb. Bot. Upsal. 14(2): 1-131.

102. Hagerup, O., 1932, Über Polyploidie in Beziehung zu Klima, Ökologie und Phylogenie. Hereditas 16: 19-40.

103. Robertson, P.A., 1974, Morphological variation and chromosome numbers of North American populations of *Koeleria cristata*. Bull. Torrey Bot. Club 101: 124-129.

104. Skalińska, M., 1947, Polyploidy in *Valeriana officinalis* Linn. in relation to its ecology and distribution. J. Linn. Soc. Bot. 53: 159-186.

105. Semple, J.C., 1978, The cytogeography of *Aster pilosum* (Compositae): Ontario and the adjacent United States. Canad. J. Bot. 56: 1274-1279.

106. Rehweder, H., 1937, Bezichungen zwischen Chromosomengrösse und Vitalität innerhalb der Gattung *Dianthus*. Planta 27: 478-499.

107. Johnson, A.W., Packer, J.G., 1965, Polyploidy and environment in Arctic Alaska. Science 148: 237-239.

108. Packer, J.G., 1969, Polyploidy in the Canadian Arctic Archipelago. Alpine Res. 1: 15-28.

109. Löve, A., Löve, D., 1957, Arctic polyploidy. Proc. Genet. Soc. Canada 2: 23-27.

110. Löve, A., Löve, D., 1967, Polyploidy and altitude: Mt. Washington. Biol. Zentral. 86(suppl.): 307-312.

111. Hancock, J.F.,Jr., Bringhurst, R.S., 1979, Ecological differentation in perennial, octoploid species of *Fragaria*. Amer. J. Bot. 66: 367-375.

112. Jackson, R.C., 1976, Evolution and systematic significance of polyploidy. Ann. Rev. Ecol. Syst. 7: 209-234.

113. Golubovskaya, I.N., 1979, Genetic control of meiosis. Inter. Rev. Cytol. 58: 247-290.

114. Sears, E.R., 1976, Genetic control of chromosome pairing in wheat. Ann. Rev. Genet. 10: 31-51.

115. Grant, V., 1952, Cytogenetics of the hybrid Gilia millefoliata x achilleaefolia. I. Variations in meiosis and polyploidy rate as affected by nutritional and genetic conditions. Chromosoma 5: 372-390.
116. Hossain, M.G., 1978, Effects of external environmental factors on chromosome pairing in autotetraploid rye. Cytologia 43: 21-34.
117. Grun, P., 1951, Variations in the meiosis of alfalfa. Amer. J. Bot. 38: 475-482.
118. Timmis, J.N., Rees, H., 1971, A pairing restriction at pachytene upon multivalent formation in autotetraploids. J. Heredity 26: 269-275.
119. Sybenga, J., 1972, Chromosome-associated control of meiotic pairing differentiation. Variation with Secale cereale. Chromosoma 39: 351-360.
120. Denison, M.F., 1976, Populational variation in Oxalis hernandesii. Bull. Torrey Bot. Club 103: 73-76.
121. Gilles, A., Randolph, L.F., 1951, Reduction of quadrivalent frequency in autotetraploid maize during a period of 10 years. Amer. J. Bot. 38: 12-17.
122. Aastveit, K., 1968, Variation and selection for seed set in tetraploid rye. Hereditas 60: 294-316.
123. Hossain, M.G., Moore, K., 1975, Selection in tetraploid rye. I. Effects of selection on the relationships between seedset, meiotic regularity and plant vigour. Hereditas 81: 141-152.
124. deWet, J.M.J., Harlan, J.R., 1970, Apomixis, polyploidy and speciation in Dichanthium. Evolution 24: 270-277.
125. Dickinson, H., Antonovics, J., 1973, Theoretical considerations of sympatric divergence. Amer. Nat. 107: 256-274.
126. Gottschalk, W., 1971, The phenomenon of "asymmetric genomic reduction." J. Indian Bot. Soc. 50A: 308-317.
127. Noggle, G.R., 1946, The physiology of polyploidy in plants. I. Review of the literature. Lloydia 9: 153-173.
128. Gustafson, F.G., 1944, Growth hormone studies of some diploid and autotetraploid plants. J. Heredity 35: 269-272.
129. Chen, S.-L., Tang, P.S., 1945, Studies on colchicine-induced autotetraploid barley. Amer. J. Bot. 32: 177-181.
130. Jinno, T., 1958, Cytogenetic and cytoecological studies on some Japanese species of Rubus IV. Relation of polyploid to flowering time, and to growth rate. Bot. Mag. (Tokyo) 71: 359-365.
131. Schlösser, L.A., 1937, Grenzen und Möglichkeiten der Ausnutzung von Polyploidie in der Pflanzen-züchtung. Forschungsdienst 3: 69-82.
132. Baldwin, J.T.,Jr., 1943, Polyploidy in Sedum pulchellum--I. Cytogeography. Bull. Torrey Bot. Club 70: 26-33.
133. Clausen, R.T., 1975, "Sedum of North America North of the Mexican Plateau," Cornell University Press, Ithica, NY. 742 p.

134. Yang, T.W., Lowe, C.H., 1968, Chromosome variation in ecotypes of Larrea divaricata in the North American desert. Madrono 19: 161–164.

135. Yang, T.W., 1968, A new chromosome race of Larrea divaricata in Arizona. West. Reserve Acad. Nat. Hist. Mus. 2: 1–4 (special publication).

136. Mauer, J., Mayo, J.M., Denford, K., 1978, Comparative ecophysiology of the chromosome races in Viola adunca J.E. Smith. Oecologia 35: 91–104.

137. Tal, M., Gardi, I., 1976, Physiology of polyploid plants: water balance in autotetraploid and diploid tomato under low and high salinity. Physiol. Pl. 38: 257–261.

138. Tal, M., 1977, Physiology of polyploid plants: DNA, RNA, protein, and abscisic acid in autotetraploid and diploid tomato under low and high salinity. Bot. Gaz. 138: 119–122.

139. Tal, M., 1980, Physiology of polyploids. This volume, p.61.

140. Hall, O., 1972, Oxygen requirement of root meristems in diploid and autotetraploid rye. Hereditas 70: 69–74.

141. Mears, J.A., The chemistry of polyploids: a summary with comments on Parthenium L. (Asteraceae-Ambrosiinae). This volume, p. 77.

142. Murray, B.G., Williams, C.A., 1973, Polyploidy and flavonoid synthesis in Briza media L. Nature 243: 87–88.

143. Murray, B.G., Williams, C.A., 1976, Chromosome number and flavonoid biosynthesis in Briza L. (Gramineae). Biochem. Genet. 14: 897–904.

144. Levy, M., 1976, Altered glycoflavone expression in induced autotetraploids of Phlox drummondii. Biochem. Syst. Ecol. 4: 249–259.

145. Levin, D.A., Torres, A.M., Levy, M., 1979, Alcohol dehydrogenase activity in diploid and autotetraploid Phlox. Biochem. Genet. 17: 35–43.

146. DeMaggio, A.E., Lambrukos, J., 1974, Polyploidy and gene dosage effects on peroxidase activity in ferns. Biochem. Genet. 12: 429–440.

147. Roose, M.L., Gottlieb, L.D., 1976, Genetic and biochemical consequences of polyploidy in Tragopogon. Evolution 30: 818–830.

148. Rowson, J.M., 1944, Increased alkaloidal contents of induced polyploids of Datura. Nature 154: 81–82.

149. Rowson, J.M., 1945, Increased alkaloidal contents of induced polyploids of Datura, Atropa and Hyoscyamus. Quart. J. Pharm. Pharmacol. 18: 175–193.

150. Jackson, B.P., Rowson, J.M., 1953, Alkaloid biogenesis in tetraploid stramonium. J. Pharm. Pharmacol. 5: 778–793.

151. Spurna, V., Plchova, S., Karpfel, Z., 1970, Study of some biotypes in the genus Achillea. Naturwissenschaften 4: 196–197.

152. Barber, H.N., 1970, Hybridization and the evolution of plants. Taxon 19: 154–160.

POLYPLOIDY IN PLANT EVOLUTION: SUMMARY

Walter H. Lewis

Department of Biology
Washington University
St. Louis, MO 63130

Six speakers give a fresh perspective of the role of polyploidy in the evolutionary process described over half a century
ago and considered by many biologists well-known and thoroughly
understood. One need only examine discussions on the subject in
general texts, that usually begin and end with hybridization of
species followed by chromosomal doubling of a sterile hybrid to
give rise to a tetraploid, to realize how little data on genome
multiplication discovered in recent years has impacted the
scientific world. Ironically, this type of neopolyploid formation
may not be as generalized as once assumed, and in fact may occur
only occasionally in nature.

As expounded by deWet, the common mode of polyploidy is not
by spontaneous chromosomal doubling from a diploid to a tetraploid
condition but rather through the formation of sexual functioning
of cytologically unreduced gametes in species populations. Often
polyploidy via unreduced gametes is a two step process by which a
diploid (2n) female gamete is fertilized by a haploid (n) male
gamete to produce a triploid (3x). In turn this organism produces
cytologically unreduced triploid (3n) female gametes that are
fertilized by haploid (n) gametes of the diploid parents that
result in tetraploid (4x) offspring. Spontaneous development of
unreduced gametes occur naturally in populations, but a quantitative study of frequency is wanting except for a few species.

The addition of genomes from different individuals that may
represent three or more differently adapted genomes is of profound
relevance for the success of polyploids. The enhanced allelic
heterozygosity may be an important advantage of neopolyploids
depending on the genetic combinations formed and the particular
needs of the individual as it grows and develops in consort with

environmental demands. Appropriate combinations of multiple
genomes could lead to the formation of highly competitive and
adaptive polyploid biotypes both in species populations and in
the production of new, vigorous, and variously adapted cytotypes
among crop plants (see Bingham later in the Conference). Agricultural research has been primarily on a single tract, and in
many instances on the wrong tract as Dewey suggests, for it has
ignored by and large the opportunities afforded by using unreduced
gametes and naturally-occurring neopolyploid cytotypes with
concomitant high heterozygosity for immediate genome duplication
induced by chemicals and other means with consequent limits to
heterozygosity.

Jackson and Casey stress fundamental features that should be
considered in cytogenetic analyses of polyploids. Too often
karyotype, chiasma frequency, male and female fertility, pachytene
analysis, and univalent, bivalent, and multivalent frequencies
are not available, though basic to an understanding of behavior
and perhaps success or failure of polyploids as incipient species.

Ehrendorfer further characterizes polyploids in relation to
ecology, habitat, and distribution. Continuing a discussion of
successful adaptation, he finds that neopolyploids tend to originate
under unstable environmental conditions and in areas of contact
between diploid (and lower polyploidy) ancestors. Chances for
the origin, establishment, and expansion of newly-formed polyploids are best in widespread pioneer and successional to subclimax communities and in areas that are being populated by
invasion floras. They tend to be expansive, dynamic elements of
the flora. In contrast, diploids and older polyploids prevail in
balanced climax communities and tend to have reduced habitats,
distributions, and genetic diversity; in these environments
neopolyploids often are limited to marginal ecological niches.

Physiological and biochemical properties of naturally-
occurring and induced polyploids are surveyed by Tal and Mears.
Although still fragmentary, data suggest that genome multiplication
may trigger the expression of advantageous processes in the
neopolyploid. Furthermore, neopolyploid diversity may be increased
at the primary enzyme level, and it is perhaps this phenomenon
and allelic heterozygosity that lead to increased genetic adaptability of polyploids and allow under certain circumstances their
successful development in habitats occupied by their parents as
well as their extension into new environments.

Lewis examines the wide occurrence of polyploidy in species
populations. What was thought a unique diversity of plants and
some insects is now known among lower vertebrates, and as further
populational studies at the cellular level are completed ploidy
variation may be found in many more animals including higher
vertebrates (e.g., human triploid born in Sweden--Böök, J.A.,
Santesson, B., 1960, Malformation syndrome in man associated with
triploids (69 chromosomes). Lancet 1: 858-859). In retrospect
polyploidy as a common event in species populations frequently

occurs by successful cross-fertilization of unreduced gametes that, step-by-step to 3x, 4x, and higher levels, incorporates genomes from different individuals (if differently adapted they may be more successful) to form neopolyploids with greater genetic diversity than their diploid progenitors.

Although neopolyploids are often meiotically abnormal, and reduced in fertility as a consequence, meiosis can be controlled by genes that either suppress multivalent formation or elevate pairing and allow diploidization of homologous and homoeologous chromosomes.

A wide range of different physiological properties may characterize neopolyploids. Genetic duplication can trigger sufficiently advantageous processes indicating that multiplication of genetic material per se may play a significant role in the polyploid evolutionary process. Neoautoploids may increase biochemical diversity by immediate derepression of repressed genetic expressions of the diploid. This may contribute to the expanded range of environments and habitats in which successful development of polyploids will occur. Other factors may also be relevant to success of polyploids in speciation such as their gigas features that may have higher survivorships and fecundities than their diploid counterparts.

The evolutionary process of polyploidy occurring in species populations is a generalized phenomenon that is a primary mechanism of speciation in plants and perhaps animals. Texts should be expanded to reflect this more comprehensive understanding of species formation that is based on current research involving many lines of evidence from populational analyses to molecular considerations of gene action.

PART II

POLYPLOIDY IN PLANT TAXA

POLYPLOIDY IN ALGAE

H. Wayne Nichols

Department of Biology
Washington University
St. Louis, MO   63130

Examples of the occurrence of polyploidy can be found in
most major groups of algae. However, most studies have been
conducted within the Chlorophycophyta. These plants often contain
fewer chromosomes and larger cells than most other algal groups,
although some contain in excess of 500 chromosomes. Godward has
been exceptionally active in cytological work which culminated in
the publication in 1966 of her book "The Chromosomes of the
Algae" (1). Since then considerably more sophisticated approaches
in establishing the existence of polyploidy have been developed
employing an array of physical techniques and quantitative measurements of DNA constituents. Further, the development of these
techniques has enabled us to begin to evaluate the genetic nature
of certain algal groups such as the Cyanochloronta,
Euglenophycophyta, and Pyrrophycophyta, which were impossible
using older techniques of analysis.
     Polyploids are known to arise in the algae in a number of
ways. Among these are true hybrids which occur spontaneously in
nature, polyploids that are produced artificially as a result of
treatment in the laboratory by certain compounds such as colchicine
or exposure to ultraviolet radiation, polyploids produced as a
result of certain sexual processes in laboratory cultures, and
most importantly polyploids which occur spontaneously in cultures
with repeated transfer.
     It is difficult in most algal divisions to ascertain a basic
chromosome number since thorough studies of a single group are
few. However, certain groups such as those contained within the
division Chlorophycophyta contain the most thoroughly studied
plants. Oedogonium, Cladophora, certain desmids, and volvocalean
flagellates represent the best known examples of green algae in
regard to the existence of polyploids.

POLYPLOIDY IN ALGAL GROUPS

Chlorophycophyta

Sixteen is now the accepted chromosome number for
Chlamydomonas. In matings of the alga 99.8% of the fused cells
become zygotes. However, 0.2% do not undergo meiosis but divide
mitotically. They produce only two flagella although they have
the genetic information necessary to produce four. They are
always of the negative mating types since negative is dominant
over positive mating types. These negative mating types can then
be crossed with a positive type which results in a triploid
zygote. The products are always haploid. Chromosomes are small,
difficult to count, and reports of counts within the genus vary
from 8 in Chlamydomonas eugametos (2) to a high of 38±4 in the
same species (3,4). There is no diploid counts and interpretation
is based upon mating behavior. The presence of an intranuclear
spindle has hampered accurate interpretation of mitotic or meiotic
counts (Goodenough, 1979, personal communication).

Volvocales

Low haploid chromosomes are found in certain Volvox species
as well as considerably higher counts in others which probably
indicate polyploid derivations. However, chromosome numbers in
the Volvocales generally indicate an aneuploid condition. This
is particularly evident in Astrephomene gubernaculifera where
Cave and Pocock (5) have found counts of n=4, 6, 7, and 8.
Goldstein (6), working with two species of volvocalean colonial
flagellates, Eudorina elegans and E. illinoisensis, demonstrated a
haploid number of n=14 for each. Further, he was able to produce
hybrid forms in matings between the species with these having
chromosome numbers of n=24 and 28. The characteristics of these
hybrids included male forms, female forms, and selfing males.
Godward (1) has suggested that mating type genes are among those
duplicated in polysomics or polyploids with various results as
related to sexuality. These polysomics and polyploids clearly
arise with ease and systematics must be a matter of convenience
only.

Zygnematales

The evolution of chromosomal races can occur rapidly in
laboratory culture of green algae and I suspect red algae as
well. This phenomenon has been reported by several investigators
(7-9). These races are produced by mitotic irregularities and
give rise to polyploids and aneuploids. According to Godward
(1):

> "Polyploidy as a basis of species formation, is rarer in the
> Chlorophyceae than aneuploidy. The search for a basic

chromosome number is not profitable except in a few series such as the Cladophorales. A glance down the lists of chromosome numbers will show that in most series polyploidy may well have occcurred once or twice but aneuploidy has occurred far more frequently diversifying both diploid and polyploid chromosome numbers by additions and subtractions, into an almost continuous range. In Conjugales, fusion of chromosomes is also a possibility."

The Zygnematales contain several groups of algae exhibiting polyploidy. They illustrate two general characteristics in regard to ploidy changes. Firstly, they exhibit an increase in cell size and, secondly, changes which often alter their morphology (Starr, 1979, personal communication). Biebel (10) has discussed the cytological condition in this group. In general, the work of Waris and Kallio (11) over many years represents the ultimate types of detailed studies within this group. Studying Micrasterias, a placcoderm desmid, they found variations in the genus associated with radiation. The wild-type cell generally contains two wings separated by an isthmus. Although some variations occurred spontaneously, they could produce other variations by treatment with chemicals, centrifugation, cold shock, heat, and continuous illumination. These variations included uniradiate, triradiate, polyradiate, and aradiate forms. These changes were often associated with changes in ploidy, both euploid and aneuploid changes were obtained. Others have reported similar changes in different desmids: Starr (12) in Cosmarium turpinii, Brandham and Godward (13) in Cosmarium botrytis, Brandham (14) in Staurastrum dilatatum and Lind and Taylor (15) in Pleurotinium. These latter studies involved sexual matings and although diploid cells were capable of mating their tetraploid zygospores would not germinate.

Filamentous members of the Zygnematales also contain polyploid series. Allen (16) obtained a polyploid series of strains of Spirogyra in culture. These apparently arose spontaneously in a series from her homothallic clone. She recognized three differing types of subcultures based on cell diameters. They were 15.0–19.5, 21.0–25.5, and 27.0–33.0 μm. These subcultures had counts of n=11–15, 26–30, and 56–60, respectively. This was interpreted as a polyploid series of x, 2x, and 4x. Allen obtained conjugation within a group and between cells of different groups. She obtained germlings which differed more than clonal cultures. She indicated a possible partial reversion by chromosome loss which gave rise to aneuploids.

Polyploid series in Spirogyra also occur in nature. There appear to be two trends in species of this genus: a straight tendency toward polyploidy, and secondly a tendency toward aneuploidy. Godward (1) offers examples of these tendencies as follows: n=6 in S. triformis and S. jugalis; n=12 in S. crassa, S. X, and S. fuellibornei; and n=24 in S. columbiana. These

species have two N.O. (nucleolar organizer) chromosomes only,
where the number is known, which means that there are not cases
of simple polyploidy. Others, however, could be apparently straightforward polyploid series, e.g., S. punctulata, n=2x=16 (2 N.O.
chromosomes); S. majuscula, n=4x=32 (4 N.O. chromosomes);
and S. pratensis, n=x=11-15, (1 N.O. chromosome), n=2x=26-30, (2
N.O. chromosomes), and n=4x=56-60, (3 N.O. chromosomes + 1?, 4
would be expected). Aneuploidy would be suspected in the ten
species, all with two N.O. chromosomes and chromosomes numbers
ranging from n=4 to 70. We have, however, to bear in mind that
these non-centric chromosomes can fragment or fuse and yet survive,
so that the peculiar form of polyploidy which has been termed
"agmatoploidy" can exist here. A quite remarkable fact nevertheless
is that despite the ease with which new karyotypes can arise and
persist in culture, there must be a stabilizing factor of some
force operating in nature, since S. crassa, whose chromosomes
were first counted by Molle (17) and Strasburger (18), was at
that time and later (1,19,20) always found to have n=12. Similarly,
S. britannica collected by Godward (1) from several localities,
Newnham (20) from more than one, and also Jordan (unpublished),
was always found to have n=10 of the same number of long, medium,
and short chromosomes. Spirogyra triformis collected only by Van
Wisselingh (21) and Godward (22) was found to have n=6 of which
two chromosomes were N.O. Geitler's (23) S. X, with 12 chromosomes
and highly peculiar midprophase features, was rediscovered by
Newnham (20) with the same peculiar midprophase and somatic
characters, although in the absence of conjugation a specific
name cannot even be given.

Gauch (24) also observed abrupt changes in cell diameter in
another filamentous member of this group, Zygnema. However, he
was unable to demonstrate an increase in ploidy.

It appears, as Beible (10) suggested, that morphological
modifications, such as those reported in the desmids involving
radiation, may be so drastic that they could only be attributed to
alterations in chromosome ploidy and hence in the balance of
genes controlling the basic cell architecture. However, based on
the non-viability of zygospores it appears that transmission is
possible but not the complex reorganization required for completion
of the sexual cycle.

Cladophorales

Certain species within this order have been thoroughly
investigated (25). The basic chromosome number in the group is
six, a haploid number frequently of 12 and obvious polyploidy
series in certain species such as Cladorphora glomerata. Reported
variations in chromosome number are n=12, 24, 36, 48, 72, and 96.

Oedogoniales

Mainx (26) was the first investigator to obtain polyploids
of Oedogonium. He produced these by germination of an unreduced
zygotic nucleus. The resulting plant had both male and female
genes with females predominant. Hoffman (27) has also obtained
similar polyploids. Additionally, polyploids can be artifically
induced with colchicine treatment (28).

Charophyta

Proctor (29) has recently reviewed the nature of the genetics
and occurrence of polyploidy in the charophytes as follows.
Although charophytes today flourish in a wide variety of aquatic
habitats, as apparently they have for the past 350 million years,
there is no indication that members of the group play any vital
role in the lives of most geneticists. Far less is known about
the genetics of Charophyta than of most vascular groups. The
basic difficulty has been one of ensuring controlled crosses
between monoecious, i.e., bisexual, clones. No such difficulties
hinder attempted crosses of dioecious, i.e., unisexual, clones,
or of a dioecious female fertilized by sperm of a monoecious
plant, which need only be cultured in a common container. However,
most charophytes are monoecious, with small and conjoined gametangia. The challenge arises when one attempts to fertilize
female gametes of such plants by sperm of a second, be it monoecious or dioecious.

For the better part of two centuries, students of the Charophyta have been seeking a generally acceptable basis for delimiting
taxonomic groupings, so far with little success. For the most
part, classification has been subjective and subject to change
on the basis of personal preferences. Few of the morphological
features long assumed to be of systematic significance have ever
been subjected to even the most cursory genetic analysis.

Polyploidy is of widespread occurrence among monoecious,
though not among dioecious, species of Chara and Nitella (30-32).
Chromosome numbers of monoecious species consistently equal or
exceed those of morphologically similar dioecious forms, supporting the general assumption that dioecism here represents the
more primitive condition. This is further supported by distributional data (33). Where complexes are represented by two or more
dioecious species together with a number of morphologically similar
monoecious forms, the dioecious strains are usually restricted in
their geographical range. Controlled crosses among different chromosomal races of a single complex (e.g., in the species Chara "zey-
lanica" n=28, 42; C. "hispida" n=28, 42; C. "globularis" n=28, 42;
C. "vulgaris-contraria" n=14,28,42), have often led to the production of mature oospores but rarely to viable offspring, and even
less frequently have such offspring proved self-fertile (32;
Proctor, unpublished). However, from the cross X-064 (n=42,

India)/415 (n=28, Texas) more than 1,000 hybrid oospores were
obtained. Only two of these germinated. Offspring W-1 is vegetatively almost normal, P.S-F, and has about 70 chromosomes indicating
that it is probably an allodiploid. Through self-fertilization
W-1 has yielded about 50 oospores and in turn 34 viable offspring.

Recent genetic studies of controlled crosses among different
chromosome races of a single complex should serve to provide
firmer and more objective bases on which to establish the taxonomy
of this remarkable order of algae.

Euglenophycophyta

Several species of Euglena can exhibit a process of nuclear
fragmentation ("amitosis") in biophasic culture which results in
occasional binucleate cells (34). At subsequent mitoses in E.
acus and E. spirogyra the half-nuclei divide simultaneously.
Cell cleavage produces two binucleate cells, though occasional
miscleavage results in cells with either one half-nucleus or
three half-nuclei. These cells are viable and their asexual
progeny retain the characteristics of the species. This suggests
that these species of Euglena are highly polyploid, cells being
fully viable with much less than the normal chromosome complement.
Normal cells of E. spirogyra have 86 chromosomes; the "half-
nuclei" in a binucleate cell contain 40 to 45 chromosomes.

According to Godward (1), Grell's (35) difficulty in recon-
ciling these observations of amitosis and mitosis in the same
species is apparently due to his misinterpretation of the significance of the amitotic process. It should be emphasized that
amitosis in Euglena is merely a nuclear fragmentation, occurring
as a rare phenomenon in response to unfavourable conditions of
growth. The process is not connected with reproduction.

Euglena gracilis has been shown to contain from 45-50 chromosomes per cell (36). It also has a relatively large amount of DNA
per cell (3pg) (37). Based on these data Schiff et al. (38)
suggested that the alga is polyploid. Rawson (39) characterized
the DNA of this species by its reassociation kinetics and found
three kinetically definable fractions: a highly repetitive
fraction, a middle repetitive fraction, and a non-repetitive
fraction. He concluded that information obtained by DNA reasso-
cation studies indicated that E. gracilis is indeed a diploid
organism. He further suggested that perhaps genetic recombination
occurs in the organism, although this has never been reported.

Rhodophycophyta

Although there are few truly critical cytological studies of
members of the Rhodophycophyta, Drew (40-42) demonstrated the
occurrence of polyploidy in Plumaria elegans and Spermothamnion
repens. More recently Van der Meer and Todd (43) reported polyploid phases in the life history of Gracilaria a multicellular

marine red alga. Rao et al. (44) concluded from their studies
within the genus Ceramium that chromosome numbers were 2n=42 for
C. fimbiatum and C. cruciatum and 2n=84 (64-114) for C. gracillimum
var. byssoideum. Based on these studies they concluded that
hybridization and polyploidy are major factors concerned in the
evolution of this group from a plausible common ancestry with x=7
chromosomes.

Recently, in my laboratory (unpublished), we have succeeded
in producing somatic cell hybrids. These are produced from
multicellular red algae enzymatically to obtain protoplasts. The
protoplasts are then fused to give the somatic cell hybrid lines
which undergo further development.

Phaeophycophyta

Wynne and Loiseaux (45) reviewed the available information
concerning the brown algae and various aspects of their life
history. They concluded that ploidy did not always affect the
stage in development of certain genera in the order Ectocarpales
and Laminariales. However, Muller (46,47) reported a complex
scheme for the life history of Ectocarpus siliculosus in which
gametophytic and sporophytic growth forms could be distinguished.
His scheme involved haploid and diploid gametophytes as well as
haploid, diploid and tetraploid sporophytes, all interconnected
by processes of fertilization, meiosis, parthenogenesis, and
spontaneous multiplication of chromosome number. Changes in
ploidy can also occur spontaneous with altered environmental
conditions in which haploid tissue may give rise to diploid buds
which result in a change from microthalli to macrothalli in
certain Chodariales (48,49)

Pyrrophycophyta

The occurrence of polyploidy in the dinoflagellates remains
obscure due to the unusual nature of the nucleus and nuclear
behavior during cell division. These plants possess nuclear
traits not observed in bacteria or higher eukaryotic cells. The
large number of chromosomes which appear identical and permanently
condensed has suggested a polytenic or polyploid condition.
Allen et al. (50) studied the dinoflagellate Crypthecodinium
cohnii in regard to determining its true nuclear condition. They
concluded from data concerning DNA per cell. chromosome counts,
and renaturation kinetics that polyploidy was not the mode of
nuclear organization.

Cyanochloronta

This division is the only major group of algae which is
prokaryotic. Further, their DNA does not have a histone coating
and appears as fibrils. Few studies concerning ploidy levels

have been attempted. However, Roberts et al. (51) suggested that the blue-green alga <u>Agmenellum quadruplicatum</u> perhaps displays the genetics of a polyploid alga. His suggestion was based upon renaturation of the extracted DNA.

COLCHICINE AND PLOIDY

Colchicine has been used widely to induce polyploids in the laboratory. It has been successful with many algae including <u>Gonium</u> (52) and <u>Cladophora</u> (53).

SUMMARY

The green algae and the charophytes represent the most widely studied groups of algae in respect to their ploidy levels. In some genera increased size accompanies ploidy level changes as well as certain morphological modifications, but in other genera no evident obvious changes can be discerned. In the other major groups of algae, namely the Rhodophycophyta and Phaeophycophyta, few cases of polyploidy have been documented adequately. In the remaining groups, unusual nuclear phenomena and/or behavior have hampered studies and few species have adequately been studied in regard to their ploidy levels.

LITERATURE CITED

1. Godward, M.B.E., 1966, "The Chromosomes of the Algae," Edward Arnold, London.
2. Buffaloe, N.P., 1958, A comparative cytological study of four species of <u>Chlamydomonas</u>. Bull. Torrey Bot. Club 85: 157-178.
3. Shaecter, M., De Lamenter, E.D., 1954, Studies on mitosis and meiosis in <u>Chlamydomonas</u>. Trans. N.Y. Acad. Sci., Ser. 2, 16: 371-372.
4. Shaecter, M., De Lamenter, E.D., 1955, Mitosis of <u>Chlamydomonas</u>. Amer. J. Bot. 42: 417-422.
5. Cave, M.S., Pocock, M.A., 1956, Variable chromosome number in <u>Asterephomene</u> <u>gubernaculifera</u>. Amer. J. Bot. 43: 122-134.
6. Goldstein, M., 1964, Speciation and mating behavior in <u>Eudorina</u>. J. Protozool. 11: 317-344.
7. King, G.C., 1954, A cytological survey of the desmids, Ph.D. thesis, London University.
8. Brandham, P.E., 1964, Cytology, sexuality and mating type in culture of certain desmids, Ph.D. thesis, London University.

9.   Abbas, A., 1963, Cultural and cytotaxonomic studies in
     chaetophorales and two additional genera, Ph.D. thesis,
     London University.

10. Biebel, P., 1958, Genetics of Zygnematales, Chapter 9, in
     Lewin, R.A.C. (ed.), "The Genetics of Algae," University of
     California Press, Berkeley.

11. Waris, H., Kallio, P., 1964, Morphogenesis in Micrasterias.
     Adv. Morphogenesis 4: 45-80.

12. Starr, R.C., 1958, The production and inheritance of the
     tri-adiate form in Cosmarium turpinii. Amer. J. Bot. 45:
     243-248.

13. Brandham, P.E., Godward, M.B.E., 1964, The production and
     inheritance of the haploid triradiate form in Cosmarium
     botrytis. Phycologia 4: 75-83.

14. Brandham, P.E., 1965, Polyploidy in desmids. Canad. J. Bot.
     43: 405-417.

15. Ling, H.V., Tyler, P.A., 1976, Meiosis, polyploidy and
     taxonomy of the Pleurotaenium mamillatum complex (Desmidiaceae).
     Br. Phycol. J. 11: 315-330.

16. Allen, M.A., 1958, The biology of a species complex in
     Spirogyra, Ph.D. thesis. 240 pp. Indiana University,
     Bloomington.

17. Molle, E., 1870, Cytological and taxonomical studies in some
     species of Spirogyra, M.Sc. Thesis, London University.

18. Strasburger, E., 1898, Cytological and taxonomical studies
     in some species of Spirogyra, M.Sc. thesis, London University.

19. Geitler, L., 1930, Uber die kern tei hung von Spirogyra.
     Arch. Protist 71: 10-18.

20. Newnham, R.E., 1962, Cytological and taxonomical studies in
     some species of Spirogyra, M.Sc. thesis, London University.

21. Van Wisselingh, C., 1900, Uber Kernteilung bei Spirogyra.
     Flora 87: 355-377.

22. Godward, M.B.E., 1950, On the nucleolus and nucleolar-
     organising chromosomes of Spirogyra. Ann. Bot. (London) N.S.
     14: 39-53.

23. Geitler, L., 1935, Never untersuchungenvber die mitose von
     Spirogyra. Arch. Protist. 85: 10-19.

24. Gauch, H.G., 1966, Studies on the life cycle and genetics of
     Zygnema, M.S. thesis, 91 pp. Cornell University, Ithaca.

25. Sinha, J.P., 1958, Cytological and cultural study of some
     members of Cladophorales and Oedogoniales, Ph.D. thesis,
     London University.

26. Mainx, F., 1931, Physiologische und Genetische Untersuchungen
     an Oedogonium I. Zeitschr. Bot. 24: 481-527.

27. Hoffman, L., 1965, Cytological studies of Oedogonium I.
     Oospore germination in O. foveolatum. Amer. J. Bot. 52:
     173-181.

28. Tschermak, E., 1943, Vergleichende und Experimentelle Cyto-
     logische Untersuchungen ander Gattung Oedogonium. Chromosoma
     2: 492-518.

29. Proctor, V.W., 1976, Genetics of Charophyta, pp. 210-218, in R. Lewin (ed.),"The Genetics of Algae," Blackwell Scientific, Oxford.

30. Guerlesquin, M., 1967, Recherches caryoptipiques et cyto-taxonomiques ches les Charophycees d'Europe occidentale et d'Afrique du Nord. Bull Soc. Sei. Bretagne 41: 1-265.

31. Guerlesquin, M. and Corrillion, R., 1972, Recherches sur la Charophycees d'Afrique occidentale: systematique, phyto-geographique et ecologie, cytologie. Bull. Soc. Sci. Bretagne 47: 1-169.

32. Grant, M.C., Proctor, V.W., 1972, Chara vulgaris and C. contraria: 1-patterns of reproductive isolation for two cosmpolitant species complexes. Evolution 26: 267-281.

33. Proctor, V.W., Griffin, D.G., Hotchkiss, A.T., 1971, A synopsis of the genus Chara, series Gymnobasalia (subsection Willdenouia RDW). Amer. J. Bot. 58: 894-901.

34. Leedale, G.F., 1959, Amitosis in three species of Euglena. Cytologia 24: 213-219.

35. Grell, K.A., 1964, The Protozoan nucleus, in Brachet, J., Mirsky, A.E., (eds.), "The Cell," Vol. 6, Academic Press, New York.

36. Leedale, G.F., 1958, Mitosis and chromosome numbers in the Euglenineae (Flagellata). Nature 181: 502-503.

37. Parenti, Brauerman, G., Preston, J.F., Eisensteedr, M., 1969, Isolation of nuclei from Euglena gracilis. Biochim. Biophys. ACTA 95: 234-243.

38. Schiff, J.A., Lyman, H., Russell, A.K., 1971, Isolation of mutants from Euglena gracilis in methods in enzymology, pp. 143-160, in San Pietro, A., (ed.), "Methods in Enzymology," Vol. 23, New York.

39. Rawson, J.R.Y., 1975, A measurement of the fraction of chloroplast DNA transcribed in Euglena, Biochem. Biophys. Rescomm. 62: 539-545.

40. Drew, K.M., 1934, Contribution to the cytology of Spermothamnion turneri (Mert.) Aresch. I. The diploid genera-tion. Ann Bot. (London) 48: 549-573.

41. Drew, K.M., 1939, An investigation of Plumaria elegans (Bonnem.) Schmitz with special reference to triploid plants bearing parasporangia. Ann. Bot. (London) N.S. 3: 347-367.

42. Drew, K.M., 1943, Contributions to the cytology of Spermothamnion turneri (Mert.) Aresch. II. The haploid and triploid generations. Ann. Bot. (London) N.S. 7: 23-30.

43. Van Der Meer, P., Todd, R., 1977, Genetics of Gracilaria sp. (Rhodophyceae, Gigartinales). IV Mitotic recombination and its relationship to mixed phases in the life history. Genetics 86(S): 66.

44. Rao, B.G.S., Mantha, S., Rao, M.U., 1977, Chromosome behaviour at meiosis and its bearing on the cytotaxonomy of Ceramium species. Bot. Marina 21: 123-129.

45. Wynne, J. Loiseaux, S., 1976, Recent advances in life history
     studies of the Phaeophyta. Phycologia 15: 435-452.
46. Muller, D.G., 1976, Generation suechsel, Kernphasenwechsel
     und Sexualitat der Ectocarpus siliculosus im Koltorversuch.
     Planta 75: 39-54.
47. Muller, D.G., 1974, Sexual reproduction and isolation of a
     sex attractant in Cutleria multifida (Smith) Grev.
     (Phaeophyta). Biochem. Physiol. Planta 165: 212-215.
48. Hoek, C. Van Den, Cortel Breeman, A.M., Rietema, H., Wanders,
     J.B.W., 1972, L'interpretation des donnees obtenues, pardes
     cuitures unialgales, surles cycles evolutifs desalgues.
     Quelquer exemples tires des recherches conduites ai
     laboratoire de Groninque. Mem. Soc. Bot. Fr. 1972: 45-66.
49. Wanders, J.B.W., Hoek Van Den, C., Schillern Van Nes, E.N.,
     1972, Observations on the life-history of Elachista stellaris
     (Phaeophyceae) in culture. Neth. J. Sea Res. 5: 458-491.
50. Allen, J.R., 1975, Characterization of the DNA from the dino-
     flagellate Cryptothecodinium cohnii and implications for
     nuclear organization. Cell 6: 161-169.
51. Roberts, T.M., Loeblich, R., Klotz, C., 1975, Studies on the
     DNA of the blue-green alga Agmenellum quadruplicatum. J.
     Phycology 11(Suppl.): 16.
52. Shyam, R., Sarma, Y.S.R.K., 1976, Effects of colchicine on
     the cell division of a colonial green algal Flagellate
     Gonium pectorale Muller. Caryologia 2a: 27-33.
53. Patel, R.J., 1971, Effects of colchicine on Pithophora,
     oedogonium and Cladophora flexuosa, Ph.D. thesis, London
     University.

POLYPLOIDY IN FUNGI

James Maniotis

Department of Biology
Washington University
St. Louis, MO 63130

Although traditional evolutionary studies in plants commonly have focussed on chromosomal changes in karyotype, recent work in molecular biology emphasizes the key role that repetitive DNA sequences play in phylogeny (1).

Genome size and complexity have been measured in relatively few fungi (2). The values obtained suggest that fungal nuclear DNA is ca. 5 to 10 times larger than bacteria (3). The yeast-fungus, Saccharomyces cerevisiae, has the smallest eukaryotic genome, about 3 times the size of Escherichia coli (2). Most chromatins of multicellular eukaryotes have a nucleosome repeat-size of 200 base pairs. The DNA content of fungal nucleosomes is in the range of 30-50 base pairs smaller than those for higher eukaryotes (1,4).

Fungi seem to stand in a zone intermediate between prokaryotes and the multicellular animals and plants with respect to their genome size and complexity. "If indeed the fungi possess limited evolutionary potential because of limited genetic material, any means to increase the quantity of DNA should provide a means to escape this restriction. The best known mechanism for this would be polyploidization" (2).

Polyploidy in fungi and fungoid organisms has been the subject of several reviews (5-8).

Polyploidy in fungi has been considered to be non-existent or rare (2,9-13), and this assumption would indicate that polyploidy as an evolutionary mechanism for fungal speciation has not assumed the same sort of role accorded it in the evolution of vascular plants (14-16). Evidence which has been adduced in a review of the subject (8) to consider polyploidy as a widespread, or at least an important, factor in fungal speciation, is still not very convincing. This is because knowledge of the phenomenon in fungi is still fragmentary, and, except in a few concrete instances, only suggestive that polyploidy may have functioned as a general mode of speciation.

DIFFICULTIES IN ESTABLISHING FUNGAL KARYOTYPES

There are a number of major reasons which may be cited to indicate why our knowledge of fungal polyploidy is still fragmentary (5,9,17-20).

1.   Haploid chromosome numbers in most of the true fungi probably are generally low. Chromosome counts of fungi performed by many of the earlier cytologic workers have been summarized or references listed (7, 21-24). Olive (7) concluded that haploid chromosome counts range mostly from 3 to 28 (up to 90 in plasmodial myxomycetes), with numbers of 8 or less predominating. A recent compilation of chromosome numbers (3,25) in 78 fungi indicates that haploid chromosome counts in most fungal groups are low, in the range of 2 to 18, with haploid counts of 4, 7, and 8 predominating. Such haploid chromosome counts would appear to offer meager support for the notion of widespread polyploid evolution, unless one were to hypothesize ancestral fungal forms having chromosome numbers of n=2. In this connection, some fungal cytologists contend that chromosome numbers of n=2, reported before the orcein squash technique was applied in Neurospora in 1945 (26), are probably erroneous. Workers who used stained, sectioned material may have misinterpreted telophase figures (7,27,28). Fixation solutions tend to clump chromosomes at each pole at telophase into two groups, possibly by compressing spindle fibers together during anaphase. Numerous instances now exist showing that many earlier counts were indeed erroneous.
Counts of about 31 fungi and 15 plasmodial slime molds were listed in 1973 (8) which are reported or suspected to be polyploid. Except for relatively few instances cited below, most of these counts (for fungi) are higher than average counts reported earlier (7,28) by a factor of about two or three. The problem with these data was stated by Rogers (8) thusly: "High chromosome numbers alone, however, seldom do more than suggest polyploidy."
2.   Fungal nuclei and chromosomes are generally small. One need only recall the spirited long-term controversy on what actually constituted the nucleus of yeasts to appreciate one of the fundamental problems in fungal cytology (29). The degree to which fungal karyotypic analysis has been carried is conceded to be at the lowest level of sophistication, e.g., "alpha" karyology (13). The exception is Neurospora crassa (see below). It is estimated that somewhat less than 400 chromosome counts are available in the literature, many probably erroneous. This should be compared to the approximately 121,000 counts available for vascular plants (30).

3.   Certain features attending fungal nuclear and chromosome behavior, morphology, and organization during mitosis promote uncertainty in providing unequivocal chromosome counts (20,31-36). Some groups of fungi maintain a nuclear membrane (closed nuclear division) during mitotic division, some do not (open nuclear division); controversy still prevails regarding the organization of fungal chromosomes during mitosis, whether it is a variation of normal eukaryotic mitosis, or quite different (37): Many reports indicate the frequent absence of a typical metaphase plate during mitosis in higher fungi--a so-called "two-track" configuration of chromatin being reported (38); some fungal groups have centrioles functioning in division, some do not; microtubule-chromatin interactions are not observed in some fungi (34); and it is reported that plasmodial myxomycetes have closed and noncentric division in diplophase and open and centric in haplophase (39).

The diploid meiotic nucleus is the largest nucleus in the life cycle of most fungi, and it is this phase which has provided the most detailed information on fungal cytology (7). However, even in meiotic division fungal chromosomes are notorious for their small size and extreme state of contraction during metaphase and anaphase, promoting ambiguity in chromosome counting. Indeed, smut fungi and yeasts have chromosomes so small that they cannot be resolved with confidence with the light microscope. The exception is Neurospora crassa. Its meiotic chromosomes have been intensively studied (26,40-46) so that the n=7 chromosomes are each familiar with respect to its length, arm ratios, chromomere patterns, and a variety of chromosomal aberrations.

Caution about accuracy of reported chromosome counts in fungi prevails, however. The case of Schizophyllum commune is illustrative. This mushroom has been intensively studied, from genetic, cytologic, physiologic, and biochemical points of view. The haploid number of chromosomes in basidia was reported to be n=3 in 1949 (47), using sectioned material embedded in paraffin and stained with haemotoxylin, and, using smear techniques, as n=8 in 1974 (48), as n=4 in 1976 (49), and as n=8 in 1978 (from mitotic figures, 50). The linkage map, constructed from genetic markers in 1977, indicates the haploid number is at least n=7 (51). Three dimensional reconstructions of pachytene nuclei revealed 11 distinct synaptinemal complexes, demonstrating a haploid chromosome number of 11 (52). If quantification is the holy grail of chromosome counts in the study of polyploid evolution, that holy grail in fungal cytogenetics is still under quest!

4.   Certain inherent features of fungi provide uncertainty or promote difficulty in providing accurate chromosome counts. Because of their small size, fungal chromosomes must be spread apart to facilitate counting. Fungal cells are highly resistant to simple mechanical pressure, and often are treated with enzymes and acids to promote spreading of chromosomes.

5.   The site of meiosis and where haplo- or diplo-phase
prevails in some fungal groups is still under dispute.   The
history of the concept of brachymeiosis, that colored ascomycete
cytology for a number of years, has been summarized (7,23,53).
This notion held that two nuclear fusions took place, one occurring
at plasmogamy, and the other occurring in the ascus, followed by
a normal reductional division and then an abnormally short, or
brachymeiotic (meiosis I only), division.   This notion affected
karyotype determinations until it was finally laid to rest by
1950.   Another long-term misinterpretation in fungal cytology is,
similarly, being discarded.
      Nuclei in hyphae of a number of families of biflagellate
water molds are now considered diploid, rather than haploid,
since cytologic work (54-58), and DNA-microspectrophotometry
(66,67) indicate that meiosis takes place in gametangia, not the
germinating oospore, as held previously (68).   The development of
cytologic and genetic theory in this group has been reviewed
(69,70).   Little or nothing is known about life cycles relative
to sites of meiosis in a number of other families in biflagellate
water molds.
      Only recently has it been established that the intensively
studied chytrid, Blastocladiella emersonii, has a meiotic phase
(71).
      Meiotic events in zygospores of Mucorales are still incompletely
understood (72-74).   Meiosis was only recently demonstrated
genetically in the cellular slime molds (75).   Meiosis may take
place in completely formed spores of some plasmodial slime molds,
and not before their formation (39).   Certain strains of slime
molds apparently produce haploid plasmodia (76-79).
      The phenomenon of parasexuality, including heterokaryosis,
formation of diploid nuclei in normally haploid fungi (diploidization), with subsequent chromosome loss yielding aneuploids and
ultimately haploid nuclei (haploidization) found in a number of
asexual and sexual fungi (17) provides a source of uncertainty in
attempts to ascribe chromosome numbers to fungi with the prospect
that syngamy might occur between nuclei of variable chromosome
number.   Aneuploids were observed to arise as frequently as 1 in
50 mitotic divisions in Aspergillus nidulans   (80).   Pseudowild
(disomic) strains (n + 1) are well known in Neurospora; their
formal genetics is well defined (6,81).
      A large number of fungi (Deuteromycetes) lack a sexual
phase.   Although linkage groups in these could be defined using
parasexual analyses, the prospect remains dim that we could
proceed rapidly to obtain a satisfactory number of linkage group
counts for a variety of species and even related ones in order to
construct a phylogeny based on ploidy changes.
      Life cycles in a particular group of fungi often are assumed
to be the same as that derived from a few intensively studied
forms, as, for example, in the mushroom, Schizophyllum commune.
It is interesting to note that in a recent report (82), in which

microspectrophotometry of nuclear DNA was applied, the data were
interpreted to support the hypothesis that the mushroom,
Armillariella mellea, has a predominantly diploid life cycle with
a possibility of tetraploidy existing in gill tissues. Alternatively, genetic studies of A. mellea were interpreted to indicate
that nuclei in cells of dikaryotic hyphae regularly fuse, then
promptly undergo (an unspecified kind of) division to yield
haploids which segregate into monokaryotic sectors (83). Cytological work suggests the possibility of diploidy in the fungus
(84). These interpretations are at variance with the haploid-
dikaryotic life cycle usually promulgated in characterizing
mushrooms (85). Variation in nuclear behavior in life cycles of
Homobasidiomycetes recently has been assessed (86,87).

     6. No comprehensive reliable study of chromosome numbers
of closely related genera, or of a number of species of the same
genus which would denote a polyploid series, has been made,
except in a few instances.

FUNGAL POLYPLOIDY

Allomyces

     The classic study in fungi, which unequivocally demonstrated
that species in the uniflagellate water-mold genus, Allomyces,
consists of a polyploidy series, was reported in the 1950's
(88,89). In the subgenus Euallomyces (90), there is a regular
alteration of generations between a haploid gametophytic (n) and
a diploid sporophytic (2n) phase. The 2n phase is derived from
fusion of gametes from gametangia of the n phase. Meiosis takes
place in resting sporangia in the 2n phase to produce meiospores
which form the n phase. A haploid series of 8, 16, 24, and 32
chromosomes were found in different geographic isolates of gametophytes of A. arbuscula, and 14, 28, and ca. 56 in A. macrogynus.
A. javanicus was shown to be a natural hybrid between these two
species. When A. arbuscula (n=16) and A. macrogynus (n=28) were
crossed, the F_1 hybrids (which displayed the characteristics of
naturally occurring A. javanicus) had from 44 to 55 chromosomes
as the diploid number. Subsequent progeny derived from F_1
hybrids had variable chromosome numbers. A question which might
be raised is: Do A. arbuscula and A. macrogynus constitute
distinct species? Both are warm latitude forms with A. arbuscula
being widespread (90). A. macrogynus is relatively rare in
nature. The two species are distinguished mainly on the basis of
male gametangium location relative to female on hyphae of gametophytes. A. javanicus has a similar, but more limited, geographic
distribution as does A. arbusculus, and, as in A. macrogynus,
possesses epigynous female gemetangia. A number of minor morphological features distinguish these three taxa. Most significantly,
percentage of viable F_1 meiosporangia in the artificially produced
hybrid, A. arbuscula X macrogynus, is ca. 0.11%, and a number of

viable meiospores produce abnormal cultures. Such results support
the notion that the two parental forms, having different ploidy,
are "good" species, despite the fact that complete isolation did
not prevail.

It was shown later (91) that A. macrogynus, n=56, is an
autotetraploid (actually 2n=4x=56). Continuous cultivation of 4x
sporophytes at high temperatures, or in the presence of para-
fluorophenylalanine (see section on diploidy in fungi), resulted
in production of stable sporophytes having half the initial
chromosome number (2n=2x=28). Thus, the basic chromosome number
of A. macrogynus is 14.

Colchicine, when applied to resting sporangia of the tetraploid, blocked meiosis; meiospores were formed with the same
ploidy number. These produced gametophytes of the same ploidy
number which yielded gametes that fused to form sporophytes of
greater ploidy than the parental tetraploid. These colchicine-
induced polyploids were unstable (91). Polyploid strains also
were induced in A. macrogynus by forming abnormal multinucleated
gametes under conditions of oxygen starvation, in the presence of
dilute lactic acid, etc. (92). Nuclear fusions within gametes
were observed to occur. Gametes developed into sporophytes
apogamously, and had ploidy numbers higher than the parental
strain.

A chromosome number of n=12-22 has been reported (93) in
strains of an isolate in the subgenus, Brachyallomyces, closely
related to the three previously discussed species but characterized by lack of a sexual phase. Rogers (8) points out that
these results with Brachyallomyces suggest the occurrence of both
aneuploidy and polyploidy. It has been suggested (94) that a
polyploid series also exists in A. neomoniliformis (=A. cytogenes)
with x/2x and 2x/4x strains with the basic number being x=7.

As emphasized by Rogers (8), Allomyces is the only fungal
genus where enough species and their isolates have been studied
to the degree that would support the contention that polyploidy
unequivocally has played a role in its speciation.

Oömycetes

Probable polyploid series are found in biflagellate water-
molds. A number of closely related species in the Saprolegniaceae
and Pythiaceae were studied (95). Multiple chromosome associations
at first metaphase with unequal divisions at first telophase or
second metaphase suggested that autopolyploidy is found in several
species. Allopolyploidy was suspected at intermediate levels of
ploidy. Haploid chromosome numbers observed were: for 8 species
of Achlya, n=3; for 4 species in a different subsection of the
genus, n=6; for 3 additional species of Achlya, n=ca.12; for
Saprolegnia ferax, S. furcata, Pythiopsis cymosa, and Apodachlyella
completa, n=ca.8-12. Pythium multisporum, P. torulosum, and P.
ultimum were observed to have a chromosome number of n=10, while

Table 1. Haploid chromosome numbers in the Oömycetes.

Taxon	Haploid Number	Material Examined	Chromo- some Associa- tion	Refer- ence
SAPROLEGNIALES				
<u>Achlya</u> spp.				
A. <u>ambisexualis</u>	3	antheridium	---	54
	3	oogonium	---	95
A. <u>inflata</u>	3	gametangia	---	70
A. <u>flagellata</u>	3	oogonium	---	95
A. <u>caroliniana</u>	3	oogonium	---	95
A. <u>colorata</u>	3	oogonium	---	95
A. <u>apiculata</u>	3	oogonium	---	95
A. <u>treleaseana</u>	3	oogonium	---	95
A. <u>benekei</u>	3	oogonium	---	95
A. <u>radiosa</u>	6	antheridium	---	95
A. <u>recurva</u>	6	oogonium	---	95
A. <u>hypogyna</u>	6	gametangea	---	95
A. <u>americana</u>	6-8	oogonium	---	95
A. sp. (Ghana)	ca.8	gametangia	---	58
A. <u>klebsiana</u>	12	gametangia	---	55
A. <u>racemosa</u>	ca.11-12	?	---	96
A. <u>sparrowii</u>	ca.12-13	?	---	96
<u>Saprolegnia</u> spp.				
S. <u>terrestris</u>	5	oogonia	yes	66
S. <u>ferax</u>	10	hyphae, gametangia	---	55
	ca.12(?)	oogonium	---	95
S. <u>furcata</u>	ca.12	oogonium	yes(?)	95
<u>Thraustotheca</u>				
<u>clarata</u>	ca.6	antherial "axial elemeats"	---	97
<u>Pythiopsis</u>				
<u>cymosa</u>	ca.10	antheridium	---	95
LEPTOMITALES				
<u>Apodachlyella</u>				
<u>completa</u>	ca.8	oogonium	---	95

PERONOSPORALES

Table 1 (continued)

Albugo spp.				
A. candida				
-- on Capsella	25–40	oogonia	---	98
-- on Lunaria	25–30	gametangia	yes	98
Sclerospora				
graminicola	14	oogonia	---	99
	14–16	oogonia	---	64
Peronospora				
parasitica	18–20	oogonia	---	98
Pythium spp.				
P. multisporum	10	gametangia	---	95
P. torulosum	10	oogonium	---	95
P. ultimum	ca.10	oogonium	(?)	95
P. debaryanum	ca.18	oogonia	yes	57
	ca.20	gametangia	yes	56
	ca.20	oogonia	yes	95
Phytophthora spp.				
P. parasitica	5	oogonia	---	100
P. palmivora				
Large chromosome				
type	ca.5–6	gametangia	yes	101
Small chromosome				
type	ca.9–12	gametangia	---	101
P. cinnamomi	9 or 10	gametangia	---	102
P. infestans	9 or 10	gametangia	yes	102
	9 ± 1	gametangia	yes	103
British isolate	ca.18–20	oogonium	yes	104
P. capsici	9	oogonia	yes	105
P. cambivora	ca.9	oogonia	---	104
P. cactorun	ca.9	gametangia	---	56
	ca.9	oogonia	---	58
P. erythroseptica	ca.9	gametangia	---	58
P. drechsleri	9–12	gametangia	yes	102
P. nicotianae				
var. parasitica	ca.9	oogonium	---	104
P. megasperma				
var. sojae	ca.10–13	gametangia	yes	106
var. megasperma	ca.22–27	gametangia	yes	106

[a] Multiple associations of chromosomes observed (trivalents, quadrivalents, or possibly translocation configurations).

P. debaryanum had n=ca.20. When these results, and those by other workers (Table 1), are considered, it seems likely that several polyploid series exist in the Saprolegniaceae (x=3) and Pythiaceae (x=10).

Large and small oogonial (female gametangial) forms of Phytophthora in the same taxonomic complex were studied cytologically (106). The haploid count in the larger form (P. megasperma) was determined to be n=ca.22-27, while that for the smaller was n=ca.10-13. This is one of the few instances in fungi where use of haploid chromosome number has been used (in addition to other characteristics) to establish varietal status of a fungus. The smaller form (formerly P. sojae) now is recognized as P. megasperma var. sojae. Earlier work had recognized these forms as two species of a larger taxonomic complex.

Similarly, two distinct interfertile varieties of Phytophthora palmivora have been defined, based on the one variety having large chromosomes and a haploid number of ca.5-6, and the other having small chromosomes and a haploid number of ca.9-12 (101).

Haploid chromosome numbers for Peronospora parasitica (n=18-20) and Albugo candida (n=25-40) were recently reported (98). Determination of exact numbers was hampered by the presence of multivalents.

These observations in the Oömycetes readily support a notion that polyploidy has played a role in evolution of this group of fungi.

Ascomycetous Yeasts

Giant, or "gigas" strains, of several yeasts have been induced by camphor vapor (107-111). Polyploid nuclei were reported to be observed in treated material in some reports, but no accurate chromosome counts could be made. Polygametic zygotes have been proposed to be the origin of some polyploidy (112). Nuclear and cell sizes have been studied in a ploidy series (113). Earlier chromosome counts of putative ploidy series in Saccharomyces cerevisiae are inaccurate (114). Based on current linkage group data, at least 17 linkage groups for the normal haploid strain have been constructed since then (115). Electron microscopy of diploid and tetraploid strains indicated that the diploid had ca.17 synaptinemal complexes, while the tetraploid had 31 (116).

Genetic segregation studies of polyploid strains have been reported in S. cerevisiae (114,117-124) and in Schizosaccharomyces pombe (125). Polyploid series up to octoploids were produced. Pentaploid and hexaploid cultures were obtained through selection of rare matings between triploids (126). Stable triploids and tetraploids were constructed for gene dosage studies (127-129) and for recombination studies (130). Certain nonsporulating clones were considered to be triploid (131). A critique of earlier work on genetic analyses of polyploids in yeast is available (132). X-ray sensitivity has been compared in haploids, diploids, and hexaploids (133). Comparative growth and aging studies have been performed using cells of different ploidy (134-136). Physiological and biochemical studies of yeasts of different ploidy are accumulating (137-143) which report increased

or decreased specific biochemical capabilities as the ploidy
level is raised. Without the rigorous marker employment used in
contemporary genetic analyses, some of these reports may hold
little validity. Evidence for polyploidy in S. cerevisiae is
based on genetic work, DNA content, and electron microscopy. DNA
content of fungal nuclei in putative polyploid strains were
studied and were proportional to the number of proposed chromosome
sets (144). This was 2.4, 4.8, 6.5, and 9.9 x 10^{14} g per nucleus
in x, 2x, 3x, and 4x strains, respectively. Ultraviolet irradiation of a ploidy series in yeast indicated that the average rate
of logarithmic inactivation for each ploidy class was greater the
greater the degree of ploidy (145). An extensive study of DNA
content for haploid and diploid cells is available (146).

Formulae have been derived relating frequencies of different
ratios of markers in asci of tetraploids to frequencies of crossing-
over between loci involved and their centromeres (120,124,147).

The significance of polyploidy in yeasts is not clear.
Perhaps the results of a recent report have bearing here. Conven-
tionally stained smears of protoplasts of Schizosaccharomyces
pombe were examined by a combined technique using light and
electron microscopy (148). Other than showing the efficacy of
the technique (n=ca.8), and the inaccuracies afforded by light
microscopy, the results indicated the possibility that polyploid
nuclei (having counts of 21-36 chromosomes) were present in 14%
of the division figures examined. The whole issue of endopolyploidy, now demonstrated in angiosperms (1), has not been considered in modern fungal polyploid studies.

Rusts

Some data exist indicating the possibility of polyploidy in
the rust fungi (Uredinales). A number of species in the genus
Puccinia were studied in mitotic division (149-151). Numbers of
n=4 were observed in homothallic species. Counts of n=3 or 6
were interpreted in heterothallic species. The possibility that
these species of Puccinia studied constituted a polyploid series
was raised. Abnormal chromosome pairing was observed. The
following chromosome numbers for species of Puccinia have been
reported: P. graminis, n=6 (149,152); (152); P. coronata, n=3
(150); P. recondita, n=6 (153); and P. striiformis, n=3 (154).
Aneuploid cells were observed in the latter species. Chromosome
numbers for several other species of Puccinia, in the range of
n=4,5, or 6, have been reported (151). P. kraussiana was studied
in meiotic division (155), and it was reported that n=20, 21, or
22. Division aberrations were observed, and the possibility of
polyploidy also was raised in the light of previous counts for
Puccinia spp.

Four species of Ravenelia were studied (156) for their
haploid complement in germinating teliospores. Results reported
were: R. taslimii, n=8; R. breyniae, n=6; R. hobsonii and

R. emblicae, n=5. Karyotypes of these species suggested some
homologies between chromosomes. It was proposed that species of
Ravenelia might have evolved via polyploidy and aneuploidy. n=4
was considered the primitive number, from which n=8 was derived
through chromosome doubling, and the other species arising as a
result of aneuploidy.

Stable somatic diploids have been reported in the rusts
(152,157,158).

Smuts

Polyploidy has been reported in the Ustilaginales, or smut-
fungi. Strains with ploidy from haploid to tetraploid have been
fabricated in Ustilago violacea (159-161), as evidenced by
genetic and DNA analyses. Mating-type reactions of strains of
various ploidy have been studied (161). Triploids also have been
synthesized in genetic crosses between haploids and diploids in
U. maydis (162). "Gigas" forms have been described (160).
Strains with high ploidy were reported as being unstable. Certain
strains of smuts known in field and genetic studies are diploid--
these are "solopathogenic" strains, causing infections and telio-
spore formation without fusions with other strains (69). Diploids
have been used with great success in mitotic crossing-over studies
in smuts (162,163).

Cyathus

It was reported (164) that the chromosome number in basidia
of Cyathus olla is n=ca.12. Abnormal pairing at pachytene and
diplotene was observed and it was suggested that the possibility
of a reciprocal translocation was present. A related species, C.
stercoreus, was reported earlier (165) to have n=12. Some chromosomes of the haploid complement at pachytene resembled one
another in pairs; these at diplotene formed quadrivalent configurations or exhibited secondary associations (166). The high frequency of their occurrence suggested the possibility that C.
stercoreus is a tetraploid. Alternative explanations (aneuploidy
and translocations) are possible, however. C. olla was suggested
to be a tetraploid as well, and it was suggested that C. stercoreus
may have evolved by allotetraploidy from species which may have
evolved from a single ancestor (166).

Plasmodial Slime Molds

Haploid chromosome counts for a number of myxomycetes have
been summarized (7,8,167,168). These vary from 4-12 in groups of
unrelated species to 20 to 300 in others. Polyploidy could be
interpreted to have been operative as a mode of speciation in
some genera, based upon the sheer magnitude of some chromosome
counts. For example, Physarum flavicomum, n=35$\pm$2; P. polycephalum,

n=90+3. The work is summarized elsewhere (8,167,169).
Even different clones in the same species in this group may
have different chromosome numbers (77,78,167,169,170-174).
Extended periods of laboratory culture may result in ploidy
changes (175). Other than promoting variation, the significance
of this variability in chromosome number is not at all clear. It
has been suggested (169) that such chromosomal variability might
account for the various types of mating systems reported. High
frequency of somatic nuclear fusions in plasmodia of Physarum
polycephalum to form giant nuclei has been reported (175). It is
possible that plasmodial slime molds may have endopolyploid
cycles of the type demonstrated in angiosperms (1).

Other Fungi Described as Being Polyploid

Other reports of fungi having ploidy levels higher than
diploid include Aspergillus oryzae (176), A. niger (177), A.
nidulans (178), and Neurospora crassa (179). A series of papers
dealing with the morphology, physiology, biochemistry and genetics
of stable induced polyploid strains of Candida spp., and especially
Leucosporidium (Candida) scottii, are of interest (180-190).
Some of these polyploid forms apparently provide higher yields of
fermented end-products than the parent cultures from which they
were derived. The giant forms are reported to have higher rates
of activity of the Kreb's cycle dehydrogenases. Mitochondria
were reported to be larger in one polyploid strain than its
parent culture. Induced mutants with affected respiratory systems
were produced at higher frequency in polyploids than in the
parental strain. Increased ploidy levels increased the sensitivity
of strains to the antibiotic, nystatin.

Rogers (8) lists a number of fungi which in his view suggests
that polyploidy may have functioned in their evolution. However,
counts typically do not cover a number of closely related taxa,
or even species in the same genus. Observations of frequent
multivalents or complex associations of chromosomes at pachytene
hardly supports a doctrine of polyploid evolution, even if the
fungus has a high (for the fungi) chromosome number. For example,
Xylaria curta was reported (191) to have a chromosome number of
n=8 or 9. Multivalents and complex associations of chromosomes
seen at pachytene suggested to the author the possibility that X.
curta is a segmental allopolyploid.

CHEMICAL INDUCTION OF POLYPLOIDY

Colchicine and colcemid seem to be ineffective as general
agents in inducing polyploidy in fungi (18,111,192-195). It
works well in Allomyces (91,196), however, and in one report
(197), contrary to results by other workers who applied it to the
Oömycetes, inhibition of meiosis was obtained in young oögonia

of Saprolegnia. Colchicine-binding components are present in
fungi (198). Colchicine effects on fungi have been reviewed
extensively (18,192).

Natural (dextrorotary) camphor vapor seems to be very effective in inducing apparent polyploidy, based on numerous morphological studies in a variety of fungi, including Oömycetes (58,64,
199), yeasts, Penicillium and Aspergillus (176,194,200-202), and
possibly in Neurospora (179). These induced forms often display
increased cell and nuclear sizes, and often are termed "gigas"
forms. Cytological confirmation of polyploidy has been difficult
to demonstrate, however. Camphor induction of apparent polyploidy
has been used to determine the place of meiosis in life cycle
studies (199,203), and to induce diploids preparatory to genetic
analysis by use of the parasexual cycle (200). Camphor-induced
putative polyploids typically are unstable, undergoing chromosome
loss during successive mitotic divisions (64,194,204). Antimitotic
agents for fungi have been reviewed (18,193).

OTHER MODES OF DETERMINING FUNGAL KARYOTYPES

Because of inherent difficulties in establishing fungal
karyotypes, techniques other than straightforward cytological
examination have been applied to establish basic haploid numbers,
or at least relative degrees of ploidy.

1.   Electron microscopy of the synaptinemal complex (SC).
Use of the SC as a diagnostic indication of paired homologous
chromosomes of meiotic prophase (205) has been successful in
delineating the site of meiosis or chromosome number in several
fungi or fungoid organisms (33,52,71,97,116,206-210). Exemplary
of this work is that performed with Labyrinthula sp. (209).
Serial sections through meiotic prophase material of this net
slime-mold indicated there were 9 separate and distinct SC's.
Since each SC represents a set of paired homologous chromosomes,
n=9 is the haploid number of this species. Similar work has been
performed for Neurospora crassa (211,212), where 7 SC's were
determined in prophase asci. Since the haploid chromosome
number of N. crassa is unequivocally n=7, based on extensive
cytological and genetical linkage studies, this technique would
appear to be ideal to establish chromosome numbers in situations
where ambiguity in counting is encountered.

The reported absence of SC's in meiotic sites in Saprolegnia
furcata (213), Schizosaccharomyces pombe (214), Podospora anserina,
and P. setosa (215) is puzzling and difficult to evaluate.

2.   Microspectrophotometry of nuclear DNA. This method has
been used to confirm the site of meiosis and relative ploidy
number in several Oömycetes (66,67), in Ascomycetes (53), and in
a deuteromycete (216). The technique also has been applied to
ploidy studies in plasmodial myxomycetes (76,78,79,167,173,175,
217,218).

3.   Cytofluorometry of nuclear DNA. This method, simpler and less expensive that the previous, has been used to determine relative ploidy of different phases in the life-history of Phytophthora drechsleri (219), Physarum polycephalum (220), and to ascertain diploidy in a variant strain of Puccinia graminis f. sp. tritici (158). It has been used with some success to verify chromosome counts in a few fungi (221).

4.   DNA content per cell. A fungus with uninucleate cells in its life-cycle readily may be analyzed for DNA content per cell, and degree of ploidy may be determined. This technique was used initially to establish the diploid nature of diploids early in the development of parasexual analyses in Aspergillus nidulans (222), and has been applied widely in studies of ploidy in a variety of fungi, as in Allomyces (91), in Cryptococcus albidus (223), in a polyploid series of yeasts (118,143,144,224), in Aspergillus (222), and in a smut (160). A very extensive study of the DNA content per nucleus for Saccharomyces cerevisiae haploids and diploids is available (146). Values of DNA content per haploid genome have been summarized for about 16 fungi (2).

5.   Electron microscopy of chromosomes using conventional smears of protoplast preparations. Although samples prepared for electron microscopy provide poor resolution of chromosomes, some success may be obtained by a combination approach. Chromosomes of Schizosaccharomyces pombe were discerned by preparing proto-plasts of the yeast, staining using a smear method, and examining by light microscopy. The identical material was then transferred to grids and examined by electron microscopy (148). Counts fell into two main groups, the first ranging from 7-9 with a sharp peak at 8, and the second from 13-17 with peaks at 14 and 16. These groups were interpreted to be the chromosome counts of the n and 2n states respectively, and the haploid number was suggested to be N = ca. 8. Counts ranging from 21-36 were interpreted as polyploid cells (148). Comparison of results by light microscopy and the combination method indicated that previous results using light microscopy were inaccurate (n=5-7).

6.   Other techniques have been used singly or in conjunction with some of the previous to establish ploidy levels in a fungus (5). These include measurements of cell and nuclear volumes, ultraviolet light mutagenesis and inactivation kinetics, and photoreactivation rates (71,84,113,118,132,145,152,157,160,223, 225-227).

DIPLOIDY IN FUNGI

Discovered in Aspergillus nidulans, essential steps of the parasexual cycle (80,178,228) are: formation of heterokaryons, fusion of unlike nuclei in hyphae, mitotic recombination, and haploidization of recombinant nuclei. Diploid strains, often fabricated in studies of mitotic crossing-over, have been estab-lished in a number of fungi (17,204). These include many sexual

and asexual filamentous molds, Ascomycetes, smuts, rusts, mushrooms, and cellular slime molds. Azygosporic Mucorales may be
diploid (229). Most diploids appear to be unstable, a fortuitous
feature permitting parasexual analysis.

There is little evidence for widespread occurrence of diploidy
in nature in haploid fungi, other than when the zygotic nucleus
is formed in the normal life-cycle. This diploid nucleus soon
undergoes meiosis. Exceptions are the biflagellate water molds,
a number of yeasts, and plasmodial myxomycetes, all of which have
dominant diplophases in their life-cycles.

An interesting example of a stable diploid fungus in a group
(Deuteromycetes) considered to consist of haploids or heterokaryons, is the pathogenic mold Verticillium dahliae var. longi-
spora. Isolated from diseased horseradish in 1961, it was suspected to be a stable diploid (230). The variety differs from V.
dahliae in having spores almost twice as long, but otherwise the
variety is morphologically identical to it. Using DL-para-
fluorophenylalanine (which promotes haploidization in diploids
studied in parasexual analysis (163,231), sectors were derived
from the variety having smaller spores (230). By introducing
auxotrophic mutations in subcultures of the sectors, stable,
long-spored, diploid strains were reconstructed by permitting
heterokaryosis to occur between different auxotrophic strains,
and selecting diploid prototrophs.

Solopathogenic strains of smuts have been found in nature,
which appear to be stable. Occasionally, stable diploids of
normally haploid species have been reported from nature (177,226).
Diploidy in fungi has been reviewed (69,232).

But for these exceptions, it is haploidy, with its variations:
the coenocytic (multinucleate) haploid condition, and the dikaryon
of the Basidiomycetes (wherein a dikaryotic haploid condition,
n + n, is found in each cell) which seems to prevail in the
fungi. We may generalize that most fungi, numerically speaking,
seem to favor the haploid condition, and the only diploid phase
is established when the zygote nucleus is formed, which undergoes
meiosis to produce haploid meiospores again.

WHY DO FUNGI FAVOR HAPLOIDY?

Burnett (17) states that it is desirable that selection
should operate on spores which are as variable as possible; hence
the widespread occurrence of meiosis prior to spore production in
most fungi; and the inevitable loss, or non-achievement, of a
prolonged diploid phase.

As Raper (233) pointed out, because most fungi lack the
mutational buffering system of diploids, that can mask genetic
deficiencies during vegetative phases, effects of natural selection
are more immediate and more rigorous in fungi than in most other
organisms. This view would explain why, amongst eukaryotes, one
of the distinguishing features of fungi is their enormous

capabilities for sexual and asexual haploid spore production and their short generation times. Selection acts on multitudes of haploid spores; this is followed by re-establishment of the zygote nucleus between heroic survivors, to be followed by meiosis again and abundant spore production. These features account for the amazing genetic diversity and versatility of the fungi.

Additionally, there is the possibility that some sort of nuclear/ cytoplasmic interaction favors haploidy (17). Consider a fungus mycelium extending for 10 to 15 feet in diameter hori- zontally in the soil, all of its hyphae interconnected, with an incalculable number of haploid nuclei flowing through its hyphal filaments. Asexual reproduction or fragmentation may disperse the fungus readily. Where is the traditional concept of the individual here? Or the population? Fungal coenocytism, then, is conceived as an alternative life style increasing the genome in the coenocyte, favoring haploidy, and fostering heterokaryosis, which is a reasonable substitute for heterosis.

On the other hand, some evidence from work performed with yeast (234) indicates that ploidy levels favored by an organism are not as significant a factor determining fitness as is the surface area of its cells. Under conditions where fitness is determined by the activity of a surface-bound enzyme, diploid cells (with a lower surface-area/volume ratio) would be expected to have a lower fitness than haploids, and experimental work confirms this (235).

Superimposed on the haploid state in many fungi is the emergence of complex, genetically determined self-incompatibility systems, in themselves rigid isolating mechanisms, which necessi- tate fusion of haploid hyphae with other specific haploid genotypes before sexual reproduction may occur (2,85,233).

The origins of diploidy are difficult to fathom, but obviously are of importance to understanding the evolution of polyploidy. It is interesting to note (12) that the polyploid series reported in this review are observed in those organisms (Allomyces, Oömycetes, yeasts) which have a dominant or lengthy diplophase in their life cycles.

As for the rest of the fungi, their karyalagic situations may represent, as Raper and Flexer said (232), "a detour in the road to diploidy."

SUMMARY

There is evidence supporting a concept of polyploid evolution in a number of groups of fungi. These typically have dominant diploid phases in their life-histories. There are a number of reports of suspected polyploidy in other fungi, but these should be considered speculative at this time.

LITERATURE CITED

1. Nagl, W., 1977, Replication: organization and replication of the eukaryotic chromosome. Prog. Bot. 39: 132-152.
2. Ullrich, R.C., Raper, J.R., 1977, Evolution of genetic mechanisms in fungi. Taxon 26: 169-179.
3. Storck, R., 1972, DNA of fungi, Pp. 371-393, in Smith, H.H., (ed.), "Evolution of Genetic Systems," Gordon and Breach, New York.
4. Horgen, P., Silver, J.C., 1978, Chromatin in eukaryotic microbes. Ann. Rev. Microbiol. 32: 249-284.
5. Esser, K., Kuenen, R., 1967, "Genetics of Fungi," Transl. by E. Steiner, Springer, New York.
6. Fincham, J.R.S., Day, P.R., 1971, "Fungal Genetics," ed. 3, Blackwell Scientific Publications, Oxford.
7. Olive, L.S., 1953, The structure and behavior of fungus nuclei. Bot. Rev. 19: 439-586.
8. Rogers, J.D., 1973, Polyploidy in fungi. Evolution 27: 153-160.
9. Burnett, J.H., 1975, "Mycogenetics," John Wiley & Sons, New York and London.
10. Dawson, G.W.P., 1962, "An Introduction to the Cytogenetics of Polyploids," Blackwell Scientific Publications, Oxford.
11. Lederberg, J., 1948, Problems in microbial genetics. Heredity 2: 145-198.
12. Stebbins, G.L., 1950, "Variation and Evolution in Plants," Columbia University Press, New York.
13. White, M.J.D., 1978, "Modes of Speciation," W. H. Freeman, San Francisco.
14. deWet, J.M.J., 1971, Polyploidy and evolution in plants. Taxon 20: 29-35.
15. Jackson, R.C., 1976, Evolution and systematic significance of polyploidy. Ann. Rev. Ecol. Syst. 7: 209-234.
16. Stebbins, G.L., 1966, Chromosomal variation and evolution. Science 152: 1463-1469.
17. Burnett, J.H., 1976, "Fundamentals of Mycology," Edward Arnold, London.
18. Heath, I.B., 1978, Experimental studies of mitosis in fungi, Chapter 3, pp. 89-176, in Heath, I.B., (ed.) "Nuclear Division in the Fungi," Academic Press, New York.
19. Webster, R.K., 1974, Recent advances in the genetics of plant pathogenic fungi. Ann. Rev. Phytopathol. 12: 331-353.
20. Wells, K., 1977, Meiotic and Mitotic division in the Basidiomycotina, pp 337-374, in Rost, T.L., Gifford, E.M., Jr. (eds.), "Mechanism and Control of Cell Division," Dowden, Hutchinson & Ross, Stroudsberg, PA.
21. Delay, C., 1953, Nombres chromosomiques chez les cryptogames. Rev. Cytol. Biol. Vég. 14: 59-107.
22. Kamat, M.N., Pande, A., 1971, Chromosome complements in Ascomycetes. J. Shivaji Univ. 4: 49-57.

23. Martens, P., 1946, Cycle de développement et sexualité des
     Ascomycètes. La Cellule 50: 17-310.
24. Moreau, F., 1952, "Les Champignons. Physiologie, Morphologie,
     Développement et Systématique," Vol. 1, Paul Lechevalier,
     Paris.
25. Storck, R., Anderson, L.E., Ahmadjian, V., Robinow, C.F.,
     contributors, 1972, Chromosome Numbers: Plants. Part I.
     Nonvascular, pp. 9-11, in Altman, L., Dittmer, D.S., (eds.),
     "Biology Data Book," Vol. 1, ed. 2, Fed. Amer. Soc. Exp.
     Biol., Bethesda, MD.
26. McClintock, B., 1945, Neurospora. I. Preliminary observa-
     tions of the chromosomes of Neurospora crassa. Amer. J.
     Bot. 32: 671-678.
27. Olive, L.S., 1942, Nuclear phenomena involved at meiosis in
     Coleosporium helianthi. J. Elisha Mitchell Sci. Soc. 58:
     43-51.
28. Olive, L.S., 1965, Nuclear behavior during meiosis, Chapter
     7, pp. 143-161, in Ainsworth, G.C., Sussman, A.S., (eds.),
     "The Fungi," Vol. 1, Academic Press, New York.
29. Cutter, V.M., Jr., 1951, The cytology of fungi. Ann. Rev.
     Microbiol. 5: 17-34.
30. Moore, D.M., 1978, The chromosomes and plant taxonomy,
     Chapter 3, pp. 39-56, in Street, H.E., (ed.), "Essays in
     Plant Taxonomy," Academic Press, London.
31. Fuller, M.S., 1976, Mitosis in Fungi. Inter. Rev. Cytol.
     45: 113-153.
32. Heath, I.B. (ed.), 1978, "Nuclear Division in the Fungi,"
     Academic Press, New York.
33. Heywood, P., Magee, P.T., 1976, Meiosis in protists. Some
     structural and physiological aspects of meiosis in algae,
     fungi, and protozoa. Bact. Rev. 40: 190-240.
34. Kubai, D.F., 1975, The evolution of the mitotic spindle.
     Inter. Nat. Rev. Cytol. 43: 167-227.
35. Robinow, C.F., Bakerspiegel, A., 1965, Somatic nuclei and
     forms of mitosis in fungi, Chapter 6, pp. 119-142, in
     Ainsworth, G.C., Sussman, A.S. (eds.), "The Fungi," Vol. 1,
     Academic Press, New York.
36. Tanaka, K., 1977, Mitosis in fungi, pp. 229-254, in Ishikawa,
     T., Maruyama, Y., Matsumiya, H. (eds.), "Growth and Differen-
     tiation in Microorganisms," University of Tokyo Press,
     Tokyo.
37. Girbardt, M., 1978, Historical review and introduction,
     Chapter 1, pp. 1-20, in Heath, I.B. (ed.), "Nuclear Division
     in the Fungi," Academic Press, New York.
38. Day, A.W., 1972, Genetic implications of current models of
     somatic nuclear division in fungi. Canad. J. Bot. 50:
     1337-1347.
39. Aldrich, H.C., 1969, The ultrastructure of mitosis in myxa-
     moebae and plasmodia of Physarum flavicomum. Amer. J. Bot.
     56: 290-299.

40. Barry, E.G., 1966, Cytological techniques for meiotic chromo-
    somes in Neurospora. Neurospora Newsletter 10: 12-13.
41. Barry, E.G., 1967, Chromosome aberrations in Neurospora, and
    the correlation of chromosomes and linkage groups. Genetics
    55: 21-32.
42. Barry, E.G., 1969, The diffuse diplotene stage of meiotic
    prophase in Neurospora. Chromosoma 26: 119-129.
43. Barry, E.G., Perkins, D.D., 1969, Position of linkage group
    V markers in chromosome 2 of Neurospora crassa. J. Heredity
    60: 120-125.
44. Perkins, D., 1974, The manifestation of chromosome rearrange-
    ments in unordered asci of Neurospora. Genetics 77: 459-489.
45. Perkins, D., Barry, E.G., 1977, The cytogenetics of Neurospora.
    Adv. Genetics 19: 133-285.
46. Singleton, J.R., 1953, Chromosome morphology and the chromo-
    some cycle in the ascus of Neurospora crassa. Amer. J. Bot.
    40: 124-144.
47. Ehrlich, H.G., McDonough, E.S., 1949, The nuclear history in
    the basidia and basidiospores of Schizophyllum commune
    Fries. Amer. J. Bot. 36: 360-363.
48. Radu, M., Steinlauf, R., Koltin, Y., 1974, Meiosis in
    Schizophyllum commune. Chromosomal behavior and the syna-
    ptinemal complex. Arch. Microbiol. 98: 301-310.
49. Haapala, O.K., Nienstedt, I., 1976, Chromosome ultrastructure
    in the basidiomycete fungus Schizophyllum commune. Hereditas
    84: 49-60.
50. Wessels, J.G.H., 1978, Incompatibility factors and the
    control of biochemical processes, pp. 81-104, in Schwald, M.N.,
    Miles, P.G. (eds.), "Genetics and Morphogenesis in the
    Basidiomycetes," Academic Press, New York.
51. Frankel, C., Ellingboe, A.H., 1977, New mutations and a 7-
    chromosome linkage map of Schizophyllum commune. Genetics
    85: 417-425.
52. Carmi, P., Holm, P.B., Koltin, Y., Rasmussen, S.W., Sage,
    J., Zickler, D., 1978, The pachytene karyotype of Schizo-
    phyllum commune analyzed by three dimensional reconstruction
    of synaptonemal complexes. Carlsberg Res. Commun. 43:
    117-132.
53. Rossen, J.M., Westergaard, M., 1966, Studies on the mechanism
    of crossing over. II. Meiosis and the time of meiotic
    chromosome replication in the ascomycete Neottiella rutilans
    (Fr.) Dennis. C. R. Trav. Lab. Carlsberg 35: 233-260.
54. Barksdale, A., 1968, Meiosis in the antheridium of Achlya
    ambisexualis E87. J. Elisha Mitchell Sci. Soc. 84: 187-194.
55. Flanagan, P.W., 1970, Meiosis and mitosis in Saprolegniaceae.
    Canad. J. Bot. 48: 2069-2076.
56. Sansome, E., 1961, Meiosis in the oogonium and antheridium
    of Pythium debaryanum Hesse. Nature 191: 827-828.

57. Sansome, E., 1963, Meiosis in Pythium debaryanum Hesse and its significance in the life history of the Biflagellatae. Trans. Brit. Mycol. Soc. 46: 63-72.

58. Sansome, E., 1965, Meiosis and diploid and polyploid sex organs of Phytophthora and Achlya. Cytologia 30: 103-117.

59. Barksdale, A., 1966, Segregation of sex in the progeny of a selfed heterozygote of Achlya bisexualis. Mycologia 58: 802-804.

60. Elliot, C.G., MacIntyre, D., 1973, Genetical evidence on the life history of Phytophthora. Trans. Brit. Mycol. Soc. 60: 311-316.

61. Khaki, I.A., Shaw, D.S., 1974, The inheritance of drug resistance and compatibility type in Phytophthora drechsleri. Genet. Res. (Cambridge) 23: 75-86.

62. Lasure, L.L., Griffin, D.H., 1974, Evidence for diploidy in Achlya bisexualis based on inheritance of cycloheximide resistance. Mycologia 46: 391-396.

63. Mullins, J.T., Raper, J.R., 1965, Heterothallism in biflagellate fungi: preliminary genetic analysis. Science 150: 1174-1175.

64. Sansome, E., 1966, Meiosis in the sex organs of the Oömycetes, pp. 77-83, in Darlington, C.D., Lewis, K.R. (eds.), "Chromosomes Today," Vol. 1, Oliver & Boyd, Edinburgh.

65. Shaw, D.S., Khaki, I.A., 1971, Genetical evidence for diploidy in Phytophthora. Genet. Res. (Cambridge) 17: 165-167.

66. Bryant, T.R., Howard, K.L., 1969, Meiosis in the Oömycetes: I. A microspectrophotometric analysis of nuclear deoxyribonucleic acid in Saprolegnia terrestris. Amer. J. Bot. 56: 1075-1083.

67. Howard, K.L., Bryant, T.R., 1971, Meiosis in the Oömycetes. II. a microspectrophotometric analysis of DNA in Apodachlya brachynema. Mycologia 63: 58-68.

68. Ziegler, A.W., 1953, Meiosis in the Saprolegniaceae. Amer. J. Bot. 40: 60-66.

69. Caten, C.E., Day, A.W., 1977, Diploidy in plant pathogenic fungi. Ann. Rev. Phytopathol. 15: 295-318.

70. Dick, M.W., Win-Tin, 1973, The development of cytological theory in the Oomycetes. Biol. Rev. 48: 133-158.

71. Olson, L.W., Reichle, R., 1978, Synaptonemal complex formation and meiosis in the resting sporangium of Blastocladiella emersonii. Protoplasma 97: 261-273.

72. Cerdá-Olmedo, E., 1975, The genetics of Phycomyces blakesleeanus. Genet. Res. (Cambridge) 25: 285-296.

73. Eslava, A.P., Alvarez, M.I., Delbrück, M., 1975, Meiosis in Phycomyces. Proc. Nat. Acad. Sci. USA 72: 4076-4080.

74. Gauger, W.L., 1977, Meiotic gene segregation in Rhizopus stolonifer. J. Gen. Microbiol. 101: 211-217.

75. Macinnes, M.A., Francis, D., 1974, Meiosis in Dictyostelium mucoroides. Nature 251: 321-323.

76. Cooke, D.J., Dee, J., 1974, Plasmodium formation without change in nuclear DNA content in Phsarum polycephalum. Genet. Res. (Cambridge) 23: 307-317.

77. Mohberg, J., 1977, Nuclear DNA content and chromosome numbers throughout the life cycle of the Colonia strain of the myxomycete, Physarum polycephalum. J. Cell Sci. 24: 95-108.

78. Therrien, C.D., Collins, O.R., 1976, Apogamic induction of haploid plasmodia in a myxomycete Didymium iridis. Dev. Biol. 49: 283-287.

79. Yemma, J.J., Therrien, C.D., 1972, Quantitative micro-spectrophotometry of nuclear DNA in selfing strains of the myxomycete Didymium iridis. Amer. J. Bot. 59: 828-835.

80. Käfer, E., 1961, The processes of spontaneous recombination in vegetative nuclei of Aspergillus nidulans. Genetics 46: 1581-1609.

81. Threlkeld, S.F.H., Stoltz, J.M., 1970, A genetic analysis of nondisjunction and mitotic recombination in Neurospora crassa. Genetic Res. (Cambridge) 16: 29-35.

82. Peabody, D.C., Motta, J.J., Therrien, C.D., 1978, Cytophoto-metric evidence for heteroploidy in the life cycle of Armillaria mellea. Mycologia 70: 487-498.

83. Korhonen, K., Hintikka, V., 1974, Cytological evidence for somatic diploidization in dikaryotic cells of Armillariella mellea. Arch. Microbiol. 95: 187-192.

84. Tommerup, I.C., Broadbent, D., 1975, Nuclear fusion, meiosis, and the origin of dikaryotic hyphae in Armillariella mellea. Arch. Microbiol. 103: 279-282.

85. Raper, J.R., 1966, "Genetics of Sexuality in Higher Fungi," Ronald Press, New York.

86. Duncan, E.G., Galbraith, M.H., 1972, Post-meiotic events in the Homobasidiomycetidae. Trans. Brit. Mycol. Soc. 58: 387-392.

87. Kühner, R., 1977, Variation of nuclear behavior in the Homobasidiomycetes. Trans. Brit. Mycol. Soc. 68: 1-16.

88. Emerson, R., Wilson, C.M., 1954, Interspecific hybrids and cytogenetics and cytotaxonomy of Euallomyces. Mycologia 46: 393-434.

89. Wilson, C.M., 1952, Meiosis in Allomyces. Bull. Torrey Bot. Club 79: 139-159.

90. Emerson, R., 1941, An experimental study of the life cycles and taxonomy of Allomyces. Lloydia 4: 77-144.

91. Olson, L.W., Borkhardt, B., 1978, Polyploidy and its control in Allomyces macrogynus. Trans. Brit. Mycol. Soc. 71: 65-76.

92. Olson, L.W., Rønne, M., 1975, Induction of abnormal male gametes and androgenesis in the aquatic phycomycete Allomyces. Protoplasma 84: 327-344.

93. Wilson, C.M., Flanagan, P.W., 1968, The life cycle and cytology of Brachyallomyces. Canad. J. Bot. 46: 1361-1367.

94. Olson, L.W., 1974, Mitosis in the aquatic phycomycete Allo-
    myces neo-moniliformis. C. R. Trav. Lab. Carlsberg 40:
    125-134.
95. Win-Tin, Dick, M.W., 1975, Cytology of Oomycetes. Evidence
    for meiosis and multiple chromosome associations in
    Saprolegniaceae and Pythiaceae, with an introduction to the
    cytotaxonomy of Achlya and Pythium. Arch. Microbiol. 105:
    283-293.
96. Green, B.R., Dick, M.W., 1972, DNA base composition and the
    taxonomy of the Oomycetes. Canad. J. Microbiol. 18: 963-968.
97. Heath, I.B., 1974, Mitosis in the fungus Thraustotheca
    clavata. J. Cell Biol. 60: 204-220.
98. Sansome, E., Sansome, F.W., 1974, Cytology and life-history
    of Peronospora parasitica on Capsella bursa-pastoris and of
    Albugo candida on C. bursa-pastoris and on Lunaria annua.
    Trans. Brit. Mycol. Soc. 62: 323-332.
99. McDonough, E.S., 1937, The nuclear history of Sclerospora
    graminicola. Mycologia 29: 151-173.
100. Huguenin, B., Boccas, B., 1970, Étude de la caryocinèse
    chez le Phytophthora parasitica Dastur. C.R. Acad. Sci.
    Paris 271: 660-663.
101. Sansome, E., Brasier, C.M., Griffin, M.J., 1975, Chromosome
    size differences in Phytophthora palmivora, a pathogen of
    cocoa. Nature 255: 704-705.
102. Brasier, C.M., Sansome, E., 1975, Diploidy and gametangial
    meiosis in Phytophthora cinnamomi, P. infestans, and P.
    drechsleri. Trans. Brit. Mycol. Soc. 65: 49-65.
103. Sansome, E., Brasier, C.M., 1973, Diploidy and chromosomal
    structural hybridity in Phytophthora infestans. Nature 241:
    344-345.
104. Sansome, E., 1977, Polyploidy and induced gametangial for-
    mation in British isolates of Phytophthora infestans. J.
    Gen. Microbiol. 99: 311-316.
105. Sansome, E., 1976, Gametangial meiosis in Phytophthora
    capsici. Canad. J. Bot. 54: 1535-1545.
106. Sansome, E., Brasier, C.M., 1974, Polyploidy associated with
    varietal differentiation in the Megasperma complex of Phyto-
    phthora. Trans. Brit. Mycol. Soc. 63: 461-467.
107. Bauch, R., 1941, Experimentelle erzeugte Polyploidreihe bei
    der Hefe. Naturwiss. 29: 687-688.
108. Levan, A., 1947, Studies on the camphor reaction of yeast.
    Hereditas 33: 457-514.
109. Levan, A., Sandwall, C.G., 1943, Quantitative investigations
    on the reaction of yeast to biologically active substances.
    Hereditas 29: 164-178.
110. Subramaniam, M.K., 1945, Induction of polyploidy in Saccharo-
    myces cerevisiae. Curr. Sci. 14: 234.
111. Thaysen, A.C., Morris, M., 1943, Preparation of a giant
    strain of Torulopsis utilis. Nature 152: 526-528.

112. Ahmad, M., Khan, A., 1954, Polygametic zygotes as a source
     of polyploidy and irregular ratios in yeast. Nature 173:
     133.
113. Mundkur, B.D., 1953, Interphase nuclei and cell sizes in a
     polyploid series of Saccharomyces. Experientia 9: 373-374.
114. McClary, D.O., Williams, M.A., Lindegren, C.C., Ogur, M.,
     1957, Chromosome counts in a polyploid series of Saccharomyces.
     J. Bact. 73: 360-364.
115. Mortimer, R.K., Hawthorne, D.C., 1973, Genetic mapping in
     Saccharomyces IV. Mapping of temperature-sensitive genes
     and use of disomic strains in localizing genes. Genetics
     74: 33-54.
116. Byers, B., Goetsch, L., 1975, Electron microscopic observa-
     tions on the meiotic karyotype of diploid and tetraploid
     Saccharomyces cerevisiae. Proc. Nat. Acad. Sci. USA 72:
     5056-5060.
117. Duntze, W., MacKay, V., Manney, T.R., 1970, Saccharomyces
     cerevisiae: a diffusible sex factor. Science 168: 1472-1473.
118. Gunge, N., Nakatomi, Y., 1972, Genetic mechanisms of rare
     matings of the yeast Saccharomyces cerevisiae heterozygous
     for mating type. Genetics 70: 41-58.
119. Leupold, U., 1956, Tetraploid inheritance in Saccharomyces.
     J. Genetics 54: 411-426.
120. Lindegren, C.C., Lindegren, G., 1951, Tetraploid Saccharomyces.
     J. Gen. Microbiol. 5: 885-893.
121. Pomper, S., Daniels, K.M., McKee, D.W., 1954, Genetic analysis
     of polyploid yeast. Genetics 39: 343-355.
122. Roman, H., 1952, Polyploidy and phenotypic ratios in Saccharo-
     myces. Genetics 37: 620.
123. Roman, H., Hawthorne, D.C., Douglas, H.C., 1951, Polyploidy
     in yeast and its bearing on the occurrence of irregular
     genetic ratios. Proc. Nat. Acad. Sci. USA 37: 79-84.
124. Roman, H., Phillips, M.M., Sands, S.M., 1955, Studies of
     polyploid Saccharomyces I. Tetraploid segregation. Genetics
     40: 546-561.
125. Leupold, U., 1956, Some data on polyploid inheritance in
     Schizosaccharomyces pombe. C. R. Lab. Carlsberg 26: 221-251.
126. Mortimer, R.K., 1958, Radiobiological and genetic studies on
     a polyploid series (haploid to hexaploid) of Saccharomyces
     cerevisiae. Radiation Res. 9: 312-326.
127. Hilger, F., 1973, Construction and analysis of tetraploid
     yeast sets for gene dosage studies. J. Gen. Microbiol. 75:
     23-31.
128. Ho, K.S.Y., 1975, The gene dosage effect of the rad 52
     mutation on X-ray survival curves of tetraploid yeast strains.
     Mutation Res. 33: 165-172.
129. Reichert, V., Winter, M., 1975, Gene dosage effects in
     polyploid strains of Saccharomyces cerevisiae containing
     gui-1 wild-type and mutant alleles. J. Bact. 124: 1041-1045.

130. Riley, M.I., Manney, T.R., 1978, Tetraploid strains of
     Saccharomyces cerevisiae that are trisomic for chromosome
     III. Genetics 89: 667-684.
131. Vezinhet, F., Pellecuer, M., Galzy, P., Pasero, J., 1975,
     Study of some anomalies of copulation in Saccharomyces
     cereviseae Hansen. Heredity 35: 109-114.
132. Winge, Ö., Roberts, C., 1958, Life history and cytology of
     yeast, Chapter 3, pp. 93-122, in Cook, A.H., (ed.), "The Chemi-
     stry and Biology of Yeasts," Academic Press, New York.
133. de Langguth, E.N., Beam, C.A., 1973, The effects of ploidy
     upon cell cycle dependent changes in X-ray sensitivity of
     Saccharomyces cerevisiae. Radiation Res. 55: 501-506.
134. Johnston, J.R., 1966, Reproductive capacity and mode of
     death of yeast cells. Antonie van Leeuwenhoek 32: 94-98.
135. Mortimer, R.K., Johnston, J.R., 1959, Life span of individual
     yeast cells. Nature 183: 1751-1752.
136. Müller, I., 1971, Experiments on ageing in single cells of
     Saccharomyces cerevisiae. Arch. Mikrobiol. 77: 20-25.
137. Hennaut, C., Hilger, F., Grenson, M., 1970, Space limitation
     for permease insertion in the cytoplasmic membrane of Saccharo-
     myces cerevisiae. Biochem. Biophys. Res. Comm. 39: 666-671.
138. Kosikov, K.V., 1977, Polyploid hybrids of Saccharomyces
     cerevisiae differing in enzymatic activity during molasses
     fermentation. Mikrobiologiya 46: 372-375.
139. Kosikov, K.V., Lyapunova, T.S., Raevskaya, O.G., Semikhatova,
     N.M., Kochkina, I.B., Meisel, M.N., 1976, Ergosterol synthesis
     by yeast hybrids and strains of the genus Saccharomyces of
     different ploidy. Mikrobiologiya 46: 86-91.
140. Kosikov, K.V., Raevskaya, O.G., 1976, Biological productivity
     of hybrids and strains of yeast of different ploidy. Mikro-
     biologiya 45: 1040-1044.
141. Kosikov, K.V., Raevskaya, O.G., Khoroshutina, E.B.,
     Perevertailo, G., 1975, Polyploid hybrids of industrial
     yeast races and prospects for their practical application.
     Mikrobiologiya 44: 682-688.
142. Mitra, K.K., 1952, Physiological consequences of polyploidy
     in yeasts. I. Fermentation characteristics of a diploid
     brewery yeast and its autotetraploid. Biochem. Biophys.
     Acta 8: 615-624.
143. Shkidchenko, A.N., Orlova, V.S., Rylkin, S.S., Korogodin,
     V.I., 1978, Comparative study of physiology and biochemistry
     of Saccharomyces cerevisiae strains of different ploidy
     during their growth. Mikrobiologiya 47: 711-716.
144. Ogur, M., Minckler, S., Lindegren, G., Lindegren, C.C.,
     1952, The nucleic acids in a polyploid series of Saccharomyces.
     Arch. Biochem. Biophys. 40: 175-184.
145. Sarachek, A., Lucke, W.H., 1953, Ultraviolet inactivation of
     polyploid Saccharomyces. Arch. Biochem. Biophys. 44: 271-279.

146. Lauer, G.D., Roberts, T.M., Klotz, L.C., 1977, Determination of the nuclear DNA content of Saccharomyces cerevisiae and implications for the organization of DNA in yeast chromosomes. J. Mol. Biol. 114: 507-526.

147. Leupold, U., 1956, Tetrad analysis of segregation in auto-tetraploids. J. Genetics, 54: 427-439.

148. Fischer, P., Binder, M., Wintersberger, V., 1975, A study of the chromosomes of the yeast Schizosaccharomyces pombe by light and electron microscopy. Exp. Cell Res. 96: 15-22.

149. McGinnis, R.C., 1953, Cytological studies of chromosomes of rust fungi. I. The mitotic chromosomes of Puccinia graminis. Canad. J. Bot. 31: 522-526.

150. McGinnis, R.C., 1954, Cytological studies of chromosomes of rust fungi. II. The mitotic chromosomes of Puccinia coronata. Canad. J. Bot. 32: 213-214.

151. McGinnis, R.C., 1956, Cytological studies of chromosomes of rust fungi. III. The relationship of chromosome number to sexuality in Puccinia. J. Heredity 47: 255-259.

152. Maclean, D.J., Tommerup, I.C., Scott, K.J., 1974, Genetic status of monokaryotic variants of the wheat stem rust fungus isolated from axenic culture. J. Gen. Microbiol. 84: 364-378.

153. Valkoun, J., Bartŭs, P., 1974, Somatic chromosome number in Puccinia recondita. Trans. Brit. Mycol. Soc. 63: 187-189.

154. Wright, R.G., Leonard, J.H., 1978, Mitosis in Puccinia striiformis 1. Light microscopy. Trans. Brit. Mycol. Soc. 70: 91-98.

155. Sansome, E., 1959, Pachytene in Puccinia kraussiana Cook, on Smilax Kraussiana. Nature 184: 1820-1821.

156. Singh, U.P., 1972, Morphology of chromosomes in Ravenelia species. Mycologia 64: 205-207.

157. Williams, P.G., 1975, Evidence for diploidy of a monokaryotic strain of Puccinia graminis f. sp. tritici. Trans. Brit. Mycol. Soc. 64: 15-22.

158. Williams, P.G., Mendgen, K.W., 1975, Cytofluorometry of DNA in uredospores of Puccinia graminis f. sp. tritici. Trans. Brit. Mycol. Soc. 64: 23-28.

159. Cummins, J.E., Day, A.W., 1977, Genetic and cell cycle analysis of a smut fungus (Ustilago violacea), Chapt. 27, pp. 445-469, in Prescott, D.M. (ed.), "Methods in Cell Biology," Vol. 15, Academic Press, New York.

160. Day, A.W., 1972, The isolation and identification of polyploid strains of Ustilago violacea. Canad. J. Genet. Cytol. 14: 925-932.

161. Day, A.W., 1972, Dominance at a fungus mating type locus. Nature, New Biol. 237: 282-283.

162. Holliday, R., 1961, Induced mitotic crossing-over in Ustilago maydis. Genet. Res. (Cambridge) 2: 231-248.

163. Day, A.W., Jones, J.K., 1971, p-Fluorophenylalanine-induced mitotic haploidization in Ustilago violacea. Genet. Res. (Cambridge) 18: 299-309.

164. Lu, B.C., Brodie, H.J., 1964, Preliminary observations of meiosis in the fungus Cyathus. Canad. J. Bot. 42: 307-310.

165. Lu, B.C., Brodie, H.J., 1962, Chromosomes of the fungus Cyathus. Nature 194: 606.

166. Lu, B.C., 1964, Polyploidy in the basidiomycete Cyathus stercoreus. Amer. J. Bot. 51: 343-347.

167. Collins, O.R., Therrien, C.D., 1976, Cytophotometric measurements of nuclear DNA in seven heterothallic isolates of Didymium iridis, a myxomycete. Amer. J. Bot. 63: 457-462.

168. Gray, W.D., Alexopoulos, C.J., 1968, "Biology of the Myxomycetes," Ronald Press, New York.

169. Collins, O.R., Therrien, C.D., Betterley, D.A., 1978, Genetical and cytological evidence for chromosome elimination in a true slime mold, Didymium iridis. Amer. J. Bot. 65: 660-670.

170. Kerr, S., 1968, Ploidy level in the true slime mold Didydmium nigripes. J. Gen. Microbiol. 53: 9-15.

171. Koevening, J.S., Jackson, R.C., 1966, Plasmodial mitosis and polyploidy in the myxomycete Physarum polycephalum. Mycologia 58: 662-667.

172. Mohberg, J., Babcock, K.L., Haugli, F.B., Rusch, H.P., 1973, Nuclear DNA content and chromosome numbers in the myxomycete Physarum polycephalum. Dev. Biol. 34: 228-245.

173. Mulleavy, P., 1979, Genetic and cytological studies in heterothallic and non-heterothallic isolates of the myxomycete, Didymium iridis. Ph.D. Dissertation, Univ. of California, Berkeley.

174. Ross, I.K., 1966, Chromosome numbers in pure and gross cultures of Myxomycetes. Amer. J. Bot. 53: 712-718.

175. Lane, E.B., Carlile, M.J., 1979, Post-fusion somatic incompatibility in plasmodia of Physarum polycephalum. J. Cell Sci. 35: 339-354.

176. Ishitani, C., Ikeda, Y., Sakaguchi, K., 1956, Hereditary variation and genetic recombination in Koji-molds (Aspergillus oryzae and A. sojae). VI. Genetic recombination in heterozygous diploids. J. Gen. Appl. Microbiol. (Tokyo) 2: 401-430.

177. Nga, B.H., Teo, S.-P., Lim, G., 1975, The occurrence in nature of a diploid strain of Aspergillus niger. J. Gen. Microbiol. 88: 364-366.

178. Käfer, E., 1977, Meiotic and mitotic recombination in Aspergillus and its chromosomal aberrations. Adv. Genetics 19: 33-131.

179. Sansome, E., 1956, Camphor-induced gigas forms in Neurospora. Trans. Brit. Mycol. Soc. 39: 67-78.

180. Imshenetskii, A., Kondrat'eva, T.F., 1968, Dehydrogenase
     activity of a polyploid form of Candida scottii. Mikro-
     biologiya 37: 784-787.
181. Imshenetskii, A., Kondrat'eva, T.F., 1972, Determination of
     the frequency of formation of induced auxotrophic mutants in
     polyploid strains of Candida scottii. Mikrobiologiya 41:
     494-499.
182. Imshenetskii, A., Kondrat'eva, T.F., 1973, Determination of
     the frequency of reversions to prototrophy in polyploid
     strains of Candida scottii. Mikrobiologiya 42: 497-500.
183. Imshenetskii, A., Kondrat'eva, T.F., 1974, Spontaneous and
     ultraviolet-induced variability in biomass production of
     polyploid strains of Candida scottii. Mikrobiologiya 43:
     884-887.
184. Imshenetskii, A., Kondrat'eva, T.F., 1976, Frequency of
     mutants with modified respiratory activity in polyploid
     strains of Candida scottii. Mikrobiologiya 45: 142-145.
185. Imshenetskii, A., Kondrat'eva, T.F., 1977, Variability of
     polyploid strains of Candida scottii in accumulation of
     riboflavin in the medium. Z. Allgemeine Mikrobiol. 17: 7-10.
186. Imshenetskii, A., Kondrat'eva, T.F., 1977, Frequency of
     arisal of nystatin-resistant mutants in polyploid strains of
     Candida scottii. Mikrobiologiya 46: 71-74.
187. Imshenetskii, A., Solntseva, L.I., Kuranova, N.F., 1963,
     Polyploid yeast-like fungi of the genus Candida. Doklady
     Akad. Nauk SSSR 152: 212-214.
188. Popova, L.S., 1966, Production of polyploids of various
     species of Candida by the action of mitotic poisons. Mikro-
     biologiya 35: 271-278.
189. Popova, L.S., 1966, Morphological and biochemical properties
     of polyploid forms of Candida scottii. Mikrobiologiya 35:
     448-457.
190. Popova, L.S., 1966, Growth and development of parent and
     polyploid cultures of Candida scottii on complex and synthetic
     media. Mikrobiologiya 35: 978-986.
191. Rogers, J.D., 1968, Xylaria curta: cytology of the ascus.
     Canad. J. Bot. 43: 1337-1340.
192. Eigsti, O.J., Dustin, P., Jr., 1955, "Colchicine - in Agri-
     culture, Medicine, Biology, and Chemistry," Iowa State
     College Press, Ames.
193. Heath, I.B., 1975, The effect of antimicrotubule agents on
     the growth and ultrastructure of the fungus Saprolegnia
     ferax and their ineffectiveness in disrupting hyphal micro-
     tubules. Protoplasma 85: 147-176.
194. Sansome, E., 1949, Spontaneous mutation in standard and
     "gigas" forms of Penicillium notatum strain 1249 B 21.
     Trans. Brit. Mycol. Soc. 32: 305-314.
195. Sansome, E., Bannon, L., 1946, Colchicine ineffective in
     inducing polyploidy in Penicillium notatum. Lancet 2: 828-831.

196. Sost, H., 1955, Über die Determination des Generationswechsels von <u>Allomyces</u> <u>arbuscula</u> (Butl.) (Polyploidieversuche). Archiv. Protistenkunde 100: 541-564.

197. Slifkin, M.K., 1967, Nuclear division in <u>Saprolegnia</u> as revealed by colchicine. Mycologia 59: 431-445.

198. Heath, I.B., 1975, Colchicine and colcemid binding components of the fungus <u>Saprolegnia</u> <u>ferax</u>. Protoplasma 85: 177-192.

199. Sansome, E., Harris, B.J., 1962, Use of camphor-induced polyploidy to determine the place of meiosis in fungi. Nature 196: 291-292.

200. Barron, G.L., 1962, The parasexual cycle and linkage relationships in the storage rot fungus <u>Penicillium</u> <u>expansum</u>. Canad. J. Bot. 40: 1603-1613.

201. Kostoff, D., 1946, Gigantism in <u>Penicillium</u>, experimentally produced. Bull. Chambre Culture Nationale, Ser. Biol., Agric. Silvic., Sophia 1: 239-240.

202. Sansome, E., 1946, Induction of "gigas" forms of <u>Penicillium</u> <u>notatum</u> by treatment with camphor vapour. Nature 157: 84-844.

203. Olson, L.W., Reichle, R., 1978, Meiosis and diploidization in the aquatic phycomycete <u>Catenaria</u> <u>anguillulae</u>. Trans. Brit. Mycol. Soc. 70: 423-437.

204. Roper, J.A., 1966, Mechamism of inheritance. 3. The parasexual cycle, Chapter 10, pp. 589-617, <u>in</u> Ainsworth, G.C., Sussman, A.S. (eds.), "The Fungi," Vol. 2, Academic Press, New York.

205. Westergaard, M., von Wettstein, D., 1972, The synaptinemal complex. Ann. Rev. Genetics 6: 71-110.

206. Aldrich, H.C., Mims, C.W., 1970, Synaptinemal complexes and meiosis in the myxomycetes. Amer. J. Bot. 57: 935-941.

207. Engels, F.M., Croes, A.F., 1968, The synaptinemal complex in yeast. Chromosoma 25: 104-106.

208. Haskins, E.F., Hinchee, A.A., Cloney, R.A., 1971, The occurrence of synaptonemal complexes in the slime mold <u>Echinostelium</u> <u>minutum</u> de Bary. J. Cell Biol. 51: 898-903.

209. Moens, P.B., Perkins, F.O., 1969, Chromosome number of a small protist: accurate determination. Science 166: 1289-1291.

210. Zickler, D., 1977, Development of the synaptonemal complex and the "recombination nodules" during meiotic prophase in the seven bivalents of the fungus <u>Sordaria</u> <u>macrospora</u> Auersw. Chromosoma 61: 289-316.

211. Gillies, C.B., 1972, Reconstruction of the <u>Neurospora</u> <u>crassa</u> pachytene karyotype from serial sections of synaptonemal complexes. Chromosoma 36: 119-130.

212. Gillies, C.B., 1979, The relationship between synaptinemal complexes, recombination nodules and crossing over in <u>Neurospora</u> bivalents and translocation quadrivalents. Genetics 91: 1-17.

213. Beakes, G.W., Gay, J.L., 1977, Gametangial nuclear division and fertilization in Saprolegnia furcata as observed by light and electron microscopy. Trans. Brit. Mycol. Soc. 69: 459-471.

214. Olson, L.W., Eden, U., Egel-Mitani, M., Egel, R., 1978, Asynaptic meiosis in fission yeast? Hereditas 89: 189-199.

215. Zickler, D., 1973, Fine structure of chromosome pairing in ten Ascomycetes: Meiotic and premeiotic (mitotic) synaptonemal complexes. Chromosoma 40: 401-416.

216. Davies, J.M.L., Jones, D.G., 1970, The origin of a diploid "hybrid" of Cercosporella herpotrichoides. Heredity 25: 137-139.

217. Haskins, E.F., 1977, The occurrence of nuclear fusion in the amoebal phase of the slime mold Echinostelium minutum: a reinterpretation of the significance of this phenomenon. Canad. J. Bot. 55: 3020-3022.

218. Therrien, C.D., Bell, W.R., Collins, O.R., 1977, Nuclear DNA content of myxamoebae and plasmodia in six non-heterothallic isolates of a myxomycete, Didymium iridis. Amer. J. Bot. 64: 286-291.

219. Mortimer, A.M., Shaw, D.S., 1975, Cytofluorimetric evidence for meiosis in gametangial nuclei of Phytophthora drechsleri. Genet. Res. (Cambridge) 25: 201-205.

220. Laffler, T.G., Dove, W.F., 1977, Viability of Physarum polycephalum spores and ploidy of plasmodial nuclei. J. Bact. 131: 473-476.

221. Lemke, P.A., Ellison, J.R., Marino, R., Morimoto, B., Arons, E., Kohman, P., 1975, Fluorescent Feulgen staining of fungal nuclei. Exp. Cell Res. 96: 367-373.

222. Heagy, F.C., Roper, J.A., 1952, Deoxyribonucleic acid content of haploid and diploid Aspergillus conidia. Nature 170: 713-714.

223. Van der Walt, J.P., de Leeuw, J., 1970, Ploidy differences in Cryptococcus albidus. Mycopathol. Mycol. Applicata 42: 17-24.

224. Grewal, N.S., Miller, J.J., 1972, Formation of asci with two diploid spores by diploid cells of Saccharomyces. Canad. J. Microbiol. 18: 1897-1905.

225. Lenhart, K., Hejtmánková, N., 1972, Parasexual cycle in dermatophytes. Experientia 28: 711.

226. Typas, M.A., Heale, J.B., 1977, Analysis of ploidy levels in strains of Verticillium using a Coulter counter. J. Gen. Microbiol. 101: 177-180.

227. Warshaw, S.D., 1952, Effect of ploidy in photoreactivation. Proc. Soc. Exp. Biol. Med. 79: 268-271.

228. Pontecorvo, G., Käfer, E., 1958, Genetic analysis by means of mitotic recombination. Adv. Genetics 9: 71-104.

229. Gauger, W.L., 1975, Further studies on sexuality in azygosporic strains of Mucor hiemalis. Trans. Brit. Mycol. Soc. 64: 113-118.

230. Ingram, R., 1968, *Verticillium dahliae* var. *longisporum*, a stable diploid. Trans. Brit. Mycol. Soc. 51: 339-341.

231. Lhoas, P., 1961, Mitotic haploidization by treatment of *Aspergillus niger* diploids with *para*-Fluorophenylalananine. Nature 190: 744.

232. Raper, J.R., Flexer, A.S., 1970, The road to diploidy with emphasis on a detour, pp. 401-432, *in* "Organization and Control in Prokaryotic and Eukaryotic cells," 20th Sym. Soc. Gen. Microbiol., Cambridge Univ. Press, London.

233. Raper, J.R., 1968, On the evolution of fungi: Chapt. 27, pp. 677-693, *in* Ainsworth, G.C., Sussman, A.S. (eds.), "The Fungi," Vol III, Academic Press, New York.

234. Adams, J., 1974, Fitness and the single genome: does ploidy matter? Genetics 77: S1.

235. Adams, J., Hansche, P.E., 1974, Population studies in microorganisms I. Evolution of diploidy in *Saccharomyces cerevisiae*. Genetics 76: 327-338.

POLYPLOIDY IN BRYOPHYTES WITH SPECIAL EMPHASIS ON MOSSES

Marshall R. Crosby

Missouri Botanical Garden
P.O. Box 299
St. Louis, MO 63166

Bryophytes are a group of about 14,000 species of non-vascular, green, land plants. Included in the group are mosses, liverworts, and hornworts. The group has long been treated as monophyletic, but recent evidence from a variety of sources, including cytology, indicates that this may not be so. For purposes of this discussion three classes of bryophytes are recognized: Musci--mosses, with six subclasses and some 800 genera and 9,000 species (1); Anthocerotae--hornworts, with about five genera and 300 species (2); and Hepaticae--liverworts, with about 400 genera and 5,500 species (2,3). Polyploidy is rare in Anthocerotae and Hepaticae, is apparently of little significance in those groups, and will be discussed here only briefly, to contrast them with mosses.

Data concerning the chromosome numbers of bryophytes have been accumulating for nearly 90 years (4). Many pre-1930 counts are erroneous, mainly because observations were made using paraffin-embedded material. The squash techniques first introduced in the late 1920's (5), and refined since then, have led to the rapid accumulation of many accurate counts of bryophyte chromosome numbers: the number of counts of mosses increased from about 120, representing about 90 species and infraspecies, in the late 1940's (6) to about 2,200, representing about 1,000 species and infraspecies, today. In the past 35 years bryologists have done a good job of producing up-to-date catalogs of the chromosome numbers known for bryophytes (6-8). Using these catalogs, together with the primary literature and their own results, bryologists have produced an excellent series of review articles discussing the significance of bryophyte chromosomes, including polyploidy (8-12). The most recent (12) contains an excellent review of polyploidy in bryophytes, considering the phenomenon as it relates to most levels of classification from that of class to various infraspecific ranks. This paper will, for the most part, summarize and comment on this recent review.

POLYPLOIDY IN THE SUBCLASSES OF MOSSES

Mosses are generally classified into six major groups, and the interrelationships of these are fairly well agreed upon by muscologists, though the groups are given different rank in different schemes of classification. The scheme used here recognizes six subclasses and has been discussed in more detail elsewhere (1). The first two subclasses represent separate lines which are isolated from each other and from the last four subclasses, and within these latter four, the first two are similarly isolated from each other and the last two subclasses.

Comments concerning the level of ploidy refer to the gametophyte, and x is used to refer to basic haploid numbers, n being used to refer to functional haploid numbers.

Andreaeideae: Two genera, 50–100 species. n=10,11.
Polyploidy: Three species have been counted, and no polyploidy is known in this subclass. There is evidence of aneuploidy.
General: Cytologically the Andreaeideae resemble neither the Sphagnideae nor the Bryidae in the broadest sense, that is in the sense which includes the last four subclasses recognized here in a single subclass. There is no cytological evidence to support the suggestion (13) that Andreaeidae are intermediate between these two groups.

Sphagnidae: One genus, 100 species. x=19 (+ m).
Polyploidy: 22 species have been counted, and three are polyploid species. Aneuploidy is unknown. The polyploid species tend to be more robust and coarser than the haploid species.
General: The number 19 is very rare among mosses, and this number together with the unique morphology of the Sphagnidae isolate the group from the other subclasses of mosses.

Tetraphidae: One or two genera, three or four species. n=7,8.
Polyploidy: One species counted. Polyploidy is unknown, and there is some aneuploidy.
General: Cytology supports the placement, based on peristome structure, of the Tetraphidae near the Polytrichidae: the basic chromosome number is the same or nearly the same; chromosomes are large, resembling those of Polytrichidae; bivalents remain more or less rounded as in Polytrichidae; and, though the sample is small, aneuploidy is unknown in the group.

Polytrichidae: 25 genera, 300 species. x=7.

Polyploidy: 70 species have been counted. There are seven known polyploid species, and infraspecific polyploidy is known in eleven species. Aneuploidy is unknown in the subclass.

General: If this is an ancient group, as has often been suggested, the chromosome number seems to have stabilized early. Based on what we know about the cytology of the group, processes other than polyploidy, aneuploidy, and gross morphological changes in chromosomes have played a role in differentiation of taxa. Most of the species of Polytrichidae are dioicous. The few monoicous species have arisen from dioicous ones mostly through apospory. For example, in <u>Atrichum</u> morphologically related monoicous/dioicous species pairs have been shown to have haploid and diploid chromosome complements, respectively, with the diploid complement being morphologically similar to the haploid one (14,15), though one exception to this is known (16).

Buxbaumiidae: Four genera, 35 species. n=8,9.

Polyploidy: Five species have been counted, but polyploidy has not been found in the Buxbaumiidae. There is some aneuploidy.

General: The relationships of the Buxbaumiidae remain obscure, some authors placing them with the arthrodont mosses, those with articulate peristome teeth (Bryidae) (1), and others placing them with the nematodont mosses, those with solid peristome teeth (Tetraphidae and Polytrichidae) (12). The large, rounded chromosomes are similar to those of the Polytrichidae.

Bryidae: About 770 genera, 8,500 species. x=6-8.

Polyploidy: Chromosome numbers have been counted for approximately 900 species of Bryidae. As long as 25 years ago, when considerably less than 200 species had had their chromosomes counted, the idea that most mosses are polyploid in nature was put forth (17). This conclusion was graphically represented in a histogram which plotted the number of species of mosses on the vertical axis against the number of chromosomes on the horizontal axis. Major peaks in the numbers of species occurred at 6-8 and 10-14 chromosomes, with smaller peaks at 20-21, 24-26, and 26-30 chromosomes. A similar histogram was prepared in the late 1960's, when the number of species known cytologically had increased by a factor of about four (18). Plotting the number of counts against gametophytic chromosome number, it was found that 12% of the species had n=6-8; 57% had n=10-14, 8% had n=18-22; and 5% had n=26-28. This suggests that the basic chromosome number for the Bryidae is x=6-8, and that the vast majority of species are functionally polyploid, with most being diploid.

Since the Bryidae are such a large and diverse group, more detailed analyses of chromosomes' variation within the group, based on histograms, have been made, as more chromosome numbers have accumulated. Thus, in the late 1960's it was shown that chromosome numbers among acrocarpous mosses, those producing gametangia on stem tips and having basically upright growth forms, are much more variable than among pleurocarpous mosses, those producing gametangia on lateral branches and having basically prostrate growth forms. Among the Bryidae many taxonomically difficult groups are acrocarpous, for example the families Pottiaceae, Bryaceae and Funariaceae, and these groups tend to occupy disturbed habitats, where physical damage to sporophytes may induce autopolyploids. Other acrocarpous groups, for example Grimmiaceae, occur in exposed habitats which may induce disturbances in meiosis. As noted, as a group the acrocarpous mosses display greater variation in chromosome numbers than do the pleurocarps, which tend to occupy more stable and less rigorous habitats (18).

A more refined analysis of the variation in chromosome numbers of Bryidae avoids the somewhat artificial division of the subclass into acrocarpous and pleurocarpous groups and analyzes the subclass on the basis of haplolepidous peristomes, those derived from two concentric cell layers, and diplolepidous peristomes, those derived from three concentric cell layers (12). All haplolepidous mosses are acrocarpous in habit, but among diplolepidous mosses there are large numbers of families which are either acrocarpous or pleurocarpous in habit. When only haplolepidous mosses are considered, nearly 40% are found to have n=13, and smaller peaks are found at n=12,14, and 26. The general shape of the histogram for haplolepidous mosses is similar to that of pleurocarpous mosses, all of which are diplolepidous, though the curve has been shifted somewhat to the left in the case of the diplolepidous mosses: among them the main peak, representing 40% of the counts, is at n=11, with smaller peaks at n=10,18, and 20. The peaks in the area of n=6-8 have disappeared (18), because most mosses with chromosome numbers in this range belong to the final group, the acrocarpous/diplolepidous mosses. In this group major peaks are found at n=6,10-11, and 21. This group is thus responsible for the large amount of variation found among all acrocarpous mosses in the late 1960's (18).

If the basic number for the Bryidae is interpreted as x=6-8, which seems reasonable, then the acrocarpous/haplolepidous mosses and the pleurocarpous/diplolepidous mosses appear to be derived groups which are now basically diploid in nature. The acrocarpous/ diplolepidous mosses appear to contain more groups with the primitive, x=6-8, chromosome number. Although this group has often been treated as containing some of the more advanced members of the Bryidae, some members of it, specifically Bryaceae and Funariaceae, have been suggested as representing the most primitive, generalized forms of Bryidae living today on the basis of morphological characteristics (1,19).

The assumption that most Bryidae are functionally polyploid in the gametophytic generation makes sense in the light of several observations concerning the biology of mosses (18):

1) Aneuploidy is a common occurrence in mosses. If gametophytes are at diploid or higher ploidy levels, deletions of

genetic material through the loss of chromosomes would not be severe, due to the masking effect of the polyploid complement.

2) Mosses easily regenerate leafy plants from sporophytic material, giving rise to autopolyploids.

3) Mosses possess a variety of means of vegetative reproduction, which allow them to tide over periods of meiotic irregularities brought about by increased ploidy levels. It has been demonstrated experimentally that artificially produced polyploids regain their ability to produce viable spores through successive vegetative generations.

In contrast to the situation in mosses, polyploidy (and aneuploidy) is rare among Hepaticae: 85% of the species have n=8-10, 2% have n=4-6, and 9% have n=16-18 (18). The rareness of aneuploidy suggests that loss of chromosomes is deleterious. And this would be true if gametophytes are functionally haploid. This leads to the suggestion that for the Hepaticae x=8-10 and that the smaller peaks at smaller and greater numbers represent anueploidy and polyploidy respectively.

Again, in contrast to mosses, Hepaticae do not commonly demonstrate aneuploidy, do not reproduce vegetatively from sporophytic material, thus lacking the means to tide themselves over during periods of meiotic irregularities, and do not regenerate from sporophytic material, thus lacking the means for easily producing autopolyploids.

LITERATURE CITED

1. Crosby, M.R., The diversity and relationships of mosses, in Taylor, R.J. (ed.), "North American Mosses: a symposium," Amer. Assoc. Adv. Sci. (in press).

2. Schuster, R.M., 1966, "The Hepaticae and Anthocerotae of North America east of the Hundredth Meridian," Vol. 1, Columbia University Press, New York and London. xvii + 802 pp.

3. Schuster, R.M., 1978, Personal communication.

4. Kruch, O., 1891, Appunti sullo sviluppo degli organi sessuali e sulla fecondazione della Riella clausonis Les. Malpighia 4: 403-423.

5. Heitz, E., 1926, Der Nachweis der Chromosomen. Zeitschr. Bot. 18: 625-681.

6. Lowry, R.J., 1948, A cytotaxonomic study of the genus Mnium. Mem. Torrey Bot. Club 20(2). 42 pp.

7. Anderson, L.E., 1962, Chromosome numbers: Bryophyta, pp. 45-57, in Altman, P.L., Dittmer, D.S. (eds.), "Growth, including Reproduction and Morphological Development," FASEB Biol. Handb. Ser., Washington, D.C.

8.   Fritsch, R., 1972, Chromosomenzahlen der Bryophyten, eine
     Übersicht und Diskussion ihres Aussagewertes für das System.
     Wiss. Zeitschr. Friedrich-Schiller Univ. Jena, Math.-Naturwiss.
     Reihe. 21: 839-944.
9.   Anderson, L.E., 1964, Biosystematic evaluations in the
     Musci. Phytomorphology 14: 27-51.
10. Anderson, L.E., 1974, Bryology: 1947-1972. Ann. Missouri
     Bot. Gard. 61: 56-85.
11. Steere, W.C., 1972, Chromosome numbers in bryophytes. J.
     Hattori Bot. Lab. 35: 99-125.
12. Smith, A.J.E., 1978, Cytogenetics, biosystematics and evolu-
     tion in the Bryophyta, pp. 195-276, in Woolhouse, H.W.,
     (ed.), "Advances in Botanical Research," Vol. 6, Academic
     Press, New York.
13. Steere, W.C., Murray, B.M., 1976, Andreaeobryum macrosporum,
     a new genus and species of Musci from northern Alaska and
     Canada. Phytologia 33: 407-410.
14. Lowry, R.J., 1954, Chromosome numbers and relationships in
     the genus Atrichum in North America. Amer. J. Bot. 41:
     410-414.
15. Ireland, R.R., 1969, Taxonomic studies on the genus Atrichum
     in North America. Canad. J. Bot. 47: 353-368.
16. Vaarama, A., 1953, Some chromosome numbers of Californian and
     Finnish moss species. Bryologist 56: 169-177.
17. Steere, W.C., Anderson, L.E., Bryan, V.S., 1954, Chromosome
     studies on California mosses. Mem. Torrey Bot. Club 20(4).
     75 pp.
18. Smith, A.J.E., Newton, M.E., 1968, Chromosome studies on
     some British and Irish mosses. III. Trans. Brit. Bryol.
     Soc. 5: 463-522.
19. Edwards, S.R., 1979, Taxonomic implications of cell pattern
     in haplolepidous moss peristomes, in "Modern Approaches to
     Bryophyte Systematics," Academic Press, New York (in press).

W. H. Wagner, Jr. and Florence S. Wagner[1]

Department of Botany
University of Michigan
Ann Arbor, MI   48109

Chromosome studies of pteridophytes had their major impetus
in the work of Irene Manton (1) who was the first to show the
far-reaching significance of polyploidy in these plants. Her
work was followed not only by numerous investigations by her own
students at the University of Leeds but by researchers in many
parts of the world, including especially India, Japan, New Zealand,
Costa Rica, United States, Canada, Germany, Italy, and Hungary.
Two major works have appeared in the past couple of years, namely
the very thorough analysis of "Evolutionary Patterns and Processes
in Ferns" by J.D. Lovis (2) and "A Cytotaxonomical Atlas of the
Pteridophyta" by Á Löve, D. Löve, and R.E.G. Pichi-Sermolli
(3,4).
The "polyploid pteridophytes" of our title refer to homosporous taxa, which are the bulk of living forms, and which are
generally believed to have been influenced by polyploidy in two
ways -- (a) ancient genome multiplications associated with the
early origins of the modern lines at the level of genera and
families, and (b) more recent, additional genome reduplications
associated with processes of auto- and allopolyploidy at the
level of species and varieties. For the most part, heterosporous
pteridophytes tend to have low chromosome numbers like those
found in seed plants. Homosporous types have high base numbers,
such as the woodferns, Dryopteris, with x=41 and polypodies,

---

[1]Paper prepared under National Science Grant INT78-19909.
We acknowledge the aid of Craig A. Ludwig in writing the manuscript and Luis Diego Gómez P. for his contributions to our
studies of polyploidy.

with x=37, in contrast to the heterosporous types with lower
numbers, like water-clovers, <u>Marsilea</u> with x=20 and quillworts
with x=11. It may be speculated that the former are at least
hexaploids or octoploids, while the latter are diploids and
tetraploids.

The special features of homosporous pteridophytes, as opposed
to heterosporous pteridophytes and seed plants, include peculiarities of the life cycle. Homosporous pteridophytes bear both
types of gametangia on their gametophytes; they are thus monoecious.
Heterosporous vascular plants have separately borne sex organs:
the male gametes are produced by microspores and the female
gametes are produced by megaspores. Recent work by Klekowski
(5,6,7,8) shows that not only are individual gametophytes capable
of producing both types of gametes but they can produce them at
the same time and thus accomplish fertilization by genetically
identical gametes. This has a number of important genetic implications. Selfing of a single gametophyte is obviously not comparable genetically to the selfing of seed plants. In the former
the gametes are genetically alike, but in the latter, even though
they come from the same sporophyte originally, the gametes are
genetically different; each gamete represents a different product
of meiosis.

Other peculiarities of homosporous pteridophytes include
their base chromosome numbers, already mentioned above, and the
pairing behavior of the chromosomes as observed at the time of
early metaphase. The base chromosome numbers of homosporous
pteridophytes are the highest known in vascular plants, averaging
somewhere around x=35-40. Some genera have much higher base
numbers, like <u>Psilotum</u> with x=52, <u>Cibotium</u> with 68, <u>Equisetum</u>
with 108 and <u>Ophioglossum</u> with 120. Workers with seed plants,
used as they are to much lower numbers, express skepticism about
the accuracy of our observations, but the fact is that except for
their high numbers ferns have rather easily studied chromosomes.
They are very uniform in size, as a rule, and not nearly as tiny
as many of those found in seed plants. Furthermore, it has
become customary to accompany chromosome interpretations with
actual photographs, a policy developed by Manton (1) to insure
high standards of accuracy. "What cannot be photographed cannot
be used as evidence." It is true, of course, that some pteridophytes do have difficult chromosomes. For example, some of the
clubmosses, <u>Lycopodium</u>, are hard to interpret because of odd
configurations.

Another boon to the cytotaxonomist is the fact that most
pteridophytes apparently form only singles and pairs where there
is irregular pairing at metaphase, as in hybrid complexes. It is
usually very simple to tell the differences between a univalent
and a bivalent, and where a unit appears to be a trivalent or
tetravalent it usually proves to be two or more units lying on
top of each other. Sterile hybrids of the constitution AB or ABC
commonly have no pairing at all as seen at metaphase. The entire

field is made up of singles. Likewise (and almost invariably) allopolyploid backcrosses of the constitution AAB show n pairs and n singles.

Lovis (2) has reviewed the fossil record of ferns, and he concludes that practically all modern ferns arose between the Cretaceous and the Paleocene periods, and he suggests that the radiation of angiosperms may have had something to do with it. In his words: "... the angiosperm radiation and expansion, with the drastic changes this produced in the structure of the world's vegetation, involving the evolution of ecosystems more complex than any seen previously in the history of the earth, most probably provided the trigger or stimulus for the production of the dennstaedtiaceous radiation, and may well have promoted or accelerated the adiantaceous and polypodiaceous (s.s.) radiations. ... The appearance of the main "polypodiaceous" radiations does seem to constitute the most recent major innovation in the evolution of the world's flora."

This does not mean that paleopolyploidy necessarily arose at the time of the evolutionary explosion of the modern ferns. Evidence for this lies among the primitive ferns, such as the Marattiaceae with x=40, Ophioglossaceae with x=45 and 120, and Osmundaceae with x=22, which on morphological and (or) chronological grounds are considered to be very ancient. Also, Lycopodiaceae (see Table 1 for chromosome numbers) run back to the Upper Devonian, and Equisetaceae (today known only as high paleopolyploids with x=108) to the Upper Carboniferous (9). Just when

Table 1. Gametophytic denominators in Lycopodium.

Polyploidy	Aneuploidy	Actual No.	Taxon
G R O U P I			
12X11	None	132	Huperzia
G R O U P II			
2X11	22+1	23	Diphasiastrum
3X11	33+1	34	Lycopodium
7X11	77+1	78	Lycopodiella

the paleopolyploidy at the levels of family and genus arose in homosporous pteridophytes can only be guessed at.

Before pursuing the subject of the origins of paleoploidy, we should, in fairness, consider the possibility that the original vascular land plants may have had high chromosome numbers, and

that what we see today is a vestige of the time in the past when
they were first beginning their evolution. The question is this:
Are the high numbers of homosporous pteridophytes actually
primitive and have they been mistakenly interpreted as derivative?
In support of an affirmative answer is the curious observation
that those pteridophytes with the most specialized morphology,
viz. the heterosporous taxa, have the low (presumably diploid)
numbers. Also, the fact that the chromosomes of homosporous
pteridophytes tend to be very uniform in size and structure (in
spite of efforts to karyotype them; see below) favors a positive
answer. The general picture seems to fit into the old tradition
that numerous like parts precede few unlike parts, both in animals
and plants. Indeed we know that in certain groups where strong
aneuploid reductions have taken place, e.g. Lomariopsis and
Hymenophyllum (2) variations in size between chromosomes do
develop. Certainly the fact that, with rare exceptions, all
homosporous pteridophytes have high numbers is significant.
Applying the general rule for deducing primitive states by
comparing all of the taxa and finding the common condition would
seem to endorse the idea that the condition of many chromosomes
is primitive. Included in this comparison are such extraordinarily
diverse elements as Lycopodiales, Equisetales, Psilotales, Ophi-
oglossales, Marattiales, and Polypodiales -- all of which have
high numbers. Either the high numbers are traceable back to a
common ancestor and aneuploid changes have reduced them, or there
is some adaptive factor that makes it advantageous for the homosporous pteridophytes to multiply their genomes.
      To resolve the question of whether the high chromosome
numbers of homosporous pteridophytes are primitive or derived

Table 2.   Primitive chromosome numbers, heterosporous genera.

Genus	n =	Denominator
Azolla	22	11
Salvinia	9	9
Marsilea	20, 22	10, 11
Pilularia	10	10
Regnellidium	19	9, 10
Isoetes	11	11
Selaginella	7[a], 8[a], 9, 10	7[a], 8[a], 9, 10

Generalized: 7[a], 8[a], 9, 10, 11

[a] Numbers found in only one genus.

Table 3.   Probable base numbers.

Magnoliophytes	7 – 9
Gnetophytes	7 – 12
Coniferophytes	10 – 13
Cycadophytes	8 – 13
Pteridophytes	9 – 11

there is actually at present no definitive evidence. We base
our ideas upon the outside evidence entirely: As shown in Tables 2
and 3, the numbers found in heterosporous pteridophytes and in
seed plants are basically low. We assume, therefore, that the
homosporous vascular plants became specialized and had to undergo
polyploidization to achieve their present high numbers. This
assumption, whether correct or not, will provide the groundwork
for the discussion to follow. The "paleopolyploid" condition
will represent the presumed ancient numbers that today constitute
the base numbers for which no lower denominators are known. The
"neopolyploid" condition is that in which lower denominators do
exist.

The basic chromosome numbers have proved to be extremely
valuable in the interpretation of families and genera of pteridophytes -- perhaps more significant in these plants than in any
others. The Genera Filicum of Copeland (10) tried to update
fern classification, and presented a complete review of the
genera as he saw them. It was not long, however, before Manton
(1) began establishing the broad outlines of the chromosome
evidence, and soon it became apparent that a number of changes
would be necessary. Prominent among these was the breaking apart
of Copeland's "Pteridaceae." In particular the adiantoid ferns
(including Vittarioideae, Adiantoideae, and Pteridoideae), which
he had placed together with a wide variety of other fern groups,
showed up as distinct, with x=30 (and apparent aneuploids based
upon this). The correlations of chromosome numbers with various
systems of classification have been reviewed in considerable
detail by Lovis (2). Among the many striking findings was that
the Asplenium group so long associated with the Athyrium group
proved to have a different basic number, 36 in the former and 40
in the latter. The Thelypteris group, so long associated with
the Dryopteris group, has 36 in the former and 41 in the latter.
And Pteris and its relatives, associated with Pteridium, was
shown to differ from it, with 29 and 26 respectively.

As discussed below, the segregates of Lycopodium, based
largely upon morphological considerations, turned out to have
very distinctive chromosome numbers, so distinct that many authors
today regard the old genus Lycopodium as actually made up of four
valid genera. However, Equisetum, out of which some authors

would like to carve a segregate genus Hippochaete, has proved
monotonously to have x=108 throughout. The Psilotales, the
relationships of which have been controversial (11), comprise two
very different-appearing genera, Psilotum and Tmesipteris;
nevertheless, their chromosome complements support their close
relationship, both having x=52.

Extensive aneuploid changes do occasionally occur. There
are some clear-cut examples among several groups of obviously
related ferns. The group presently construed as comprising a
single genus Blechnum displays the series 36,34,33,32,29, and 28.
In the case of Thelypteris, traditionally considered a single
genus, an even more complete series is present: 36,35,34,32,31,30,
29,28, and 27; however, critical work currently being carried out
by R.E. Holttum in England and Alan R. Smith in the United States
is leading to a clearer definition of the components of the
thelypterid group, and there seem to be good correlations of
chromosome numbers with the segregates. In the case of the
traditional large genus Lindsaea we find numbers as different as
·82,47, and 34. The most extensive aneuploid series is probably
that in the filmy ferns (Hymenophylloideae)-36,34,33,32,28,26,22,21,
18,13,11.

The attempt to find low base numbers for homosporous ferns
has included efforts to karyotype somatic genomes by Tatuno and
his co-workers (12,13,14). However, the results have proved to
be inconclusive. Duncan and Smith (15) analyzed the karyological
data and concluded that unreasonable inferences had been made,
and indeed that karyotypic analysis in ferns is a "dubious
practice." Using quantitative techniques they found numerous
sources of error, and they wrote as follows: "We conclude that
although polyploidy may very well be a part of the evolutionary
history of ferns, the karyological data thus far presented do not
show this. We believe, therefore, that it is premature to postulate
primary basic chromosome numbers for ferns."

A number of workers have come up with imaginative arithmetical
schemes attempting to deduce the original low chromosome numbers
of the ancestral vascular plants, most of them based upon common
denominators with more or less aneuploidy hypothesized. We
present in Table 1 as an example of such deduction the genus
Lycopodium and its segregates. Using the simplest explanation of
this situation, and assuming that all the taxa had a common
ancestor, a base number of x=11 seems likely. The numbers 10 and
11 seem to appear most often in schemes based upon arithmetical
considerations. Whatever the base numbers are, no one seems to
have questioned that the family-genus polyploidy in homosporous
pteridophytes involves different levels, from tetraploid up to at
least as high as duodecaploid. Thus Diphasiastrum and Osmunda
with x=23 and 22 respectively represent a low level, and the
cyatheoids with present day lowest numbers in the 50's and 60's
represent a high level. If we can in fact accept the idea that

all or most homosporous pteridophytes are paleopolyploids of
various ploidal levels, then it would seem most useful to obtain

Table 4.   Estimated levels of polyploidy.

Genome Composition	x=	Example
	17	
2X9........................	18	
	19	
2X10.......................	20	Gleichenia
	21	
2X11.......................	22	Osmunda, Gleichenia
	23	Diphasiastrum
	24	
	25	
	26	Matonia, Pteridium
3X9....................	27	
	28	
	29	Pteris
3X10...................	30	Vittaria, Adiantum, Lygodium
	31	
	32	
3X11..................	33	Dipteris
	34	Gleichenia, Lycopodium
	35	
4X9................	36	Polypodium, Grammitis, Asplenium, Thelypteris
	37	
	38	Anemia
	39	
4X10..............	40	Marattia, Athyrium
	41	Dryopteris, Polystichum
	42	
	43	
4X11..............	44	
5X9..........	45	Botrychium
	46	Dennstaedtia
	47	
	48	
	49	
5X10..........	50	Loxsoma

outside evidence from heterosporous pteridophytes which are diploids. Also comparisons may be made with the known base numbers of the different lines of seed plants, the ancestors of which were themselves presumably once pteridophytes.

If we do this we learn that the base chromosome numbers or common denominators now known among living heterosporous pteridophytes are x=9,10, and 11, as shown in Table 2. The low numbers of 7 and 8 are found in a few spikemosses, Selaginella, but the other numbers are more widespread and reappear in two or more genera. These three numbers seem remarkably persistent, in view of the wide diversity of plants involved, belonging to strongly differentiated lines of evolution, including two or three major lines of ferns and two major lines of lycopsids. For comparison of modern-day seed plants we used Raven's (16) numerical estimates for the angiosperms (x=7 for angiosperms at large and x=9 for Caryophyllidae); and several sources for the numbers of the various classes of gymnosperms. Table 3 shows the base number ranges for seed plants in comparison with those for the heterosporous pteridophytes. The average range in base numbers of living seed plants is 8-12, slightly wider than that of the heterosporous pteridophytes at 9-11. If we can assume that the latter numbers do have a probable validity for the original diploid conditions of the homosporous ferns, then we can obtain estimates like those in Table 4. Osmunda and Diphasiastrum would most likely be paleotetraploids; the adiantoid ferns paleohexaploids; and the dryopteroids paleooctoploids. Gleichenia may have two origins: tetraploid and hexaploid or octoploid. The high level found in cyatheoid ferns may represent 10-ploid or 12-ploid origins.

Although we do agree with Duncan and Smith (15) that it is premature to postulate basic numbers for ferns, we do not believe that we should not form any hypotheses about them. The important questions of (a) whether homosporous pteridophytes are truly polyploid in the first place, (b) the reasons for polyploidization if they are, (c) the systematic significance of present-day base numbers, and (d) the relationship of high chromosome numbers to variability, life cycle, and evolutionary potential -- all of these are involved in our understanding the structure and genetic nature of the genome. So long as the limits of reliability are always kept in mind we should continue to pursue any sources of data that will clarify our understanding of the paleopolyploidy of homosporous pteridophytes.

Most of the work on polyploid pteridophytes has involved description of chromosome observations, tabulating records, and working out reticulate patterns of taxonomic relationships. Relatively little attention has been paid to the significance of paleopolyploidy and its over-all biological relevance. The leading theorist in this area has been Edward J. Klekowski, Jr., whose ideas have been rather controversial. His first statement regarding the adaptive significance of polyploidy in homosporous

pteridophytes (8) contained the germ of his ideas, which were
subsequently developed in a series of papers (see bibliography).
In essence the theory has to do with the genetic consequences of
gametophytic selfing, and the basic premises run as follows:
   a. The gametophytes of homosporous pteridophytes have the
   ability to self-fertilize (which he calls "intragametophytic
   mating"), as evidenced by various controlled experiments
   using single gametophytes.
   b. The further away the spore shower gets from the mother
   sporophyte, the more likely that only a single spore will
   reach a suitable germination site. [This is supported by
   numerous observations by researchers on pollen dispersal.]
   c. Accordingly it is to be expected that a very large
   number of colonies of homosporous pteridophytes begin as
   single spores; the resultant solitary gametophytes, therefore,
   must either self-fertilize to produce a sporophyte or simply
   perish.
The genetic consequence of this leads to problems of variability:
   d. The result of such habitual intragametophytic mating
   leads to homozygosity and consequent effects involving
   genetic load (e.g., deleterious alleles) as well as evolutionary potential.
   e. The problems of homozygosity may be solved by redupli-
   cating chromosome sets, so that every gene undergoes repe-
   tition and it is possible to maintain stored variability in
   the multiple genomes.
   f.   Accordingly, in evolution of modern homosporous pteridophytes, paleopolyploidy arose not as a mere passive
   accumulation of genomes but as an adaptation to counteract
   the commonly homozygotizing effects of the mating system and
   to maintain variability.
   g.   Another means of maintaining variability now possible
   in polyploid gametophytic selfers is homeologous pairing
   between the corresponding members of the several genomes.
   For criticisms of these ideas, see Lovis (2). Clearly much
further work is called for by the stimulating theory proposed by
Klekowski, including not only laboratory research but field
studies of natural populations as well, the latter aimed to
determine just what percentage of new populations is in fact
initiated by single spores.
   In spite of their apparent high polyploid numbers, the
homosporous pteridophytes appear to be evolving actively today.
A number of genera (or generic groups made of slightly differentiated elements) contain from 200 to 700 species (e.g.,
Lycopodium segregate Huperzia, Grammitis, Pteris, Cyathea,
Elaphoglossum, Athyrium, Blechnum, and Asplenium). If according
to genetic theory, polyploidy has a depressing effect on evolutionary change, then it seems reasonable to postulate that in the
pteridophytes mechanisms do exist that promote variability.
There is no question that most of the present-day "higher ferns"

appear to be undergoing active evolution, especially in the
extensive tropical rain forests of the world.

Artificial doubling of chromosome numbers in ferns is a
simple procedure involving merely the sowing of spores. The
first experimental use of this technique was apparently reported
in 1957 (17), when a sterile AB type of hybrid spleenwort,
Asplenium ebenoides R.R. Scott, was doubled by sowing large
numbers of spores, some of which had failed to undergo meiosis
properly. The diploid gametophytes fertilized either themselves
or other diploids and thus produced the fertile AABB form.
DeBenedictis (18) used this technique extensively to determine
whether "sterile hybrids" could produce viable spores and gametophytes, and she found that almost all of the fifty hybrids she
studied produced spores from unreduced spore mother cells or
sporocytes. She called them sporocytic spores. Gametophytes
with doubled chromosome numbers involving sterile hybrids are
much easier to detect, of course, than those involving fertile,
normal species; only the doubled spores will germinate from the
hybrids, but both doubled and normal undoubled spores will germinate in species. There is no reason to believe that this
process does not occur also in nature. In higher plants, Harlan
and deWet (19) concluded that almost all polyploids arise by way
of unreduced gametes, and that the most common origin is 2n + n,
the resulting triploid giving tetraploids on backcrossing and
hexaploids in selfing. The situation in homosporous pteridophytes
is different: the familiar "hybridization followed by chromosome
doubling" is probably the usual route for allopolyploids, mediated
by unreduced spores and self-fertilization, and this may apply
also to autopolyploids.

Pteridophytes very likely run the complete gamut from strict
autopolyploids of the sort that one produces in the laboratory to
extreme allopolyploids in which the parents, as judged by physiological and morphological characteristics, are sharply and
extensively differentiated genetically. The latter involve
hybrids between distinct taxa at the level of species and genera.
Most of the so-called autopolyploids reported in natural populations of pteridophytes have proved to have at least some degree
of differentiation. For example, the U.S.A.-Canada representative
of hart's tongue fern, Phyllitis scolopendrium, is a tetraploid
(n=72). It differs subtly both ecologically and anatomically
from its European counterpart which is a diploid (n=36). More
and more of these "autopolyploid" complexes are being discovered,
both in the tropics and in the temperate zones. In the tropics --
thus far at least -- the tendency has been to treat the diploids
and tetraploids as the same species, but in the temperate regions
they are being treated increasingly as separate species or
subspecies. This is probably due to more intensive study of the
temperate forms which leads to the detection of fine differences.
Among the troublesome temperate genera, in which the elements are
poorly differentiated except for levels of polyploidy, are such

complexes as those of the maidenhair spleenwort, Asplenium tri-
chomanes, the brittle fern, Cystopteris fragilis, and the common
polypody, Polypodium vulgare.

Allopolyploidy in ferns includes a number of very well known
and striking examples. In North America alone we have splendid
illustrations in the spleenworts, Asplenium (20), woodferns,
Dryopteris (21), and holly ferns, Polystichum (22), in which
allopolyploid complexes have arisen based upon three or more
original diploids. Sometimes both diploid sterile forms and
tetraploid fertile forms of the hybrids are found in the same
habitat (e.g., Polystichum scopulinum, P. californicum), and in
other cases, the allopolyploid forms have been produced experimentally in the laboratory. In some cases (e.g., Asplenium
bradleyi) the allopolyploid is much more common in nature than
the allodiploid; in others (e.g. A. ebenoides) the hybrid diploid
is much more common than the hybrid tetraploid. Why these
varying balances between the sterile and fertile forms should
exist is not clear. Not surprisingly, the polyploid fertile
hybrids have received much more attention than have the diploid
sterile hybrids. A real question is why there are so many,
relatively common hybrids of AB and the ABC cytogenetic composition
that have not doubled their chromosomes to become fertile. In
nature, there are far more allodiploids than allopolyploids.[2]

In at least two cases, the diploid Asplenium ebenoides (17)
and the triploid A. kentuckiense (unpublished), we have found it
extremely easy to produce allopolyploids simply by sowing spores
on culture media and permitting the unreduced ones to develop
into sexual gametophytes. Why does this not happen in nature?
For example, such a fern as Dryopteris boottii (D. cristata X
intermedia) has the cytogenetic formula ABC and is common in
swamps everywhere in northeastern North America. Asplenium
ebenoides, an AB hybrid occurs reliably with intermixed colonies
of its parents (A. platyneuron and A. rhizophyllum) but has
doubled its chromosomes in only a single locality. It seems to
us that there are two places in the life cycle where the cause or
causes may lie: meiosis and syngamy. There is nothing about the

------

[2]Some idea of the extent of the problem can be found in
North American Dryopteris alone, in which the following hybrids
would be expected to double and form fertile allopolyploids: D.
cristata X intermedia (formula ILS), celsa X intermedia (GIL),
goldiana X intermedia (GI), clintoniana X intermedia (IGLS),
expansa X marginalis (DM), campyloptera X marginalis (IDM),
intermedia X marginalis (IM), marginalis X spinulosa (IMS),
marginalis X cristata (LMS), celsa X marginalis (GLM), clintoniana
X marginalis (GLMS), and fragrans X marginalis (RM). Although
some of these are rare, a number of them are common hybrids
spready widely over eastern North America.

vegetative appearance of the plants that suggests hybrid weakness. In fact, most of the hybrids are quite vigorous and grow well not only in the wild but in the garden as well.

Of the two points in the life cycle where new allopolyploids may break down, we suggest that meiosis and sporogenesis may constitute the bottleneck. One possibility is that after the new allopolyploid plant forms, homeologous pairing occurs, thus mixing up the genomes and forming unbalanced combinations of the parental chromosomes. Instead of having complete genomes of each of the parents, the progeny have random combinations which are inviable or weakened to the extent that the allopolyploid derivatives soon die out.

There is probably much yet to be learned about pairing controls and other meiotic processes in polyploid pteridophytes. It is possible that in some cases there are simple genetic controls of pairing rather than complex intrachromosomal differentiation that are responsible for the observed behavior of hybrid genomes. Hybrids between taxonomically closely related or even conspecific populations may show no pairing at all; all of the chromosomes are in the form of univalents. On the contrary, hybrids between extremely distinctive taxa belonging to different genera may show high levels of pairing (23). As most of our conclusions regarding genome homologies are based upon observations in late diakinesis and in metaphase, is it possible that our assessments are not complete? Perhaps valuable data are awaiting discovery by our investigation of premeiotic associations and synaptonemal complexes as well as conditions in the stages of anaphase.

One of the methods of assessing the significance in terms of ecological success of neopolyploids is to determine their abundance in the wild relative to diploids. So far this approach has not been widely used, but a few years ago we made such a comparison in the eastern United States (24). We analyzed the pteridophytic floras of Virginia and Michigan using the most objective estimates we could make of over-all abundance. In the "abundant" category we found that only 15-20% are polyploids, but in the "rare to very rare" category 35-55% are polyploids. In addition to absolute abundance, future geographical studies should emphasize the boundaries of ranges of polyploids, especially allopolyploids in relation to their diploid ancestors. It is our impression that in general the longitudinal distribution is not necessarily intermediate between the parents, but that the latitudinal distribution is intermediate. Such comparisons must take into consideration altitude, of course, and its effect on climate with relation to north-south distribution.

Finally, we should note the correlation of polyploidy with apomixis. Obligate apogamy is well known in ferns and tends to be associated with polyploidy. Roughly three-quarters of apogamous ferns are polyploids, and most of these are triploids. With very few exceptions (25), the apogamous life cycle follows a monotonously uniform pattern. The plants involved are cytogenetically

like ABC hybrids. Meiosis is irregular and results in abortive
spores unless chromosome doubling occurs at the time of spor-
genesis. If sporocytic chromosome doubling does take place to
AABBCC then meiosis becomes normal and there are usually only
half as many spore mother cells and half as many spores, but
these spores are viable (ABC) and form the gametophytes. The
gametophytes which have the same chromosome number as the sporophyte, do not perform normal syngamy; instead the new sporophytic
plant arises directly by proliferation. The sporophyte grows up
and repeats the life cycle. This type of alternation of generations
is found widely scattered in the groups of higher ferns (e.g.,
polypodioid, asplenioid, dryopteroid) but is especially common in
the adiantoid ferns, usually species of dry habitats, and is
believed to be a possible means of counteracting the problems of
the xeric environment where free water for fertilization is
usually absent. Detailed accounts of apogamy, including the
historical development of our knowledge of the subject, are
presented by Irene Manton (1) from her classical studies. There
are several questions about apogamy that remain unanswered. One
is why so many apogamous ferns are 3x (ca. 60%) rather than
diploid or tetraploid. Another is why certain ferns (especially
species of Pellaea [26]) occur both as sexual diploids and apogamous tetraploids, sometimes even in the same population. And
finally, why apogamous ferns, especially those of mesic habitats,
simply do not double their sporophytic chromosome number for the
entire generation, and have normal meiosis, normal sexual gametophytes, and normal syngamy. It may be that in apogamous ferns
the bottleneck in attainment of sexual allopolyploidy involves
the stage of syngamy.

SUMMARY

     In less than thirty years, research on pteridophyte cytology
has become a very active endeavor. The polyploid pteridophytes
discussed here are the homosporous ones with high chromosome
numbers (x=ca.20-70), unlike the heterosporous pteridophytes with
x=7-11. The gametophytes are capable of self-fertilization with
consequent homozygotizing effects. The chromosomes do not normally
form multivalents, only pairs and singles. In spite of their
high numbers, the chromosomes are not difficult to interpret.
Although usually considered to be very ancient, a number of
modern groups did not arise until the time of the angiosperms or
later.
     On the basis of widespread occurrence of high numbers of
chromosomes in homosporous pteridophytes, combined with the
fairly uniform structure, one may speculate that the original
land plant numbers were actually high, and that the low numbers
of today (of heterosporous pteridophytes and seed plants) were
derived. This matter is not resolved, and this paper assumes
that we really are dealing with polyploidy -- of two kinds:

ancient (paleopolyploids) and recent (neopolyploids). The former
involve taxa at high levels, families and genera, and (with
aneuploid changes) provide the base numbers. The latter involve
changes at the levels of species and varieties.

If we use outside comparisons of modern homosporous pteridophytes with heterosporous ferns and fern allies and with seed
plants, we conclude that the base numbers may have been 7-13,
and more likely 9-11. If the latter is true then most living
genera are tetraploid, hexaploid, and octoploid, but some groups
(e.g., cyatheoids) may be 10- or 12-ploid.

One explanation for paleopolyploidy is that it is adaptive,
a response to the homozygotizing effect of intragametophytic
mating, as has been suggested in various papers of Klekowski.
Reduplication of genomes may store variability and also make
possible homoeologous pairing. Although not universally accepted,
these ideas have heuristic value in suggesting lines of research.
That homosporous ferns and fern allies, although presumably
polyploid in origin, are capable of active evolution is demonstrated in a number of large genera, especially in the tropical
rainforest.

Chromosome numbers may be experimentally doubled simply by
sowing spores; unreduced spores will yield polyploid gametophytes,
these capable of forming zygotes. Strict autopolyploids are
probably rare in nature, but a number of fern species are made up
of polyploid sectors which, upon close study, reveal subtle
differences in morphology and physiology. Allopolyploid ferns
are well known, and some exist in the wild both as sterile diploids
and fertile polyploids. However, the presence of so many AB
sterile hybrids, which far outnumber AABB fertile hybrids, brings
up a number of questions. One possibility is that upon assuming
the AABB constitution, the subsequent progeny receive inviable
genetic combinations due to homeologous pairing between alien
genomes. Polyploids in general may be less common in nature than
diploids (using modern x numbers as the base). Allopolyploids
tend to occur in latitudes intermediate between the parental
ranges.

Polyploidy is associated with apomixis, and the apogamous
ferns tend to be 3x. The usual apogamous life cycle involves
plants which are cytogenetically hybrids; doubling occurs in
sporocytes just prior to spore formation, thus producing gametophytes with the same number as the sporophytes. The new sporophytes are produced by direct bud proliferation. It is curious
that apogamous ferns do not simply transform to sexual allopolyploids with n and 2n alternation of generations. Perhaps inter-
ferences in syngamy explain this paradox.

LITERATURE CITED

1. Manton, I., 1950, "Problems of Cytology and Evolution in the Pteridophyta," University Press, Cambridge. ix + 316 p.

2. Lovis, J.D., 1977, Evolutionary patterns and processes in ferns, pp. 229-440, in Preston, R.D., Woolhouse, H.W., "Advances in Botanical Research," Academic Press, London.

3. Löve, A., Löve, D., Pichi Sermolli, R.E.G., 1977, "Cytotaxo-monic Atlas of Pteridophyta," J. Cramer, Vaduz. xviii + 398 p.

4. Smith, A.R., 1977, Review of Löve, A., Löve, D., Pichi Sermolli, R.E.G., "Cytotaxonomical Atlas of the Pteridophyta." Sys. Bot. 2: 86.

5. Klekowski, E.J.,Jr., 1971, Ferns and genetics. BioScience 21: 317-322.

6. Klekowski, E.J.,Jr., 1972, Genetical features of ferns as contrasted to seed plants. Ann. Missouri Bot. Gard. 59: 138-151.

7. Klekowski, E.J., Jr., 1973, Sexual and subsexual systems in homosporous pteridophytes: a new hypothesis. Amer. J. Bot. 60: 535-544.

8. Klekowski, E.J.,Jr., Baker, H.G., 1966, Evolutionary signi-ficance of polyploidy in the pteridophyta. Science 153: 305-307.

9. Emberger, L., 1968, "Les Plantes Fossiles," Masson et Cie, Paris, 758 p.

10. Copeland, E.B., 1947, "Genera Filicum," Chronica Botanica, Waltham, MA. xvi + 247 p., pl. 1-10.

11. White, R.A. (ed.) 1977, Taxonomic and morphological relation-ships of the Psilotaceae. A symposium. Brittonia 29: 1-68.

12. Tatuno, S., Kawakami, S., 1969, Karyological studies on Aspleniaceae. I. Karyotypes of three species in Asplenium. Bot. Mag. Tokyo 82: 436-444.

13. Tatuno, S., Takei, M., 1969, Karylogical studies in Hymeno-phyllaceae I. Chromosomes of the Genus Hymenophyllum and Mecodium in Japan. Bot. Mag. Tokyo 82: 121-129.

14. Tatuno, S., Yoshida, H., 1967, Karyological studies on Osmundaceae II. Chromosome of the genus Osmundastrum and Plenasium in Japan. Bot. Mag. Tokyo 80: 130-138.

15. Duncan, T., Smith, A.R., 1979, Primary basic chromosome numbers in ferns: facts or fantasies? Syst. Bot. 3: 105-114.

16. Raven, P.H., 1975, The bases of angiosperm phylogeny: Cytology. Ann. Missouri Bot. Gard. 62: 724-764.

17. Wagner, W.H., Jr., Whitmire, R.S., 1957, Spontaneous produc-tion of a morphologically distinct fertile allopolyploid by a sterile diploid of Asplenium ebenoides. Bull. Torrey Bot. Club 84: 79-89.

18. DeBenedictus, V.M.M., 1961, Apomixis in Ferns with special reference to Sterile Hybrids. Doctoral Thesis, University of Michigan.

19. Harlan, J.R., deWet, J.M.J., 1976, On Ö. Winge and a prayer: the origins of polyploidy. Bot. Rev. 41: 361–390.

20. Wagner, W.H., Jr., 1954, Reticulate evolution in the Appalachian Aspleniums. Evolution 8: 103–108.

21. Wagner, W.H., Jr., 1970, Evolution of Dryopteris in relation to the Appalachians, in P.C. Holt (ed.), "The Distributional History of the Biota of the Southern Appalachians, Part II: Flora," Virginia Polytechnic Institute and State Univ. Research Division Monogr. 2: 147–192.

22. Wagner, W.H., Jr., 1973, Reticulation of Holly ferns (Polystichum) in the western United States and adjacent Canada. Amer. Fern J. 63: 99–115.

23. Wagner, W.H., Jr., Wagner, F.S., Gómez P, L.D., 1978, The singular origin of a Central American Fern, Pleuroderris michleriana. Biotropica 10: 254–264.

24. Wagner, W.H. Jr.., 1969, The role and taxonomic treatment of hybrids. BioScience 19: 785–789, 795.

25. Evans, A.M., 1964, Ameiotic alternation of generations: a new life cycle in the ferns. Science 143: 261–263.

26. Wagner, W.H., Jr., Farrar, D.R., Chen, K.L., 1965, A new sexual form of Pellaea glabella var. glabella from Missouri. Amer. Fern J. 55: 171–178.

POLYPLOIDY IN GYMNOSPERMS

T. Delevoryas

Department of Botany
University of Texas
Austin, TX 78712

A discussion in gymnosperms as a group is somewhat meaningless
so far as discerning trends or ascertaining general principles. It
is now generally recognized (1, 2) that gymnosperms as a class probably never existed, and that gymnospermy should be regarded as a way
of life rather than suggesting that the plants possessing naked
seeds are somehow closely related. So before surveying the occurrence of polyploidy in gymnosperms, it might be appropriate to
indicate the kinds and degree of relationships of plants that are
loosely included in the group.

Gymnospermous plants appeared early in the fossil record, with
the first seedlike bodies reported from late Devonian rocks. The
kinds of plants that bore them have not been identified with certainty, but because the ovules were exposed, the plants that bore
them must be regarded as gymnospermous.

Seed ferns, an important group of gymnospermous plants, were
abundant in the late Paleozoic, and plants also referred to as
seed ferns persisted into the Mesozoic. The latter, however, may
not have had much to do with the Paleozoic forms, and there may
not even have been any close relationship at all. Seed ferns, by
an apparently arbitrary definition, were plants with fernlike
leaves with seeds borne on foliar structures. It has not even
been agreed upon that seed-bearing structures in the so-called
Mesozoic pteridosperms were foliar.

Conifers and coniferlike plants also appeared in the late
Paleozoic. Seed ferns and coniferlike plants are thought to have
originated from a group of progymnospermous plants that were important during the Devonian period. Members of the Cycadales,
probably having originated from seed fern ancestors, are known
first from the Permian, but were widespread during the Mesozoic.
Cycadeoidales, cycadlike plants that seem to have been confined to

the Mesozoic, probably were only remotely related to the Cycadales.
The glossopterids, an enigmatic group of seed plants (some consider
them seed ferns), were most common in the Permian period. The time
of appearance of the Gnetophyta is uncertain, with unconvincing
fossil remains.

Thus, in such a diverse group with apparently unrelated or,
in some instances, distantly related forms, to say as a general
statement that polyploidy is or is not frequent is meaningless.

In spite of that introduction, it may now be generalized that
polyploidy in gymnosperms is indeed rare. Fewer than 5% of the
species have been shown to be polyploid, but, of that, only 1.5%
are conifers.

The Gnetophyta, considered to represent a single group of
gymnospermous plants by many workers, are better regarded as three
distinct groups with uncertain affinities among them. One species
of Gnetum was once considered to be tetraploid, but only on uncertain bases. Also, Welwitschia was at one time presumed to be
hexaploid (2n=42) but it most likely has only 2 sets of 21 chromosomes rather than a multiple of x=7 as seen in Ephedra (3). Now
that Ephedra and Welwitschia are considered to be quite distinct
morphologically and not closely related, that argument loses even
more potency. The question of polyploidy in Welwitschia remains
unsettled.

Ephedra, however, shows polyploidy in eight species, the most
of any gymnospermous genus (4-7). Eames (8) considered it to be an
ancient genus, with ancestry among the cordaite-conifer stock.
Ephedra altissima, E. intermedia, E. likiagensis, E. saxatilis, E.
sinica, and the tetraploid form of E. americana (= E. andia) are
thought to be allotetraploids. Source of polyploidy in E. breana
and E. distachya is undetermined. Apparently intraspecific polyploidy occurs in E. americana (sensu lato) and E. breana. In
summary, 44.4% of the Ephedrales demonstrate polyploidy.

Polyploidy has not been demonstrated in the Cycadales and
Ginkgo.

Conifers typically have a basic chromosome number of x=12,
with aneuploidal variations of n=10 in Sciadopitys (Taxodiaceae),
n=11 in most Taxodiaceae, Cupressaceae, and n=13 in Pseudotsuga
(Pinaceae) and Pherosphaera (Podocarpaceae) (9).

Polyploidy in members of the Coniferales occurs very sporadically. It is found occasionally in seedlings, but these are often
aberrant, slow-growing, and do not establish themselves as trees.
Christianson (10) reported one tree of Larix decidua in Denmark with
a chromosome number of 2n=48. This autotetraploid exhibited growth
irregularities and deviating chromosome numbers in the pollen grains.
Stiff (11) described a single tree of Juniperus virginiana as being
triploid, with 2n=33. This autotriploid had larger features, including stomatal size, and greater nuclear volume.

The best known naturally occurring polyploid is Sequoia
sempervirens (Taxodiaceae), considered to be hexaploid with 2n=66.

It is the only known hexaploid gymnosperm (12). On the basis of
stomatal measurements, Miki and Hikita (13) concluded that Sequoia
must have been polyploid for some time in the geologic past.
Sequoia (2n=66) has an everage stomatal length of 58 μm and
Metasequoia, of the same family, has a chromosome number of
2n=22, with an average stomatal length of 42 μm. These differences
in stomatal length between the two genera are recognizable in
fossils as old as Pliocene.

Cupressaceae show more polyploids than any other conifer
family (14). In Thuja plicata 'Excelsa,' 2n=33 (15). Juniperus
chinensis 'Pfitzeriana' is thought to be an allotetraploid, with
2n=44 (16). Source of polyploidy in another species, J. squamata
'Meyeri' (17), has not been determined. Hair (18) reported
polyploidy in another member of the Cupressaceae, Fitzroya cupres-
soides, with 2n=44.

In the Pinaceae, only Pseudotsuga aurabilis (2n=44) is a
naturally occurring polyploid (19). A puzzle here is that the
usual situation in the Pinaceae is x=12.

According to Darlington (20,21) division is difficult in
cells with large chromosomes in a polyploid state. Pinus, with
no naturally occurring polyploids, has large chromosomes.

In Dacrydium of the Podocarpaceae, somatic chromosome numbers
vary from 1830, and in Podocarpus, of the same family, chromosome
range is from 20-38. It is felt that this situation represents
aneuploidy (9). Other instances of aneuploidy occur in the
Coniferales.

In summary, it is apparent that polyploidy in gymnosperms is
rare, and except for Ephedra and a few members of the Cupressaceae,
does not seem to be pronounced in any one group.

LITERATURE CITED

1.   Arnold, C.A., 1948, Classification of gymnosperms from the
      viewpoint of phylogeny. Bot. Gaz. 110: 2-12.
2.   Bold, H.C., 1973, "Morphology of Plants," ed. 3, Harper &
      Row, New York.
3.   Fernandes, A., 1936, Sur la caryologie de Welwitschia mirabi-
      lis Hook. f. Bol. Soc. Bot. Brot. 11: 267-282.
4.   Florin, R., 1932, Die chromosomenzahlen bei Welwitschia und
      einigen Ephedra Arten. Svensk Bot. Tidskr. 26: 205-214.
5.   Hunziker, J.H., 1953, Número de cromosomas de varias especies
      sudamericanas de Ephedra. Res. Argent. Agron. 20: 141-143.
6.   Hunziker, J.H., 1955, Morfología cromosómica de nueve especies
      Argentinas del género Ephedra. Rev. Investig. Agricolas
      9: 201-209.
7.   Mehra, P.N. 1946, A study of the karyotypes and the occurrence
      of diploid male gametophytes in some species of the genus
      Ephedra. Proc. Nat. Acad. Sci. India 16: 259-286.

8.   Eames, A.J. 1952, Relationships of the Ephedrales. Phytomor-
     phology 2: 79–100.
9.   Grant, W.F. 1976, The evolution of karyotype and polyploidy
     in arboreal plants. Taxon 25: 75–84.
10. Christianson, H., 1950, A tetraploid Larix decidua Miller.
     Det. Kgl. Danske Vidensk. Selsk 19: 19.
11. Stiff, M.L., 1951, A naturally occurring triploid juniper.
     Va. J. Sci. 2: 317.
12. Stebbins, G.L. 1948, The chromosomes and relationships of
     Metasequoia and Sequoia. Science 108: 95–98.
13. Miki, S., Hikita, S., 1951, Probable chromosome number of
     fossil Sequoia and Metasequoia found in Japan. Science 113:
     34.
14. Khoshoo, T.N., 1959, Polyploidy in gymnosperms. Evolution
     13: 24–39.
15. Pohlheim, F., 1970, Triploids bei Thuja plicata excelsa
     Timm. Biol. Rundschau 8: 402–403.
16. Sax, K., Sax, H.J., 1934, Chromosome number and morphology
     in conifers. J. Arnold Arb. 15: 255–262.
17. Jensen, H., Levan, A., 1941, Colchicine induced tetraploidy
     in Sequoia gigantea. Hereditas 27: 220–224.
18. Hair, J.B., 1968, The chromosomes of the Cupressaceae. I.
     Tetraclineae and Actinostrobeae (Callitroideae). New Zealand
     J. Bot. 6: 277–284.
19   Hall, M.T., Mukherjee, A., Crowley, W.R., 1973, Chromosome
     counts in cultivated junipers. J. Arnold Arb. 54: 369–376.
20. Darlington, C.D., 1932, "Recent Advances in Cytology," ed.
     1, Churchill, London.
21. Darlington, C.D., 1937, "Recent Advances in Cytology," ed.
     2, Churchill, London.

POLYPLOIDY IN ANGIOSPERMS: MONOCOTYLEDONS[1]

Peter Goldblatt[2]

Missouri Botanical Garden
P.O. Box 299
St. Louis, MO 63166

Several different estimates of polyploid frequency in angiosperms have been made, including G.L. Stebbins' (1,2) figure,
first published in 1950, of 30-35%, and suggestions by M.J.D.
White in 1942 (3) of at least 40%, and by Grant in 1963 (4) of
47%. These figures represent different ways of calculating
polyploidy and different interpretations of the meaning of the
word in the context of plant systematics. Stebbins' estimate
includes as polyploid those species which have gametic chromosome
numbers that are multiples of the basic diploid number found in
their genus, in other words, intrageneric polyploidy. White's
figure is based on the simple observation that even haploid
numbers exceed odd by about 40% and he thus assumed this 40% to
be largely attributable to a polyploid origin. Grant postulated
that species with haploid numbers in excess of n=13 would mainly
be polyploid and those with n=13 or less, predominantly diploid.
Grant's study also included the only estimate I have encountered
of polyploidy in each of the two subclasses of angiosperms. He
calculated a frequency of 43% in Dicotyledonae and a much higher
58% in Monocotyledonae. These figures were based on chromosome
data accumulated by 1955 for some 17,138 species. Since this time,
approximately an equal number of additional species have been
counted and the proportion of tropical as compared with north
temperate species has increased substantially. The large number
of counts now available allows an increasingly critical appraisal
of the significance of polyploidy from the systematic viewpoint.

---

[1]This work was supported by grant DEB 78-10655 from N.S.F.

[2]I thank G. Davidse, T. Croat, R.W. Faden, and H.E. Moore
for their advice on particular groups.

MATERIALS AND METHODS

The main sources of information on chromosome numbers used here are the compendium edited by Fedorov (5), which includes published counts up to 1966, and the annual "Index to Plant Chromosome Numbers," the most recent of which summarizes reports for the years 1973 and 1974 (6). A scattering of publications of more recent date have been consulted and some unpublished data have been included where relevant.

For reasons explained by Raven (7) many counts made prior to 1920 are faulty, and these, as well as more recent and obviously incorrect reports, have simply been disregarded. I have also tried to account for synonomy wherever possible, but in some large groups, counts for the same species under different names will have inadvertently been included in my analysis.

The question of what to include under the heading polyploid has posed some problems. Intrageneric polyploidy is most easily calculated, though there are considerable problems in cytologically complex groups in which a range of aneuploid numbers occurs. Some taxonomic insight is usually helpful in resolving such examples. Frequency of intrageneric polyploidy is nevertheless the most readily comparable figure when viewing different taxa. However, it is clear that intrageneric polyploidy presents only a partial analysis of the phenomenon of polyploidy, as it excludes taxa above species rank that are polyploid and many monocot and dicot genera, tribes, and families are obviously polyploid when compared with haploid numbers in their relatives at the same rank.

The recognition of polyploidy at generic level and above is often difficult to gauge due partly to gaps in the cytological record, and to insufficient or conflicting systematic data, even assuming the naturalness of groups, and so is much more subjective than the calculation of intrageneric polyploidy. I think, however, it may be fair to suggest that almost all angiosperms with haploid numbers above n=9 and 10 probably have polyploidy in their evolutionary history, those with n=11 or more almost certainly, while even some plants with lower numbers are derived from polyploid ancestors. In Table 1, I have provided figures only for intrageneric polyploidy, and for species with numbers in excess of n=13. The latter provides a rough guide to total polyploidy, but, if anything, errs on the low side. The frequency of haploid numbers in monocot species is given in Fig. 1. In the discursive review that follows, I have provided more data than the bare table allows, and have made suggestions about numbers of polyploid genera and ancestral basic numbers for families. Some of the latter information is derived from a comprehensive review of base numbers in angiosperm families by Raven (7), but may be self-evident in other families.

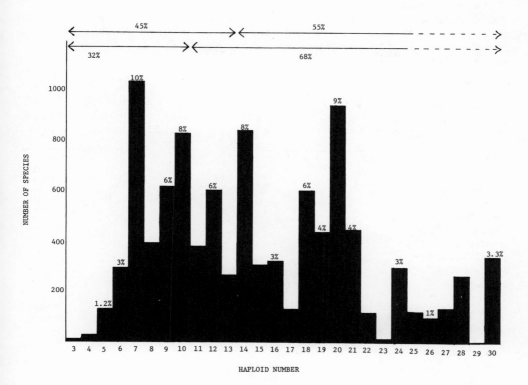

Fig. 1.   Frequency of haploid numbers between n=3 and n=30
in species of monocots.   Less than 5% of the species counted have
numbers higher than n=30, and thus do not appear on the graph.

RESULTS: GAPS IN THE RECORD

Following Raven's example (7), I will point out important
gaps in the chromosome record for monocots.   At the family level
Ecdeiocoleaceae (1/1), Geosiridaceae (1/1), Mayacaceae (1/10),
Petrosaviaceae (1/3), and Thurniaceae (1/3) are unknown cytologically.   The following, if recognized, can be added to this
list: Hanguanaceae (1/2), Joinvilleaceae (1/2), Petermanniaceae
(1/1), Posidoniaceae (1/3), and Stenomderidaceae (1/2).   Poaceae
(= Gramineae) are perhaps best understood, with over 40% of the
species known from at least one count.   Liliaceae, Alliaceae,
Commelinaceae, and Iridaceae, in which 40-50% or more of the
species have been counted, are also comparatively well sampled,
but are cytologically complex and require much more investigation.
For the remaining families, on average less than one species in
six has been examined.   Rapateaceae (16/80) and Stemonaceae

Table 1. Summary of polyploid frequencies in monocot families, calculated as percentage of intrageneric polyploidy and percentage of species with numbers greater than n=13. {Figures in parentheses after family names are estimated total species in each, mainly after Airy Shaw (8).}

Family	Number of species counted	Number of Intrageneric polyploid species	% of total counted	Number of species n=>13	% of total counted
Alismatales					
Butomaceae (1)	1	0	0	0	0
Liminocharit- aceae (12)	3	0	0	0	0
Alismat- aceae (70)	50	7	16%	8	16%
Hydrocharitales					
Hydrocharit- aceae (100)	43	16	37%	26	60%
Najadales					
Aponogeton- aceae (40)	5	3	60%	3	60%
Scheuchzeri- aceae (1)	1	0	0	0	0
Juncagin- aceae (18)	12	10	83%	8	67%
Najadaceae (35)	12	6	5%	0	0
Potamogeton- aceae (90)	66	49	74%	49	74%
Ruppiaceae (4)	4	2	50%	2	50%
Zannichelli- aceae (7)	4	2	50%	0	0
Zosteraceae (30)	12	2	17%	0	0
Triuridales					
Petrosavi- aceae (3)	--	--	--	--	--
Triuridaceae (70)	3	2	67%	3	100%
Commelinales					
Rapateaceae (80)	1	0	0	0	0
Xyridaceae (250)	21	4	19%	4	19%
Mayacaceae (10)	--	--	--	--	--
Commelin- aceae (700)	307	112	36%	154	50%
Eriocaulales					
Eriocaul- aceae (1,150)	13	12	92%	13	100%

Table 1 (continued)

Family	Number of species counted	Number of Intrageneric polyploid species	% of total counted	Number of species n=>13	% of total counted
Restionales					
Flagellari-aceae (3)	2	0	0	2	100%
Anarthri-aceae (5)	3	2	67%	2	67%
Ecdeiocole-aceae (1)	--	--	--	--	--
Restion-aceae (450)	39	13	33%	3	8%
Centrolepid-aceae (40)	4	2	50%	2	50%
Juncales					
Junc-aceae (400)	104	70	°67%	70	67%
Thurni-aceae (3)	--	--	--	--	--
Cyperales					
Cyper-aceae (4,000)	500	386	77%	363	73%
Poaceae (10,000)	3,900	2,192	55%	2,338	60%
Typhales					
Typhaceae (15)	6	2	33%	6	100%
Spargani-aceae (20)	14	0	0	14	100%
Bromeliales					
Bromeli-aceae (1,700)	122	14	11%	122	100%
Zingiberales					
Strelitzi-aceae (7)	4	0	0	0	0
Lowiaceae (2)	2	0	0	0	0
Heliconi-aceae (80)	12	0	0	0	0
Musaceae (42)	33	0	0	0	0
Zingiber-aceae (700)	126	45	36%	92	73%
Costaceae (200)	27	2	7%	5	19%
Cannaceae (55)	20	1	5%	1	5%
Marant-aceae (400)	62	8	5%	9	15%

Table 1 (continued)

Family	Number of species counted	Number of Intrageneric polyploid species	% of total counted	Number of species n=>13	% of total counted
Arecales					
Arec-aceae (3,500)	268	1	<1%	249	93%
Cyclanthales					
Cyclanth-aceae (80)	3	2	67%	2	67%
Pandanales					
Pandan-aceae (900)	24	0	0	24	100%
Arales					
Araceae (1,800)	344	72	21%	278	82%
Lemnaceae (30)	13	1	8%	13	100%
Liliales					
Philydr-aceae (6)	4	0	0	3	75%
Pontederi-aceae (30)	13	7	54%	10	77%
Lili-aceae (3,700)	1,498	281	19%	346	23%
Amaryllid-aceae (1,100)	328	49	15%	60	18%
Hypoxid-aceae (120)	13	9	69%	8	62%
Agavaceae (300)	116	15	15%	116	100%
Xanthorrhoe-aceae (66)	17	5	29%	3	18%
Iridaceae (1,470)	811	186	23%	275	34%
Vellozi-aceae (200)	13	0	0	7	54%
Haemodor-aceae (75)	30	16	53%	7	23%
Taccaceae (10)	2	0	0	2	100%
Tecophilae-aceae (20)	6	1	17%	0	0
Cyanastraceae (2)	1	0	0	0	0
Stemonaceae (25)	1	0	0	0	0
Smilac-aceae (375)	27	1	4%	16	67%
Dioscoreaceae (750)	45	33	73%	35	77%
Alliaceae (650)	333	65	20%	55	17%

Table 1 (continued)

Family	Number of species counted	Number of Intrageneric polyploid species	% of total counted	Number of species n=>13	% of total counted
Orchidales					
Geosirid- aceae (1)	--	--	--	--	--
Burmanni- aceae (125)	6	3	50%	3	50%
Corsiaceae (29)	2	0	0	0	0
Orchidaceae (18,000)	1,114	70	6%	1,050	94%
Total	10,580	3,750	36%	5,863	55%
{excl. Poaceae	6,680	1,568	23%	3,525	53%}

(1/25) are known from single counts only, while Cyclanthaceae (11/80), Centrolepidaceae (4/40), Eriocaulaceae (13/1150), and Xyridaceae (2/250) are especially poorly sampled for their size. The situation in Burmanniaceae (17/125) is particularly confused, with very different early and recent counts. The large families, Orchidaceae, Bromeliaceae, and Arecaceae, are relatively poorly known owing to particular difficulties in studying them. Nevertheless the cytological pattern in these families presents a coherent picture, although Orchidaceae in particular still require much study.

RESULTS: REVIEW OF POLYPLOIDY IN MONOCOT FAMILIES

The following survey is based on the sources mentioned above, and is arranged in general according to the system of Cronquist (9). I have made changes only in the Liliales, where I think it is useful to deal separately with several families included by Cronquist in the Liliaceae, namely Amaryllidaceae, Alliaceae (including Apaganthus and Tulbaghia), Hypoxidaceae, and Tecophilaeaceae. My reasons are purely utilitarian, and do not reflect a judgement that these families merit separation from Liliaceae any more than do other groups within this diverse family.

I. Alismatidae

I-1. Alismatales. In the monotypic Butomaceae, B. umbellatus probably has x=13 (7), although there are some early counts of n=8, 11, and 12. Triploidy is suggested by reports in the range

2n=39, ca.40, and 42. There is no polyploidy in the related Limnocharitaceae, which have n=10, 8, and 7 in different genera. In the largest family of the order, Alismataceae, n=7 and 11 are most frequent, with polyploidy recorded in six of the 12 species of Alisma counted and one of two in Echinodorus. The only counts in Luronium and Damasonium are n=14 and 21, suggesting on available data, that they are polyploid. Including the species in these polyploid genera, there are some 10 polyploid species of 50 counted in Alismataceae. The high number in Butomaceae relative to counts in the other families of Alismatales indicates palaeo-polyploidy and a possible polyploid origin here.

I-2. Hydrocharitales. Sixteen of 42 species counted are polyploid in Hydrocharitaceae, almost 40%, when compared to the basic numbers in their genera. Several genera, however, have high base numbers and must on available information also be considered polyploid. These include Bootia (n=33), Ottelia (n=22), Trianea (n=24), and, if recognized as distinct from Elegia, also Egeria (n=24). Including species in these genera, polyploidy in Hydrocharitaceae is 50%.

I-3. Najadales. Aponogetonaceae with a base number of x = 8 have two species 2n = 16 and two more with 2n = ca.80. Both diploid and tetraploid counts have been recorded in A. distachyus. Scheuchzeriaceae have x=11 and no recorded polyploidy, while the related Juncaginaceae have x=6, with n=6 only, in Lilaea, and n=6 as well as 12, 18, 24, and 30 in Triglochin maritima. Polyploidy is clearly important in Triglochin with a range of numbers from n=12, 16, 18, 24, 48, 60, and 72 recorded in the remaining nine species counted. Potamogetonaceae with x=7 (assuming two early reports of n=7 are correct) and a secondary base of x=13, exhibit a considerable polyploid range: 75% of the ca. 66 species counted have numbers above n=14; if x=7 is regarded as the basic number, polyploidy is recorded for all species (the two in which n=7 have been found to also have polyploid forms). In Ruppiaceae, x=10, of five species counted two are tetraploid and a third, Ruppia maritima, has diploid and tetraploid counts, and in Zannichelli-aceae two of the four species counted exhibit polyploidy. Only two of the ten species of Zosteraceae known cytologically are polyploid.

I-4. Triuridales. Of the two families of Triuridales, Petrosaviaceae (1/3) is unknown cytologically, while in Truirid-aceae (7/70) only Sciaphila has been counted. Reports give two species with numbers in the range n=24-22 and one n=14-12, suggesting some polyploidy in this poorly studied order.

II. Commelinidae

II-1. Commelinales. The only count available in Rapateaceae
is n=11, for the sole African species of this otherwise New World
family. In Xyridaceae, Xyris has n=9 in North American species,
n=13 and 26 in Australian, and n=17 in African and Asian species.
Only two cases of polyploidy have been reported on any of these
bases. Mayacaceae are unknown chromosomally. Commelinaceae are
cytologically complex (10) and exhibit an unusually wide range of
chromosome morphology and base numbers. Interpretation of the
patterns of chromosome evolution is complicated by well-developed
aneuploid sequences, for example, in Cyanotis (n=14-8) (11),
Commelina (n=15-10), Aneilema (n=16-9) (12), and by intricate
patterns of chromosome rearrangement, very well documented by
Jones (13,14) for Gibasis and Cymbispatha. In the latter, C.
geniculata and C. commelinoides both have n=7, but C. geniculata
has 7 acrocentrics and C. commelinoides 7 metacentrics, and twice
the amount of chromosome material, and is in fact polyploid with
respect to C. geniculata though the numbers alone disguise this.
Clearly, cytological patterns in Commelinaceae need careful and
detailed study before a clear picture can be assembled. Pro-
visionally, some 112 species can be regarded as intrageneric
polyploids of 307 Commelinaceae counted, 36%. Less specialized
genera of the family tend to have high basic numbers suggesting
perhaps a palaeotetraploid origin for the family. Nevertheless,
several genera should probably also be considered polyploid on a
palaeotetraploid base, even in the absence of known ancestral
base numbers for the family or tribes. At least genera with
numbers in the range x=17-20 (in Palisota, Colchliostemma,
Dichorisandra, and a few more) appear secondarily polyploid.

II-2. Eriocaulales. The only report at the diploid level
in Eriocaulon is n=9 in E. sieboldianum (15) which, if correct,
suggests x=9 for Eriocaulaceae. The remaining twelve species of
this genus known cytologically have n=15, 16, and 20 as well as
higher numbers. A polyploid frequency of above 90% is indicated.
No other genus of Eriocaulaceae has been studied, and the family
is at present really too poorly known for cytological conclusions
to be of much value.

II-3. Restionales. Flagellariaceae have n=19 in the two
species counted of the three species of Flagellaria, the sole
genus, and the family appears to be of polyploid origin. Anarthria
(Anarthriaceae) has x=11 with two species tetraploid, 2n=44 and
one diploid, 2n=22. In the related Restionaceae, x=7 or 6 has
been suggested as an original base number for the family with
early tetraploidy and subsequent aneuploidy to give the predominant
numbers of n=7, 13, 12, 11, and 9 (7,16,17). If this is correct,
all numbers above n=7 may be of polyploid origin, and thus 29 of
the 39 species of the family counted to date, 74%, could be

considered polyploid. Intrageneric polyploidy is less, with only
thirteen polyploid species, 36%, so far known, if species of
Restio with numbers other than n=7 are regarded as derived tetraploids. Ecdeiocoleaceae are uncounted. Centrolepidaceae are
poorly known with reports of n=10 and n=13 in two species of
Centrolepis, and n=20 and n=ca.24 in another two, apparently
polyploid.

   II-4. Juncales. In Juncaceae,[3] Juncus may have x=10 as
basic, if the count of n=10 in J. decipiens from Taiwan (18) is
correct. The only other count at this ploidy level is n=9 in the
South African annual species J. capitatus (19). Most species of
Juncus, however, have n=20, and there is evidently a decreasing
aneuploid series, n=19, 18, 15, derived from this number and
several higher polyploid species based on x=20. Based on a
single count, the Andean Oxychloe has x=8, while Luzula with x=6
has an extensive polyploid sequence but a majority of species
n=6. The low number in L. elegans (syn. L. purpurea) n=3 is
almost certainly derived, as already suggested (7). The other
family of Juncales, Thurniaceae, is unknown cytologically.

   II-5 Cyperales. The two families of Cyperales are both
large, and exhibit the highest frequencies of polyploidy among
angiosperms excluding some of the smaller families. Cyperaceae[3]
have some 390 species polyploid with respect to apparent base
numbers in their genera, of a total of nearly 500 species counted,
i.e., over 75% polyploid. Several small genera or those with few
counts also have very high numbers: Blysmus and Dichromena x=20;
Elyna and Eriophorum x=30, 29; Juncellus x=ca.42; Uncinia x=44;
and species of these genera, if added to the number of polyploids,
would raise the polyploid level to about 90%. Poaceae are the
second largest family of monocots, and because of their economic
importance, as well as cytological diversity, the family is
unusually well sampled. Some 4,000 of the estimated 10,000
species of Poaceae have been counted at least once and this
represents nearly 40% of the species of monocots counted. Almost
2,200 species of Poaceae have numbers that are multiples of the
basic diploid number in their genera, 55%, and a substantial
number of species have both diploid and polyploid races. The
figure of 55% polyploidy would be raised to 64% if species belonging to obviously polyploid genera are added to the total. The

---

[3]Many Juncaceae and Cyperaceae are agmatoploids, i.e., organisms having polycentric chromosomes (with diffuse or multiple
centromeres) that lead to an increase of chromosome number by
chromosomal fragmentation, or pseudopolyploidy. This phenomenon is
often combined with true polyploidy in these families. (Editor)

number of apparently polyploid genera is too many to list, but
includes notably many Bambusoid genera, e.g., <u>Arundinaria</u>, <u>Sasa</u>
x=24; <u>Dendrocalamus</u>, <u>Ochlandra</u> x=36; etc.

A base number of x=12 has been suggested for Poaceae on the
grounds that this number is basic for the primitive Bambusoideae
and Oryzoideae (7). An alternative hypothesis (20) of x=7 or 6
has also been proposed based in the occurrence of these numbers
in Arundinoideae including <u>Danthonia</u>, and in the Pooideae (=
Festuciodeae), both unspecialized subfamilies of predominantly
temperate distribution. If the latter is correct, at least
Bambusoideae-Oryzoideae-Olyroideae are polyploid in origin, and
the more specialized tropical subfamilies with x=10 and 9 predominantly, appear to have been derived by aneuploid reduction from
ancestors of polyploid origin. Intrageneric polyploidy seems as
important in tropical as in temperate areas.

Polyploidy has been studied extensively in Poaceae (e.g.,
21,22), and it is widely known that polyploidy has played an
important role in the evolution of the family. It is less well
known that this situation is unusual in the monocots, and the
apparently high frequency of intrageneric polyploidy in monocots
is strongly affected by the large contribution to the total made
by species of Poaceae.

II-6 <u>Typhales</u>. The presence of x=15 in both families of
the order, Typhaceae and Sparganiaceae, suggests that Typhales
may be polyploid in origin. Two species of <u>Typha</u> of six counted
are tetraploid, n=30.

II-7. <u>Bromeliales</u>. In Bromeliaceae x=25 is the most important number and the only one in the primitive Pitcairnioideae
(23,24). Other numbers have been reported in more specialized
subfamilies, notably n=17 in <u>Cryptanthus</u> and n=21 in <u>Aechmea</u>
<u>tillansioides</u> while Sharma and Ghosh (24) have found in addition
n=23, 24, 26, and 27 in a few genera, mostly those in which
Marchant (23) had established n=25. Although these numbers need
to be verified, there seems little reason to doubt that x=25 is
basic for Bromeliaceae, and the family may be of polyploid origin.

II-8. <u>Zingiberales</u>. <u>Heliconia</u>, only genus of Heliconiaceae,
has n=12 with 11 in a few species. In Musaceae, <u>Musa</u> has n=11
and 10, while <u>Ensete</u> has n=9, and <u>Orchidantha</u> (Lowiaceae) also
n=9. Numbers are similar in Strelitziaceae with n=11 in <u>Ravenala</u>
and the arborescent <u>Strelitzia alba</u> (syn. <u>S</u>. <u>augusta</u>) but surprisingly n=7 in <u>S</u>. <u>nicolai</u>, also arborescent, and in the subherb-
aceous species, all of temperate southern Africa. The available
evidence clearly supports Mahanty's (25) suggestion of a high
base number for this basal group of families of Zingiberales, but
although x=11 is most frequent, it may have been derived from a
somewhat higher number. Thus x=12, basic for Heliconiaceae, may
also be ancestral for the whole Musaceae alliance. The low

number of n=7 in some species of Strelitzia is most probably
derived, but the situation here needs further investigation.
There are no recorded polyploid species in this reasonably well-
known group, although the fairly high base number suggests a
significant role for polyploidy in its early evolution.

Zingiberaceae, largest family of Zingiberales and rather
poorly known cytologically, have some 45 intrageneric polyploids
of 125 species counted, 36%. Ancestral base number for the
family is likely in the x=14-12 range, x=12 having been postulated
by Mahanty (25). In this light several genera must be regarded
as polyploid including at least Aframomum, Amomum, Burbidgea,
Elletaria, and Nicolaea, all n=24; and Curcuma and Hitchenia,
n=21. Hedychium, n=17, should perhaps be included among the
polyploid genera. More counts in these genera may well reveal
species with numbers at the diploid level which would change
substantially our present view of polyploidy in the family. In
Costaceae, Costus has n=9, possibly also 8 (26,27), and of 24
species counted there are only three with polyploidy, two of
these also having diploid forms. The derived Dimerocostus and
Monocostus both have n=14 (27), and are most likely tetraploid
based on x=7. Cannaceae have n=9 in the 20 species of Canna
counted, while one species has diploid and polyploid forms.

Marantaceae, a large family and poorly known cytologically,
have only five intrageneric polyploid species, of 62 counted, or
8%. Species of Calathea with n=8 are probably derived aneuploids
rather than relict diploids. Other base numbers in Calathea are
n=13, 12, 11, and 9, while C. taeniosa, n=26, is regarded as the
only polyploid in the genus. The only comparable low count in
the family, in Ischnosiphon, also n=8, has been shown by Andersson
(28) to be erroneous. Ancestral base number for Marantaceae may
be x=13 as proposed by Mahanty or at least in the range x=14-12.
Phrynium, n=18, appears, from available data, the only polyploid
genus.

III. Arecales

III-1. Arecaceae. Arecaceae may have an ancestral basic
number of n=18 (7,29), universal throughout the primitive subfamilies Arecoideae and Phoenicoideae. A decreasing aneuploid
series is evident, lower numbers appearing in more specialized
lines, with n=16 most frequent, n=14 less so, n=17 and 15 poorly
represented, and n=13 in only one genus, Chamaedorea (also n=16).
Only one polyploid palm has been recorded, Arenga caudata, n=32.
There are a few low chromosome numbers in the cytological record,
mostly shown to be incorrect by the excellent work of Read (30,31)
and the few still standing, notably in Licuala, n=14 and n=8;
Pritchardia, n=18, but n=8 in P. "grandis hort"; and Butia n=16,
but n=8 in B. paraguayensis, all require confirmation. Given the
very uneven frequency of numbers in the family, n=18 and 16

predominating, and n=17 and 15 so infrequent, an alternative hypothesis, that x=9 is basic for Arecaceae with early aneuploidy to n=8 and 7 and subsequent polyploidization to 18, 17, 16, 15, and 14 appears possible.

III-2. Cyclanthales. There are no counts for Cyclanthaceae, only family of this order.

III-3. Pandanales. All 22 species of Pandanus counted have n=30 while the two species of Freycinetia for which there are chromosome data have numbers in the n=28-29 range. Available information suggests x=30 for Pandanaceae, the only family of Pandanales.

III-4. Arales. Araceae, which comprises the majority of species in the order have some 72 species, or 21% polyploid in their genera out of 337 species counted, indicating only a small role for polyploidy in speciation in the family. However, the distribution of generic base numbers in the subfamilies and tribes presents a picture suggesting that an unusual number of genera are polyploid when compared with other genera of each grouping. Thus in Monsteroideae generic base numbers are x=15, 14, 30, 28, 56; in Lasioideae, x=14, 13, 30, 26, 21, 20; Philo-dendroideae, x=17, 16, 13, 24, 21, 20, etc. The lowest numbers in the family (excluding a few early and almost certainly incorrect counts) are in the specialized subfamily Aroideae, where Typhonium has n=13, 9, and 8, and Biarum, n=13, 12, 11, 8, and these sequences are interpreted as decreasing aneuploidy given the predominance of higher numbers in the n=14 and 13 range in the subfamily. Most counts for the very reduced Pistia, sole member of Pisteae, indicate n=14 palaeopolyploidy in this tribe also. However, there is also an interesting, unpublished report of n=7 in Pistia in North America by Huttleston fide Jones (32), which, if correct, is remarkable.

All genera of Araceae appear to have base numbers of x=11 or higher, but the distribution of these numbers within several sub-families and tribes make it seem likely that they were derived from ancestors with lower numbers rather than directly from one another by polyploidy and subsequent aneuploid changes. For example, in Pothoideae base numbers of x=17, 15, 12, and 21 seem likely to have arisen from ancestors with x=9, 8, 7, and 6. Similarly, the pattern in Lasioideae, x=14, 13, 21, and 20 may have arisen from ancestors having x=7, 6, and perhaps even 5. To summarize, intrageneric polyploidy is of limited importance in speciation in Araceae. However, the family appears to have undergone earlier cycles of polyploidy, having arisen from diploid ancestors, all possibly extinct, a conclusion also reached by others (7,32,33,34). This would explain the present prepon-derance of base numbers at the tetraploid, x=16-13, and hexaploid-octoploid levels with several genera x=20, 21, 24, 26, 27, 30,

and above in different subfamilies, all of which indicates substantial significance for polyploidy in Araceae. The other
family of the order, Lemnaceae, is clearly polyploid, with n=22-
20 predominant. Intrageneric polyploidy in Lemnaceae is represented
by two species of Lemna which have forms with n=20, 30, and 40.

IV. Liliidae

IV-1. Liliales. Philydraceae have x=8 in Philydrum, x=17
in Helmholtzia, and x=16 in Othothylax, which suggests x=9 or 8
as ancestral for the group and a possible polyploid derivation
for the latter two genera. In Pontederiaceae, two genera,
Pontederia and Eichhornia have species n=8 and n=16, while the
other genera counted have x=15 and 14, respectively. With x=8
likely, on available evidence for the family, two of the four
genera counted appear polyploid. Intrageneric polyploidy is
known in seven species or 54% of those counted.

Liliaceae, the largest family in the order, is variously
constituted by different phylogenists. I find it convenient to
depart from the Cronquist system here, and will discuss several
families as separate from the main core of Liliaceae, still a
large and diverse group. In Liliaceae, excluding Amaryllidaceae,
Alliaceae, and Hypoxidaceae, some 1500 species are known cytologically, and of these some 280, or 19%, are intrageneric polyploids. Intrageneric polyploidy is unimportant in most of the
larger tribes including Aloineae (5%), Tulipeae (9%), Polygonateae
(12%), but assumes importance in Scilleae (27%) notably in its
Eurasian representatives, and in Colchiceae (58%) in which most
counts available are also for Eurasian taxa. Liliaceae are
diverse cytologically and relationships between groups are often
obscure so that basic numbers for the family, or for some larger
tribes, cannot readily be gauged. It is, however, clear that
certain genera and tribes are polyploid, notably Rusceae x=20,
Convalarieae x=19, and Aspidistreae x=19 or 18.

In Amaryllidaceae (senu stricto) n=11 occurs in almost all
tribes and is the most frequent number. A base number of x=11
thus seems a likely candidate for the ancestral number. In any
case, it was clearly established early and much evolution seems
to have proceeded from this point. The extensive aneuploid
sequences in some genera, e.g., Lycoris, n=11, 9, 8, 7, 6;
Narcissus, n=11, 10, 7, and 5; Leucojum, n=11, 10, 9, 8, 7 should
probably be read as have proceeded from the higher numbers (35,36)
rather than the reverse as proposed by Stern (37) for Leucojum.
Fernandez's (39) suggestion that n=5, found only in N. serotinum
(also n=10, 15) is basic in Narcissus is questionable given the
fairly specialized position of this species. Viewing x=11 as
most likely basic, intrageneric polyploidy in Amaryllidaceae is
low, about 15% of the estimated 328 species known cytologically.
A few genera appear polyploid on the assumed family base, mostly
New World and mainly tropical, including Stenomesson, Pamianthe,

n=23; Hymenocallis, Phaedranassa, and Eustephia, n=26; and
Sprekelia, n=56. A few more appear polyploid from derived base
numbers such as Tapeinanthus, n=14. Species counted in these
genera number only 14, so the view of generally low polyploidy in
the family is maintained. Hypoxidaceae, a small family, have
relatively high polyploidy, mainly in the genus Hypoxis, based
upon an apparent aneuploid series n=9, 8, and 7. The situation
is still unclear in this family owing to conflicting counts and
some early and evidently incorrect records. Alliaceae have about
20% polyploidy, about the mean for monocots excluding grasses.
Aneuploid changes from base numbers in the x=10-8 range appear
important in almost all genera of this family. The southern
African genus Agapanthus, probably x=15, seems out of place in
the family. Agavaceae are interesting cytologically. A group of
genera around Agave have n=30 with the bimodal karyotype of 5
large and 25 small chromosomes (39,40). The apparently related
Doryanthes and Hesperocallis have n=24, while the group of genera
including Cordyline and Nolina have n=19. Sanseviera has n=20,
and Dracaena probably also n=20 (41,42), and perhaps n=19, although
the record for Dracaena is confused by a range of counts from
plants, all of horticultural origin, by Sharma and Datta (43),
who record n=8, 14, 16, 17, 19, 21, and 42. Their findings
conflict with counts of n=20 for several of the same species.
The genus clearly further requires investigation. Lastly, Phormium
alone has n=16 and it may well be misallied in Agavaceae. In the
family intrageneric polyploidy is important only in Agave, where
half the species counted are polyploid, but for the family accounts
for 15% of those known cytologically. The origin of the distinctive karyotype in Agave and its allies is puzzling, but clearly
polyploidy was involved in the history of this cytologically
diverse family.

Xanthorrhoeaceae, a Pacific family, have about average
intrageneric polyploidy with five species, all Lomandra, tetraploid,
of 17 species counts in three genera of the family. In the
African and South American Velloziaceae, no intrageneric polyploidy
has been recorded by Goldblatt et al. (44), but only Vellozia has
numbers at a diploid level, n=8 and 7 {not 9 as reported previously
(7)}, while Barbacenia, n=17 (not 16), and Xerophyta and Talbotia,
n=24, appear, from the few available counts, polyploid genera,
indicating a very significant role for polyploidy in the early
evolution of this family. There is a remarkable situation in
Haemodoraceae where the Australian Conostylis has n=4 in the
least specialized species (45), while the remaining species are
polyploid with n=8, 7, 5, and 14. The related Anigosanthus has
n=6. All genera outside Australia have higher base numbers with
n=ca.20, 18, and 15 in South Africa, and n=24 and 21 in North
America (46). Tecophilaeaceae, often included in Haemodoraceae,
may have x=12; Ornduff (47) having found n=12 and 24 in the South
African Cyanella, while Tecophilaea, Chilean, has n=12 and
Odontostomum, Californian, n=10. Cyanastraceae, perhaps allied

to Tecophilaeaceae, have n=11 and 12 reported for the same species. Polyploidy is obviously important in the evolution of the Haemodoraceae-Tecophilaeaceae-Cyanastraceae group, the majority of genera of which have high base numbers, but intrageneric polyploidy is significant only in Conostylis.

Some 23% of 811 species counted in Iridaceae are intrageneric polyploids, an average figure for monocots. Distribution of polyploidy is, however, very uneven, being concentrated in north temperate taxa such as Iris (40% polyploid); Eurasian species of Gladiolus and Romulea; and Sisyrinchium where most north temperate species are polyploid. In other areas, polyploidy at species level is much rarer. Ancestral base number in Iridaceae is probably in the x=11-9 range. Descending aneuploidy probably led to the establishment of x=7 and 6 characteristic of many genera, and secondary polyploidy was clearly involved in the evolution of the primitive Libertia, x=19; in Tigridia and its close allies x=14; the relatively primitive African Aristea and its shrubby relatives x=16; and in genera of Ixioideae such as Pillansia x=20, Gladiolus x=15, perhaps Hesperantha and Geissorhiza x=13, and Romulea x=12-14, amongst others. The significance of polyploidy is unclear in Crocus, which has a bewildering range of chromosome numbers in a series (48) running from n=14 to 3 (excluding a few obvious high polyploid species).

Smilax, cytologically best known genus of Smilacaceae, has basic numbers in the x=16-13 range with most species so far counted either n=16 or 13. Polyploidy is reported in S. china only, which has n=15 as well as 30. There are single counts in Lapageria, n=15, Eustrephus, n=10, and Philesia, n=19. The latter count, apparently polyploid, is unusual in the family.

In Dioscoreaceae, the primitive, hermaphroditic and relictual Trichopus (49) has n=14, which may be basic for the family. The Mediterranean Tamus has n=24, while Old World Dioscorea species have x=10 except D. pyrenaica which has n=12, suggesting its segregation as Borderia may have merit. New World Dioscorea species and Rajania have n=18 and 27 and appear entirely polyploid. They are perhaps polyploid derivatives from aneuploid ancestors with n=9, a number not so far discovered. Intrageneric polyploidy is well developed, and if New World Dioscorea species are treated as polyploid, the frequency is above 75%. The above interpretation of chromosome evolution in Dioscoreaceae suggests that, with x=14, the whole family may be polyploid in origin. Its closest relatives are Stemonaceae, x=7, and Taccaceae, in which n=14 has been reported in one species and n=15 in another. Taccaceae may also have x=14.

IV-2. Orchidales. Burmanniaceae appear to have a base number in the range x=9-6, if some early reports for Burmannia and Thisma are correct. Assuming this, three of the six species counted are polyploid. Corsiaceae, counted for the first time by Kores et al. (50) have n=9 in two species of Corsia. The mono-

typic Madagascan Geosiridaceae are unknown cytologically. Orchidaceae, the largest monocot family, are cytologically complex and
relatively poorly studied, owing in part to the difficulty in
working with their chromosomes (51). Intrageneric polyploidy
appears unusually low, some 70 species, only 6% are polyploid of
over 1,100 counted. However, some of the highest generic base
numbers in the angiosperms occur in Orchidaceae. Basic number
for the family is unknown, but in the less advanced Diandreae,
Cypripedium has x=10 and Paphiopedilum perhaps x=13, the former
comparable with apparent basic numbers for Corsiaceae and Burmanniaceae. Most genera of Orchidaceae have much higher numbers
(51,52) with n=19, 20 and 21 most frequent and several specialized
tropical tribes have base numbers above x=19, excluding obviously
derived aneuploid species. Polyploid ancestry for most genera of
Orchidaceae is apparent and, although the family is still poorly
known cytologically, the role of polyploidy in its evolution
cannot be overemphasized.

DISCUSSION

From the foregoing, it is clear that polyploidy can be viewed
in several different ways. Perhaps the most important is intrageneric polyploidy (neopolyploidy), which provides a measure of
the role of polyploidy in the origin of modern species and
perhaps a few genera. It must be understood, however, that at
this level by no means all polyploid species arose from diploid
progenitors, and some (perhaps many) originated from other
polyploid ancestors.

Grant's (4) method of calculating polyploidy, by assuming
all species with numbers above n=13 to be polyploid, is a rough
measure of total polyploidy, ancient and recent, which includes
both polyploid species and higher taxa. Interestingly, his
figure for monocots, 58%, has changed only three points to 55%
with the addition of as many more species counts as he had available in 1955 when his analysis was made. The suggestion by Grant
that the frequency of species with haploid numbers above n=13
gives a fair indication of overall polyploidy is, I believe,
conservative and the impression gained from my analysis is that
at least species with numbers of n=11 and above, have polyploidy
in their evolutionary history and probably many of those with
n=10 and even n=9 appear to be aneuploid derivatives of ancestors
with higher numbers. For this reason, I think it is fair to say
that at least 70%, and most likely above 80% of monocots are in
some sense polyploid. It is difficult to guage whether families
which appear entirely polyploid today are actually of polyploid
origin or whether they are derived from now extinct diploid
relatives. The uneven distribution of generic base numbers in
Araceae and Arecaceae, for example, suggests that the modern
genera were derived from diploid, and not from some unknown

polyploid ancestors. In contrast, basic numbers in families are
genera of Bromeliales, Zingiberales, and Typhales are consistently
high and these entire orders may have evolved from polyploid
ancestors.

Available data present an interesting situation in several
families such as Juncaceae, Potamogetonaceae, Eriocaulaceae, and
perhaps Haemodoraceae, of only a few species palaeodiploid and
the majority polyploid with radiation from a tetraploid base.
Large and cytologically complex families like Orchidaceae,
Iridaceae, Liliaceae, and Commelinaceae are characterized by
extensive aneuploid sequences accompanied by karyotype rearrangements, and speculation on the chromosomal history of these is
difficult. Their example indicates that numerical change from
tetraploid to diploid levels can be rapid, and provides a cautionary
note in speculating about cytological patterns in other groups.

The frequency of intrageneric polyploidy is by far the
highest in the two families of Cyperales, Cyperaceae (77%) and
Poaceae (55%) alone contribute some 2,192 polyploid species or
races of species to the total of 3,750 polyploid monocots. Thus the
overall frequency of polyploidy in monocots, 36%, is strongly
influenced by this order, and especially by Poaceae. When the
latter is excluded, the frequency of polyploidy for the remaining
monocot families drops to only 23% and, when Cyperaceae are also
excluded, to 19%. Intraspecific polyploidy, not dealt with in
this review, is also a notable characteristic of Poaceae. It
occurs in other families, but to a much smaller degree. More
often, it appears from the counts available that polyploidy is a
characteristic of a species which sets it apart from its relatives.

Poaceae may in fact owe their success, in part, to the
evident facility with which races or forms of species become
polyploid, and thus are able to adapt to a wider range of habitats.
This difference in intraspecific polyploid frequencies between
Poaceae and most other monocot families suggests that examples in
Poaceae on the origin and role of polyploidy in evolution may not
be universally applicable.

The overall frequency of intrageneric polyploidy in monocots,
36%, is strikingly similar to Stebbins' (1) estimate of 30-35%
for angiosperms. Stebbins' figures were based on selected examples
of genera for which several species at least were known cytologically, and the sample included many dicots as well as monocots
(Stebbins, personal communication). The concurrence of the
figures quoted above suggests comparable significance of polyploidy in dicots and monocots if taken at face value, but as in
the monocots the frequency of polyploidy varies tremendously
between different families of dicots.

LITERATURE CITED

1. Stebbins, G.L., 1959, "Variation and Evolution in Plants,"
    Columbia University Press, New York.
2. Stebbins, G.L., 1971, "Chromosomal Evolution in Higher
    Plants," Edward Arnold, London.
3. White, M.J.D., 1952, "The Chromosomes," ed. 2, Methuen,
    London.
4. Grant, V., 1963, "The Origin of Adaptations," Columbia
    University Press, New York.
5. Fedorov, A.N., 1969, "Chromosome Numbers of Flowering Plants,"
    Acad. Nauk, Leningrad.
6. Moore, R.J., 1975, Index to Plant Chromosome Numbers for
    1973-1974. Regnum Vegetabile 96: 1-257.
7. Raven, P.H., 1975, The bases of angiosperm phylogeny: cytology.
    Ann. Missouri Bot. Gard. 62: 724-764.
8. Airy Shaw, H.K., 1973, J.C. Willis' "A Dictionary of the
    Flowering Plants and Ferns," ed. 8, University Press,
    Cambridge.
9. Cronquist, A., 1968, "The Evolution and Classification of
    Flowering Plants," Houghton Mifflin, Boston.
10. Jones, K., Jopling, C., 1972, Chromosomes and the classifi-
    cation of the Commelinaceae. Bot. J. Linn. Soc. 65: 129-
    162.
11. Lewis, W.H., 1964, Meiotic chromosomes in African Commelin-
    aceae. Sida 1: 274-293.
12. Faden, R.W., 1975, A biosystematic study of the genus Aneilema
    R. Br. (Commelinaceae). Ph.D. Dissertation, Washington
    University.
13. Jones, K., 1974, Chromosome Evolution by Robertsonian change
    in Gibasis (Commelinaceae). Chromosoma 45: 353-368.
14. Jones, K., 1977, The role of Robertsonian change in karyotype
    evolution in higher plants. Chromosomes Today 6: 121-129.
15. Mehra, P.N., Sachdeva, S.K., 1971, in IOPB Chromosome number
    reports 34. Taxon 20: 609-614.
16. Briggs, B.G., 1963, Chromosome numbers in Lapyrodia and
    Restio in Australia. Contr. N.S.W. Nat. Herb. 3: 228-232.
17. Briggs, B.G., 1966, Chromosome numbers in some Australian
    monocotyledons. Contr. N.S.W. Nat. Herb. 4: 24-34.
18. Hsu, C., 1971, Preliminary chromosome studies on the vascular
    plants of Taiwan (IV). Counts and systematic notes on some
    monocotyledons. Taiwania 16: 123-136.
19. Snogerup, S., 1963, Studies in the genus Juncus III. Bot.
    Not. 116: 142-156.
20. Brown, W.V., Smith, B.N., 1972, Grass evolution, the Kranz
    syndrome, $^{13}C/^{12}C$ ratios and continental drift. Nature 239:
    345-346.
21. Stebbins, G.L., 1975, The role of polyploid complexes in the
    evolution of North American grasslands. Taxon 24: 91-106.

22. Harlan, J.R., deWet, J.M.J., 1975, On Ö. Winge and a prayer: the origins of polyploidy. Bot. Rev. 41: 361-390.

23. Marchant, C.J., 1968, Chromosome evolution in the Bromeliaceae. Kew Bull. 21: 161-168.

24. Sharma, A.K., Ghosh, I., 1971, Cytotaxonomy of the family Bromeliaceae. Cytologia 36: 327-427.

25. Mahanty, H.K., 1970, A cytological study of the Zingiberales with special reference to their taxonomy. Cytologia 35: 13-49.

26. Maas, P.J.M., 1972, Costoideae. Flora Neotropica Monograph 8: 1-139.

27. Maas, P.J.M., 1977, Renealmia & Costoideae Additions. Flora Neotropica Monograph 18: 1-218.

28. Anderson, L., 1977, The genus Ischnosiphon (Marantaceae). Opera Bot. 43: 1-113.

29. Moore, H.E., Uhl, N.W., 1973, Palms and the origin and evolution of monocotyledons. Quart. Rev. Biol. 48: 414-436.

30. Read, R.W., 1965, Chromosome numbers in the Coryphoideae. Cytologia 30: 385-391.

31. Read, R.W., 1966, New chromosome counts in the Palmae. Principes 10: 55-61.

32. Jones, G.E., 1957, Chromosome numbers and phylogenetic relationships in the Araceae. Ph.D. Dissertation, Univ. of Virginia.

33. Marchant, C.J., 1970, Chromosome variation in Araceae I. Pothoeae to Stylochitoneae. Kew Bull. 24: 315-322.

34. Marchant, C.J., 1973, Chromosome variation in Araceae: V. Acoreae to Lasieae. Kew Bull. 28: 199-210.

35. Traub, H.P., Moldenke, H.N., 1947, The tribe Galantheae. Herbertia 14: 85-116.

36. Traub, H.P., Moldenke, H.N., 1949, Amaryllidaceae: Tribe Amarylleae. Amer. Pl. Life Soc., Stanford.

37. Stern, F.C., 1956, "Snowdrops and Snowflakes," Royal Horticultural Soc., London.

38. Fernandes, A., 1967, Contribution à la connaissance de la biosystématique de quelques espèces du genre Narcissus L. Portug. Acta Biol. ser. B. 9: 1-42.

39. Whitaker, T.W., 1934, Chromosome constitution in certain monocotyledons. J. Arnold Arb. 15: 135-142.

40. Gomez-Pompa, A., Villalobos-Pietrini, 1971, Studies in Agavaceae. I. Chromosome morphology and number of seven species. Madroño 21: 208-221.

41. Borgen, L., 1967, Chromosome numbers of vascular plants from the Canary Islands with special reference to polyploidy. Nyt. Mag. Bot. 16; 81-121.

42. Gadella, T.W.J., 1972, Cytological studies on some flowering plants collected in Africa. Bull. J. Bot. Nat. Belg. 42: 393-402.

43. Sharma, A.K., Datta, P.C., 1960, Chromosome studies in
    species of Dracaena with special reference to their means of
    speciation. J. Genetics 57: 43-76.
44. Goldblatt, P., Poston, M.E., Ayensu, E.S., 1980, Observations
    on chromosome cytology of Velloziaceae. (In preparation.)
45. Green, J.W., 1960, The genus Conostylis II. Taxonomy.
    Proc. Linn. Soc. N.S.W. 85: 334-373.
46. Ornduff, R., 1979, Chromosome numbers and relationships of
    certain African and American genera of Haemodoraceae. Ann.
    Missouri Bot. Gard. 66 (in press).
47. Ornduff, R., 1979, Chromosome numbers of Cyanella (Tecophil-
    aeaceae). Ann. Missouri Bot. Gard. 66 (in press).
48. Brighton, C.A., Mathew, B., Marchant, C.J., 1973, Chromosome
    counts in the genus Crocus. Kew Bull. 28: 451-464.
49. Burkill, I.H., 1960, The organography and the evolution of
    Dioscoreaceae, the family of the yams. J. Linn. Soc. (Bot.)
    56: 319-412.
50. Kores, P., White, D.A., Thien, L.B., 1978, Chromosomes of
    Corsia (Corsiaceae). Amer. J. Bot. 65: 584-585.
51. Jones, K. 1974, Cytology and the study of orchids, pp. 383-
    392, in Wither, C.L., (ed.), "The Orchids: Scientific Studies,"
    John Wiley & Sons, New York.
52. Duncan, R.E., 1959, Orchids and cytology, pp. 189-260, in
    Wither, C.L., (ed.), "The Orchids, A Scientific Survey,"
    Ronald Press, New York.

POLYPLOIDY IN ANGIOSPERMS: DICOTYLEDONS[1]

Walter H. Lewis

Department of Biology
Washington University
St. Louis, MO   63130

As summarized by Goldblatt (1) in the previous article,
"Polyploidy in angiosperms: monocotyledons," recent estimates of
polyploid frequency among angiosperms vary from 30-35% to 47%.
The highest value is based on the postulation that haploid numbers
in excess of n=13 would be mainly polyploid and those with n=13
or less would be predominantly diploid (2). On this basis 43% of
dicotyledons and 58% of monocotyledons from a sample of 17,138
species were considered polyploid. Goldblatt (1) believes,
however, that limiting polyploidy to haploid numbers over n=13 is
too conservative and that at least species with numbers of n=11
and above have polyploidy in their evolutionary history, and
perhaps also many of those with n=10 and n=9 may be aneuploid
derivatives of ancestors with higher numbers. He suggests that
at least 70% and most likely above 80% of monocotyledons are in
some sense polyploid.

MATERIALS AND METHODS

Chromosomal data have been gleaned to 1966 from compilations
of Federov (3) and to 1974 from Moore (4-6). Original reports
have also been studied through 1974 and a limited number subsequently. Liberal use has also been made of a number of important

---

[1]As it was not possible for the speaker assigned this topic
to attend the Conference, the Editor has written a synopsis,
largely to give the reader an overall background and to provide
sufficient reference for a more detailed study.

general discussions of basic chromosome number (7-14), notably by
Ehrendorfer and Raven. All comments on polyploidy are obviously
predicated by counts presently known. Terms used include primary
diploids (commonly x=5-9) that may be original base numbers or
base numbers derived largely by aneuploid loss of ancestral or
early polyploids that are generally paleopolyploids (x=11+),
secondary polyploids that are multiples of earlier polyploids and
may be paleopolyploids, mesopolyploids, or neopolyploids, and
infraspecific polyploids (summarized in the Appendix, p. 263, and
also discussed by Lewis, p. 103) that are mostly if not exclusively
neopolyploids. An abbreviation, Px, is used to indicate a polyploid state at any level of ploidy (3x+).

    The classification followed is basically that of Thorne (15-
17) modified into 11 phylogenetic groups (18).

                    POLYPLOIDY IN DICOTYLEDON FAMILIES

1. Superorder Annoniflorae (phylogenetic group 1)

    Annonales. Assuming an original base number of 7 for this
primitive order (7-13), most members are paleopolyploids that
reach 24x levels in Magnolia and Zygogynum. The following familial
numbers are known: Winteraceae x=13 and 43; Illiciaceae and
Schisandraceae x=14; Magnoliaceae x=19; Degeneriaceae, Himantandraceae (19), and Lauraceae (20) x=12; Eupomatiaceae x=10; Myristi-
caceae x=19 and 21; Amborellaceae, Aristolochiaceae p.p. (21),
and Canellaceae x=13; Antherospermataceae, Austrobaileyaceae, and
Siparunaceae x=22; Chloranthaceae p.p. x=14 and 15; Monimiaceae
(22) x=18,19,22, and 39; Calycanthaceae and Saururaceae x=11;
Lactoridaceae x=20 (or 21); Gomortagaceae (23) x=21; Hernandiaceae
x=20; and Piperaceae (24,25) x=11 and 12. All are of undoubted
polyploid origin. They represent paleotetraploids (10?,11,12,13,
14,15 by primarily descending aneuploidy and infrequently ascending
aneuploidy from 14), paleohexaploids (18,19,20,21,22, also by
primarily descending aneuploidy and secondarily ascending aneuploidy from 21), and paleododecaploids (39,43). Secondary polyploidy also occurs in some genera, notably Magnolia (x=19, 4x and
8x), Hernandia (x=20, 4x), and Piper (x=12, to 10x), but by and
large additional polyploidy is rare. Likewise infraspecific
polyploidy is infrequent, being reported once in only eight
genera and two or three times in Magnolia, Peperomia, and Piper.
Primary diploids among Annonales are not common. Paleodiploids
(x=8) are known in Trimeniaceae (26) and diploids are common in
Annonaceae (x=7,8,9) (27) and Aristolochiaceae (x=6,7) although
polyploids particularly in the latter are frequent (e.g., Aristolochia with 13 2x and 9 4x species). It is among these families,
especially Trimeniaceae having paleodiploid species in Trimenia
and Piptocalyx, where those arguing that the first angiosperms
were successful because they possessed a homomorphic multiple

allele selfincompatibility system that breaks down when polyploids
occur (11) and therefore should not be encountered among the
relictual primitive families, toward which this research ought to
focus.

Berberidales. Lardizabalaceae with x=14-16 are all of
polyploid origin; there are no known secondary polyploids.
Menispermaceae with x=12 and 13 are also all of early polyploid
origin, but in both Cocculus and Menispermum secondary polyploids
occur. In contrast, primary diploids are found throughout
Ranunculaceae (x=7,8,9) although derived polyploid bases exist
(e.g., x=13) (28). For most modern genera diploid species are
more common than polyploid ones: Actaea, Cimicifuga, Hepatica,
Lycoctonom, and Nigella having only 2x species; Aquilegia,
Clematis, Isopyrum, Pulsatilla, and Trollius mostly with 2x
species, Px rare or infrequent; Anemone and Delphinium about
2.5:1 2x:Px species; Adonis and Batarachium with 2x and Px species
about equal in number; Acotinum and Callianthemum somewhat more
Px species than 2x; Ranunculus having about 55% species 2x and
45% Px from a total of 175 species counted, the polyploidy to 16x
and including frequent infraspecific cytotypes; and Thalictrum,
of 67 species studies, with 19% 2x, 60% 4x or 6x, and 21% having
2x and Px cytotypes. For Caltha and Helleborus polyploid species
are primary, the latter perhaps totally polyploid based on 16.
For many Ranunculaceae polyploidy has not been a factor in evolution, but for Caltha, Helleborus, Ranunculus, and Thalictrum in
particular it has been and continues to be important. Likewise
among Papaveraceae (29,30) many genera have primary diploid bases
and secondarily few to numerous polyploids (Corydalis, Fumaria,
Papaver); additionally, early polyploidization is indicated for
Eschscholtzia (x=17) and Argemone (x=14), the latter also evolving
in conjunction with secondary polyploidy to the 8x level and
infraspecific polyploidy.

Nymphaeales. Primary diploid and polyploid genera are found
in Nymphaeaceae: Nelumbo (x=8) is diploid while Cabomba (x=12),
Nuphur (x=17), and Nymphaea (x=14) are probably paleotetraploids
with Nymphaea continuing the process via secondary polyploidy
(species to 8x and many others with infraspecific polyploidy).
Ceratophyllaceae (x=12) are paleotetraploids.

2.   Superorder Hamamelidiflorae (phylogenetic group 2)

Hamamelidales. Primary diploids are infrequent, the more
common basic numbers being paleopolyploids as for Trochodendraceae
(x=20), Tetracentraceae (x=24,23?), Hamamelidaceae (x=12,16) but
also paleodiploid Disanthus with x=8 (31), Cercidiphyllaceae
(x=19), and Eucommiaceae (x=14). Platanaceae have extant primary
diploids with numerous polyploids based on 7.

Casuarinales. Casuarina (Casuarinaceae) (32) has a wide
range of base numbers (x=8-14) that are diploid or polyploid, of
which x=9,10,11,12, and 14 are most common, but with x=8 among

the more primitive members of the genus. The occurrence of
similar base numbers in Hamamelidaceae and Casuarinaceae now
allows for a plausible relationship between the families on
cytological evidence (31).

Fagales. Ancestral polyploid base numbers are fundamental
to Fagaceae (x=12,13); primary diploids and secondary polyploids
are absent. In Betulaceae paleotetraploids are also common (Alnus,
Betula, Corylus x=14), although secondary polyploids occur.
However, primary diploids are fundamental to Carpinus, Ostrya,
and Ostryopsis where x=8, a base number now common to the three
major orders of this phylogenetic group.

Balanopales. Balanops, the only genus of Balanopaceae, is
x=21 (33) and paleohexaploid.

3. Superorder Caryophyllidae (phylogenetic group 3)

Chenopodiales. Phytolaccaceae (x=9) are predominantly
polyploids. Nyctaginaceae are also polyploids, but they are
fundamentally paleopolyploids with x=13 (Boerhavia), 17 (Bougainvillea), and 29 (Allionia, Mirabilis, Oxybaphus). Like Phytolaccaceae, Aizoaceae (34) are based widely on 9 (excepting
Tetragonia x=16, Trianthema x=8,13), but are more fundamentally
diploid than polyploid (about 30% of species). Cactaceae are
x=11 (35), probably paleotetraploids. Only 14% of known species
are secondary polyploids although well-developed in Opuntia where
40% of the species are 2x, 20% are both 2x and Px (3x-10x), and
in Mammillaria (35). Few counts are known for Didiereaceae, but
they suggest high polyploidy. Diverse primary and secondary base
numbers and widespread paleo- and neopolyploidy are found in
Portulacaceae (37-38) as exemplified by Calandrinia (x=12),
Claytonia (x=5,8), Naiocrene (x=11), Oreobroma (x=17), Portulaca
(x=8,9), and Talinum (x=12). Basellaceae are all fundamentally
polyploid (x=11,12) including secondary polyploidy superimposed
on these bases. Polyploidy is also well-developed in Chenopodiaceae (x=6,9) (39-40) where 2x species number 55%, those with
2x and Px cytotypes total 14%, and Px species include 31% of
those counted. Primary diploid base numbers and derived polyploid
bases typify genera in Amaranthaceae where Amaranthus (x=16,17)
has remained diploid, but Alternanthera (x=7-9) has evolved many
polyploids. With base numbers of 9-12, 15-17, and 23, Caryophyllaceae (41,42) are, however, primarily early polyploids, the commonest bases being 12 and 15. Additionally, secondary polyploidy
and infraspecific polyploidy are common in that family.

Polygonales. Both primary diploid and early polyploid bases
are known in Polygonaceae (x=7-9, more commonly 10-12). Rumex
having x=7-10 is about 1/2 polyploid with species to 20x and
infraspecific polyploidy is common (43); a similar situation
prevails in Eriogonum (x=9-12,16,17,20), Polygonum (primarily
x=10-12), and Rheum (x=11), in contrast to Calligonum where x=9

and only about 1/3 of species are polyploids limited to the 4x level.

Balanopales. Batis (Batidaceae) is x=11 with no known secondary polyploidy. The order does not fit well in Caryophyllidae based on recent chemical and cytological data (44); affinities may be closer to Capparidales.

4. Superorders Theiflorae and Sarraceniiflorae (phylogenetic group 4)

Theales. Dilleniaceae (12) are primarily paleopolyploids from an extinct base of 7 with modern genera represented frequently by x=12 and 13, but Dillenia is known with n=8; Paeoniaceae, x=5, are more frequently diploid than polyploid; Actinidiaceae are high polyploids; Theaceae are perhaps all paleotetraploids with x=15 predominating, but in Camellia secondary polyploidy to 6x is also well-developed (45); Aquifoliaceae are high polyploids; Clethraceae are diploids and tetraploids with x=8; Cyrillaceae, x=10, are diploid (Cliftonia) and tetraploid (Cyrilla); Ochnaceae are fundamentally polyploid (x=12,14) with very few neopolyploids; Scytopetalaceae, x=11 and 18, are of polyploid origin; Dipterocarpaceae include primary diploids (x=6,7) and commonly x=10 that may be of polyploid origin, but secondary polyploids on these bases are very rare; Dioncophyllaceae, x=18 from a single count, are polyploid; Clusiaceae, x=7-10 and 12, have many polyploids, e.g., Hypericum (x=12) of polyploid origin with speciation involving both descending aneuploidy (x=12,10,9,8,7) and secondary polyploidy in all but the last aneuploid line (46); Elatinaceae are x=9 and 12 with polyploidy dominant in the few counts available; and Lecythidaceae, x=13 and 16-18, are all derived polyploids with secondary polyploidy on these bases frequent.

Sarraceniales. Sarraceniaceae (47), x=13,15 and 21, are all of polyploid origin; there is no known secondary polyploid.

Nepenthales. Nepenthaceae, x=39, are paleohexaploids with no known secondary polyploid based on limited counts.

Ericales. Ericaceae, including Pyrolaceae (x=11-13 most common), are largely early polyploids possibly from an original base of 6. Secondary polyploids are not common, except in Rhododendron (18% of species Px) and particularly in Vaccinium (40% Px). Diploids are reported for Calluna, Monotropa, and Pterospora, all x=8. Diploids are, however, common in Epacridaceae (48) (x=4,6,7-9); there are few polyploids, but Andersonia, Richea, and Woollsia, all x=13, are polyploid in derivation. The base number of 13 is also shared by Empetraceae at both diploid and tetraploid levels.

Ebenales. Ebenaceae, x=15, and Symplocaceae, x=11, probably arose from early polyploidization, though lacking secondary polyploidy based on known counts; Sapotaceae have x=13 predominating; and Styracaceae, x=8 and 12, originated at least in part by polyploidy but with limited secondary polyploidy.

Primulales. Myrsinaceae, x=10,12 and 23, and Theophrastaceae, x=13 and 18, by and large represent early polyploids with limited subsequent polyploidy. Primulaceae (49), commonly x=12, have few primary diploids, the majority of taxa being of polyploid origin. Secondary and infraspecific polyploidy in Dodecatheon are frequent.

Plumbaginales. Plumbaginaceae, x=7-9, are exclusively of primary diploid bases having frequent euploidy (e.g., Statice with 30% polyploid species). Lacking a polyploid origin is a fundamental difference between Plumbaginales and other orders of this phylogenetic group. The possibility exists, however, that these bases are terminals of a very old descending aneuploid series from even more ancient polyploid stocks.

5. Superorder Cistiflorae (phylogenetic group 5)

Cistales. Flacourtiaceae, x=10 but primarily 11 and 12, probably arose by polyploidy early; additionally, species of Abatia, Casearia, Hydnocarpus, Idesia, and Lindackeria are secondarily polyploid. Scyphostegiaceae based on a single count are diploid with x=9. In Violaceae (50) x=12 is the commonest base number although dysploidy to x=4 is found in Hybanthus and Viola. Even some of these may be of polyploid origin prior to aneuploid reduction and with subsequent secondary polyploidy; aneuploid increase from x=12 to 13 may also have occurred in some species of Viola. Bixaceae are diploid with x=7(8) in Bixus and x=6 in Cochlospermum. Cistaceae (51) include Tuberaria with x=12 and Fumana with x=16, undoubtedly both of polyploid origin, as well as the diploid based Cistus and Halimum (x=9). The x=5 and particularly the x=9-12 of Helianthemum perhaps represents a descending aneuploid series from 12; it is the only Cistaceae having widespread secondary polyploidy. Turneraceae are x=7 and 10 with limited secondary polyploidy. Malesherbiaceae are diploid (x=7). Passifloraceae, x=9,11, and 12 with descending dysploids, are of polyploid origin at least in part; species of Adenia (x=12), additionally, are about 50% secondary polyploids (4x). Carica (Caricaceae) is diploid based on 9. Cucurbitaceae have x=12 as the commonest base and are therefore largely of polyploid derivation; secondary polyploidy is scattered throughout the family but nowhere is dominant. The most frequent base number in Begonia (52) (Begoniaceae) is 14 and most species are thus originally polyploid; about 1/4 of the species are secondary polyploids and infraspecific polyploidy is also frequent. Datiscaceae, x=11(23?), are also polyploid derivatives. Loasaceae (53) have basic numbers of 7-14 and 37; many genera are of polyploid origin and some have secondary polyploid species as well. Caiophera, x=7 and 8, appears to be diploid, an unusual chromosomal level in the family.

Salicales. All genera of Salicaceae (54) are based on 19 and are derived, perhaps tribasic, polyploids. Populus has few secondary polyploids but about 1/3 of $\underline{Salix}$ species are secondary polyploids and infraspecific polyploidy is common.

$\underline{Tamaricales}$. All Tamaricaceae are x=12 and are derived polyploids; no secondary polyploid is known. $\underline{Frankenia}$ (Frankeniaceae) has x=5, the majority of species polyploid to 6x.

$\underline{Capparidales}$. In Capparidaceae basic numbers of 10 and 11 are most frequent with secondarily higher bases, x=12,15-18,21, and 29 and more occasionally lower ones as x=8 in $\underline{Atamisquea}$ and $\underline{Cadaba}$. The majority are therefore of polyploid origin. Brassicaceae (55,56) with x=4-15 may have an original base number of 12 or 14, and ascending and primarily descending aneuploidy to form other lines of evolution. Secondary polyploidy is widespread, although not particularly common in $\underline{Lesquerella}$ (57), $\underline{Raphanus}$, or $\underline{Thlaspi}$; infraspecific polyploidy is also frequent (the Appendix lists 45 genera where it has been reported) and together with aneuploidy emphasize that change at the chromosomal level has been and continues to be very important in the evolution of the family. In Resedaceae, where x=6 and 10, polyploidy and diploidy occur about equally. Moringaceae and Tovariaceae are based on 14 and are of polyploid origin, perhaps from an ancestral x=7.

6.   Superorder Malviiflorae (p.p.) (phylogenetic group 6)

$\underline{Malvales}$. A base number of 10 with euploidy is common in Sterculiaceae, although much lower (x=7 in $\underline{Melochia}$ and $\underline{Waltheria}$) and higher (x=9 in $\underline{Pentapetes}$ and $\underline{Pterygota}$, and x=21(20) in $\underline{Cola}$) bases exist. Many are obviously of polyploid origin; the diploid genera may be primary diploids or diploids derived by aneuploid reduction from polyploids. Elaeocarpaceae, x=13 and 14 primarily, are also fundamentally polyploid; more recent superimposed polyploidy is unknown. In Tiliaceae $\underline{Corchorus}$ (x=7), $\underline{Glyphae}$ (x=8), $\underline{Duboscia}$ (x=9), and $\underline{Grewia}$ (x=9) are primary diploid genera, whereas $\underline{Triumfetta}$ (x=16), $\underline{Clappertonia}$ (x=18), and $\underline{Tilia}$ (x=41) are of polyploid ancestry. Moreover, about 25% of $\underline{Tilia}$ species are also secondary polyploids with 4x. Bombacaceae are also all derived from polyploid bases with some super-imposed secondary polyploid based on x=36 (58), perhaps ancestrally from x=12. Malvaceae (59), possibly from an early base of 7, are highly diverse and complex cytologically: $\underline{Nototriche}$ forms a euploid series based on 5 with 41% of species 2x and, of the remaining polyploids, 35% are 4x, 12% 6x, and 12% 8x; $\underline{Spaeralcea}$ and $\underline{Tarasa}$ are both x=5, the latter having about 50% polyploid species, the former with a high frequency of infraspecific polyploidy; $\underline{Wissadula}$ (x=7) is diploid; and $\underline{Abutilon}$ and $\underline{Sida}$ have x=7 and 8 with about 1/3 species polyploid. To these fundamentally diploid genera can be added those derived from polyploid ancestry: $\underline{Hibiscus}$ (60,61) with x=11-20 and a high frequency of secondary polyploidy, $\underline{Gossypium}$ with x=13 and about 50% secondary polyploidy, $\underline{Anoda}$ with x=15 and some secondary polyploidy, and $\underline{Alcea}$, $\underline{Althaea}$,

and <u>Malva</u> with x=21 and increasing frequency of secondary polyploidy to 6x in <u>Malva</u>.

    <u>Urticales</u>. Ulmaceae, x=10 and 14, have few polyploid species
in <u>Ulmus</u>, but nearly 50% of <u>Celtis</u> species are polyploid. Moraceae
(62), primarily x=12-14, are probably all of polyploid origin and
secondary polyploids are few. Cannabaceae are based on 10: they
likely are derived by reduction from a higher (polyploid) ancestral
number. Infraspecific polyploidy is known in both <u>Cannabis</u> and
<u>Humulus</u>. For Urticaceae x=13 and 14 predominate with few secondary
polyploids formed from these ancestral polyploid bases.

    <u>Euphorbiales</u>. In Euphorbiaceae (63,64) x=13 is prevalent
among primitive taxa of subf. Phyllanthoideae (65) and x=9-11
common among subf. Euphorbioideae, x=10 being predominant in
<u>Euphorbia</u>. The majority of taxa therefore arose from early
polyploid bases with secondary polyploidy occasional to frequent
in <u>Euphorbia</u> and <u>Phyllanthus</u>, respectively. Mehra and Choda
(66), for example, concluded that the large number of polyploids
and incidence of higher levels of polyploids in <u>Euphorbia</u> indicate
that chromosomal multiplication has played an important role in
the evolution and speciation among the euphorbias. Pandaceae are
x=15 on limited data, and Dichapetalaceae are x=10 on equally few
counts. Thymelaeaceae with x=9 are fundamentally diploid (but
perhaps by aneuploid reduction from a polyploid base), although
polyploidy has been important in the evolution of <u>Pimella</u>.
Buxaceae with x=10,13, and 14 are largely derived from ancestral
polyploidy; secondary polyploidy is infrequent.

7. <u>Superorder Rosiflorae (phylogenetic group 7)</u>

    <u>Rosales</u>. Subfamilies of Rosaceae (67) typically have the
following base numbers: Spiraeoideae x=9, Prunoideae x=8, Ro-
soideae x=7 predominately with x=8 and 9 in several phylads, and
Maloideae x=17 including anomolous genera from the unnatural
Quillajeae (68). Base numbers of 7 and 9 are postulated, euploid
series are widespread, and as the subf. Maloideae is evidently of
paleotetraploid origin, polyploidy has been of evolutionary
significance in the family for a long time. It continues to be
as evidenced by the high frequency of infraspecific polyploidy in
such genera as <u>Potentilla</u> and <u>Rubus</u>. The allied families
Chrysobalanaceae have x=10 and 11 and Neuadaceae x=7, the former
at least in part ancestrally polyploid, and neither with known
secondary polyploidy. Crassosomataceae (x=12) and Connaraceae
(x=14) are of polyploid origin and they also lack secondary polyploids. Subfamilies of Fabaceae (69,70) with their base numbers
are: Mimosoideae frequently with x=13 and 14 and evidently of early
tetraploid origin, perhaps <u>Calliandra</u> (x=8) arising as a consequence of descending aneuploidy; Caesalpinioideae with x=7 in
one line that appears basic (e.g., <u>Cercis</u> a paleodiploid), and in
another line x=14 and 12 that are fundamentally polyploid, an
early event in the evolution of the subfamily; and Faboideae with

primitive Sophoreae polyploid having x=14 (possibly diploid x=7 with early establishment of polyploidy), and other tribes formed as polyploid derivates often with high base numbers. Secondary waves of polyploidy account for high levels of polyploidy in Erythrina (71) where x=21, Genisteae (Genista 75% polyploid species, Lupinus 98%, Ulex 80%, Cytisus 85%+), Galegeae (Astragalus, Oxytropis), Trifolieae (Medicago, Ononis, Trifolium), and Loteae (Lotus), including infraspecific polyploidy known among 55 genera. Mimosoideae and Caesalpinioideae do not possess high frequencies of secondary polyploidy. Crassulaceae (72-74) are x=7-9 and also x=15 in Aichryson and x=15 and 17-19 in Sempervivum at diploid and polyploid levels. Infraspecific polyploidy is also important: 32 species of Sedum are known with diploid and polyploid cytotypes or two or more polyploid forms. Saxifragaceae (75) have many polyploid base numbers (x=11-13,17,18); secondary polyploid between and within species is particularly relevant in Saxifraga. Similarly, Stylidiaceae commonly have the derived x=15, but also x=5-16; secondary polyploidy occurs on bases of 13,14, and 15 (76). Droseraceae have wide-range x=13,14,16,17,19, and 23, but x=10 with euploidy is most frequent, perhaps having arisen by aneuploid reduction from a polyploid base. Podostemaceae are x=10 also with euploidy. Diapensiaceae have x=6, apparently a primary base number; all are paleodiploids with Galax exhibiting infraspecific tetraploidy. Cunonaceae have x=12,15 and 16, all secondary basic numbers of polyploid origin. High base numbers also exist in Davidsoniaceae (x=16), Eucryphiaceae (77) (x=15), Staphyleaceae (x=13), Corynocarpaceae (x=22), and Coriariaceae (x=20); these fundamentally polyploid families have little superimposed secondary polyploidy. High base numbers are more or less typical of Rosales and on this basis these families fit well here.

   Pittosporales. Daphniphyllaceae (x=16) and Pittosporaceae (x=12,18) in so far as data exist have base numbers of early polyploid origin. However, Byblidaceae (x=7,12) and Bruniaceae (x=11) each have base numbers either of primary origin or of descending aneuploid origin from higher ancestral bases. Many families in the order are unknown chromosomally.

8. Superorders Proteiflorae and Myrtiflorae (phylogenetic group 8)

   Proteales. Proteaceae (78) with a prototypic x=7 (represented by Persoonia and Placospermum) involved early polyploidy to n=14 that is basic to subfamilies Grevilleoideae and Persoonioideae. This was followed in both subfamilies by aneuploid reduction from x=14-10, now basic, for example, in Agastachys (x=13), Protea (x=12), Aulax (x=11), and Grevillea (x=10). The latter is a prime example of x=10 being of polyploidy origin. There is little secondary polyploidy.

   Myrtales. Lythraceae are basically primary diploids with x=5,6, and 8. Euploidy is general in Lythrum (x=5) where most species are polyploid. Punicaceae (x=8) are diploids in so far

as known. Trapaceae are highly polyploid (x=24), perhaps from a
base of x=12 as found in Combretaceae, the majority of which are
also fundamentally polyploid with subsequent dysploidy but with
little secondary polyploidy. Myrtaceae are based on 11 (79),
probably via polyploidy from an original primitive genome with
x=6 (80). There is limited polyploidy among species of Lepto-
spermum, and Psidium species are about equally divided between
diploidy and polyploidy, but the majority of genera are diploid
as typified by Eucalyptus and Melaleuca. Melastomataceae (81)
are basically diploid, as illustrated by Memecylon x=7, Heeria
x=8, and Guyonia x=9, with limited polyploidy, and secondarily of
polyploid origin, as exemplified by Dissotis and Tristemma, both
x=17, Rhexia, x=11, and perhaps Osbeckia, x=10. The family
combines to fundamental modes of chromosomal evolution: the
first represented by extant diploids usually with polyploidy, and
the second in which diploids are extinct but with early evolution
involving polyploidy followed by dysploidy and often secondary
polyploidy. Onagraceae are x=11 with new basic numbers formed by
descending aneuploidy (13) and still others by polyploid increases
as in Epilobium (predominantly x=18), or by ascending aneuploidy
as in Zauschernia (x=15).

9. Superorders Geraniiflorae and Rutiflorae (phylogenetic group 9)

Geraniales. Linaceae, as represented by Linum, fundamentally
are x=9 with aneuploid reduction to 6, and with widespread polyploidy (n=18) followed by aneuploid reduction of polyploids to
n=15 and 13 (82,83), and ultimately higher polyploidy on these
bases. In this primarily temperate family, the tropical Hugonia,
x=6, may prove basic. Houmiriaceae and Erythroxylaceae are both
x=12. Zygophyllaceae have Tribulus based on 6 with a euploid
series, Larrea based on 13, and Zygophyllum based on 11, suggesting
x=6 or 12 as basic with aneuploid increase and decrease. Somewhat
paralleling Zygophyllaceae, Oxalidaceae (84) possess primary
diploid and early polyploid genera: herbaceous Oxalis has x=5-12
with 7 predominant and including euploidy, herbaceous Biophytum
has x=9, and woody Averrhoa has x=11. Like Tribulus, modern
Oxalis species could represent a series based on aneuploid reduction from an ancient polyploid of x=±12 with more primitive
genera retaining base numbers close to the original. Core genera
of Geraniaceae have x=10-14; only for Erodium is additional
polyploidy frequent with about 25% of species 4x. Likewise
Tropaeolaceae have derived base numbers with x=14 predominant and
little additional polyploidy. Segregates from Geraniaceae such
as Vivianiaceae (x=7) and Ledocarpaceae (x=9) are lower (33,85),
and may prove of primary origin, as indeed may representatives
among the remaining families of the order, Balsaminaceae (36)
x=7 predominant and Limnanthaceae x=5 (87), both with limited
polyploidy.

Polygalales. In Malpighiaceae x=9 and 10 predominate with
polyploidy meager; too few counts are available to suggest base
number and significance of polyploidy in the evolution of the
family. Polygalaceae parallel Oxalidaceae in that Oxalis and
Polygala are represented by scarce (relictual?) x=7 (and 8), yet
with widespread base number diversity at the polyploidy level.
Bases of 12,14,17, and 19 predominate in Polygala (88,89) with
secondary polyploidy also well-developed and important in speciation. Monnina is x=5 and primarily polyploid. Krameriaceae (90)
with x=6 and no polyploidy differ from other members of the
order, whereas Trigoniaceae (x=ca.10) and Vochysiaceae (x=11)
(33) derived partly or totally from polyploid bases are more
characteristic.
        Rutales. Ehrendorfer (12) summarized three evolutionary
phases in Rutaceae: primary diploid radiation by ascending
aneuploidy from x=7 to 9 represented now by relictual paleopolyploid genera with these genomes as basic (Toddalioideae, Zanthoxy-
leae, and some Flindersioideae); genetic and some polyploid
radiation based on 9 (Aurantioideae, Rutoideae); and secondary
aneuploid and polyploid explosive evolution in Boronieae. This
parallels that of a number of other (sub)tropical woody families:
Simaroubaceae are all early polyploids with the lowest base
numbers x=12-14 most common but extending to x=25, Cneoraceae
with x=14, Meliaceae (91-98) having high base numbers, the lowest
about 11, Burseraceae having primarily x=13, and Anacardiaceae
fundamentally x=14-16 but also higher as illustrated by Mangifera
with x=20. However, Podoaceae sometimes segregated from Anacardiaceae are x=7. This pattern of meager frequencies of primary
diploids and extensive radiation at paleopolyploid levels with
little secondary polyploidy is found also in woody tropical
families sometimes segregated in Sapindales, such as Sapindaceae
with x=12,14, and 16 common, Sabiaceae with x=12 and 16, and
Melianthaceae with x=19. Likewise temperately and tropically
distributed Hippocastanaceae having Aesculus based on 20 and
temperate Aceraceae with x=13 fit this pattern.
        Juglandales. Juglandaceae (94) are paleopolyploids with
x=16; only in Carya is secondary polyploidy well-developed.
        Myricales. Muricaceae are fundamentally x=8 having both
diploid and polyploid taxa; n=16 is widespread.
        Leitneriales. Leitneriaceae have x=16. All three orders
fit well with the concept of an ancient x=18, still extant in
Myricales, and x=16 fundamental to all and of early origin.

10. Superorders Santaliflorae, Rafflesiiflorae, and Corniflorae
        (phylogenetic group 10)

        Santalales. Common base numbers in Celastraceae are 16 for
Euonymus (95) with secondary polyploidy and 23 for Celastrus.
The predominant number in Stackhousiaceae is 10 with some secondary
polyploidy, for Icacinaceae x=10 and 11 with euploidy, Olacaceae

x=19 and 20, Opiliaceae x=10, Santalaceae x=5-7 common but Thesium
having x=6,7,10 and 13 illustrating both primary (or derived)
diploid and fundamentally polyploid bases, Loranthaceae (96-98)
subf. Loranthoideae basically x=12 with subsequent aneuploid
reduction to x=8 and subf. Viscoideae x=14-10 also of polyploid-
aneuploid origins, a loranthaceous segregate Eremolepidaceae x=13
and 10, Balanophoraceae x=9 predominating with euploidy common,
and Cynomoriaceae x=12. The order is characterized by early
polyploid-formed base numbers between 12 and 14 with subsequent
aneuploidy and limited secondary polyploidy on these bases.

Oleales. Salvadoraceae are x=12. Oleaceae (99,100) subf.
Jasminoideae are x=11,13, and 14, and subf. Oleoideae x=23, the
latter likely derived by additional polyploidy from a Jasminoideae-
like base.

Rafflesiales. Rafflesiaceae have x=12,16, and 20 and the
segregated Mitrastemonaceae (101) x=10.

Cornales. Rhizophoraceae have x=16 and 18 with secondary
polyploidy, Vitaceae x=11 and 12 with additional polyploid bases
of x=19 and 20, Nyssaceae x=22, Davidiaceae x=21, Cornaceae subf.
Cornoideae primarily x=11 but Aucuba x=8 with polyploidy, subf.
Mastixioideae x=11 and 13 and subf. Curtisioideae x=13 (102),
Alangiaceae x=11, Garryaceae x=11, Haloragidaceae x=7 with euploidy
common in Haloragis and Myriophyllum but derived polyploid x=17
in Gunnera, and Hippuridaceae x=16. All families have polyploid
origins; extant primary diploids occur only in Haloragidaceae.
Continuing a ± fundamental theme of early polyploidy around a
basic number of 12, often with additional polyploidy, are Araliaceae (103) with x=12 and many species either 4x or 8x, and the
allied Apiaceae with x=11 and 10 (104,105) and well-developed
polyploidy. The latter perhaps represents an early aneuploid
reduction from an ancestral 12 now common to the Araliaceae.

Dipsacales. Caprifoliaceae (106) are often x=8 and 9, a
secondary base of x=18 being modal for Sambucus and Symphoricarpos.
Adoxaceae have x=18, and Valerianaceae have x=7 (Valerianella),
x=7 and 8 with euploidy (Valeriana), and x=11 (Patrinia). Dipsacaceae parallel Valerianaceae with x=8,9 and 10 predominant.

11. Superorders Gentianiflorae, Malviiflorae (p.p.), Lamiiflorae,
    and Asteriflorae (phylogenetic group 11)

Gentianales. Loganiaceae (107) are commonly x=11 with a
high percent of secondary polyploidy, less commonly x=13 and 19
(the last typical of Buddleja segregated as a family and sometimes
included in the next order, 101), or 10,8, and 7. Rubiaceae
(108) are also fundamentally x=11 in woody tropical tribes, but
predominantly herbaceous and derived tribes are either x=14 as in
Spermacoceae (ascending aneuploidy), or x=13, and 11-6 in Hedyo-
tideae (ascending but largely descending aneuploidy among temperate
representatives). Many herbaceous genera have diploid and polyploid species, as Asperula and Rubia, but many woody genera, as

Psychotria, Ixora, and Gardenia, only rarely if at all have
diploid and polyploid species. Apocynaceae (109) commonly are
x=11 and 10, although descending aneuploidy to x=6 exists with
secondary polyploidy rare in some genera (Strophanthus, x=10),
while important in others (Rauwolfia, x=11). Asclepiadaceae are
x=11 with secondary polyploidy rare in Asclepias but common in
Stapelia. Whereas x=11 is a unifying element of these four large
families, Gentianaceae (110,111) are predominantly x=9 and 13
with x=11 less frequent; about 58% of species are polyploids.
Menyanthaceae (112) have predominantly x=9 with euploidy common.
    Bignoniales. High basic polyploid numbers as well as some
secondary polyploidy characterize the first part of the order:
Bignoniaceae (113) have mostly x=20 (with limited euploidy),
Pedaliaceae have x=18 and euploidy, Martyniaceae have x=15 and
16, and Myoporaceae have x=18 with euploidy. Scrophulariaceae
(114,115), however, have genera such as Hebe (x=20,21) that
conform to this mode, but others are known with lower polyploid
bases, such as Digitalis (x=14), and still others with diploid
levels (Collinsia, Gratiola, Lindernia, Dopatrium, all n=7).
Polyploidy is a continuing mechanism of speciation, however,
judging from the high frequency of infraspecific polyploidy
(Appendix). Even lower diploid numbers typify Plantaginaceae
(116) with x=6,5, and 4; radiating from these bases 46% of Plantago
species are known to be polyploid and 17% of additional species
have both diploid and polyploid cytotypes. Orobanchaceae (117)
have x=12 and 19 in Orobanche with secondary polyploidy, as well
as additional high base numbers in other genera. Lentibulariaceae
are x=8 (in Pinguicula) and x=9 (in Utricularia), the latter
highly euploid. Acanthaceae (118) are x=7-9 with widespread
euploidy and some polyploid base numbers as in Ruellia (x=17).
Gesneriaceae (119) may have a basic number of x=9, although the
dysploids 8 and 10 are common; polyploidy is sporadic and sometimes
rare as in Columnea where 34 of 35 species counted are n=9.
    Solanales. Nolanaceae are x=12. Solanaceae (120) are also
largely x=12, particularly in Solaneae with euploidy and little
aneuploidy. This contrasts with Cestreae where bases are various,
but not usually x=12, and where aneuploidy is present, as for the
remarkable reduction series from 12 to 7 in Petunia. Infraspecific
polyploidy is well-marked especially in Solanum where, for example,
S. tuberosum has five distinct euploid series ranging from 2x to
6x with the tetraploid the most successful in terms of yield and
cultivation (121). In Convolvulaceae (122,123) Cuscuta has
primary diploid species based on 7 with an extensive euploid
series. Elsewhere in the family x=14 and 15 are dominant and
these bases may have arisen by early polyploidy from x=7 with
subsequent aneuploid reduction in Porana (x=13), Evolvulus (x=13,
12), Calystegia (x=11), and Jacquemontia (x=9), all essentially
tetraploid in origin excepting perhaps the last. Secondary
polyploidy is well represented throughout the family. The basic
number in Polemoniaceae (124,125) is 9 represented in ancient

genera such as <u>Cobaea</u> by x=26 and <u>Cantua</u> by x=27 (both paleopolyploids) and found in each tribe of the family; x=8,7 and 6 are
derived by aneuploid reduction. Polyploidy may be important in
speciation, as in <u>Gilia</u>, or it may be irrelevant as in <u>Polemonium</u>.
Primary diploids are also fundamental in Fouquieriaceae where
x=8.

    <u>Lamiales</u>. The most frequent basic numbers in Hydrophyllaceae
(126) are 7 (<u>Nama</u>), 9 (<u>Hydrophyllum</u>, <u>Nemophila</u>), and 11 (<u>Phacelia</u>
The latter as well as <u>Turricula</u> (x=13), <u>Eriodictyon</u> (x=14), <u>Codon</u>
(x=17), <u>Emmenanthe</u> (x=18), and <u>Wigandia</u> (x=19) are of polyploid
origin. The basic number of Boraginaceae may have been 12 with
early aneuploid reduction (13), although Britton (127) suggests
x=8, while noting that almost all species of Cynoglosseae are
x=12, a number also found in <u>Symphytum</u> (128). Lennoaceae have
x=9 with polyploidy. Primary diploid numbers are also common in
Verbenaceae (x=7,8,9) (129), but these may have arisen at least
in part by aneuploid reduction from early polyploid base numbers
that are fundamental to so many genera in the family. Infrageneric
polyploidy is frequent in <u>Verbena</u> (130) subg. <u>Verbena</u> (x=7) with
63% of species 2x and 37% Px and subg. <u>Glandularia</u> (x=5) with 50%
2x and 50% Px, the hexaploids more common than tetraploids in
both lines. Callitrichaceae have low primary numbers (x=3,5 are
common) and about 1/2 of <u>Callitriche</u> species are polyploid. High
polyploid bases typify Lamiaceae; x=14 may be basic (13). <u>Hedeoma</u>
(131), for example, has x=18 for most sections.

    <u>Campanulales</u>. As for the preceding order, high base numbers
combined with primary diploid numbers are found in Campanulaceae
(132). <u>Lobelia</u> has x=7 with an extensive euploid series, yet
<u>Campanula</u> and its allies commonly are polyploid-derived (x=17)
with secondary polyploidy common (n=68). Goodeniaceae (133) have
x=7,8, and 9 and little infrageneric polyploidy (14%) in contrast
to its significance in Campanulaceae, although infraspecific
polyploidy is unusually high and may prove important in current
speciation.

    <u>Asterales</u>. In Asteraceae when the modal group at the tribal
level is not x=9, it is either x=10 or x=17 with the sole exception
of Mutisieae (x=12) (134). There is considerable base number
variation at the subtribal level as exemplified by the three main
evolutionary lines in Heliantheae (135): Verbesininae x=15,16,17,
Galinsoginae x=8,9, and Coreopsidinae-Fitchiinae x=12. Polyploidy
continues to be important in evolution and speciation as the
occurrence of infraspecific polyploidy among 122 genera suggests.
Genomic diversity is particularly frequent in <u>Chrysanthemum</u> and
<u>Senecio</u> (at least 25 species each).

SUMMARY

    A number of generalized trends relative to polyploidy are
apparent throughout the dicotyledons. Those taxa with polyploid

base numbers whether known to be paleopolyploids or not have few
secondary and infraspecific polyploids. In contrast, those with
extant primary diploid bases commonly have extensive euploid
series and infraspecific polyploidy is a much more common phenomenon.

1. <u>Annoniflorae</u>. Assuming an ancestral $x=7$, paleopolyploids
dominate the superorder with many families represented only by
ancestral hexaploid and higher base numbers. Infrageneric and
infraspecific polyploidy are not common, and there are obvious
gaps in the chromosome number series. All of these aspects can be
taken as evidence of great age, a high rate of extinction, and
evolutionary stagnation (12).

2. <u>Hamamelidiflorae</u>. The most recent cytological data show
that the superorder is held together by more than parallel adaptations to anemophily, for diploids based on 8 are common to Hamamelidales, Casuarinales, and Fagales. Their existence suggests that
if not somewhat younger than the Annoniflorae then at least a
reduced elimination of cytologically fundamental elements has
characterized the superorder. In common with the Annoniflorae,
paleopolyploids clearly dominate (12) with probably the same
ancestral base number of 7, early aneuploid reduction to $x=6$
followed by polyploidy, and early aneuploid increase to $x=8$ (31)
to establish the only extant primary diploid species.

3. <u>Caryophyllidae</u>. A base number of 9 in widespread,
presumably by early aneuploid increase from $x=7$ (13) and perhaps
decrease to $x=6$, with ancestral polyploidy fundamental to the
origin of taxa in Nyctaginaceae, Aizoaceae, Cactaceae, Portulacaceae, Amaranthaceae, Caryophyllaceae, Polygonaceae, Batidaceae,
and much less so in Chenopodiaceae. Secondary polyploidy is also
of wide significance.

4. <u>Theiflorae and Sarraceniiflorae</u>. An early polyploid
origin characterizes members of these superorders that, like the
preceding, probably arose from an ancestral $x=7$. Only Plumbaginales is out of phase, where primary diploid bases are typical
and euploidy frequent.

5. <u>Cistiflorae</u>. Many orders are characterized by an ancestral base of 12, or less generally 14, and probably arose in
consort with polyploidy early in their evolution. Dysploidy is
very frequent by aneuploid decrease, and secondarily increase,
from $x=12$ (or 14) with subsequent secondary polyploidy. A few
families, such as Bixaceae and Malesherbiaceae, apparently are
primary diploids without polyploid ancestry.

6. <u>Malviiflorae</u>. As for the preceeding, ancestral polyploid
base numbers are common among the Malviiflorae with many genera
typified by descending dysploidy from $x=12-14$. There are probably
instances both of genera with primary diploid basic numbers and
others with the same number that evolved by aneuploid reduction
from polyploids. Euploidy is frequent particularly where primary
diploids are extant.

7. <u>Rosiflorae</u>. Whereas many families or subfamilies have high secondary base numbers that have a polyploid origin, many others characteristically have primary diploid base numbers (x=7-9) with euploidy. This dichotomy is well represented in the Rosales and is a feature of many of the more advanced phylogenetic groups discussed below.

8. <u>Proteiflorae and Myrtiflorae</u>. Proteiflorae are fundamentally polyploid based on 7 with widespread dysploidy. As for Rosales, Myrtiflorae combine the primary diploid mode between x=6 and 9 with the more frequent ancestral polyploid mode with subsequent, often descending, dysploidy. Secondary polyploidy is not common.

9. <u>Geraniiflorae and Rutiflorae</u>. Geraniales and Polygalales are perhaps derived from a base of 7 and secondarily from x=12 or 14. Aneuploid reduction and polyploidy are common. Among the more woody Rutiflorae x=7 and 8 are primary with early polyploidy and further radiation by dysploidy and secondary polyploidy common (12). High base numbers are typical of both tropical and temperate woody elements of the superorder.

10. <u>Santaliflorae, Rafflesiiflorae, and Corniflorae</u>. Throughout these superorders the most frequent and widespread base number is 12 with descending (x=11,10,9) and ascending (x=13,14) dysploidy common. Only Dipsacales are widely represented with diploid basic numbers (x=10,9,8,7); however, these bases may have arisen by descending dysploidy similar to, but more extensive than, that found among other taxa.

11. <u>Gentianiflorae, Malviiflorae (p.p.), Lamiiflorae, and Asteriflorae</u>. Gentianales have primarily ancestral polyploid bases around x=11 with secondary dysploidy to x=13 and 9; Bignoniales have both old and high polyploid bases and apparently primary diploid basic numbers as found in some Scrophulariaceae and all Plantaginaceae; Solanales, Lamiales, and Campanulales, have x=12 and higher polyploids with aneuploid reduction widespread and often greatly reduced to perhaps x=6, although lower diploid bases may also be of primary origin; and Asterales have x=9 with great variation. Polyploidy, including ancestral, secondary, and infraspecific, have been and continue to be of major importance in the evolution of this phylogenetic group.

Although lacking explicit counts by taxa, my survey supports the conclusion of Goldblatt (1) for monocotyledons that the frequency of polyploidy (sensu lato) closely approximates 70% for dicotyledons and may reach 80%, indicating that the incidence of polyploidy in flowering plants has been underestimated and that its significance in evolution is greater than had been assumed.

LITERATURE CITED

1.   Goldblatt, P., 1980, Polyploidy in angiosperms: monocotyledons. This volume, p. 219.

2.   Grant, V., 1963, "The Origin of Adaptations," Columbia University Press, New York. 606 p.

3.   Fedorov, A.N. (ed.), 1969, "Chromosome Numbers of Flowering Plants," Acad. Nauk, Leningrad. 926 p.

4.   Moore, R.J. (ed.), 1973, "Index to Plant Chromosome Numbers 1967-1971," Regnum Vegetabile 90. 539 p.

5.   Moore, R.J. (ed.), 1974, "Index to Plant Chromosome Numbers for 1972," Regnum Vegetabile 91. 108 p.

6.   Moore, R.J. (ed.), 1977, "Index to Plant Chromosome Numbers for 1973/74," Regnum Vegetabile 96. 257 p.

7.   Raven, P.H., Kyhos, D.W., 1965, New evidence concerning the original basic chromosome number of angiosperms. Evolution 19: 244-248.

8.   Ehrendorfer, F., Krendl, F., Habeler, E., Sauer, W., 1968, Chromosome numbers and evolution in primitive angiosperms. Taxon 17: 337-353.

9.   Ehrendorfer, F., 1970, Evolutionary patterns and strategies in seed plants. Taxon 19: 185-195.

10. Raven, P.H., 1971, Chromosome numbers and relationships in Annoniflorae. Taxon 20: 479-483.

11. Ratter, J.A., Milne, C., 1973, Chromosome numbers of some primitive angiosperms. Notes Roy. Bot. Gard. Edinburgh 32: 423-428.

12. Ehrendorfer, F., 1976, Evolutionary significance of chromo-somal differentiation patterns in gymnosperms and primitive angiosperms, in Beck, C.B. (ed.), "Origin and Early Evolution of Angiosperms," Columbia University Press, New York; Ehrendorfer, F., 1980, Polyploidy and distribution. This volume, p. 45.

13. Raven, P.H., 1975, The bases of angiosperm phylogeny: cyto-logy. Ann. Missouri Bot. Gard. 62: 724-764.

14. Grant, W.F., 1976, The evolution of karyotype and polyploidy in arboreal plants. Taxon 25: 75-83.

15. Thorne, R.F., 1968, Synopsis of a putatively phylogenetic classification of the flowering plants. Aliso 6: 57-66.

16. Thorne, R.F., 1973, The "Amentiferae" or Hamamelidae as an artificial group: a summary statement. Brittonia 25: 395-405.

17. Thorne, R.F., 1974, A phylogenetic classification of the Annoniflorae. Aliso 8: 147-209.

18. Lewis, W.H., Elvin-Lewis, M.P.F., 1977, "Medical Botany: Plants Affecting Man's Health," Wiley-Interscience, New York. Appendix 1.

19. Sauer, W., Ehrendorfer, F., 1970, Chromosomen, Verwandtschaft und Evolution tropischer Holzpflanzen, II. Himantandraceae. Österr. Bot. Z. 118: 38-54.

20. Okada, H., Tanaka, R., 1975, Karyological studies in some species of Lauraceae. Taxon 24: 271-280.

21. Gregory, M.P., 1956, A phyletic rearrangement in the Aristo-lochiaceae. Amer. J. Bot. 43: 110-122.

22. Lorence, D., 1979, Personal communication.
23. Goldblatt, P., 1976, Chromosome number in Gomortega Keule.
    Ann Missouri Bot. Gard. 63: 207-208.
24. Smith, J.B., 1966, Chromosome numbers in Peperomia Ruiz and
    Pav. (Piperaceae) and a note on chromosome number of Piper
    magnificum Trelease. Kew Bull. 20: 521-526.
25. Dasgupta, A., Datta, P.C., 1976, Cytotaxonomy of Piperaceae.
    Cytologia 41: 697-706.
26. Goldblatt, P., 1974, A contribution to the knowledge of
    cytology in Magnolialaes. J. Arnold Arb. 55: 453-457.
27. Bowden, W.M., 1948, Chromosome numbers in the Annonaceae.
    Amer. J. Bot. 35: 377-381.
28. Gregory, W.C., 1941, Phylogenetic and cytological studies in
    the Ranunculaceae. Trans. Amer. Phil. Soc. n.s. 31: 443-521.
29. Ownbey, G.B., 1958, Monograph of the genus Argemone for
    North America and the West Indies. Mem. Torrey Bot. Club
    21(1): 1-159.
30. Ernst, W.R., 1959, Chromosome numbers of some Papaveraceae.
    Contr. Dudley Herb. 5: 137-139.
31. Goldblatt, P., Endress, P.K., 1977, Cytology and evolution
    in Hamamelidaceae. J. Arnold Arb. 58: 67-71.
32. Barlow, B.A., 1959, Chromosome numbers in the Casuarinaceae.
    Austral. J. Bot. 7: 230-237.
33. Goldblatt, P., 1979, Miscellaneous chromosome counts in
    angiosperms, II. Including new family and generic records.
    Ann. Missouri Bot. Gard. (in press).
34. Riley, H.P., Varney, D.R., 1967, Some new chromosome numbers
    in the Mesembryanthemae. Cytologia 32: 346-349.
35. Spencer, J.L., 1955, A cytological study of the Cactaceae of
    Puerto Rico.   Bot. Gaz. 117: 33-37.
36. Remski, M.F., 1954, Cytological investigations in Mammillaria
    and some associated genera. Bot. Gaz. 116: 163-171.
37. Steiner, E., 1944, Cytogenetic studies on Talinum and Por-
    tulaca. Bot. Gaz. 105: 374-379.
38. Swanson, J.R., 1966, A synopsis of relationships in Mon-
    tioideae (Portulacaceae). Brittonia 18: 229-241.
39. Mehra, P.N., Malik, C.P., 1963, Cytology of some Indian
    Chenopodiaceae. Caryologia 16: 67-84.
40. Sharma, A.K., Dey, D., 1967, A comprehensive cytotaxonomic
    study on the family Chenopodiaceae. J. Cytol. Genet. 1:
    114-127.
41. Blackburn, K.B., Morton, J.K., 1957, The incidence of poly-
    ploidy in the Caryophyllaceae of Britain and of Portugal.
    New Phytol. 56: 344-351.
42. Ratter, J.A., 1964, Cytogenetic studies in Spergularia. I.
    Cytology of some Old World species. Notes Roy. Bot. Gard.
    Edinburgh 25: 293-302.
43. Löve, A., Kapoor, B.M., 1968, A chromosome atlas of the
    collective genus Rumex. Cytologia 32: 328-342.

44. Goldblatt, P., 1976, Chromosome number and its significance in Batis maritima (Bataceae). J. Arnold Arb. 57: 526-530.

45. Bezbaruah, H.P., 1971, Cytological investigations in the family Theaceae--I. Chromosome numbers in some Camellia species and allied genera. Caryologia 24: 421-426.

46. Robson, N.K.B., Adams, P., 1968, Chromosome numbers in Hypericum and related genera. Brittonia 20: 95-106.

47. Bell, C.R., 1949, A cytotaxonomic study of the Sarraceniaceae of North America. Elisha Mitchell Sci. Soc. 65: 137-166.

48. Smith-White, S., 1955, Chromosome number and pollen types in the Epacridaceae. Austral. J. Bot. 3: 48-67.

49. Kress, A., 1963, Zytotaxonomische untersuchungen an Primu-laceen. Phyton (Austria) 10: 225-236.

50. Clausen, J., 1927, Chromosome number and the relationship of species in the genus Viola. Ann. Bot. 41: 677-714.

51. Atsmon, D., Feinbrun, N., 1960, Chromosome counts in Israeli Cistaceae. Caryologia 13: 240-246.

52. Sharma, A.K., Bhattacharyya, U.C., 1961, Cytological studies in Begonia--II. Caryologia 14: 279-300.

53. Thompson, H.J., Lewis, H., 1955, Chromosome numbers in Mentzelia (Loasaceae). Madroño 13: 102-107.

54. Suda, Y., 1963, The chromosome numbers of salicaceous plants in relation to their taxonomy. Sci. Rep. Tôhoku Univ. ser. 4. (Biol.) 29: 413-430.

55. Mulligan, G.A., 1964, Chromosome numbers of the family Cruciferae. I. Canad. J. Bot. 42: 1509-1519.

56. Mukherjee, P., 1973, Chromosome study as an aid in tracing the evolution in Cruciferae. Cytologia 40: 727-734.

57. Rollins, R.C., Shaw, E.A., 1973, "The genus Lesquerella (Cruciferae) in North America," Harvard University Press, Cambridge, MA. 288 p.

58. Baker, H.G., Baker, I., 1968, Chromosome numbers in the Bombacaceae. Bot. Gaz. 129: 294-296.

59. Bates, D.M., Blanchard, O.J.,Jr., 1970, Chromosome numbers in the Malvales. II. New or otherwise noteworthy counts relevant to classification in the Malvaceae, tribe Malveae. Amer. J. Bot. 57: 927-934.

60. Menzel, M.Y., Wilson, F.D., 1963, Cytotaxonomy of twelve species of Hibiscus section Furcaria. Amer. J. Bot. 50: 262-271.

61. Menzel, M.Y., Wilson, F.D., 1969, Genetic relationships in Hibiscus section Furcaria. Brittonia 21: 91-125.

62. Condit, I.J., 1964, Cytological studies in the genus Ficus. III. Chromosome numbers in sixty-two species. Madroño 17: 153-155.

63. Perry, B.A., 1943, Chromosome number and phylogenetic relation-ships in the Euphorbiaceae. Amer. J. Bot. 30: 527-543.

64. Hans, A.S., 1963, Chromosomal conspectus of the Euphorbia-ceae. Taxon 22: 591-636.

65. Webster, G.L., 1967, The genera of Euphorbiaceae in the
     southeastern United States. J. Arnold Arb. 48: 303-430.
66. Mehra, P.N., Choda, S.P., 1978, Cyto-taxonomical studies in
     the genus Euphorbia L. Cytologia 43: 217-235.
67. Robertson, K.R., 1974, The genera of Rosaceae in the south-
     eastern United States. J. Arnold Arb. 55: 303-332, 344-401,
     611-662.
68. Goldblatt, P., 1976, Cytotaxonomic studies in the tribe
     Quillajeae (Rosaceae). Ann. Missouri Bot. Gard. 63: 200-206.
69. Bandel, G., 1974, Chromosome numbers and evolution in the
     Leguminosae. Caryologia 27: 17-32.
70. Goldblatt, P., Cytology and the evolution of Leguminosae, in
     Polhill, R.M., Raven, P.H. (eds.), "Advances in Legume
     Systematics," Royal Bot. Gard., Kew (in press).
71. Lewis, W.H., 1974, Chromosomes and phylogeny of Erythrina
     (Fabaceae). Lloydia 37: 460-464.
72. Uhl, C.H., 1948, Cytotaxonomic studies in the subfamilies
     Crassuloideae, Kalanchoideae, and Cotyledonoideae of the
     Crassulaceae. Amer. J. Bot. 35: 695-706.
73. Uhl, C.H., 1961, The chromosomes of the Sempervivoideae
     (Crassulaceae). Amer. J. Bot. 48: 114-123.
74. Sharma, A.K., Ghosh, S., 1967, Cytotaxonomy of Crassulaceae.
     Biol. Zentralb. 86(suppl.): 313-336.
75. Skovsted, A., 1934, Cytological studies in the tribe Saxi-
     frageae. Dansk Bot. Arkiv 8(5): 1-52.
76. James, S.H., 1979, Chromosome numbers and genetic systems in
     the trigger plants of Western Australia (Stylidium; Stylidia-
     ceae). Austral. J. Bot. 27: 17-25.
77. Hamel, J.L., 1959, Contribution a l'étude caryo-taxonomique
     des Eucryphiacées. Bull. Mus. (Paris), series 2, 31: 526-535.
78. Ramsay, H.P., 1963, Chromosome numbers in the Proteaceae.
     Austral. J. Bot. 11: 1-20.
79. Atchison, E., 1947, Chromosome numbers in the Myrtaceae.
     Amer. J. Bot. 34: 159-164.
80. Smith-White, S., 1948, Cytological studies in the Myrtaceae.
     II. Chromosome numbers in the Leptospermoideae and Myrioideae.
     Proc. Linn. Soc. New South Wales 73: 16-36.
81. Favarger, C., 1962, Nouvelles recherches cytologiques sur
     les Mélastomatacées. Bull. Soc. Bot. Suisse 72: 201-305.
82. Ray, C.,Jr., 1944, Cytological studies of the flax genus,
     Linum. Amer. J. Bot. 31: 241-248.
83. Harris, B.D., 1968, Chromosome numbers and evolution in
     North American species of Linum. Amer. J. Bot. 55: 1197-1204.
84. Mathew, P.M., 1958, Cytology of Oxalidaceae. Cytologia 23:
     200-210.
85. Goldblatt, P., 1978, Chromosome number in two cytologically
     unknown New World families, Tovariaceae and Vivianiaceae.
     Ann. Missouri Bot. Gard. 65: 776-777.
86. Jones, K., Smith, J.B., 1966, The cytogeography of Impatiens
     L. (Balsaminaceae). Kew Bull. 20: 63-72.

87. Ornduff, R., 1971, Systematic studies of Limnanthaceae.
    Madroño 21: 103–111.
88. Lewis, W.H., Davis, S.A., 1962, Cytological observations of
    Polygala in eastern North America. Rhodora 64: 102–113.
89. Sharma, M.L., Mehra, P.N., 1978, Chromosome numbers in some
    north west Indian species of Polygala. Cytologia 43: 589–593.
90. Turner, B.L., 1958, Chromosome numbers in the genus Krameria:
    evidence for familial status. Rhodora 60: 101–106.
91. Styles, B.T., Vosa, C.G., 1971, Chromosome numbers in the
    Meliaceae. Taxon 20: 485–499.
92. Mehra, P.N., Sareen, T.S., Khosla, P.K., 1972, Cytological
    studies on Himalayan Meliaceae. J. Arnold Arb. 53: 558–568.
93. Datta, P.C., Samanta, P., 1977, Cytotaxonomy of Meliaceae.
    Cytologia 42: 197–208.
94. Stone, D.E., 1961, Ploidal level and stomatal size in the
    American hickories. Brittonia 13: 293–302.
95. Nath, J., Clay, S.N., 1972, Cytogenetic studies on some
    species of Euonymus. Caryologia 25: 417–427.
96. Barlow, B.A., 1963, Studies in Australian Loranthaceae. IV.
    Chromosome numbers and their relationships. Proc. Linn.
    Soc. New South Wales 88: 151–160.
97. Barlow, B.A., Wiens, D., 1971, The cytogeography of the
    loranthaceous mistletoes. Taxon 20: 291–312.
98. Wiens, D., Barlow, B.A., 1971, The cytogeography and relation-
    ships of the viscaceous and eremolepidaceous mistletoes.
    Taxon 20: 313–332.
99. Taylor, H., 1945, Cyto-taxonomy and phylogeny of the Oleaceae.
    Brittonia 5: 337–367.
100. Johnson, L.A.S., 1957, A review of the family Oleaceae.
    Contr. New South Wales Nat. Herb. 2: 395–418.
101. Cronquist, A., 1968, "The Evolution and Classification of
    Flowering Plants," Houghton Mifflin, Boston. 396 p.
102. Goldblatt, P., 1978, A contribution to cytology in Cornales.
    Ann. Missouri Bot. Gard. 65: 650–655.
103. Sharma, A.K., Chatterji, A.K., 1964, Cytological study as an
    aid in the interpretation of the systematic status of the
    different genera of Araliaceae. Cytologia 29: 1–12.
104. Moore, D.M., 1971, Chromosome studies in the Umbelliferae,
    pp. 233–247, in Heywood, V.H. (ed.), "The Biology and
    Chemistry of the Umbelliferae," Academic Press, London.
105. Constance, L., Chuang, T.-I., Bell, C.R., 1976, Chromosome
    numbers in Umbelliferae. V. Amer. J. Bot. 63: 608–625.
106. Lewis, W.H., Fantz, P.R., 1973, Tribal classification of
    Triosteum (Caprifoliaceae). Rhodora 75: 120–121.
107. Moore, R.J., 1947, Cytotaxonomic studies in the Loganiaceae.
    I. Chromosome numbers and phylogeny in the Loganiaceae.
    Amer. J. Bot. 34: 527–538.
108. Lewis, W.H., 1962, Chromosome numbers in North American
    Rubiaceae. Brittonia 14: 285–290.

109. Tapadar, R., 1964, Cytotaxonomic studies in Apocynaceae and deliniation of the different evolutionary tendencies operating within the family. Caryologia 17: 103-138.
110. Rork, C.L., 1949, Cytological studies in the Gentianaceae. Amer J. Bot. 36: 687-701.
111. Löve, D., 1953, Cytotaxonomical remarks on the Gentianaceae. Hereditas 39: 225-235.
112. Ornduff, R., 1974, Cytotaxonomic observations on Villarsia (Menyanthaceae). Austral. J. Bot. 22: 513-516.
113. Goldblatt, P., Gentry, A.H., 1979, Cytology of Bignoniaceae. Bot. Not. 132: 475-482.
114. Heckard, L.R., 1968, Chromosome numbers and polyploidy in Castilleja (Scrophulariaceae). Brittonia 20: 212-226.
115. Cooperrider, T.S., McCready, G.A., 1970, Chromosome numbers in Chelone (Scrophulariaceae). Brittonia 22: 175-183.
116. Fernandes, A., Franca, F., 1972, Contribution à la connaissance cytotaxonomique des Spermatophyta du Portugal. VI. Plantaginaceae. Bol. Soc. Broteriana 46(series2): 465-501.
117. Heckard, L.R., Chuang, T.I., 1975, Chromosome numbers and polyploidy in Orobanche (Orobanchaceae). Brittonia 27: 179-186.
118. Grant, W.F., 1955, A cytogenetic study in the Acanthaceae. Brittonia 8: 121-149.
119. Ratter, J.A., 1975, A survey of chromosome numbers in the Gesnerianceae of the Old World. Notes Roy. Bot. Gard. Edinburgh 33: 527-543.
120. D'Arcy, W.G., 1975, The Solanaceae: an overview. Solanaceae Newsletter 2: 8-10.
121. Hawkes, J.G., 1979, Evolution and polyploidy in potato species, pp. 637-645, in Hawkes, J.G., Lester, R.N., Skelding, A.D. (eds.), "The Biology and Taxonomy of the Solanaceae," Academic Press, London.
122. Sharma, A.K., Chatterji, A.K., 1957, A cytological investigation of some Convolvulaceae as an aid in understanding their lines of evolution. Phyton (Argentina) 9: 143-157.
123. Vij, S.P., Singh, S., Sachdeva, V.P., 1977, Cytomorphological studies in Convolvulaceae. II. Ipomoea and allied genera. Cytologia 42: 451-464.
124. Flory, W.S., 1937, Chromosome numbers in the Polemoniaceae. Cytologia (Fujii Jubilee Volume): 171-180.
125. Grant, V., 1959, "Natural History of the Phlox Family," Volume 1, Martinus Nijhoff, The Hague. 280 p.
126. Constance, L., 1963, Chromosome number and classification in Hydrophyllaceae. Brittonia 15: 273-285.
127. Britton, D.M., 1951, Cytogenetic studies on the Boraginaceae. Brittonia 7: 233-266.
128. Grau, J., 1971, Cytologische Untersuchungen an Boraginaceae II. Mitt. Bot. München 9: 177-194.
129. Sharma, A.K., Mukhopadhyay, S., 1963, Cytotaxonomic investigations with the aid of an improved method on the family

Verbenaceae with special reference to the lines of evolution. J. Genetics 58: 358-386.

130. Lewis, W.H., Oliver, R.L., 1961, Cytogeography and phylogeny of the North American species of Verbena. Amer. J. Bot. 48: 638-643.

131. Irving, R.S., 1976, Chromosome numbers of Hedeoma (Labiatae) and related genera. Syst. Bot. 1: 46-56.

132. Gadella, T.W.J., 1966, Some notes on the deliminitation of genera in the Campanulaceae. I. Koninkl. Nederl. Adad. Weterschappen, series C, 69: 502-521.

133. Peacock, W.J., 1963, Chromosome numbers and cytoevolution in the Goodeniaceae. Proc. Linn. Soc. New South Wales 88: 8-27.

134. Solbrig, O.T., 1977, Chromosomal cytology and evolution in the family Compositae, pp. 267-281, in Heywood, V.H., Harborne, J.B., Turner, B.L. (eds.), "The Biology and Chemistry of the Compositae," Academic Press, London.

135. Stuessy, T.F., 1977, Heliantheae--systematic review, pp. 621-671, in Heywood, V.H., Harborne, J.B., Turner, B.L. (eds.), "The Biology and Chemistry of the Compositae," Academic Press, London.

APPENDIX

Genera with reported infraspecific polyploidy (through 1974), the number of species following each genus.

Phylogenetic Group 1.

Annonales. MAGNOLIACEAE: Magnolia 2. ANNONACEAE: Asimina 1. ARISTOLOCHIACEAE: Aristolochia 1; Asarum 1; Heterotropa 1. CHLORANTHACEAE: Chloranthus 1. CALYCANTHACEAE: Calycanthus 1; Chimonanthus 1. PIPERACEAE: Peperomia 3; Piper 3. SAURURACEAE: Houttuynia 1.

Berberidales. MENISPERMACEAE: Cocculus 1. RANUNCULACEAE: Aconitum 8; Actaea 2; Adonis 1; Anemone 21; Aquilegia 2; Batrachium 2; Caltha 9; Cimicifuga 1; Clematis 3; Delphinium 14; Eranthis 1; Ficaria 1; Helleborus 2; Hepatica 2; Myosurus 1; Pulsatilla 8; Ranunculus 47; Thalictrum 17; Trollius 1. BERBERIDACEAE: Achlys 1; Berberis 2; Bongardia 1. PAPAVERACEAE: Argemone 8; Corydalis 6; Dicentra 1; Eschscholtzia 1; Fumaria 3; Hunnemannia 1; Meconopsis 1; Papaver 10.

Nymphaeales. NYMPHAEACEAE: Cabomba 1; Nymphaea 6. CERATO-PHYLLACEAE: Ceratophyllum 1.

Phylogenetic Group 2.

Hamamelidales. PLATANACEAE: Platanus 3.
Casuarinales. CASUARINACEAE: Casuarina 8.

Fagales.   BETULACEAE: Alnus 7; Betula 7.

Phylogenetic Group 3.

Chenopodiales. NYCTAGINACEAE: Boerhavia 1; Bougainvillea 1.
AIZOACEAE: Delosperma 1; Gibbaeum 3; Hymenocyclus 1; Ruschia 2;
Sesuvium 1.   CACTACEAE: Cephalocereus 1; Mammillaria 2; Myrtil-
locactus 1; Opuntia 19; Rhipsalis 1.   PORTULACACEAE: Calandrinia
4; Claytonia 9; Claytoniella 1; Montia 1; Portulaca 4; Talinum 3.
BASELLACEAE: Boussingaultia 1; Ullucus 1.   CHENOPODIACEAE: Atriplex
6; Beta 3; Camphorosma 1; Chenopodium 8; Obione 1;   Salicornia 3;
Salsola 1; Suaeda 2.   AMARANTHACEAE: Achyranthes 2; Aerua 1;
Alternanthera 1; Amaranthus 3; Celosia 1; Pupalia 1.   CARYOPHYLLA-
CEAE: Agrostemma 1; Arenaria 7; Cerastrium 13; Corrigiola 1;
Dianthus 30; Gypsophila 1; Herniaria 2; Honkenya 2; Kahlrauschia
1; Lychnis 1; Melandrium 3; Merckia 1; Minuartia 5; Paronychia 2;
Petrorhagia 1; Sagina 1; Scleranthus 2; Silene 15; Spergularia
10; Stellaria 10; Tunica 1; Vaccaria 1.
Polygonales. POLYGONACEAE: Calligonum 3; Coccoloba 1;
Eriogonum 2; Fagopyrum 2; Oxyria 2; Persicaria 1; Polygonella 1;
Polygonum 20; Rheum 8; Rumex 24.

Phylogenetic Group 4.

Theales. DILLENIACEAE: Dillenia 1; Hibbertia 1.   PAEONIACEAE:
Paeonia 5.   ACTINIDIACEAE: Actinidia 2.   THEACEAE: Camellia 3.
DIPTEROCARPACEAE: Dipterocarpus 1.   CLUSIACEAE: Hypericum 2.
Ericales. ERICACEAE: Arctostaphylos 2; Gaultheria 1; Harri-
manella 1; Kalmia 1; Moneses 1; Monotropa 1; Oxycoccus 1; Phyl-
lodoce 1; Pyrola 3; Rhododendron 16; Vaccinium 5.   EPACRIDACEAE:
Epacris 1; Lissanthe 1.
Ebenales. EBENACEAE: Diospyros 1.
Primulales. MYRSINIACEAE: Ardisia 1.   PRIMULACEAE: Anagallis
2; Androsace 2; Cyclamen 6; Dodecatheon 5; Gregoria 1; Lysimachia
2; Naumburgia 1; Primula 16; Soldanella 1; Trientalis 1; Vitaliana
1.
Plumbaginales. PLUMBAGINACEAE: Armeria 2; Goniolimon 1;
Limonium 1; Statice 1.

Phylogenetic Group 5.

Cistales. VIOLACEAE: Hybanthus 3; Viola 16.   CISTACEAE:
Helianthemum 1; Tuberaria 1.   TURNERACEAE: Turnera 1.   PASSIFLORA-
CEAE: Adenia 1; Passiflora 2.   CARICACEAE: Carica 1.   CUCURBITACEAE:
Bryonia 1; Coccinia 1; Cucumis 1; Cucurbita 3; Echinocystis 1;
Trichosanthes 1; Trochomeriopsis 1.   BEGONIACEAE: Begonia 7.
LOASACEAE: Mentzelia 1.
Salicales. SALICACEAE: Populus 5; Salix 14.
Capparidales. CAPPARIDACEAE: Cadaba 1; Cleome 1.   BRASSICA-
CEAE: Aethionema 2; Alliaria 1; Alyssum 9; Arabis 18; Biscutella 1;

Brassica 3; Brassicella 2; Braya 1; Bunias 1; Cakile 1; Calepina 1; Camelina 1; Capsella 1; Cardamine 14; Cardaminopsis 4; Carrichtera 1; Clypeola 1; Cochlearia 1; Crambe 2; Dentaria 2; Descurainia 3; Diplotaxis 1; Draba 13; Ermania 1; Erophila 1; Erysimum 9; Eutrema 1; Hesperis 2; Iberis 1; Kernera 1; Leaven-worthia 1; Lepidium 3; Lesquerella 2; Lunaria 1; Malcolmia 1; Nasturtium 1; Parrya 2; Peltaria 1; Physaria 2; Rhynchosinapis 1; Rorippa 6; Sisymbrium 2; Standleya 1; Thlaspi 2; Turritis 1. RESEDACEAE: Oligomeris 1.

Phylogenetic Group 6.

Malvales. TILLIACEAE: Corchorus 2; Triumfetta 1. BOMBACACEAE: Adansonia 1; Ochroma 1; Pseudobombax 1. MALVACEAE: Abelmoschus 1; Abutilon 3; Altheae 1; Anoda 3; Callirhoe 1; Eremalche 1; Gossypium 1; Hibiscus 12; Malva 1; Modiolastrum 1; Pavonia 1; Sida 4; Sidalcea 3; Sphaeralcea 8; Thespesia 1; Urena 1.

Urticales. ULMACEAE: Celtis 1; Ulmus 1. MORACEAE: Artocarpus 1; Broussonetia 1; Ficus 4; Morus 4. CANNABACEAE: Cannabis 1; Humulus 1. URTICACEAE: Boehmeria 1; Pilea 1; Urtica 3.

Euphorbiales. EUPHORBIACEAE: Acalypha 1; Aleurites 1; Antidesma 1; Breynia 1; Codiaeum 1; Euphorbia 14; Hevea 3; Mallotus 1; Mercurialis 2; Micrococca 1; Phyllanthus 7; Poinsettia 1; Synadenium 1. THYMELAEACEAE: Daphne 1; Edgeworthia 1; Wikstroemia 3.

Rhamnales. RHAMNACEAE: Ziziphus 3. ELAEAGNACEAE: Elaeagnus 1; Hippophae 1.

Phylogenetic Group 7.

Rosales. ROSACEAE: Acomastylis 1; Agrimonia 1; Alchemilla 11; Amelanchier 1; Aruncus 5; Comarum 1; Cotoneaster 22; Crataegus 7; Duchesnea 1; Filipendula 3; Fragaria 2; Geum 3; Malus 13; Photinia 1; Potentilla 60; Prunus 10; Pyrus 2; Rosa 32; Rubus 39; Sanguisorba 4; Sorbocotoneaster 1; Sorbus 5; Spiraea 5; Waldsteinia 2. FABACEAE: Acacia 12; Adesmia 2; Albizia 1; Amorpha 1; Anthyllis 1; Arachis 1; Arthrosamanea 1; Astragalus 18; Bauhinia 2; Cajanus 1; Canavalia 2; Caragana 1; Carmichaelia 1; Cassia 12; Chamaespar-tium 1; Cicer 2; Coronilla 4; Crotalaria 3; Cytisus 7; Delonix 1; Derris 2; Dorycnium 1; Entada 1; Erythrina 1; Glycine 2; Hedysarum 3;, Hippocrepis 1; Indigofera 9; Lathyrus 3; Leucaena 1; Lotus 15; Lupinus 9; Medicago 10; Melilotus 3; Mucuna 1; Onobrychis 4; Ononis 3; Oxytropis 8; Phaseolus 1; Piliostigma 1; Pisum 1; Prosopis 1; Pultenaea 1; Samanea 1; Sarothamnus 1; Scorpiurus 1; Sesbania 3; Sophora 1; Tephrosia 1; Trifolium 20; Trigonella 4; Ulex 3; Vicia 9; Wisteria 4. CRASSULACEAE: Aeonium 2; Cotyledon 1; Crassula 13; Dudleya 10; Graptopetalum 3; Greenovia 1; Hassean-thus 1; Kalanchoe 4; Monanthes 1; Orostachys 2; Pachyphytum 4; Sedum 32; Sempervivum 4. SAXIFRAGACEAE: Chrysosplenium 2;

Deutzia 1; Heuchera 1; Hydrangea 1; Mitella 1; Parnassia 2; Saxifraga 28. DROSERACEAE: Drosera 3. DIAPENSIACEAE: Galax 1.

Phylogenetic Group 8.

Proteales. PROTEACEAE: Macadamia 1.
Myrtales. LYTHRACEAE: Cuphea 3; Lythrum 2. TRAPACEAE: Trapa 1. COMBRETACEAE: Terminalia 2. MYRTACEAE: Callistemon 3; Eugenia 3; Psidium 1. MELASTOMATACEAE: Rhexia 3; Tibouchina 1. ONAGRACEAE: Camissonia 6; Chamaenerion 1; Epilobium 6; Fuchsia 1; Gaura 3; Gayophytum 1; Godetia 1; Lopezia 1; Ludwigia 1; Oenothera 16; Zauschneria 3.

Phylogenetic Group 9.

Geraniales. LINACEAE: Hugonia 1; Linum 7. ZYGOPHYLLACEAE: Larrea 2; Nitraria 1; Peganum 1; Tribulus 1; Zygophyllum 1. OXALIDACEAE: Oxalis 7. GERANIACEAE: Erodium 4; Geranium 9; Pelargonium 4. BALSAMINACEAE: Impatiens 2.
Polygalales. MALPIGHIACEAE: Hiptage 1. POLYGALACEAE: Epirrhizanthes 1; Polygala 2.
Rutales. RUTACEAE: Aegle 1; Boronia 2; Citrus 14; Dictamnus 1; Fortunella 1; Poncirus 1; Ruta 1; Zanthoxylum 1; Zieria 1. MELIACEAE: Cedrela 1; Entandophragma 2; Sandoricum 1; Turraeanthus 1. ACERACEAE: Acer 2. HIPPOCASTANACEAE: Aesculus 1.

Phylogenetic Group 10.

Santalales. STACKHOUSIACEAE: Stackhousia 1. LORANTHACEAE: Gaiadendron 1; Phoradendron 1; Phthirusa 1.
Oleales. OLEACEAE: Fraxinus 4; Jasminum 4; Menodora 1; Syringa 3.
Cornales. VITACEAE: Ampelocissus 1; Cissus 2; Vitis 2. CORNACEAE: Aucuba 1; Cornus 2; Macrocarpium 1. HALORAGIDACEAE: Myriophyllum 2. ARALIACEAE: Aralia 1; Fatsia 1; Hedera 1; Helwingia 2; Panax 1; Polyscias 1. APIACEAE: Aegopodium 1; Apium 1; Arracacia 1; Astrantia 1; Bupleurum 2; Centella 1; Chaerophyllum 1; Cicuta 1; Cnidium 1; Eryngium 7; Hydrocotyle 4; Mulinum 1; Perideridia 1; Pimpinella 1; Pleurospermum 1; Ptilimnium 1; Sanicula 1; Thapsia 1.
Dipsacales. CAPRIFOLIACEAE: Diervilla 1; Lonicera 7; Sambucus 2; Symphoricarpos 1; Viburnum 10. ADOXACEAE: Adoxa 1. VALERIANA-CEAE: Centranthus 2; Valeriana 7; Valerianella 1. DIPSACACEAE: Cephalaria 1; Dipsacus 1; Knautia 6; Scabiosa 3.

Phyloegenetic Group 11.

Gentianales. LOGANIACEAE: Buddleja 1. RUBIACEAE: Asperula 3; Borreria 1; Bouvardia 2; Coffea 8; Coprosma 1; Crucianella 2; Galium 43; Hedyotis 10; Leptodermis 1; Myrmecodia 1; Pentas 1;

Relbunium 1; Richardia 2; Rubia 2; Spermacoce 1. APOCYNACEAE:
Alyxia 1; Catharanthus 1; Plumeria 1; Rauvolfia 2; Tabernaemontana
1; Vinca 2. ASCLEPIADACEAE: Gomphocarpus 1; Huernia 1; Stapelia
2. GENTIANACEAE: Centaurium 4; Gentiana 2; Swertia 2. MENYANTH-
ACEAE: Menyanthes 1; Nephrophyllidium 1; Nymphoides 1; Villarsia
1.

Bignoniales. BIGNONIACEAE: Bignonia 1; Jacaranda 1; Spathodea
1. PEDALIACEAE: Sesamum 1. MYOPORACEAE: Eremophila 12.
SCROPHULARIACEAE: Alonsoa 1; Antirrhinum 1; Bartsia 1; Calceolaria
2; Castilleja 12; Chaenorrhinum 1; Chelone 2; Digitalis 4;
Euphrasia 2; Hebe 7; Lagotis 1; Linaria 1; Lindernia 2; Mimulus
4; Nelsonia 1; Nemesia 1; Odontites 2; Paederota 1; Parentucellia
1; Pentstemon 8; Petrodora 1; Pseudolysimachion 1; Scoparia 1;
Scrophularia 4; Verbascum 3; Veronica 18; Veronicatrum 1. PLANTA-
GINACEAE: Plantago 25. OROBANCHACEAE: Orobanche 2; Phacellanthus
1. LENTIBULARIACEAE: Pinguicula 3; Utricularia 1. ACANTHACEAE:
Acanthus 1; Adhotoda 1; Andrographis 1; Crossandra 1; Fittonia 1;
Hydrophila ; Justicia 1; Thunbergia 2. GESNERIACEAE: Aeschynanthus
1; Columnea 1; Ramonda 1; Saintpaulia 2; Smithiantha 1.

Solanales. SOLANACEAE: Atropa 1; Browallia 1; Capsicum 1;
Chamaesaracha 2; Datura 2; Lycium 3; Lycopersicon 3; Nicotiana 6;
Petunia 2; Physalis 5; Quincula 1; Scopolia 1; Solanum 35.
CONVOLVULACEAE: Convolvulus 2; Cuscuta 1; Ipomoea 5. POLEMONIACEAE:
Gilia 3; Linanthus 1; Phlox 5; Polemonium 1.

Lamiales. HYDROPHYLLACEAE: Eucrypta 21; Nama 3; Phacelia
10; Wigandia 1. BORAGINACEAE: Amsinckia 2; Cerinthe 1; Cryptantha
1; Cynoglossum 3; Echium 9; Eritrichium 1; Heliotropium 4; Litho-
spermum 1; Lobostemon 2; Mertensia 1; Myosotis 11; Onosma 2;
Pulmonaria 31; Symphytum 2; Trichodesma 1. VERBENACEAE: Caryopteris
1; Clerodendrum 2; Duranta 1; Lantana 3; Lippia 1; Verbena 8;
Vitex 2. CALLITRICHACEAE: Callitriche 2. LAMIACEAE: Calamintha
2; Coleus 2; Englerastum 1; Galeobdolon 1; Galeopsis 1; Glechoma
1; Hyptis 1; Lamium 1; Melissa 1; Mentha 15; Micromeria 1; Nepeta
2; Ocimum 1; Platostoma 1; Plectranthus 3; Pycnanthemum 4; Salvia
9; Satureja 1; Sideritis 2; Solenostemon 2; Stachys 4; Teucrium
5; Thymus 3.

Campanulales. CAMPANULACEAE: Adenophora 2; Asyneuma 1;
Campanula 33; Canarina 1; Isotoma 1; Jasione 1; Lobelia 4; Phyteuma
2; Platycodon 1; Wahlenbergia 1. GOODENIACEAE: Dampiera 8;
Goodenia 7; Leschenaultia 2; Scaevola 2; Selliera 1.

Asterales. ASTERACEAE: Achillea 6; Ageratum 5 Agoseris 2;
Ainsliaea 1; Ambrosia 5; Antennaria 5; Anthemis 3; Arnica 6;
Artemisia 48; Aster 20; Astranthium 1; Baeria 1; Bahia 2; Bellis
1; Bidens 8; Blumea 2; Brachycome 7; Calea 2; Calendula 4; Cal-
listephus 1; Calyptocarpus 1; Carduus 1; Carthamus 2; Centaurea
8; Chaenactis 1; Chaetopappa 1; Chondrilla 1; Chrysanthemoides 1;
Chrysanthemum 25; Chrysopsis 2; Chrysothamnus 2; Cichorium 1;
Cineraria 1; Cirsium 1; Conyza 1; Coreopsis 2; Cosmos 3; Crepis
14; Cyanus 1; Dahlia 3; Doronicum 3; Dyssodia 3; Echinacea 1;
Elephantopus 2; Emilia 2; Erechtites 1; Erigeron 17; Eriophyllum 2;

Ethulia 1; Eupatorium 13; Euryops 3; Gaillardia 2; Galinsoga 1;
Gnaphalium 3; Grindelia 5; Gutierrezia 4; Gymnaster 1; Gynura 1;
Haplopappus 6; Hedypnois 2; Helianthus 7; Helichrysum 3; Heliopsis
1; Heterotheca 1; Hieracium 18; Holozonia 1; Homogyne 1; Hymeno-
pappus 1; Hymenoxys 2; Inula 2; Isocoma 1; Iva 1; Ixeris 1;
Jaegeria 2; Kalimeris 2; Kleinia 1; Lactuca 2; Laphamia 1; Leontodon
1; Leontopodium 1; Leucanthemum 7; Liatris 4; Madia 1; Malacothrix
1; Matricaria 2; Melampodium 5; Melanthera 1; Microseris 1;
Nicolettia 1; Othonna 1; Parthenium 6; Perityle 2; Petasites 1;
Pinaropappus 1; Polymnia 1; Porophyllum 1; Pyrethrum 1; Rudbeckia
3; Santolina 1; Saussurea 2; Scorzonera 3; Senecio 25: Sigesbeckia
1; Solidago 11; Sonchus 2; Spilanthes 2; Stephanomeria 1; Stevia
5; Syneilesis 1; Tagetes 2; Tanacetum 1; Taraxacum 23; Tetradymia
2; Townsendia 4; Tragoceros 1; Tragopogon 2; Tridax 1; Tripleuro-
spermum 1; Vernonia 3; Viguiera 2; Wedelia 1; Zinnia 2.

POLYPLOIDY IN PLANT TAXA: SUMMARY

John E. Averett

Department of Biology
University of Missouri-St. Louis
St. Louis, MO 63121

The preceding seven papers deal with the distribution and evolutionary significance of polyploidy in each of the major plant taxa. Polyploidy, the multiplication of entire chromosomal complements, is the most widespread and distinctive cytogenetic process affecting higher plant evolution. Approximately 36% of the species of flowering plants have gametic chromosome numbers which are multiples of the basic diploid number found within their respective genera, but between 70 and 80 percent may, in fact, have polyploidy in their evolutionary history. The percent of intrageneric polyploidy in ferns is even higher and the occurrence of intergeneric polyploidy is equivalent to that in angiosperms. Studies to date have been largely confined to the aforementioned groups, especially the dicotyledonous angiosperms. However, the preceding papers suggest that polyploidy may be an important aspect of evolution among at least certain groups of the thallophytes. The only group in which polyploidy is conspicuously rare is the gymnosperms.

Algae. Studies of polyploidy have been most extensive in Chlorophycophyta, but examples of the occurrence of polyploidy may be found in most of the algal groups. Polyploids are known to arise in algae in several ways, among which are natural polyploids associated with natural hybridization, artificially-produced polyploids (e.g., colchicine), polyploids produced as a result of certain sexual processes in laboratory cultures, and polyploids occurring spontaneously in repeatedly transferred cultures. The latter is of particular consequence.

Oedogonium, Cladophora, certain desmids, and volvocalean flagellates represent the best known examples of green algae with respect to the occurrence of polyploidy. In Rhodophycophyta and Phaeophycophyta only a few cases of polyploidy are adequately

documented. Unusual nuclear phenomena and/or behavior have
hampered studies in the remaining divisions and few species have
been carefully studied in regard to their ploidy levels. The
study of polyploidy in all groups is complicated by the difficulty
in determining a base chromosome number for any one group.

Fungi. Polyploidy in fungi has generally been considered
rare or non-existent and, as a consequence, polyploidy as a
mechanism for fungal speciation and evolution has not assumed the
same sort of role accorded it in the evolution of vascular plants.
Recent reviews remain unconvincing that polyploidy in fungi is
either widespread or a major factor in fungal evolution. Our
knowledge of the phenomenon in fungi, however, is only fragmentary
and there are indications that polyploidy is more important than
it was once thought to be.

There are several reasons for our fragmentary knowledge of
polyploidy in fungi. Among these are the tendency of chromosomes
to clump in fixation; fungal chromosomes and nuclei are often
small; certain features attending nuclear and chromosomal behavior,
morphology, and organization during meiosis promote uncertainty
in providing unequivocal chromosome counts; the site of meiosis
in certain fungi remains in dispute; and only in a few instances
has a reliable comprehensive study of chromosome numbers of a
confined group been made. Where extensive studies have been
completed, there is evidence supporting the concept of polyploid
evolution in a number of groups of fungi, typically those that
have dominant diploid phases in their life histories. There are
a number of reports of suspected polyploidy in other fungi, but
these should be considered speculative at this time.

Bryophytes. The mosses, liverworts, and hornworts, classes
Musci, Hepaticae, and Anthocerotae, represent a diverse groups of
organisms but, because of the overall similarity of their life
cycles and general organization, they are generally treated as the
single division Bryophyta. Cytologically they differ in several
respects, particularly in the frequency of polyploidy. There is
also a difference in base chromosome numbers, x=6-8 for the
mosses and x=8-10 for the liverworts.

Polyploids are most apparent among the mosses with nearly
60% having chromosome numbers of n=10-14. About 85% of the
species of liverworts have chromosome numbers of n=8-10 and, if
this represents the base number of the group, polyploidy is not a
major feature among these plants.

An interesting feature of mosses is that unlike liverworts,
vegetative regeneration is possible from almost any portion of
the moss plant, including tissue from immature sporophytes.
Polyploidy is highest among those moss groups which occur in
unstable habitats where there is the greatest possibility for
polyploids to arise from damaged sporophytes. This appears to be
the primary means of the induction of polyploidy among mosses.
This in turn may account, at least in part, for the greater

success of mosses in numbers of species and greater ecological
adaptiveness.

Pteridophytes. Polyploidy is a major and widespread feature
in the evolution of the pteridophytes, especially among the
homosporous ferns. Although generally considered to be very
ancient, many pteridophytes appeared during and after the origin
of angiosperms. There may, in fact, be a correlation between the
radiation of angiosperms and that of the pteridophytes. For
that reason it is useful to recognize two types of polyploids:
paleopolyploids and neopolyploids.

In considering the origins of polyploidy in ferns, the
question of original base numbers emerges. It is possible that
the original vascular land plants may have had high chromosome
numbers and what is seen in the ferns today is a vestige of the
time when the pteridophytes were first beginning their evolution.
There is actually little definitive evidence; however,
numbers in the heterosporous ferns, fern allies, and seed plants
are basically low and the Wagners assume the homosporous members
have undergone polyploidization to achieve their present high
numbers. The paleopolyploid condition represents the presumed
ancient numbers that now constitute base numbers for which no
lower denominators are known and neopolyploidy is the condition
in which lower denominators do exist.

If the assumptions based on outside evidence are correct, it
may be concluded that ancestral base chromosome numbers for the
pteridophytes may have been 7-13, and more likely 9-11. If the
latter is true then most living genera are tetraploid, hexaploid,
and octoploid, but some groups may be 10-12 ploid. Further,
perhaps as many as 50% the extant pteridophytes are neopolyploids
on these paleopolyploid bases.

Allopolyploid ferns are well-documented and some exist in
the wild both as sterile diploids and fertile polyploids. Although
polyploids may be experimentally produced by simply sowing spores
and having unreduced spores yield polyploid gametophytes capable
of forming zygotes, strict autopolyploid ferns are probably rare
in nature. Polyploidy in ferns is also associated with apomixis,
tending to be 3x,4x, and 5x. New sporophytes are produced by
direct bud proliferation. Why these apogamous ferns (and also
the sterile AB hybrids which far outnumber the AABB polyploids)
do not transform to sexual allopolyploids with n and 2n alternation
of generations is an interesting question.

Gymnosperms. The gymnosperms represent an eclectic grouping
based largely on a general similarity of life cycles among the
several elements. As such, discussions discerning trends and
general principles become rather meaningless. In spite of that,
it seems apparent that polyploidy in the group as a whole is
indeed rare. Fewer than 5% of the species have been shown to be
polyploid. Polyploidy is questionable in Welwitschia, present in
eight species of Ephedra, undemonstrated in the cycads and Ginkgo,
and is sporadic in the conifers. Among the latter, more polyploids

are found in the Cupressaceae (Juniperus, Thuja, and Fitzroya)
than any other family. One of the best known naturally-occurring
polyploids is Sequoia sempervirens (Taxodiaceae) which is considered a hexaploid with n=33. It is the only known hexaploid
gymnosperm. Hence, it is clear that polyploidy among the gymnosperms is rare and not pronounced in any one group.

    Angiosperms. Although discussions regarding polyploidy in
angiosperms were divided into two presentations[1] many general
statements may be made of both groups. As indicated in the
opening paragraph of this discussion, polyploidy has played a
major role in the evolution of angiosperms. Several estimates of
polyploidy have been made, including J.D. White's 1942 suggestion
of at least 40%, G.L. Stebbins' 1950 estimate of 30-35%, and
Verne Grant's estimate in 1963 of 47%. The variance of these
figures represents different methods of calculating polyploidy
and different interpretations of the meaning of the work in the
context of plant systematics. Stebbins considered those species
having gametic chromosome numbers that are multiples of the basic
diploid number found in their respective genera ($\sim$ neopolyploids)
and has since pointed out that the percentage would be higher if
ancestral polyploidy ($\sim$ paleopolyploidy) is taken into account.
Grant includes some ancestral polyploidy in his estimates by
postulating that all species with a haploid number of n=13 or
over would be largely polyploid. He estimated a frequency of 43%
in the Dicotyledonae and 58% in the Monocotyledonae. Since
Grant's estimate, approximately twice as many species have been
counted and Goldblatt, utilizing Grant's method, arrived at a
figure of 55% polyploidy within the monocots. He believes the
method is fair but is probably conservative. He suggests that
species with n=11, and probably many of those with n=9 and 10,
have polyploidy in their evolutionary histories. The same is
probably true of the dicots at Lewis point out.

    General Conclusion. In each of the several plant groups
discussed, the question as to what to include as polyploid arises.
Intrageneric polyploidy is relatively easy to calculate. There
are problems in chromosomally complex groups in which a range of
auneploid numbers occurs but such instances can usually be resolved
with some taxonomic insight. The recognition of polyploidy at
higher levels is much more difficult and often much more subjective. Base number determinations at this level are complicated
by gaps in the cytological record, erroneous reports of chromosome numbers, and insufficient or conflicting systematic data.
Where a taxon, at any level, is made up of discordant elements,
cytological deductions within that group may well be invalid.

----

[1]Polyploidy in dicots was not presented during the symposium
but general information regarding this important group has been
summarized by Dr. W.H. Lewis for this symposium volume.

Because intrageneric polyploidy is only a partial analysis of the overall incidence of the phenomenon and because it excludes all taxa above the species rank, it is of the utmost importance to deduce the original base number of the taxon in question. The importance of the establishment of base numbers becomes apparent in the attention given the subject and the questions raised for lack of such information in each of the papers presented in this section.

PART III

POLYPLOIDY IN ANIMAL EVOLUTION

POLYPLOIDY IN INSECT EVOLUTION

Juhani Lokki and Anssi Saura[1]

Department of Genetics
University of Helsinki
Helsinki, Finland

The number of existing insect species is estimated to be of the order of between two and a half and three million. More than a third of this number has already been described. In comparison with this diversity, the list of known polyploid insect forms is exceedingly small, less than one hundred.

In contrast to the apparent success of polyploid plants, polyploid insects represent rare exceptions, as the vast majority are diploid. All well documented polyploid insects reproduce parthenogenetically. Two polyploid forms represent cases of pseudogamy. In this latter mode of reproduction, a sperm is needed to activate the development of the egg, but the sperm does not contribute hereditary material to the developing egg. There have been reports (1,2) of what appears to be a polyploid series in various bisexual groups, notably in Dermaptera, in the genus Gryllotalpa, and in Lepidoptera. A closer examination of the DNA content of their nuclei has shown equal amounts of nucleic acid in these forms (3,4) and they are no longer considered polyploid.

The difference in the extent of polyploidy found in the evolutionarily highly successful insects and plants has long engaged the attention of students of evolution, and the problem is of general interest in many respects. Polyploidy is a major evolutionary factor in the plant kingdom. In insects, however, the role of polyploidy is very modest. There have been many

---

[1] We are happy to dedicate this paper to our mentor, Professor Esko Suomalainen, on the occasion of his seventieth birthday. His pioneering studies in the field of insect polyploidy have been a source of inspiration to many.

attempts to explain why polyploidy is so much rarer among insects than in plants. In this article, we first describe the documented cases of polyploidy in insects and we then shall attempt to answer the question of why polyploidy is not an evolutionary factor of consequence among insects.

DOCUMENTED CASES OF POLYPLOIDY IN INSECTS

The vast majority of insects reproduces bisexually and so we need not here be concern with hermaphroditism, which is often associated with polyploidy in diverse worms (e.g., Turbellaria, Oligochaeta). Polyploidy occurs in insects in connection with parthenogenesis. We shall here accept this established fact and shall not be concerned with the question of why there are no polyploid bisexual insects.

The evolutionary potential of parthenogenetic animals depends on the cytological mechanism of parthenogenesis. Most polyploid insects have the more advanced type of parthenogenesis, apomixis (5), in which the meiotic mechanism is suppressed. Only one maturation division takes place in the eggs and this division is an equational one. In the more primitive type, automictic parthenogenesis, the early stages of meiosis proceed in the normal fashion, and the zygoid chromosome number is restored by a fusion of two azygoid nuclei, endomitosis, or some other mechanism. This restoration of the zygoid chromosome number may, e.g., occur by a fusion of two polar nuclei (the moth _Solenobia triquetrella_) (6) or by a fusion of the first polar nucleus with the secondary oocyte, as in the case of _Solenobia lichenella_ (7). We have elsewhere (8) reviewed the various automictic mechanisms connected with the parthenogenesis of insects as well as their genetic consequences.

There are certain insect orders in which numerous parthenogenetic forms are known to occur, e.g., Ephemeroptera (9). Until cytological data are available, it may be suspected that polyploids may be found among them. The formation of stable polyploid states is particularly favorable in insects with apomictic parthenogenesis. These forms lack secondarily some of the major obstacles for polyploidy in animals, namely, normal meiosis and sex determination mechanism involving sex chromsomes (3,4).

The following list enumerates the insects in which polyploidy has been cytologically verified.

Orthoptera: Tettigoniidae. _Saga pedo_ Pallas. A tetraploid parthenogenetic species (10-12).

Homoptera: Coccidae. The scale insects exhibit a wide variety of different mechanism of parthenogenesis. At least certain individuals of _Physokermes hemicryphus_ Dalam are triploid (13). Delphacidae. _Muellerianella fairmairei_ Perris. A triploid pseudogamic race (14,15).

Lepidoptera: In this large insect order, only a few parthenogenetic forms are known (16). Psychidae. Two species, Solenobia triquetrella Hb. and S. lichenella L. have, in addition to a diploid race also a tetraploid one (6,7,17-20). There are two tetraploid parthenogenetic species, Solenobia seileri Sauter (21) and S. fennicella Suomalainen (22).

Diptera: Chironomidae. Limnophyes virgo Remm. A triploid parthenogenetic species (23,24). Simuliidae. Cnephia mutata Mall., Prosimulium ursinum Edw., P. macropyga Rubtzov, and Gymonopais sp., triploid parthenogenetic races (25). Psychodidae. Psychoda parthenogenetica Tonnoir, a triploid parthenogenetic species (26). Phytomyza crassiseta Zett. A triploid parthenogenetic race (27). Chamaemyiidae. Ochthiphila polystigma Meig. A triploid parthenogenetic species (28).

Coleoptera: Ptinidae. Ptinus clavipes f. mobilis Moore. A triploid pseudogamic race (29). Chrysomelidae. Bromius (Adoxus) obscurus L. A triploid parthenogenetic race (30), six tetraploid parthenogenetic Calligrapha species (31). Curculionidae. 38 triploid, 17 tetraploid, 5 pentaploid, and 2 hexaploid parthenogenetic races or species. Table 1 gives the degrees of ploidy, geographic distribution, and references to literature to these parthenogenetic species or races. As shown, only two of the total of 64 parthenogenetic Curculionid forms are diploid.

Hymenoptera: In this order the males are haploid and develop from unfertilized eggs. At least theoretically polyploidy could be established in this order as it lacks the chromosomal sex-determining mechanism. There are, indeed, numerous reports of evolutionary polyploidy in this order, all summarized (and found doubtful) in a recent review by Crozier (44) including the contention that all Hymenoptera are in fact diploid and tetraploid. Crozier accepts two cases as probable (44): Tenthredinidae. Diprion simile Hart. The females are tetraploid and males diploid; there are also parthenogenetic forms (45). Apoidea. Melipona quinquefasciata Lepp.; the males are diploid and females tetraploid; there is, however, also evidence against polyploidy in this case (4,44).

GEOGRAPHICAL DISTRIBUTION OF POLYPLOID INSECTS

Vandel (46) coined the term geographical parthenogenesis to describe the fact that the bisexual and parthenogenetic (and polyploid) races of a species have different distributions. In general the polyploid parthenogenetic form has a very wide distribution in comparison with the diploid bisexual race. We present in the following certain representative cases of geographic distribution of polyploid insects.

The wingless tetraploid grasshopper, Saga pedo, is widespread in the countries north of the Mediterranean. It occurs on an area extending from Portugal through southern Italy to the southern Urals. It has certain bisexual relatives with a more limited

Table 1.   Degrees of ploidy and geographical distribution of parthenogenetic weevils.

Subfamily and species	Degree of ploidy					Geographical distribution	Reference
	2x	3x	4x	5x	6x		
BRACHYDERINAE							
Polydrusus mollis Stroem.	x	x				NE,CE	32
Scepticus insularis Roelofs	x	x		x		JA	32
Naupactus peregrinus (?)		x				AU	33
Eusomus ovulum Germ.		x				CE	32
Foucartia squamulata Herbst		x				CE	34
Barynotus squamosus Germ.		x				NA	32
moerens F.		x		x		CE	32
obscurus F.			x			NE	32
Sciaphilus asperatus Bonsd		x				NA,NE,CE	32
Strophosomus melanogrammus Fürst.		x				NA,NE,CE	32
Catapionus gracilicornis Roelofs			x	x		JA	32
Blosyrus japonicus Sharp			x	x	x	JA	35
OTIORHYNCHINAE							
Otiorhynchus gemmatus Scop.		x				CE	32
ligustici L.		x				NE	32
ovatus L.		x				NA,NE	32
pauxillus Rosh.		x				CE	32
proximus Strl.		x				CE	32
rugifrons Gyll.		x				CE	32
salicis Ström.		x				NE,CE	32
singularis L.		x				NE,CE	32
subcostatus Stierl.		x				CE	32
sulcatus F.		x				NE,CE	32

Table 1. (continued)

Subfamily and species	2x	3x	4x	5x	6x	Geographical distribution	Reference
chrysocomus Gm.		x	x			CE	32
niger F.		x	x			CE	32
scaber L.		x	x			NE,CE	32
subdentatus Bach.		x	x			CE	32
dubius Ström.			x			NE	32
pupillatus Gyll.			x			CE	36
anthracinus Scop.				x		CE	32
Sciopithes obscurus Horn.			x			NA	32
Peritelus hirticornis Hbst.		x	x			CE	32
Cyrtepistomus castaneus Roelofs		x				JA	37
Myllocerus nipponicus Zumpt.		x				JA	38
fumosus Faust.		x				JA	39
Myosides seriehispidus Roelofs		x				JA	40
Trachyphloeus aristatus Gyll.		x				CE	41
scabriculus L.		x				CE	32
bifoveolatus Beck		x				NE,CE	32
Macrocorynus griseoides Zumpt.		x				JA	39
Trachyrhinus sp.		x				JA	40
EREMNINAE							
Callirhopalus minimus Roelofs		x	x			JA	42
bifasciatus Roelofs			x			JA	32
obesus Roelofs			x		x	JA	35
setosus Roelofs			x			JA	42

Table 1. (continued)

Subfamily and species	Degree of ploidy					Geographical distribution	Reference
	2x	3x	4x	5x	6x		
BAGOINAE							
Lissorhoptrus oryzophilus Kuschel		x				NA,JA	43
LEPTOPINAE							
Trophiphorus carinatus Müll.		x				CE	32
cucullatus Fauv.			x			CE	32
terricola Newm.			x			NA	32
CYLINDRORRHININAE							
Listroderes costirostris Schönherr		x				JA	32
ALOPHINAE							
Liophloeus tessulatus Müll.		x				NE	32

NA = North America, NE = North Europe (in most cases Finland), CE = Central Europe (includes Poland, Germany, Switzerland and Austria), JA = Japan, AU = Australia. Only one of the American species, Sciopithes obscurus, is native to North America, all other American forms are introduced.

distribution in the eastern Mediterranean countries (10,12).
Saga pedo lives in small isolated colonies, but the surviving
colonies are considered to be on the verge of extinction. We
should point out here that the ideas concerning the precarious
survival of S. pedo date back to the time of the early theories
concerning apomictic polyploids as evolutionary non-hopers. The
geographical data can be interpreted also to indicate that S.
pedo is a widespread and successful ecological specialist, far
more widespread than its bisexual relatives. This view is
supported by the longevity of S. pedo; it has a life cycle extending over a number of years.

The distribution of the different races of the wingless moth
Solenobia triquetrella has been studied extensively by Seiler
(47). The tetraploid parthenogenetic race is spread over most of
Europe, to central Finland in the north. Diploid races have been
found only in the Alps and adjacent areas. The diploid bisexual
race lives only on areas which were unglaciated in the last Ice
Age (Würm). Such localities may be found to the north of the
Alpine Ice sheet (and to the south of the Scandinavian Ice sheet,
which extended to northern Germany in the south) or on mountains,
which rose above the ice as nunataks. The diploid parthenogenetic
race lives, in part, sympatrically with the bisexual race. It
has also spread a little to previously glaciated areas in the
Swiss Mittelland.

In Europe the polyploid races of weevils have distributions
clearly differing from that of their presumed diploid bisexual
ancestors. In certain species the diploid bisexual races are
unknown and may well be extinct. Almost all polyploid parthenogenetic weevils are flightless forms. In spite of the restricted
mobility they have often spread wide and far. Suomalainen and
others (16,36,41,48-52) have extensively studied the geographic
distribution of polyploid weevils. In typical cases, e.g., in
the genera Otiorhynchus and Trachyphloeus, the bisexual races
live in restricted areas in the mountains of central Europe or in
southern Europe. The polyploid parthenogenetic races have spread
often all the way to northern Europe over the area exposed by the
retreating Würm ice sheet. A typical example is tetraploid
Otiorhynchus dubius, which is spread over Iceland, the British
Isles through Scandinavia to the Urals in the East. The diploid
bisexual race lives in the Alps and the Carpathians. It should
be stressed that the Pleistocene glaciations do not necessarily
have any causal connection with the origin of polyploid insects;
they are, however, the main historical factor explaining the
distribution of different forms. The polyploid forms have been
successful in colonizing northern continental Europe, whereas the
distributions of the diploid bisexual races are evidently relictual.

Takenouchi (32,35,37,53) has extensively studied the geographical distribution of polyploid weevils in Japan. Most of
the polyploid races studied by him (cf. Table 1) occur in northern
Japan: on the islands of Hokkaido or northern Honshu. Figure 1

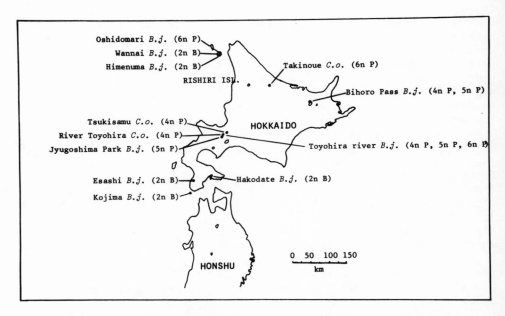

Fig. 1. Map of Hokkaido showing collecting localities and distribution of different races of Blosyrus japonicus and Callirhopalus obesus (35,54).

shows the collection localities and distribution of different races of Blosyrus japonicus and Callirhopalus obesus on Hokkaido. There are four races of B. japonicus with different degrees of polyploidy (4x, 5x, and 6x) and a diploid bisexual race. At certain localities two and, in one, three polyploid races are sympatric; on the isolated Rishiri island the bisexual race lives together with the hexaploid one. Also in Japan the bisexual diploid races are in general rarer than the polyploids. Northern Japan appears to offer an ideal geographic test situation for observing correlations between polyploidy and different ecological variables such as altitude, temperature, isolation, etc. The polyploid forms seem to have a northern distribution and occur often at higher altitudes. Takenouchi (35,42) has found evidence of historic factors in his material; furthermore he has also found two polyploid forms in southern Japan.

     Polyploid parthenogenetic insects have, apparently, been successful colonizers of vast land areas. This becomes more remarkable, when we consider that they are mostly sluggish and flightless forms. Many European polyploid weevils have been

transported to North America (32). The dispersal of parthenogenetic forms is, of course, efficient by the single reason that
the transport of a single individual at any stage of development
suffices to establish a new population. This is definitely not
the only reason for their success. The present distributions
show that the polyploid forms are able to outcompete their bisexual
ancestors and colonize areas in which the diploids very probably
would not be able to survive.

The Scandinavian tetraploid parthenogenetic individuals of
Otiorhynchus dubius have an average of 2°C lower thermal limit of
activity than the corresponding Alpine diploids (55). These data
are, of course, controversial, as the specimens studied were of
different geographical origin; precise comparisons on the ecology
of various populations remain to be made. Morphological differences certainly exist between different polyploid populations of
the same species (48,56).

THE ORIGIN OF POLYPLOIDY IN INSECTS

None of the hypotheses concerning the origin of polyploidy
in parthenogenetic insects has been experimentally verified.

Polyploid parthenogenetic insects have evidently arisen from
diploid bisexual ancestors. We have much indirect, mostly zoo-
geographic, evidence that in cases like Solenobia triquetrella
and the parthenogenetic weevils, the evolution of polyploidy has
proceeded first through a diploid parthenogenetic stage and
polyploidization has occurred after the establishment of the
parthenogenetic mode of reproduction.

Seiler (19) has demonstrated certain cytological peculiarities
in Solenobia triquetrella, which probably are connected with the
origin of parthenogenesis and polyploidy in this moth. The
oocytes of all races of this moth undergo a normal meiosis and
chromosome reduction. In the parthenogenetic eggs the chromosome
number is restored by a fusion of two central nuclei; this results
in the formation of the so-called "Richtungs-Kopulations-Kern"
(RKK). The individuals rising from parthenogenetic eggs are
always females, since the fusion of the two central polar nuclei
leads to heterogamety. A RKK is formed normally also in the eggs
of the bisexual race, but its development is inhibited through
fertilization of the egg.

The first step in the transition from bisexuality to diploid
parthenogenesis is an unstable parthenogenesis, in which all eggs
do not develop completely. The next step is a stable parthenogenesis with normal development of all eggs. Local populations
of S. triquetrella exist, which probably correspond to these
hypothetical steps. Diploid parthenogenetic populations show
many cytological differences, e.g., some have the chromosomal
constitution XY while others have lost the Y chromosome and are,
accordingly, of XO type.

Diploid parthenogenetic eggs of S. triquetrella have deficiencies in the cortical ooplasm in comparison with the eggs of the
diploid bisexual race. In certain populations the ooplasm containing the spindles of the meiotic divisions is absent. This
results in meiotic disturbances. In certain other populations
the nuclei of the embryo may fuse at the blastoderm stage or
later. Both of these mechanisms have been observed to lead to
the formation of tetraploid eggs (19).

Triploidy is by far the most common degree of polyploidy in
weevils, so that 38 out of the total of 64 known parthenogenetic
Curculionid races or species are triploid (cf. Table 1). Explaining the origin of anisoploidy (3x, 5x, etc.) appears, at first,
difficult to explain.

Practically all anisopolyploids have apomictic parthenogenesis. Suomalainen (36) suggested that as the races with
different degrees of polyploidy are often sympatric and as there
is reduction of the chromosome number, different degrees of
polyploidy could have originated by chance fertilizations of the
parthenogenetic eggs by haploid sperms. There are observations
(57) suggesting that in weevils the apomictic parthenogenesis is
preceded by an automictic mechanism. A triploid race would
result from a diploid parthenogenetic egg fertilized by a haploid
sperm. Subsequent fertilizations would add to the degrees of
polyploidy. Seiler (58) has demonstrated with Solenobia triquetrella that parthenogenetic eggs can be easily fertilized. In
Lepidoptera the female heterogamety leads to the formation of
sterile anisopolyploid intersexes. This does not apply in other
polyploid insects, where females are the homogametic sex.

Suomalainen (59) and Takenouchi (54) have observed deviating
chromosome numbers in the oocytes of polyploid weevils so that,
e.g., a hexaploid female Blosyrus japonicus may produce triploid
and tetraploid eggs. It is uncertain whether nondisjunction
processes involving whole metaphase plates are responsible for
the formation of new degrees of polyploidy in weevils, but this
is, however, a possibility. There is evidence that such processes
are real phenomena producing polyploid insects. Triploid simuliids
(60) probably arise through a nondisjunction process. Single
triploid chromosome complements are widespread in natural black
fly populations, and they probably arise through chance abnormalities in the oogenesis (61).

Stalker (28) suggests that the triploidy in Ochthiphila
polystigma has originated first through a diploid automictic
parthenogenetic state. This is followed by triploid automictic
parthenogenesis, finally resulting in triploid apomictic parthenogenesis. An automictic mechanism involving a regular fusion of
three haploid meiotic products may appear improbable. Recently,
however, Nur (13) has found evidence of such a mechanism.

Pseudogamy is the means through which a new anisopolyploid
parthenogenetic species may quite possibly arise. The triploid

pseudogamic race of <u>Muellerianella</u> <u>fairmairei</u> (<u>M</u>. 2-<u>fairmairei</u>-<u>brevipennis</u>) (15) appears to have two haploid genomes of <u>M</u>. <u>fairmairei</u> and one of <u>M</u>. <u>brevipennis</u>. A triploid phenotype identical with the wild pseudogamic form has been reconstructed experimentally in the laboratory by crosses. Pseudogamy may also (as in the case of <u>Ptinus</u> <u>clavipes</u> f. <u>mobilis</u>) lead to normal parthenogenesis, in which a sperm is no longer required to trigger the development of the egg.

Astaurov (62) has experimentally produced sexually reproducing allotetraploid silkworm moths in the laboratory. He first maintained a diploid all-female line of <u>Bombyx</u> <u>mori</u> in the laboratory by artificial parthenogenesis (heat treatment applied to unfertilized eggs at the metaphase stage; this results in normal mitosis and consequently apomictic parthenogenesis). Such females occasionally lay tetraploid eggs, which produce an all-female tetraploid line. This line can again be maintained indefinitely by the heat treatment in each generation. Sterile allotriploid moths of both sexes can be produced subsequently by crossing the autotetraploid females with males of <u>Bombyx</u> <u>mandarina</u>. Allotriploid females can again be maintained by the heat treatment of the eggs. Many females resulting from this treatment are mixoploid, being mosaics consisting of triploid and hexaploid tissues. Hexaploid eggs undergo normal meiosis and, when fertilized with a haploid <u>B</u>. <u>mandarina</u> sperm, give rise to tetraploids of both sexes. These allotetraploid individuals are, in part, fertile and can be maintained in the laboratory. Astaurov has named this allotetraploid species <u>Bombyx</u> <u>allotetraploidus</u>. It is, of course, reproductively isolated from both of its parent species.

Astaurov's experiment is a model of clear thinking connected with good experimental design. In order to produce a viable allopolyploid strain he had to proceed through several stages of apomictic parthenogenesis. Accordingly, it is unlikely that natural polyploids arise in this fashion, as the capacity for meiosis is lost in apomixis, and once lost, such complex phenomena as meiosis and sexual reproduction are unlikely be restored in later evolution. Again, as mentioned before, we have no good evidence for natural bisexual polyploid insect species.

GENETIC VARIATION IN POLYPLOID INSECTS

The evolutionary potential of a species is a function of the amount of its genetic variation. According to Fisher's fundamental theorem of natural selection the rate of increase in fitness of a species at any time is equal to its genetic variance in fitness at that time. Polyploidy is in insects always associated with parthenogenesis. Parthenogenesis is the notorious "blind alley of evolution," leading to decreased genetic variablity. The issue is of central importance in biology, as demonstrating the

evolutionary advantages of sex in comparison with asexual or
parthenogenetic reproduction remains a major unresolved aspect of
the theory of evolution. We certainly do not lack elegant hypotheses, as a recent review convincingly demonstrates (63); the
real need is for experimental data bearing on the subject.

At this point we shall make a frank value judgement. We
feel that implicit in much of the older literature on the evolutionary possibilities of polyploid and parthenogenetic insects is
the idea that such forms are doomed and on the verge of extinction.
With the evolutionary advantages of sex as a central unresolved
issue, people working on the subject are probably happier with
the traditional notion. This has probably led to a serious
underestimation of the evolutionary potential of polyploid parthenogenetic insects (8,64,65). True, there are no polyploid
parthenogenetic insect taxa above the species level, but nevertheless, the present evidence indicates that polyploid insects are
more efficient than their bisexual diploid ancestors in occupying
whatever niche is available for the species as a whole. Precise
ecological comparisons between diploid bisexual races and different
polyploid forms have not been done.

CHROMOSOMAL POLYMORPHISM

It is unfortunate that polyploid species of the Diptera are
a neglected group. Polytene chromosome studies have yield the
basic experimental groundwork of evolutionary genetics and we
hope that such studies will be made on the polyploid Diptera in
the future. We shall here briefly review the present state of
knowledge.

Phytomyza crassiseta

In addition to a triploid parthenogenetic race, this leaf-
mining fly species has a diploid parthenogenetic as well as a
diploid bisexual race (27). The different races are largely
sympatric. An interesting feature of the triploid race is its
automictic parthenogenesis with nonhomologous pairing during
meiosis. In addition to some homologous bivalents, nonhomologous
bivalents are found. This results in a variable number of chromosome units and probably accounts for the regular separation of
chromosomes. There are several structural rearrangements. These
include nine inversions, a duplication, and a deletion. A total
of four different triploid chromosomal races have been found in
Scandinavia. Two of them have arisen from a common ancestral
type through different rearrangements, which have occurred
following the establishment of triploidy. The two other types
can probably be best explained as resulting from chance fertilization of diploid parthenogenetic females by males bearing the

chromosomal inversions found in these types. Two of the types
have a southern distribution, while the two others are manifestly
northern.

Cnephia mutata

The parthenogenetic race of this simuliid, with more than
700 different chromosomal types recognized (66), approaches the
concept of an agamic complex in insects. As many as 70 different
inversion types have been found in a single locality. These
types differ from each other with regard to slightly dissimilar
inverted segments in two chromosomal elements. These inversions
are suggested to have originated through an automictic mechanism
involving crossing over and segregation (25). Details of this
mechanism are obscure.

A triploid, chromosomally monomorphic, bisexual race of this
black fly is sympatric with the triploid parthenogenetic race in
Canada. The material (25) suggests that there are three major
chromosome types. All minor inversions can be derived from
these; they may well represent recombination products. This
could be confirmed by studying the offspring of single triploid
females. If the offspring is polymorphic, there indeed is a
mechanism of recombination. The adaptive significance of the
inversion polymorphism of C. mutata is unknown. It could be
studied by collecting samples from different parts of the distribution area. The question would be whether the polymorphism is
distributed in an orderly manner and whether it is correlated
with any ecological variable.

Psychoda parthenogenetica

The triploid parthenogenetic race of this species has a
cosmopolitan distribution (there are records from Europe, Africa,
Asia, and Oceania) (26). Generally, as in this case, the distribution of related bisexual species is not as extensive as that of
the polyploid one. The parthenogenesis is apomictic. Unfortunately, the polytene chromosomes of P. parthenogenetica do
not easily offer themselves to cytological analysis. There
exist, however, other comparable parthenogenetic species, which
may well prove to be more amenable for a study on eventual chromosome polymorphism. Finally, there are numerous polyploid parthenogenetic Chironomidae. Cases of complex inversion heterozygosity
have been described in them (23,24,67), but the distributions of
these rearrangements have not been followed in different populations.

GENIC VARIATION

Standard methods of enzyme electrophoresis have been applied to study the genetic constitution of polyploid insect populations. As we are mainly responsible for these studies, we shall first express our reservations. The genetic relationships of different allozymes can in bisexual organisms (such as Drosophila) be experimentally verified by crosses and a formal genetic analysis helps to unravel any difficulties in interpretation (68). The Drosophila studies are, of course, the basis for all studies on animals, which can not be easily crossed. Much can be inferred of them in studying the polyploids; the difficulty is that we can not test the interpretation. An enzyme phenotype of a polyploid may at first glance present a formidable problem of interpretation, in particular when all enzyme alleles are different. One should, therefore, first establish the appearance of different allozyme combinations in a conspecific (or closely related) diploid bisexual population and ascertain whether the enzyme is a monomer, a multimer, etc., factors that affect the appearance of hybrid enzyme phenotype. A polyploid apparently homozygous for an enzyme allele may give a highly misleading result, as we have no way (except for a crude visual interpretation or equally crude densitometric study of enzyme activity) to quantify the amount of alleles producing enzymes with identical migration properties. Furthermore, a triploid heterozygous for two alleles has two doses of one allele and one dose of the other; we have attempted to analyze such situations (64), but more refined techniques must become available before progress can be made.

POLYPLOID CURCILIONIDAE

These weevils all have an apomictic parthenogenesis with no recombination of genes. In a polyploid situation without recombination the likelihood of mutant recessive alleles being expressed in lower than in diploid parthenogenetic forms (unless the same mutation happens three or four times in succession--a notion, which stretches one's credibility too far). All other theoretical arguments like Muller's ratchet, etc., apply for these unfortunate things (63), which should fare badly indeed in this changing world.

Suomalainen, after having studied the cytology and geographical distribution of these forms for over 20 years, published in 1961 a morphometric study on polyploid weevil populations (56). He attempted to see whether these apparently successful insects would really be as invariable in different parts of their wide European area of distribution as postulated by the theory. He measured the total length of an individual as well as the relation between the total length and the other measured parts for each individual (Fig. 2). Of the 18 populations of Otiorhynchus

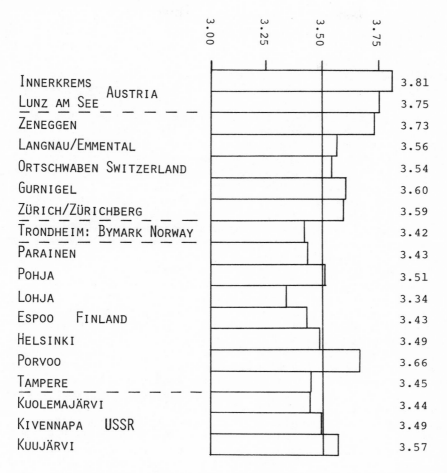

Fig. 2. The ratio of total length to length of hind tibia in the Otiorhynchus scaber populations. The values of the ordinate refer to the ratio mentioned (56).

scaber studied certain southern Finnish populations differed significantly from populations from adjacent areas. Suomalainen interpreted these observations as a result of genetic differences between these populations. Clearly, new mutations had occurred and established themselves in polyploid populations. In his words, "evolution has not come to a standstill in parthenogenetic polyploid populations, but continues, even if it may have been slowed down" (56).

This conclusion was greeted with some disbelief (66,69). It was argued that the polyploid biotypes were polyphyletic, so that the polyploid constitution had originated several times at different localities. An alternative explanation would be that both parthenogenesis and polyploidy would have originated through multiple hybridizations between Otiorhynchus scaber and diverse related species. Both processes would result in differences between populations. Both explanations also reinforced the hypothesis that polyploid parthenogenetic insects are evolutionary dead ends.

Clearly, the problem could be solved by an electrophoretic analysis of the polyploid populations. The starting point here was to find a bisexual diploid population. Such populations live in a limited area in southeastern Austria only. Even there they are sympatric with the more numerous polyploid races. The bisexual diploids were found and studied with electrophoresis (64). The results were somewhat puzzling as the degree of heterozygosity over the loci studied proved to be very high, in fact, highest ever recorded for any bisexual population. We intend to study the reasons for this high heterozygosity and the relationship of the bisexual and parthenogenetic individuals further.

The genetic constitution of both triploid central European and tetraploid Finnish O. scaber populations was determined by comparing their enzyme phenotypes with the ones of the diploid bisexual population. In general all populations proved to be variable. In particular certain loci were variable, while others were monomorphic. As there is no recombination, we may conveniently present the results over all loci studied to determine the genetic constitution of the individual. We call this enzyme phenotype (more than 20 loci have been studied) the overall genotype of an individual. Comparisons between different overall genotypes proved that there was no evidence of polyphyletic origin of different populations and degrees of polyploidy; the material suggested that parthenogenesis and polyploidy are, at least in central and northern European populations, monophyletic condition in O. scaber (64,70). Virtually all differences between individuals and populations could be explained to be due to an addition (or deletion) of a single allozyme to an otherwise invariable overall genotype. The considerable amount of genetic variability detected between and within populations may, accordingly, be assumed to be due to mutations, which have occurred in the polyploid parthenogenetic lineage following the establishment of the parthenogenetic mode of reproduction. Similar results were obtained for several other polyploid weevil species (64,70-72). A somatic recombination would be an efficient mechanism for restoring genetic variability, but we have no evidence for it.

The tetraploid race of O. scaber is widespread in Europe; it is known to occur in the mountains of central Europe (Alps, Carpathians, etc.) as well as in the boreal coniferous forests of northern Europe. It is associated with the Norway spruce (Picea abies), one of the dominant tree species in these areas.

We decided to study the extent of the genetic variability in tetraploid O. scaber populations by collecting individuals from even intervals over northwestern Europe as well as from certain central European populations. The weevils are so common that a sample can be conveniently taken from a population in a matter of minutes. We collected a total of 482 tetraploid individuals from 123 populations. The populations sampled extend from the southern limit of the boreal coniferous forests in southern Sweden all the way to the northen limit of distribution of O. scaber. In general four weevils were studied for each population. Nine loci were monomorphic in this material, i.e., all weevils had an identical allele configuration at these loci. Three were monomorphic for a heterozygous allele combination. This may be taken as a very strong argument for a monophyletic origin of tetraploidy.

There were, however, differences at certain loci, most notably those coding for leucine aminopeptidases and malic enzyme. A total of 75 different overall genotypes were detected in this material (70). A total of 27 of them were found to occur in more than one population. It is true that our method of taking a small sample only does not reveal the distribution of less common genotypes, as the aim was to establish the distribution pattern of the predominant types.

Half of the total number of weevils studied belong to three genotypes, labeled, I, VII and XVI. Type I is found in 50 populations, type VII in 34 populations and type XVI in 22 populations in northern Europe and in one population in Switzerland. The geographic distributions of these types are presented in Fig. 3–5. In addition to these three common types, the populations contain in general several other, less common genotypes. The distribution of the less common types is given in detail in our original publication (70). The situation in central European mountains is roughly similar to that in northern Europe; there are numerous types in a single population. The central European types differ from the northern types only slightly.

Polydrusus mollis

This weevil is exceptional in two ways: it can fly, and there is in addition to a triploid, a diploid parthenogenetic race (as mentioned earlier, out of total of 64 parthenogenetic weevil forms, only two are diploid). The diploid parthenogenetic race inhabits northern and eastern Europe (Finland, Sweden, Poland and all the way to Siberia), triploids are found in eastern and southern parts of central Europe (71). The bisexual diploid populations live in southern Yugoslavia and Albania. Accordingly, we have here a case in which the race with a lower degree of ploidy is more widespread than the higher (triploid) degree of ploidy.

This weevil is associated with the climax tree species of the temperate zone: oak (Quercus), on the northern margin of its

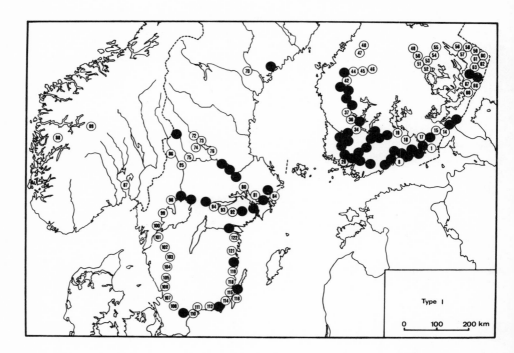

Fig. 3. The collection localities of the northern European
Otiorhynchus scaber samples. A black circle indicates a locality,
where the genotype identified with a Roman number, has been
found (70).

distribution it lives on elm (Ulmus), and hazel (Corylus). The
parthenogenetic populations are again polymorphic and the overall
pattern of variation follows that of polyploid parthenogenetic
weevil populations in general. The triploid genotypes resemble
the diploid parthenogenetic ones to the extent that one triploid
type is indistinguishable from a diploid type. Even though the
populations are variable, three loci are permanently heterozygous
for an identical allele combination in all parthenogenetic
individuals, i.e., a similar enzyme phenotype is present in all
parthenogenetic P. mollis weevils irrespective of their degree of
polyploidy. Accordingly, both triploid and diploid parthenogenesis
represent a monophyletic condition in P. mollis.
     On the northern margin of distribution of P. mollis the
plant communities typical to the temperate zone are patchy. The
P. mollis individuals from different populations differ from each
other rather sharply (at least in comparison with O. scaber
individuals). There has been considerable genetic differentiation
in different parthenogenetic lineages of P. mollis, in particular,

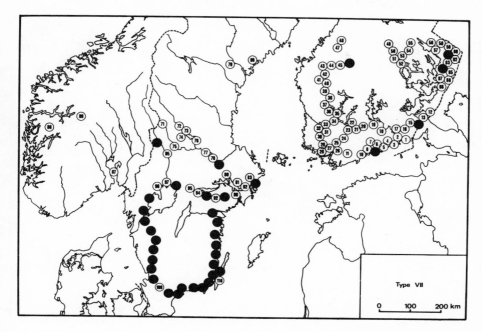

Fig. 4.   The collection localities of the northern European
Otiorhynchus scaber samples. A black circle indicates a locality,
where the genotype identified with a Roman number, has been
found (70).

as any explanations invoking a polyphyletic hybrid ancestry are
improbable in the diploid lineage.

ECOLOGICAL ADAPTATIONS OF POLYPLOID CURCULIONIDAE

        The general pattern of variability in weevil populations can
be summarized by stating that each individual population is
composed of individuals with slightly different overall genotypes.
Some of these genotypes are common and widespread, whereas some
are evidently local. Certain inferences of the relative ages of
these populations can be made on the basis of these distributions
and the genic configurations (e.g., a local type may be thought
to be younger than a widespread one). The differences between
the major overall genotypes (that is I, VII and XVI) of O.
scaber are slight, but as shown in Fig. 3-5, their geographic
distributions are strikingly different.
        The distribution of the three major types of O. scaber is
remarkably well in accord with the phytogeographic zones of
northwestern Europe illustrated in Fig. 6. The genotype XVI

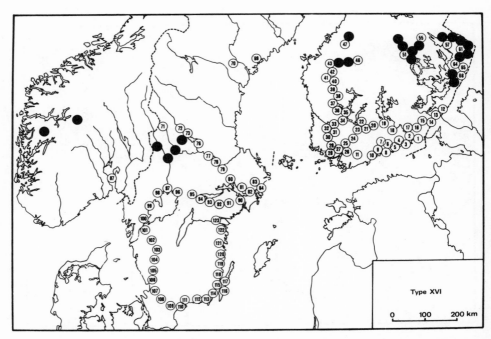

Fig. 5.   The collection localities of the northern European
Otiorhynchus scaber samples.   A black circle indicates a locality,
where the genotype identified with a Roman number, has been
found (70).

occurs in the central boreal zone in Finland and Sweden and also
on rather high country on the western coast of Norway.   A single
individual of this type has been found on the top of Zürichberg
in Switzerland.   Type I has a southern boreal distribution in
Sweden and Finland but it occurs also in some hemiboreal populations.   The distribution of the major type VII is predominantly
hemiboreal.   The distributions of these as well as the less
frequent types have not yet been worked out in detail with respect
to the ecological variables.   We are, however, analyzing these
data more extensively.   A difficulty here is that historical
factors are difficult to separate from responses to ecological
variables.
     The polyploid weevils are in general sluggish and flightless
forms and explaining why they have been able to colonize successfully a northern European climax community presents some
difficulty.   Similar genotypes are found over very large areas in
similar biotopes.   This may be taken to indicate that the dispersal
of the species has not been just passive transport of single
individuals, but rather a polymorphic colonizing population has

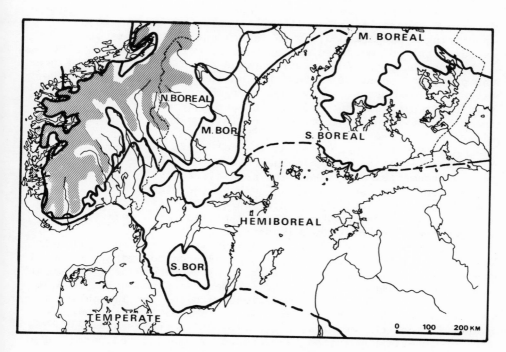

Fig. 6. The biotic zones of northwestern Europe (73). The
solid lines indicate zonal boundaries. The shading indicates
Alpine zone of the Scandinavian Range.

spread over the present area of distribution. The differences in
the relative frequencies of different types in different environments indicate the response of a polymorphic parthenogenetic
population to selection: the best genotypes are favored and
become common.

At this point we must concede that our knowledge on the
ecology of polyploid weevils is poor. The adults are collected
by shaking young trees in the spring, but these young trees are
only a temporary feeding site of females prior to oviposition.
The development of an individual weevil takes two years; the
larvae live in the roots of trees. Evidently the weevils show no
preference for young trees, the simple reason that we have
collected them from young trees is that large trees are harder to
shake.

The pattern of polymorphism in polyploid apomictic population
is orderly, as the geographic distributions of the common (as well
as many less common) genotypes indicate that they are adapted to

different environments. Many local polyploid weevil populations (e.g., of O. scaber in central Europe) consist of triploid and tetraploid parthenogenetic individuals. Takenouchi (54,74) has described several cases of different polyploid weevil races inhabiting a single locality in Japan; our preliminary studies suggest that polymorphism is the rule also in Japanese populations. In Europe the geographic distributions are differentiated, since the polyploid populations have had an opportunity to spread over extensive land areas. They have everywhere been more successful than their bisexual ancestors. In fact many ancestral bisexual races have evidently become extinct (64) or at least their present distributions are relictual.

All evidence suggests that the polyploid races have been more successful than the bisexual races in adapting themselves to new environments. The amount of gene diversity in diploid bisexual populations of these weevils is as high (or higher) than in any insect species. Yet, in spite of this variability and access to recombination, they, and not the polyploids, have been the dead end (in the sense of being, in part, extinct).

A polyploid weevil population consists of numerous slightly differing genotypes, each of which is adapted to exploit maximally some component of the niche. These components may be variable in space and in time. We may contrast the evident adaptive genetic differentiation in weevil populations with the considerably more uniform allele frequencies noted in a bisexual insect population sympatric with the weevils, e.g., Drosophila subobscura (75). A parthenogenetic population is composed of specialized forms. Due to recombination, the bisexual population is more average.

The geographically differentiated distribution of different polyploid genotypes suggests that some components of the niche are geographically separate. The geographic ranges of different genotypes overlap widely, so that a population consists of an array of genotypes. The polymorphism is maintained by the postulated differing niche preferences as well as by enviornmental changes, to each of which a population responds by a rapid multiplication of the fittest genotype.

In conclusion, a polyploid weevil population consists of an array of genotypes with different adaptive properties. Clearly, such notions as competitive exclusion do not apply here. As long as the population remains polymorphic, it has not lost evolutionary hope. Once a genotype is lost, it can be regained either by migration from other populations or through mutation. Both processes are, of course, ineffective as compared with recombination. Anyway, the sterotypic notions that polyploid insects were evolutionary dead ends are now incompatable with modern information.

Bromius obscurus

In contrast to the weevils, these triploid flying beetles
live in early successional environments. In northern Europe they
live on a plant typical of forest clearings caused by human
activity or fire, the fireweed (Chamaenerion). In North America
this beetle species is bisexual and diploid and a pest of viti-
culture. We have studied a Canadian diploid bisexual population
as well as 52 triploid apomictic populations in northern Europe
(Sweden and Finland). A single triploid genotype was found to be
present in all but five of the 52 populations sampled. Eighty per
cent of the individuals studied belonged to this genotype (out of
a total of 328 beetles studied). Only six other genotypes were
found in this material, even though the collection area was far
wider than that of O. scaber. Two of these types were common
(comprising 45 individuals). Their distributions were well
differentiated (76,77). All triploid forms of this beetle were
clearly monophyletic.

In Bromius populations the dispersal ability has led to a
situation, where single genotypes dominate in wide areas. Populations are not appreciably polymorphic, i.e., the mutual exclusion
principle holds. The vagrant host plant enforces active migration
on Bromius populations. We may briefly contrast this presumed
effect of dispersal ability with the contrasting situation in
Polydrusus mollis: in spite of its active dispersal, the populations of this species were polymorphic (71). The species is,
however, a resident of the temperate climax community. This is
fragmented at best in central Europe in these days and even more
fragmented in its outposts in the boreal zone. Yet we feel that
the reasons for Polydrusus polymorphism are not that simple as it
anyway has the complex weevil ecology. Bromius ecology is rather
straightforward: the larvae feed on the leaves of the host plant,
pupate and a partial new generation may follow already in the
autumn.

Solenobia triquetrella

This bagworm moth is flightless. It is interesting to note
that practically all parthenogenetic Lepidoptera have lost the
ability for flight (16). The bisexual Solenobia populations are
again rare and local in the Alps; the diploid parthenogenetic
populations have not done much better. In spite of its evidently
limited dispersal ability the tetraploid race has reached central
Finland in the north.

We have studied the genetic constitution of the Alpine
diploid bisexual populations and again made a corresponding
analysis on diploid and tetraploid parthenogenetic populations
(78). Again, the parthenogenetic populations are polymorphic.
A part of this polymorphism is due to a polyphyletic origin of
these populations (already postulated by Seiler on the basis of

cytological evidence). In the Alps each population differs
clearly from all other populations, so that no overall genotypes
are common to two populations. The differences within a population
can often be explained by single mutations, which have occurred
following the establishment of parthenogenesis and polyploidy.

Very probably every Alpine tetraploid population represents
a consequence of a different polyploidization event. This is
understandable, as they are sympatric with the diploid bisexual
race. In northern Europe there are, likewise, several overall
genotypes. The area studied (southern Finland) is larger than
Switzerland. Two of the northern genotypes are geographically
widespread and occur in many localities. Their geographic distributions can be explained by historical factors; no correlations
with environmental variables emerge out of these distributions.

ECOLOGICAL REMARKS

There is a remarkable correlation between flightlessness and
parthenogenesis and polyploidy in insects. Forms with active
dispersal are seldom polyploid, and if they are, they utilize
their ability for flight to feed on a plant with high seed
production and dispersal ability. The environments inhabited by
the polyploid weevils are stable and their development extends
over two (or more years). This holds true for Saga and Solenobia
as well. They probably do not need to respond to short-term
environmental changes. We have emphasized that polyploidy gives
them increased genetic homeostasis (8,77,79); they probably
exhibit wide ecological tolerance due to the buffering effects of
polyploidy. A flightless polyploid insect population is polymorphic. The extent of this polymorphism is its evolutionary
hope, as genotypes once lost are not easily replaced. A population
of flying polyploids is able to overcome environmental variability
by the means of active dispersal. We may note that Bromius has a
short life cycle in comparison with the flightless forms: the
active dispersal helps it to overcome the local short-term uncertainty. Parthenogenesis may be a valuable asset in active
dispersal over sexual reproduction, as one migrant suffices to
establish a new population at any available site. In this context
we wish to point out that we have in this study avoided stressing
the innate higher reproductive capacity of parthenogenetic forms
as a fitness component. This is intentional, as we do not have
experimental data on the subject.

THEORETICAL CONSIDERATIONS

Parthenogensis in insects seems to lead to polyploidy. In
the most extensively studied parthenogenetic insect group,
Curculionidae, out of the total of 64 known parthenogenetic
forms, only two are diploid. There is evidence that polyploidy

does not arise as a sudden event in a hybrid lineage in this group (57). Rather apomixis has an evolution of its own through automixis. In fact assuming a sudden appearance of both apomixis and polyploidy involves a combination of two improbable and separate events. In general, a parthenogenetic insect is often successful only when polyploid. The advantages conferred by the acquisition of polyploidy seem to be obvious.

Polyploidy leads to increased genetic versatility by gene duplication. In the case of polyploid weevils, the added haploid genomes are probably derived from bisexual males of the same species. This may prove to be important. A combination of foreign genetic regulatory systems, as would be expected of a species hybrid, does not necessarily lead to an improvement of the genetic homeostasis. Table 2 demonstrates the increase in heterozygosity in a polyploid through an addition of an arbitrary haploid genome. Whatever the extent of increase in heterozygosity, the heterozygosity derived from a conspecific genome should represent a balanced gene combination. These consideratons do not apply in cases like Solenobia, where a diploid genome is simply duplicated. This does, of course, not increase its heterozygosity.

Due to the accumulation of new mutations, animals with apomictic parthenogenesis should become completely heterozygous (5,80,81). When there is free recombination, parthenogenesis should again result in complete homozygosity, unless opposed by selection (82-84).

Mutations occurring in a parthenogenetic lineage affect the fitness of their bearers. The consequences of certain mutations may be selectively neutral, while others result in altered fitness, either increased or decreased. When there is no recombination, mutations producing nonfunctioning alleles may be rather neutral for the fitness of an apomictic individual. Any diploid organisms have a functional reserve of most gene products (85). Nonfunctioning is, of course, a completely recessive character. We need not be concerned with beneficial mutations here, as the effect of their accumulation in an asexual lineage is well established. Furthermore, they are probably rarer than recessive lethal or semilethal mutations.

By making certain simple assumptions (85) we may arrive at a model, which depicts the amount of heterozygosity in the course of a diploid parthenogenetic lineage (Fig. 7). The model is based on a situation, where one individual produces, on an average, one offspring. The main result is that mutation pressure alone suffices to increase the functioning heterozygosity in a parthenogenetic lineage following the establishment of this mode of reproduction.

Polyploidization offers here an immediate advantage, as heterozygosity increases very markedly within the same period of time in comparison with diploidy. Polyploids are also far better buffered against mutations producing nunfunctioning alleles.

Table 2. The frequencies of loci with identical alleles, and with different proportions of identical and dissimilar alleles in triploid and tetraploid lineages, on the assumption that polyploidy arises by chance union of gametes. h = the degree of homozygosity in the diploid ancestral population (79).

	Allele constitution	Frequency	$h=0.8$	$h=0.7$
Triploidy	all alleles are identical	h^2	0.640	0.490
	two identical/one different	$2h(1-h) + h(1-h)^2$	0.352	0.483
	all alleles are different	$(1-h)^3$	0.008	0.027
Tetraploidy	all alleles are identical	h^3	0.512	0.343
	three identical/one different	$h^2(1-h)\,(4-h)$	0.410	0.485
	two and two identical	$h^2(1-h)^2(3-h)$	0.056	0.101
	two identical/two different	$h(1-h)^3(6-4h+h^2)$	0.022	0.070
	all alleles are different	$(1-h)^6$	0.000	0.001

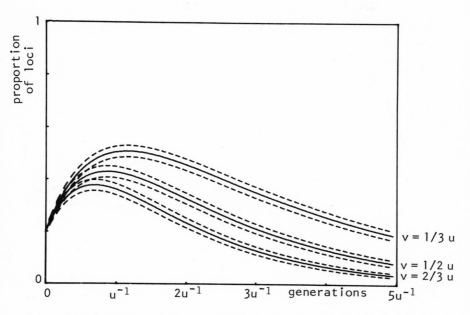

Fig. 7. The amount of functioning heterozygosity (with two functioning alleles) in a diploid parthenogenetic lineage. The dots give the theoretical standard deviations multiplied with two. This gives a confidence level of 95%. Initial heterozygosity is 0.2; u is the mutation rate to a functioning allele and v is the mutation rate to a nonfunctioning allele (85).

This gives a polyploid population an increased life expectancy in relation to a diploid parthenogenetic population. Fig. 8 and 9 show the amount of heterozygosity in a triploid and tetraploid lineage.

An inspection of the figures shows that the time span allotted for the life of populations (in terms of the mutation rate) is improbably long. We have stressed (79) that death by four consequent mutations producing nonfunctioning alleles at the same locus is a very improbable cause of death of any tetraploid parthenogenetic insect.

Polyploid parthenogenetic populations tolerate, in fact, considerable chromosomal changes. A common observation in studies on polyploid weevils is that their chromosome numbers are not exact multiples of their basic number 11 (37,42,48,51,53,59). That these discrepant chromosome counts need not be due to errors in counting the chromosomes has been shown by Suomalainen (30).

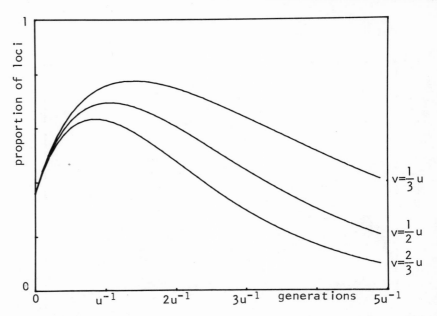

Fig. 8. The amount of functioning heterozygosity in a triploid
parthenogenetic lineage. The initial heterozygosity in diploids
is 0.2; u and v as in Fig. 7 (79).

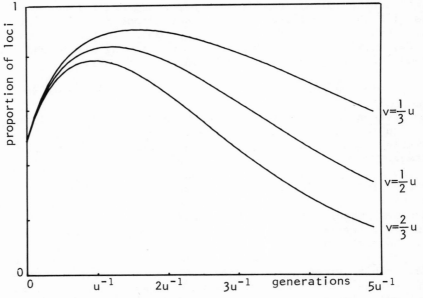

Fig. 9. The amount of functioning heterozygosity in a tetraploid parthenogenetic lineage. The initial heterozygosity in
diploids is 0.2; u and v as in Fig. 7 (79).

He noted a centric fusion of two <u>Bromius</u> chromosomes, which
produced a large chromosome absent in other populations. This
was not a chromosome loss, as the chromosome number of the aberrant
population was 23 instead of the usual 24 for parthenogenetic
triploid populations. Losses of whole chromosomes or fusions
result in a considerable loss of genetic material. Consequently,
recessive alleles in the remaining chromosomes may express themselves in situations, when a dominant allele is removed with the
loss of a whole chromosome.

Our model on the functioning heterozygosity fits well with
the observed distribution of different degrees of polyploidy in
the weevils, where out of the total of 64 parthenogenetic forms 2
are diploid, 38 are triploid, 17 are tetraploid, 5 are pentaploid
and 2 are hexaploid. The most pronounced increase in heterozygosity is conferred by an acquisition of triploidy.

Table 3 gives the degrees of heterozygosity per locus per
individual in polyploid insect populations. We may here remember
that the automictic mechanism of <u>Solenobia</u> is functionally equivalent to apomixis.

Heterozygosity has, indeed, increased in polyploid beetles
with the exception of <u>Otiorhynchus</u> <u>scaber</u>. We have, however,
pointed out earlier that the heterozygosity of diploid <u>O. scaber</u>
is exceptionally high. The heterozygosity values for diploid and
tetraploid <u>Solenobia</u> are identical (in fact there is a slight,
but insignificant increase in the Finnish as compared with the
Swiss tetraploids). This agrees well with the postulated origin
of polyploidy in <u>Solenobia</u>. It also shows that the effect of
mutations on the presumably older northern European tetraploid
populations has been negligible. The heterozygosity values for
diploid and triploid parthenogenetic <u>Polydrusus</u> are again virtually
identical. This does not fit well with the postulated origin of
polyploidy as result of a hybridization of a diploid parthenogenetic female with a bisexual male as expressed in Table 2.
Data on the Japanese polyploid weevil series would be particularly
useful here.

The polyploid parthenogenetic insects are often successful
and widespread forms. They are an apparent contradiction to the
doctrine of polyploid parthenogenetic forms as evolutionary dead
ends. Yet, their evolutionary possibilities are certainly limited.
Polyploidy confers upon previously bisexual (and parthenogenetic)
forms a higher genetic homeostasis with a buffering effect
against nonfunctioning alleles and chromosomal abnormalities.
Life spans extending over several years help polyploid insects to
survive short-term environmental changes. However, it is evident
that even if we exclude the effects of competitive communities
composed of adaptively more versatile sexual species, the loss of
homeostasis through accumulating harmful mutations will limit the
evolutionary potential of polyploid insects.

Table 3. The observed degrees of heterozygosity per locus per individual in different diploid and polyploid populations of parthenogenetic insects.

Species	Bisexual race	Parthenogenetic races			References
		2x	3x	4x	
Bromius obscurus	0.18		0.34		76
Polydrusus mollis	0.14	0.36	0.37		71
Otiorhynchus scaber	0.31		0.25	0.38	64,70
Otiorhynchus salicis	0.12		0.24		72
Otiorhynchus singularis			0.37		64
Strophosomus melanogrammus			0.30		64
Solenobia triquetrella	0.23	0.23		0.23	78

SUMMARY

Of all living organisms insects are the group with the highest number of existing species. It is, of course, true that a fraction of the total number of insects has been cytologically studied. Polyploid forms are rare exceptions among them. Polyploidy in insects is always associated with the parthenogenetic mode of reproduction. The cytologically verified cases are described. As for the geographic distribution of polyploid insects, they have successfully colonized vast land areas. Their distributions are, in general, northern and montane. The polyploid races are in general far more widespread than their diploid bisexual ancestors. The possible models of origin of polyploid insects are covered as well as data on their genetic variability. There are apparent environmental correlations in the distribution of certain forms. Most polyploid insects have life cycles extending over two (or more) years. They are also in general flightless forms. Hypotheses on the relation between heterozygosity in polyploids as well as the consequences of mutations in polyploid lineages are also presented.

LITERATURE CITED

1.   Matthey, R., 1954, La polyploidie animale naturelle, Proc. 9th Inter. Congr. Genet. 1: 302-306.
2.   Vandel, A., 1946, Le rôle de la polyploidie dans le règne animal, Arch. Julius Klaus-Stift. 21: 397-410.
3.   Suomalainen, E., 1959, On polyploidy in animals, Proc. Finnish Acad. Sci. 1958: 105-119.
4.   White, M.J.D., 1973, "Animal Cytology and Evolution," ed. 3. Cambridge University Press, Cambridge.
5.   Suomalainen, E., 1950, Parthenogenesis in animals, Advances Genet. 3: 193-253.
6.   Seiler, J., 1963, Untersuchungen über die Entstehung der Parthenogenese bei Solenobia triquetrella F.R. (Lepidoptera, Psychidae). IV. Z. Vererbungsl. 94: 29-66.
7.   Narbel-Hofstetter, M., 1950, La cytologie de la parthénogénèse chez Solenobia sp. (lichenella L.?) (Lépidoptères, Psychides). Chromosoma 4: 56-90.
8.   Suomalainen, E., Saura, A., Lokki, J., 1976, Evolution of parthenogenetic insects, pp. 209-257, in Hecht, M., Steer, W., Wallace, B. (eds.), "Evolutionary Biology," Vol. 9, Plenum, New York.
9.   Degrange, C., 1960, Recherches sur la reproduction des Éphéméroptères. Trav. Lab. Hydrobiol. Piscicult. (Grenoble) 50-51: 7-193.
10. Goldschmidt, E. 1946, Polyploidy and parthenogenesis in the genus Saga. Nature 158: 587-588.

11. Matthey, R., 1941, Étude biologique et cytologique de Saga pedo Pallas (Orthoptères: Tettigoniidae), Rev. Suisse Zool. 48: 91-142.

12. Matthey, R., 1946, Demonstration du charactere geographique de la parthenogenese de Saga pedo Pallas et de la polyploidie, par comparison avec les espèces bisexuées S. ephippigera Fisch. et S. gracilipes Uvar. Experientia 2: 260-261.

13. Nur, U., 1979, Gonoid thelytoky in soft scale insects (Coccidae: Homoptera). Chromosoma 72: 89-104.

14. Drosopoulos, S., 1976, Triploid pseudogamous biotype of the leafhopper Muellerianella fairmairei. Nature 263: 499-500.

15. Drosopoulos, S., 1978, Laboratory synthesis of a pseudogamous triploid "species" of the genus Muellerianella (Homoptera, Delphacidae). Evolution 32: 916-920.

16. Suomalainen, E., 1978, Two new cases of parthenogenesis in moths. Nota Lepidopterologica 1: 65-68.

17. Seiler, J., 1923, Geschlechtschromosomenuntersuchungen an Psychiden. IV. Die Parthenogenese der Psychiden. Z. indukt. Abstammungs. Vererbungsl. 31: 1-99.

18. Seiler, J., 1943, Über den Ursprung der Parthenogenese und Polyploidie bei Schmetterlingen. Arch. Julius Klaus-Stift. 18: 691-699.

19. Seiler, J., 1964, Untersuchungen über die Entstehung der Parthenogenese bei Solenobia triquetrella F.R. (Lepidoptera, Psychidae). V. Chromosoma 15: 503-539.

20. Seiler, J., Schäffer, K., 1960, Untersuchungen über die Entstehung der Parthenogenese bei Solenobia triquetrella F.R. (Lepidoptera, Psychidae). II. Chromosoma 11: 29-102.

21. Seiler, J., Puchta, O., 1956, Die Fortpflanzungsbiologie der Solenobien (Lepid. Psychidae), Verhalten bei Artkreuzungen und F_1-Resultate. Roux' Arch. Entwicklungsmech. 149: 115-246.

22. Suomalainen, E., personal communication.

23. Scholl, H., 1956, Die Chromosomen parthenogenetischer Mücken. Naturwissenschaften 43: 91-92.

24. Scholl, H., 1960, Die Oogenese einiger parthenogenetischer Orthocladiinen (Diptera). Chromosoma 11: 380-401.

25. Basrur, V.R., Rothfels, K.H., 1959, Triploidy in natural populations of the black fly Cnephia mutata (Malloch.). Canad. J. Zool. 37: 571-589.

26. Troiano, G., 1978, Triploidy in the natural population of the Psychodine moth fly Psychoda parthenogenetica Tonnoir (Diptera: Psychodidae). Caryologia 31: 225-232.

27. Block, K., 1969, Chromosome variation in the Agromyzidae. II. Phytomyza crassiseta Zetterstedt - a parthenogenetic species. Hereditas 62: 357-381.

28. Stalker, H.D., 1956, A case of polyploidy in Diptera. Proc. Nat. Acad. Sci. USA 42: 194-199.

29. Sanderson, A.R., 1960, The cytology of a diploid bisexual
     spider beetle Ptinus clavipes Panzer and its triploid gyno-
     genetic form mobilis Moore. Proc. Roy. Soc. Edinb. (B) 67:
     333-350.
30. Suomalainen, E., 1965, Die Polyploidie bei dem partheno-
     genetischen Blattkäfer Adoxus obscurus L. (Coleoptera,
     Chrysomelidae). Zool. Jahrb. Syst. 92: 183-192.
31. Robertson, J.G., 1966, The chromosomes of bisexual and
     parthenogenetic species of Calligrapha (Coleoptera: Chry-
     somelidae) with notes on sex ratio, abundance and egg
     number. Canad. J. Genet. Cytol. 8: 695-732.
32. Suomalainen, E., 1969, Evolution in parthenogenetic Cur-
     culionidae, pp. 261-269, in Dobzhansky, T., Hecht, M.,
     Steere, W. (eds.), "Evolutionary Biology," Vol. 3. Appleton-
     Century-Crofts, New York.
33. Sanderson, A.R., 1973, The cytology of the parthenogenetic
     Australian weevil Listroderes costirostris Schönh. Trans.
     Roy. Soc. Edinb. 69: 71-89.
34. Petryszak, B., 1972, Chromosome numbers of Foucartia liturata
     Striel., Foucartia squamulata (Herbst) and Sciaphilus asperatus
     (Bonsd.) (Curculionidae, Coleoptera). Prac. Zool. Univ.
     Jag. 18: 27-60.
35. Takenouchi, Y., 1976, A study of polyploidy in races of
     Japanese weevils (Coleoptera: Curculionidae). Genetica 46:
     327-334.
36. Suomalainen, E., 1947, Parthenogenese und Polyploidie bei
     Rüsselkäfern (Curculionidae). Hereditas 33: 425-456.
37. Takenouchi, Y., 1970, Three further studies of the chromosomes
     of Japanese weevils (Coleoptera: Curculionidae). Canad. J.
     Genet. Cytol. 12: 273-277.
38. Takenouchi, Y., 1972, A chromosome study of a new polyploid
     parthenogenetic weevil, Myllocerus nipponicus Zumpt. (Cole-
     optera: Curculionidae), Kontyû 40: 121-123.
39. Takenouchi, Y., personal communication.
40. Takenouchi, Y., 1972, A chromosome study on two new Japanese
     parthenogenetic weevils (Coleoptera: Curculionidae). Jap.
     J. Genet. 47: 19-22.
41. Petryszak, P., 1975, Chromosome number of Trachyphloeus
     scabriculus (L.) and T. aristatus (Gyll.) (Coleoptera,
     Curculionidae), Acta Biol. Cracov. Ser. Zool. 18: 91-95.
42. Takenouchi, Y., 1976, A chromosome study on two new Japanese
     polyploid parthenogenetic weevils (Coleoptera: Curculionidae),
     pp. 341-348, in Pearson, P.L., Lewis, K.R. (eds.), "Chromo-
     some Today," Vol. 5. John Wiley & Sons, New York.
43. Takenouchi, Y., 1978, A chromosome study of the partheno-
     genetic rice water weevil, Lissorhoptrus oryzophilus Kuschel
     (Coleoptera: Curculionidae), in Japan. Experientia 34: 444-445.
44. Crozier, R.H., 1975, "Hymenoptera. Animal Cytogenetics,"
     Vol. 3, Insecta 7, Gebrüder Borntraeger, Berlin, Stuttgart.

45. Smith, S.G., 1941, A new form of spruce sawfly identified by means of its cytology and parthenogenesis. Sci. Agric. 21: 244-305.

46. Vandel, A., 1928, La parthénogenèse geographique. Contribution à l'étude biologique et cytologique de la parthénogenèse naturelle, Bull. Biol. France Belg. 62: 164-281.

47. Seiler, J., 1961, Untersuchungen über die Entstehung der Parthenogenese bei Solenobia triquetrella F.R. (Lepidoptera, Psychidae), III. Z. Vererbungsl. 92: 261-316.

48. Mikulska, I., 1960, New data on the cytology of the parthenogenetic weevils of the genus Otiorrhynchus Germ. (Curculionidae, Coleoptera) from Poland. Cytologia 25: 322-333.

49. Suomalainen, E., 1948, Parthenogenesis and polyploidy in the weevils, Curculionidae. Ann. Entomol. Fenn. 14, Suppl.: 206-212.

50. Suomalainen, E., 1953, Die Polyploidie bei den parthenogenetischen Rüsselkäfern. Verh. Deutsch. Zool. Ges. 1952; Zool. Anz., Suppl. 17: 280-289.

51. Suomalainen, E., 1954, Zur Zytologie der parthenogenetischen Curculioniden der Schweiz. Chromosoma 6: 627-655.

52. Suomalainen, E., 1955, A further instance of geographical parthenogenesis and polyploidy in the weevils, Curculionidae. Arch. Soc. "Vanamo" 9, suppl.: 350-354.

53. Takenouchi, Y., 1972, Chromosome numbers of Japanese weevils of Curculionoidea (Coleoptera). Kontyû 40: 123-132.

54. Takenouchi, Y., 1978, A further chromosome study on races of two reportedly Japanese polyploid parthenogenetic weevils (Coleoptera: Curculionidae). J. Hokkaido Univ. Educ. II B 29: 1-4.

55. Lindroth, C.H., 1954, Experimentelle Beobachtungen an parthenogenetischem und bisexuellem Otiorrhynchus dubius Stroem. Coleoptera: Curculionidae). Entomol. Tidskrift 75: 111-116.

56. Suomalainen, E., 1961, On morphological differences and evolution of different polyploid parthenogenetic weevil populations. Hereditas 47: 309-341.

57. Seiler, J., 1947, Die Zytologie eines parthenogenetischen Rüsselkäfers, Otiorrhynchus sulcatus F. Chromosoma 3: 88-109.

58. Seiler, J., 1927, Ergebnisse aus der Kreuzung parthenogenetischer und zweigeschlechtlicher Schmetterlinge. Biol. Zentralbl. 47: 426-446.

59. Suomalainen, E., 1940, Beiträge zur Zytologie der parthenogenetischen Insekten. I. Coleoptera. Ann. Acad. Sci. Fenn. A 54: 1-144.

60. Chubareva, L.A., Tzapygina, R.I., 1965, On the triploids in the natural populations of Odagmia ornata ornata (Simuliidae, Diptera). Genetika 3: 15-18.

61. Chubareva, L.A., Grinchuk, T.M., Kachvoryan, E.A., 1974, On the occurrence of triploid individuals in the natural populations of blackflies. Tsitologia 16: 253-255.

62. Astaurov, B.L., 1972, Experimental model of the origin of
     bisexual polyploid species of animals. Biol. Zbl. 91:
     137-150.
63. Maynard Smith, J., 1978, "The Evolution of Sex." Cambridge
     University Press, Cambridge.
64. Suomalainen, E., Saura, A., 1973, Genetic polymorphism and
     evolution in parthenogenetic animals. I. Polyploid Curcu-
     lionidae. Genetics 74: 489-508.
65. Webb, G.C., White, M.J.D., Contreras, N., Cheney, J., 1978,
     Cytogenetics of the parthenogenetic grasshopper Warramaba
     (formerly Moraba) virgo and its bisexual relatives. IV.
     Chromosome banding studies. Chromosoma 67: 309-339.
66. White, M.J.D., 1970, Heterozygosity and genetic polymorphism
     in parthenogenetic animals, pp. 237-262, in Hecht, M.K.,
     Steere, W.C. (eds.), "Essays in Evolution and Genetics in
     Honor of Theodosius Dobzhansky," (suppl.) "Evolutionary
     Biology," Appleton-Century-Crofts, New York.
67. Porter, D.L., 1971, Oogenesis and chromosomal heterozygosity
     in the telytokous midge, Lundstroemia parthenogenetica
     (Diptera, Chironomidae). Chromosoma 32: 333-342.
68. Lakovaara, S., Saura, A., 1972, Location of enzyme loci in
     chromosomes of Drosophila willistoni. Experientia 28:
     355-356.
69. Smith, S.G., 1971, Parthenogenesis and polyploidy in beetles.
     Amer. Zool. 11: 341-349.
70. Saura, A., Lokki, J., Lankinen, P., Suomalainen, E., 1976,
     Genetic polymorphism and evolution in parthenogenetic animals.
     III. Tetraploid Otiorrhynchus scaber (Coleoptera: Cur-
     culionidae). Hereditas 82: 79-100.
71. Lokki, J., Saura, A., Lankinen, P., Suomalainen, E., 1976,
     Genetic polymorphism and evolution in parthenogenetic animals.
     VI. Diploid and triploid Polydrosus mollis (Coleoptera:
     Curculionidae). Hereditas 82: 209-216.
72. Saura, A., Lokki, J., Lankinen, P., Suomalainen, E., 1976,
     Genetic polymorphism and evolution in parthenogenetic animals.
     IV. Triploid Otiorrhynchus salicis (Coleoptera: Curculioni-
     dae). Entomol. Scand. 7: 1-6.
73. Ahti, T., Hämet-Ahti, L., Jalas, J., 1968, Vegetation zones
     and their sections in northwestern Europe. Ann. Bot. Fenn.
     5: 169-211.
74. Takenouchi, Y., 1968, A chromosome study on bisexual and
     parthenogenetic races of Scepticus insularis Roelofs (Cur-
     culionidae: Coleoptera). Canad. J. Genet. Cytol. 10: 945-950.
75. Saura, A., Lakovaara, S., Lokki, J., Lankinen, P., 1973,
     Genic variation in central and marginal populations of
     Drosophila subobscura. Hereditas 75: 33-46.
76. Lokki, J., Saura, A., Lankinen, P., Suomalainen, E., 1976,
     Genetic polymorphism and evolution in parthenogenetic animals.
     V. Triploid Adoxus obscurus (Coleoptera: Chrysomelidae).
     Genet. Res. 28: 27-36.

77. Saura, A., Lokki, J., Suomalainen, E., 1977, Selection and
     genetic differentation in parthenogenetic populations.
     Lecture Notes in Biomathematics 19: 381-402.
78. Lokki, J., Suomalainen, E., Saura, A., Lankinen, P., 1975,
     Genetic polymorphism and evolution in parthenogenetic animals.
     II. Diploid and polyploid Solenobia triquetrella (Lepi-
     doptera: Psychidae). Genetics 79: 513-525.
79. Lokki, J., 1976, Genetic polymorphism and evolution in
     parthenogenetic animals. VIII. Heterozygosity in relation
     to polyploidy. Hereditas 83: 65-72.
80. Darlington, C.D., 1937, "Recent Advances in Cytology," ed.
     2, J. and A. Churchill, London.
81. White, M.J.D., 1945, "Animal Cytology and Evolution,"
     Cambridge University Press, Cambridge.
82. Asher, J.H.,Jr., 1970, Parthenogenesis and genetic variabi-
     lity. II. One-locus models for various diploid populations.
     Genetics 66: 369-391.
83. Asher, J.H., Nace, G.W., 1971, The genetic structure and
     evolutionary fate of parthenogenetic Amphibian populations
     as determined by Markovian analysis. Amer. Zool. 11: 381-398.
84. Templeton, A.R., Rothman, E.D., 1973, The population genetics
     of parthenogenetic strains of Drosophila mercatorum. I.
     One locus model and statistics. Theor. Appl. Genet. 43:
     204-212.
85. Lokki, J., 1976, Genetic polymorphism and evolution in
     parthenogenetic animals. VII. The amount of heterozygosity
     in diploid populations. Hereditas 83: 57-64.

ROLE OF POLYPLOIDY IN THE EVOLUTION OF FISHES

R. Jack Schultz[1]

Ecology Section, Biological Sciences Group
University of Connecticut
Storrs, CT 06268

Polyploidy is not generally believed to have played a major role in the evolution of animals. This view has been fostered principally by G. L. Stebbins and M. J. D. White, both of whom as early as the 1940's advocated that polyploidy at best has played a secondary role in evolution; neither of them has substantially altered this view in recent years (1,2). Some of the arguments against the importance of polyploidy are: (a) that the large amount of gene duplication in polyploids dilutes the effects of new mutations so significant adaptive changes are unlikely, (b) that polyploidy in animals is restricted mainly to asexual forms which are evolutionary dead ends, and (c) the number of polyploid animals relative to diploids is small.

The study of polyploidy is gradually beginning to feel the impact of new techniques which have come into use during the last 20 years. Through the use of electrophoresis, tissue graft analysis, measurement of cellular DNA levels, experimental hybridization, and advanced cytological techniques, as well as the simple accumulation of more information, new lines of reasoning have emerged. As one example, we have the view championed especially by Ohno (3, 4) that polyploidy, far from playing a secondary role in evolution, has provided the additional, uncommitted gene loci necessary for major steps in the evolution of animals.

The development of terrestrial tetrapods was one of the most dramatic events in the evolution of animals. Whereas most evolutionary changes involve simplification, including a loss of parts

[1]I thank Mrs. Ellie DeCarli for typing the manuscript. The
Poeciliopsis research is supported by the N.S.F.

and streamlining, the adaptions called for here required additions to existing form and function and presumably the additional
genetic coding to produce it. The marked increase in DNA levels
in amphibians vs. fishes, presumably provides that coding. This
increase is believed to have arisen by polyploidy. Other major
steps in evolution also appear to be accompanied by increases in
DNA which also may have been supplied by polyploidy. If Ohno's
arguments are correct, then polyploidy has played far more than a
secondary role in evolution.

        Although many of the stages of polyploidy in the evolution
of animals occurred long ago and may be irretrievable today, some
of the ingredients for a reconstruction still exist among the
fishes. Hybridization, for example, which often triggers polyploidy, runs unusually high; 3,130 different species combinations
are recorded (5); this includes reciprocal matings but not subspecies crosses. Fishes also have a wide range of DNA values,
with the lowest running only 20% that of mammals and the highest
35 times that amount (6,7).

        Assessment of the role of polyploidy in animal evolution may
come from studying groups in which the process is currently
active and within which the actual synthesis of polyploids in the
laboratory is possible. One may now, for example, investigate:
(a) how polyploidization occurs, (b) the adaptive relationships
of polyploids to parental progenitors, (c) the capacity of polyploids to evolve in spite of their duplicate loci, (d) the role
of triploid unisexual polyploids as a stepping stone to sexually
reproducing tetraploids, and (e) the relationship of DNA values
to adaptations--as generalists or as specialists.

        Before discussing the active processes of polyploidy, a
survey of where polyploidy has been found among fishes may help
to set the stage, especially so since a majority of biologists
today are still unaware that polyploid vertebrates do exist.
Even in recent evolution books (8), one reads: "The main reason
why polyploid species are rare in animals is that most animals
are not hermaphrodites capable of self-fertilization, and self-
fertilization, common in plants, is necessary for successful
species-formation by polyploidy." Only one species of fish known,
Rivulus marmoratus, is a selffertilizing hermaphrodite (9); yet,
among the many species of polyploid fishes on record, none of
them is in the same family as R. marmoratus.

                    OCCURRENCE OF POLYPLOIDY IN FISHES

Salmonids

        The first suspicion that naturally occurring polyploid
vertebrates exist came from Svärdson who in 1945 (10) proposed
that salmonids have a basic haploid number of 10 and that the

smelt (Osmerus eperlanus), the rainbow trout (Salmo gairdnerii),
and the Atlantic salmon (Salmo salar) are all hexaploids, whereas
the brown trout (Salmo trutta) is octoploid and the European
grayling (Thymallus thymallus) decaploid. Subsequently it has
been established that these levels of polyploidy, which were
based on chromosome numbers, are not accompanied by stepwise
increases in nuclear DNA content (11). The brown trout, with a
diploid chromosome number of 80, has the same DNA level as the
Atlantic salmon, which has only 60 chromosomes. Fusions or
fragmentation apparently account for differences in the chromosome numbers among salmonids.

Although Svärdson was wrong about differences in the ploid
levels among salmonids, he was not wrong about the involvement of
polyploidy in this family. All members,[2] including the trout,
whitefish, and grayling are tetraploids, whereas closely related
families such as the herrings (Clupeidae), anchovies (Engraulidae),
and smelt (Osmeridae) are not (4). This determination is based
on four types of evidence: chromosome arm number, presence of
quadrivalents, nuclear DNA content, and duplicated gene loci.

A substantial majority of the fishes of the world have a
chromosome number of 46 to 52 acrocentrics with a strong modal
number of 48 (4). This number is encountered, for example, among
such diverse groups as the primitive jawless hagfish, Eptatretus
stoutii (12), the livebearing poeciliids (14, 15), the flatfishes (6), and the sunfishes of the family Centrarchidae (16).
Although the salmonids have chromosome numbers ranging from 56 to
82 the chromosome arm numbers are less variable, 100 to 104
(Table 1), approximately twice that of most other fishes.

The argument that salmonids are tetraploids is further
supported by the consistent occurrence of quadrivalents (17) in
the rainbow trout. This has been taken as evidence that the
process of diploidization has not been completed yet and that
some of the original four homologues still retain enough affinity
for each other to form quadrivalents rather than separate bivalents. In keeping with the formation of some quadrivalents,
certain electrophoretically distinguishable alleles still show
the tetrasomic mode of inheritance; thus, at a single locus, four
different alleles can all be found. For example, in the rainbow
trout the supernatant form of NADP-dependent isocitrate dehydrogenase exhibits four alleles: A, A', A", and A'" at a single
locus (24). A similar relationship exists for NADP-dependent
sorbitol dehydrogenase in the rainbow and whitefish, but in the
brown trout, the enzyme possesses two separate gene loci, each
showing disomic inheritance (25) and indicating that diploidization
has occurred.

---

[2]Ohno (4) lists the trout, whitefish, and grayling as being
in the separate families, Salmonidae, Coregonidae, and Thymallidae;
Greenwood et al. (13) lump them in the single family Salmonidae.

Table 1.   Chromosome numbers and DNA values of salmonids and
representatives from closely related families.   Numbers in
parentheses indicate reference.

Family/Species	Haploid DNA content 10-9 mg.	Diploid Chromosome Number	Number of Chromosome Arms
Clupeidae (Herrings)			
Alosa pseudoharengus (alewife)	1.4 (18)	48 (17)	
Alosa sapidissima (American shad)	1.3 (18)		
Alosa chrysochloris (Skipjack herring)	1.1 (18)		
Clupea harengus pallosi (Pacific herring)	0.77 (18)	52 (17)	
Salmonidae (salmon, trout, whitefish, grayling)			
Oncorhynchus kisutch (coho salmon)	3.0 (18)	60 (20)	112 (20)
Oncorhynchus keta (chum salmon)	---	74 (20)	102 (20)
Oncorhynchus tshawytcha (chinook salmon)	3.3 (18)	68 (20)	104 (20)
Oncorhynchus nerka (sockeye salmon)	---	56 (20)	102 (20)
Oncorhynchus gorbusaka (pink salmon)	---	52 (20)	104 (20)
Salmo salar (Atlantic salmon)	---	60 (10)	72 (10)
Salmo gairdneri (rainbow trout)	2.8 (23)	60 (9)	104 (9)
Salmo trutta (brown trout)	---	80 (10)	98 (10)
Salvelinus fontinalis (brook trout)	3.5 (4)		
Coregonus clupeaformis (lake whitefish)		80 (19)	108 (19)
Coregonus artedii (cisco or lake herring)		86 (19)	106 (19)
Coregonus reighadi (shortnose cisco)		80 (19)	104 (19)

Table 1 (continued)

Coregonus zenithicus (shortjaw cisco)		80 (19)	98 (19)
Coregonus hoyi		80 (19)	98 (19)
Coregonus lavaretus (blaufelche whitefish)	3.2 (4)	80 (10)	96 (10)
Coregonus macerophthalmus (gangfish whitefish)	3.2 (4)	--	--
Coregonus peled		80 (22)	92 (22)
Coregonus albula		80 (10)	96 (10)
Prosopium coulteri		82 (19)	100 (19)
Prosopium cylindraceum (round whitefish)		78 (19)	100 (19)
Thymallus thymallus (grayling)	1.9 (4)	102 (10)	130 (10)
Esocidae			
Esox lucieus (northern pike)	0.97 (4)	50 (51)	50 (51)

An extensive literature has developed in this area, most of it favorable to the polyploid thesis and bringing Ohno (4) to the following conclusion:

By and large, with regard to any given enzyme or protein trout salmon, whitefish and grayling appear to be endowed with twice the gene loci present in their diploid counterparts. Such findings not only supply overwhelming evidence in favor of their tetraploid origin but also show that the process of diploidization has been completed in most cases.

The final evidence of the polyploid nature of salmonids is reflected in the nuclear DNA contents. Surveys of over 300 fishes (4, 18) reveal that the vast majority of them have haploid nuclear DNA contents of less than 1.5×10^{-9} mg. The herrings, family Clupeidae, which are related to the salmonids, have approximately twice as much DNA, ranging from 1.9×10^{-9} mg in the grayling to 3.5×10^{-9} mg in the brook trout (Table 1). Some variation in DNA levels occurs within many groups of fishes as a result of two chromosomal processes other than polyploidy. Increases in DNA can be brought about by random duplications, wherein genes or segments of chromosomes or chromatids are

duplicated through unequal crossing-over, or by redundant duplication of DNA (26). In bony fishes the range of DNA is from
0.4×10^{-9} mg to 4.4×10^{-9} mg. In terms of mammals, which
have fairly uniform genome sizes of roughly 3.5×10^{-9} mg, the
range in bony fishes is 11 to 100%.

Catostomids

The only other example of polyploidy which, like the salmonids, apparently involves an entire family, is provided by
the freshwater suckers (Catostomidae). Chromosome counts on
14 species, including 8 genera, were all within the range of
2n=96-100 (27). The family is believed to have diverged from
the family Cyprinidae (minnows) which, with only a few exceptions,
to be considered later, have a uniform chromosome number of
2n=50. Evaluation of the cyprinids is based on a survey of 60
out of the 230 known North American species and represents 74%
of the genera (29). DNA values of the sucker, Catostomus
commersoni were twice those of the cyprinid Clinostomus elongatus
(27). On the basis of the apparent doubling of the chromosome
number and DNA content of catostomid fishes and the lack of intermediate numbers, Uyeno and Smith (27) suggested that "the catostomid
karyotype evolved by tetraploidy from a cyprinid-like ancestor".
Divergence of these two families took place between the Eocene
and Paleocene (28), over 50 million years ago. All but two species
of suckers occur in North America; the most primitive genus
Myxocyprinus, restricted to China, has not been karyotyped, so
it is not certain whether the family is of polyploid origin or
whether polyploidy arose subsequent to the arrival of catostomids
in North America; the former hypothesis seems most attractive.

Cyprinids

In reporting the evidence that suckers (Catostomidae) are
tetraploids, their chromosome numbers were cited as being twice
that of most members of the closely related minnow family (Cyprinidae). Of the 60 North American cyprinids surveyed by Uyeno
(29) and 10 European and Asian cyprinids listed by Ohno et al.
(30), only four do not have a 2n chromosome number of 50. One of
these, the tench (Tinca tinca), has 48 and is diploid like all of
the others; but, one species of barb (Barbus barbis), the carp
(Cyprinus carpio), and the goldfish (Carassius auratus), have
100, 104, and 104 and apparently are all tetraploid. The DNA
values of minnows with 48 to 50 chromosomes are 20 to 38% of that
of mammals, whereas those with 100 to 104 chromosomes have 49 to
53% of that of mammals (30-32).

Biochemical evidence of gene duplication also supports the
view that some of the minnows are tetraploid. Several proteins
and enzymes in the barb, carp, and goldfish have more gene loci
than do diploid cyprinids. For example, diploid members of the

family have three loci for lactate dehydrogenase but the tetraploids have five or six loci (33). Similar duplications have
been found in carp and goldfish involving NADP-dependent isocitrate dehydrogenase (34) and NADP-dependent 6-phosphogluconate
dehydrogenase (35).

A remarkable aspect of the goldfish story is that the tetraploid level does not seem to be the end of its experimentation
with polyploidy. Having become diploidized, over an apparently
long period of existence, it has now added to its 104 chromosome
complement (30) a unisexual triploid form with 156 chromosomes
and a unisexual tetraploid with 206 chromosomes (36). Both unisexuals apparently reproduce by gynogenesis. In nature embryonic
development of eggs is stimulated by sperm supplied by the
bisexual goldfish, Carassius auratus auratus, but fusion of
maternal and paternal nuclei does not occur. Although the sperma-
tazoan enters the egg and later takes up a position next to the
female pronucleus, amphimixis does not occur. The egg undergoes the
first karyokinesis while the sperm nucleus remains as a condensed
mass in contact with the spindle. When the two blastomeres are
formed, the sperm nucleus is left in the cytoplasm of one of them
(37).

Sperm from a variety of species, as remotely related as the
loach, Misgurnus anguillicaudatus (family Cobitidae), have been
tested in hybrid crosses with the triploids with no evidence of
paternal characters being revealed in the offspring (38, 39). The
tetraploid form, however, has been tested less thoroughly; one
female has been crossed with the 2x kinbuna, a different subspecies of C. auratus from a different district. The chromosome
number and morphology of six offspring was the same as the mothers;
thus, reproduction was interpreted as being gynogenetic.

The tetraploid ginbuna does not seem to be widespread nor in
high frequency where it does occur. Thus far it has been reported
only from the Kanto district where, from a collection of 30 unisexuals, 28 were 3x and 2 were 4x (38, 39). Wider sampling from
12 localities in Japan and one in Korea included 45 triploids to
17 bisexual diploids but no tetraploids (40). At one locality,
27 specimens were taken, all of them triploids but at another
only 4 out of 10 were triploids.

Goldfish, in addition to the selected varieties used for
ornamental purposes, are cultured as a food fish. Beginning in
1946 massive introductions were made in the reservoirs of the
U.S.S.R. (41). Some of these goldfish (called Carassius auratus
gibelio) came directly from the Amur River basin near the Man-
churian border. Populations of "silver goldfish", which have
spread to Europe (42) as well as being widely dispersed in the
Soviet Union, contain males, bisexual females, and unisexual females. Cytological studies (43) on a small number of silver
goldfish from the Volma Fishery near Minsk indicate that the
bisexual forms have 94 chromosomes and the unisexuals 141 and
are, therefore, triploid. The unisexual forms in Germany, however,

unlike the Russian or Japanese forms, are diploid (42). The four
forms of goldfish, that is, the diploid bisexual and the diploid,
triploid, and tetraploid unisexuals cannot be accurately separated
morphologically, a factor which has limited assessment of how
widespread each form is and in which habitat each type is most
successful. It is possible that the diploid unisexual which, so
far, has been found in Europe, also occurs in Russia and Japan,
and that the seemingly rare tetraploid unisexual occurs outside
the Kanto district of Japan. One might even ask if all of the
bisexuals are diploid.

     The difficulty of identifying unisexual, bisexual, and poly-
ploid biotypes is especially pronounced among the goldfishes. No
single technique, simple or complex, will positively distinguish
all possible forms. From several sites in Japan, electrophoresis
and erythrocyte size were tested as a means of separating diploids
and triploids (40). At most localities both methods were reasonably accurate; but at one, from which 27 specimens were all
identified by karyotype analysis as being triploids, erythroctye
size indicated that only 10 were diploid, and electrophoresis
picked only 14 as diploid. Had the samples contained 2x and 4x
unisexuals it is difficult to say how the electrophoretic data
alone might have been interpreted. Accurate assessment of populations with the potential complexity of goldfishes, given
the present state of knowledge, seems to require at least two
methods of evaluation: hybridization progeny analysis, and karyotype analysis. To establish gynogenesis it is necessary to
demonstrate that, when goldfish eggs are fertilized by sperm of
another species or at least from a male with a radically different
genotype than the female, paternal characters are not present in
the offspring. The chromosome count is necessary to determine
the ploid level since 2x, 3x, and 4x goldfish apparently all produce offspring identical to their mothers. Small wonder that
frequencies of the various biotypes of gynogenetic goldfishes in
natural populations is not known.

     The mitotic mechanism that perpetuates the triploids both
in Russia (43) and Japan (39) is characterized by a first maturation division with a tripolar spindle; the homologous chromosomes
do not pair and ultimately the division aborts. Thus it is
essentially endomitotic. Metaphase of the equational division
contains the triploid number of chromosomes estimated at 143 to
152 (43). In the gynogenetic diploid the somatic diploid chromosome number is maintained by chromosome replication without
cytokinesis during the first mitotic cleavage (42).

Cobitids

     The spinous loach, Cobitis biwae, which lives on three of the
major islands of Japan is made up of two races of different
sizes. The smaller one which averages about 5.3 cm has 48 chromosomes and is diploid; the larger one, 8.62 cm, has 96 chromosomes

and is tetraploid (44). The erythrocyte and nuclear surface
areas of the tetraploid race, 112.8 and 21.0 micron^2, are about
twice those of the diploid race, 69.7 and 12.1 micron^2 (45).
Larger cell sizes have been reported in other polyploid fishes,
too, when comparison between closely related diploids was possible,
e.g., Carassius (43, 45), Poeciliopsis (46), Gasterosteus (47),
Pleuronectes (48), and Tilapia (49). In plants the increase in
cell size associated with polyploidy produces gigantism but in
polyploid animals, except for a few invertebrates, a compensating
decrease in cell number holds body sizes to normal limits (5).
The tetraploid spinous loach with its large erythrocytes and large
body size may be a rare example of gigantism in vertebrates.

Ancient fishes

Three fishes which might be ranked as "living fossils" show
evidence of being tetraploids. Two of these, the paddle fish
(Polyodontidae) and the sturgeon (Acipenseridae), are leftovers
of the once flourishing chondrosteians, which were the dominant
fishes of the Permian. The third fish, a gar, is a member of the
holosteans which replaced the chondrosteians and then gave way
themselves to the modern bony fishes.
One species of paddlefish or spoon bill, as they are also
called, remains in North America and one in China. Chromosome
counts on the North American species, Polyodon spathula, revealed
a mode of 2n=120. These consisted of 48 macrosomes and 72 microchromosomes which could be "easily arranged into 30 groups of
four homologs each" suggesting tetraploidy (52). These values
are within the same range of those found in the shovelnose sturgeon,
Scaphirhynchus platorhynchus, which has 112 chromosomes with 50
metacentrics, 14 acrocentrics, and 48 microchromosomes (53). The
first 64 chromosomes of the sturgeon can also be arranged into
groups of four homologues, again suggesting tetraploidy. The
third possible ancient polyploid is the spotted gar, Lepisosteus
productus, the only one of several gars for which a katyotype is
available. Here 68 chromosomes are divided into 28 metacentrics,
14 acrocentrics, and 26 microsomes (53). The argument that the
spotted gar is polyploid is less convincing than for the sturgeon
and paddle fish. Another surviving holostean, the bowfin Amia
calva, has only 46 chromosomes, 20 metacentrics, and 26 acrocentrics but no microchromosomes (53). Although DNA values are not
available on the paddle fish, Ohno (4) compared the DNA levels of
the other three to mammals; (1) the bowfin was 35%; (2) the
spotted gar, 40%; and (3) the shovelnose sturgeon, 50%. He also
listed a value of 70% for the starred sturgeon, Acipenser stellatus.
The presence of microchromosomes and high DNA values in these
ancient fishes are characteristics they have in common with
lizards, snakes, and birds. Ohno et al. (53) suggested that the
ancient crossopterygian fish which gave rise to terrestrial
vertebrates may have done so through several lineages, one of

which may have had a DNA level and chromosome complement similar
to the sturgeon and gar.

Poeciliidae

Within the family Poeciliidae, which is made up of livebearing
fishes, polyploidy has arisen in two genera, one of these
Poeciliopsis in northwestern Mexico, the other Poecilia in northeastern Mexico. In both genera hybridization has lead to formation
of diploid unisexual or all-female biotypes which gave rise to
triploid unisexual forms.

In Poeciliopsis six unisexual biotypes occur, three are
allodiploids and three are allotriploids. Each of them lives
with at least one gonochoristic or bisexual species of Poeciliopsis
and is dependent on it for sperm. By morphological analysis,
hybridization experiments (54-56), and electrophoretic analysis
(57,58), it was established that five of the seven bisexual
species of Poeciliopsis living in this region were involved in
the hybrid origin of the unisexual complex. One of the bisexual
species, P. monacha, has contributed genes to all six unisexuals.

P. monacha is an "island species" in the sense of consisting
of five disjunct populations scattered among three different
river systems, the Rios Mayo (59), Fuerte, and Sinaloa (60).
Each populations occupies its own rocky, headwater arroyo, and is
essentially isolated from the others by distance and inhospitable
habitat. At four localities, the P. monacha territory overlaps
with Poeciliopsis lucida, a widespread downstream species.
Although P. monacha and P. lucida are quite different in terms of
their dentition (56), reproductive process (61), habitat selection,
etc., they have hybridized and produced a unisexual species, P.
monacha-lucida, which has become well established and widespread,
living everywhere that P. lucida occurs (62).

In the laboratory, stocks of P. monacha-lucida, collected in
1965, have been maintained by matings with males of P. lucida for
over 25 generations and have not produced a single male. The
perpetual hybrid nature and presences of both parental genomes of
P. monacha-lucida through successive generations is accomplished
by means of an unusual reproductive mechanism known as "hybridogenesis" (56). During meiosis or just prior to meiosis, a cell
division occurs during which only one set of chromosomes (P.
monacha) aligns on the metaphase plate. These are collected by a
unipolar spindle and included in the reconstituted nucleus while
the other set of chromosomes (P. lucida) remains scattered in the
cytoplasm (63). A single equational division follows, resulting
in the production of haploid eggs which contain only maternal
chromosomes. The paternal set is either absorbed by the cytoplasm
or expelled as a polar body-like extrusion.

This peculiar mechanism is clearly reflected in the inheritance pattern of P. monacha-lucida. Although the offspring from
the unisexuals inherit characteristics of both parents, none of

the paternal genes are transmitted through the egg to the offspring (55, 57, 64, 65); all paternal traits are derived from the
father and none from the grandfather. Thus, if the P. monacha
and P. lucida genomes of a unisexual female are homozygous for
two single gene traits such as clear dorsal fin, s' and Lactate
Dehydrogenase E, and the male is homozygous for the alternative
alleles spot dorsal fin, s', and LDH, E', then a unisexual female
of the genotype ssEE X an s's'E'E' male produces all heterozygous
ss'EE' offspring. Repeated backcrosses to the same male produce
the same phenotype; yet, mating one of the heterozygous unisexuals
to a homozygous ssEE, male will result in all ssEE female off-
spring--no traits from the previous male are transmitted to the
next generation. Mating tests, wherein a substantial portion of
the paternal genome is marked by polygenes associated with morphological traits (55) or the histocompatability mechanism (65),
further demonstrate that if any paternal genes leak through the
hybridogenic system it is indeed a rare event. Furthermore, when
P. monacha-lucida females are mated to males of P. monacha, in a
single generation all P. lucida genes are lost and P. monacha
offspring of both sexes are produced (66).

     The fifth disjunct population of P. monacha is in the Rio
Mayo which is in the next river system north of the range of P.
lucida and P. monacha-lucida (59). Here P. monacha has hybridized
with Poeciliopsis occidentalis, a species closely related to P.
lucida. The P. monacha genome in combination with occidentalis
triggers hybridogenesis, as it did with P. lucida, and in so
doing, originates a second all-female, hybrid species, P. monacha-
occidentalis (54,65,67,69). With P. occidentalis as its host
species, this sexual parasite has spread northward carrying the
P. monacha genome 550 kilometers outside its matural range.

     Both of these hybridogenic species have been synthesized in
the laboratory by crossing P. monacha with P. lucida (70) on the
one hand, and P. occidentalis (71) on the other. The first cross
goes with some difficulty but the second rather easily. Two
synthesized lines of P. monacha-lucida have been maintained in
the laboratory since they were started in 1968 and 1971. They
are currently in their 11th and 10th generation of consistently
producing all-female offspring.

     A third hybridogenic unisexual of Poeciliopsis has not been
studied as carefully as the previous two but the best interpretation available, which is based on morphological analysis,
indicates that it is a P. monacha-latidens hybrid (62,69). Among
the difficulties surrounding this hybrid is the fact that attempts
to synthesize it in the laboratory have failed. Although the cross
goes well enough, so far, all of the offspring have been sterile
males (66). In nature P. monacha-latindens hybrids are mostly
females; only 6 out of thousands collected were males. From one
of the three rivers where it lives, the Rio Fuerte, all P. monacha-
lucida hybrids collected over a period of some 20 years of
sampling, have been females. Several lines have been maintained

in the laboratory by matings to P. latidens, and, none of these, including one line reared since 1965 which is in its 18th generation, has ever produced a male. From the Rio Mocorito, on the other hand, males are sometimes produced in the laboratory by P. monacha-latidens. A third bisexual species, Poeciliopsis viriosa, which is closely related to monacha and lives at a few specialized localities in the Rio Mocorito and Rio Sinaloa, may be involved. Some lines of P. monacha-latidens and P. monacha-lucida may have a few genes of P. viriosa incorporated in their P. monacha genomes; these may influence all-femaleness when P. latidens is the father. It is also likely that selection is fairly strong against P. monacha-latidens females that produce males; so, those clones or more accurately hemiclones that survive, are the ones that produce female offspring in the highest frequency and with the greatest consistency regardless of the male with which they mate.

The three additional unisexual biotypes of Poeciliopsis are triploids. The diploid chromosome number of P. lucida (64), P. monacha (56), P. occidentalis (64), P. latidens (72), P. viriosa (73) and all three hybridogens (64,72) is 48, the triploids have $3x=72$ (56,72,73). DNA cell content, as one would expect, is approximately half again as much as in the diploids (74). One of the triploids, determined by morphological analysis to consist of two genomes of monacha and one of lucida, has been named Poeciliopsis 2 monacha-lucida to reflect its hybrid origin and composition; the second, made up of one genome of P. monacha and 2 of P. lucida, is called P. monacha-2 lucida (56), the third triploid is less clearly defined but reflects traits from three species, P. monacha, P. viriosa, and P. lucida, but not necessarily in equal quantities as in the other two triploids (62).

All three triploids reproduce by gynogenesis (56,62,72). Clones of P. monacha-2 lucida have been maintained in the laboratory since 1961 and 1963, P. 2 monacha-lucida since 1968 and P. monacha-viriosa-lucida since 1963. All have been mated to males of four or five different species but the offspring are consistently the same phenotype as the mother. Tissue grafts, i.e., pieces of heart, liver, spleen, or scales, removed from daughters and implanted in the musculature of the mother or among daughters are as successful as homograft transplants.

The meiotic mechanism, whereby triploid mothers produce triploid eggs and triploid offspring, involves a premeiotic division during which the chromosome number is raised to the hexaploid level (75). Two normal meiotic divisions, including formation of bivalents, restores the number of chromosomes in the eggs to the 3n number. Although sister replicates disassociate from each other before meiosis, synapsis apparently involves pairing of sister homologues, no tri-, tetra-, or hexavalent figures occur.

The genus Poecilia in southeastern Texas and northeastern Mexico has enacted a similar scenario to that of Poeciliopsis in northwestern Mexico. Two bisexual progenitor species, Poecilia mexicana and P. latipinna, have given rise to a diploid biotype,

Poecilia formosa (76,77) and two triploid biotypes which have not been named yet by their discoverers (78-80) but might appropriately be called P. mexicana-2 latipinna and P. 2 mexicana latipinna. The major differences between Poeciliopsis and Poecilia unisexual complexes is that in Poeciliopsis diploid hybridogenic biotypes occur as well as triploid gynogens, whereas in Poecilia the diploid and two triploids are all gynogenic.

In southeastern Texas and in the coastal tributaries of Mexico, P. latipinna provides sperm for the unisexuals; in the inland tributaries, P. mexicana is the host species. The diploid P. formosa and the triploid P. 2 mexicana-latipinna are both highly successful but their abundance relative to each other and to the host species varies from one tributary to the next as well as annually and seasonally. In general, P. mexicana is most successful in the headwaters, the diploid, P. formosa, becomes the dominant form below this, while in the lower reaches, P. 2 mexicana-latipinna is most common (79). Discovery of the P. mexicana-2 latipinna triploid from several localities near Brownsville, Texas is recent (80); its abundance and range of distribution have not been worked out yet. Positive identification of the various forms of Poecilia is difficult. Although P. mexicana-2 latipinna looks more like P. latipinna than P. 2 mexicana-latipinna, clean morphological separation of all of the biotypes is uncertain and has to be supplemented by measurements of cell DNA content or chromosome counts and examination of the serum albumin phenotypes.

THE ORIGIN OF POLYPLOIDY

The tetraploid condition of salmonids, suckers, chondrosteans, and probably the initial polyploid level of the carp and goldfish, are of an antiquity that limits investigation of their origins. All of them are likely to have undergone considerable evolution since they split from their diploid ancestors, and the ancestors themselves are likely to have evolved or become extinct. In the absence of these prototypes it is not possible to establish what advantages or alternate opportunities polyploidy provides. Among the poeciliids and goldfishes, however, polyploidy appears to be an active process. Perhaps by looking here insight may be gained as to how polyploidy begins and how it gains a foothold in the face of established diploid forms.

In looking for the origin of polyploidy among vertebrates one cannot help but be impressed by the strong relationship shared by hybridization, unisexuality, and polyploidy (56). The laboratory synthesis of unisexual "species" in Poeciliopsis by crossing P. monacha with either P. lucida or P. occidentalis leaves no doubt that hybridization provides at least one route to unisexuality. Precisely what causes the all-femaleness is not certain, but crosses among various bisexual species of Poeciliopsis often result in distorted sex ratios, suggesting that sex-determining mechanisms differ in "strength" from one species to the next (64). Thus if P. monacha has a "strong" sex-determining mechanism and P. occidentalis and P. lucida are both weak, then a "strong" female X a "weak" male results in all-femaleness. In subsequent genera- tions, the strongly female-determining P. monacha genome is continuously united with a weaker male-determining genome. What induces formation of the unipolar spindle is not clear. Cimino (63) adopted the suggestion used to explain formation of a unipolar spindle in crested wheatgrass, Agropyron cristatum (81). Here each chromosome set is believed to carry its own spindle organizer. In P. monacha-lucida the paternal half-spindle may fail to form properly because of a chemical incompatibility between the paternal organizer and the ooplasm.

Although some of the details of gynogenesis as practiced by diploid and triploid Poecilia and Carassius and by triploid Poeciliopsis unisexuals are not known, the mechanism is a little better understood than hybridogenesis. The key appears to reside in a physical or chemical stimulus that induces development of eggs. The stimulus may be provided by a diversity of agents: (a) active sperm from another species, (b) irradiated sperm from the same or different species (82), or (c) from cold or heat shock (83). Gynogenesis has been experimentally induced in trout, loach, carp, goldfish, flatfishes, and others. It has been suggested (41) that the function of the sperm in gynogenesis, even though it is not transformed into a male pronucleus and does not unite with the female pronucleus, is to regulate the cleavage divisions. This seem doubtful since cold or heat shock can also initiate development which then proceeds normally in the complete absence of a sperm nucleus.

One might suspect that failure of synapsis in the gynogenetic process stems from inactivation of the sperm by the foreign cyto- plasm. Two events suggest that if inactivation occurs the sperm is not always "caught." One of these is the dramatic production of androgenic fish (83) in crosses between female carp, Cyprinus carpio, and males of the white amur, Ctenopharyngodon idella (a fish native to the Far East, also known as the grass carp). Three kinds of offspring were produced: 17 hybrids; 1 carp by gynogenesis; and 43 white amur by androgenesis. Apparently the amur sperm was sufficiently compatible in the carp cytoplasm not only to displace the carp pronucleus but to undergo cleavage on its own, producing diploid progeny. The second evidence that egg cytoplasm does not inactivate the foreign sperm comes from the occasional production (about 1%) of triploid offspring by diploid gynogenetic females of Poecilia formosa. These de novo triploids express paternal characters, have 69 chromosomes instead of 46, and have half again as much DNA as P. formosa (84,85).

Gynogenesis occurs in two forms, one which is temporary and autodiploid, the other which persists during successive generations and is allodiploid. In the temporary form failure of synapsis leads to a doubling of the maternal set of chromosomes by suppress-

ion of the second meiotic division, re-entry of the second polar
body, or suppression of the first mitotic division. The high
degree of homozygosity associated with any of these pathways
probably results in unpromising zygotes or at least offers no
special advantages, such as heterosis. Insufficient testing of
autodiploid gynogens makes an assessment of their fitness impossible
at this time.

The relationship of unisexuality to polyploidy is twofold.
First of all, it provides a newly formed reproductive mechanism
which may not be completely stabilized yet; and, thus, has the
potential for additional deviation. Secondly, the success of a
unisexual species provides millions of allodiploid or allotriploid
individuals which, because they are perpetuated for many generations,
have ample opportunity for additional rare events of polyploidization to occur. This argument is fortified by the fact that in
all three genera, Poecilia, Poeciliopsis, and Carassius, where
diploid unisexuals occur, one also finds triploids and, in Carassius,
also tetraploids.

The relationship of hybridization, unisexuality, and polyploidy in Poecilia and Poeciliopsis has already been made. It is
not certain, however, whether diploid or triploid goldfishes are
alloploids or autoploids; but some recent experiments (38) demonstrate the potential of hybridization to influence genome size
in these animals. Analysis of the progeny from an F_1 goldfish
(Carassius auratus) X crucian carp (Carassius carassius) female,
backcrossed to a male crucian carp, revealed that three of the
males and the one female examined had a diploid chromosome number
of 101 but that two males had 150 chromosomes. From the reciprocal
backcross of the F_1 female goldfish X carp hybrid to a goldfish
male, four male and two female offspring were all triploids.
Whether or not some of the F_1 or backcross progeny might have
continued to produce by hybridogenesis or gynogenesis was not
established.

The data available from the three genera actively involved
in polyploidy, i.e., Poecilia, Poeciliopsis, and Carassius,
suggest that its origin involves, as a first step, hybridization
which results in the formation of diploid gynogenic or hybridogenic
populations.

Successive populations consisting of millions of individuals
provide ample time and opportunity for the addition of a third
genome and then a fourth. This system overcomes some of the
difficulties imposed by the more popular view that the 4x state
is reached in a single leap which is preceeded by the following
rather unlikely series of events: (a) production of 2n eggs in
one individuals, (b) production of 2n sperm in another, and (c)
the union of enough of each to start a self-sustaining colony of
intrabreeding tetraploids which (d) are reproductively isolated
from surrounding diploids.

The process calling for a successive build-up of ploid
levels to the 4x stage has one weakness. So far, sexually

reproducing tetraploids have not been found together with the 2x
and 3x unisexual biotypes. It could also be argued that return to
sexual reproduction is no longer possible after generations of
unisexuality (2). One could cite the fact that 4x goldfish
reproduce gynogenetically. It should be pointed out, however,
that only two individuals have been tested so far (39).

A third possible route, which combines attributes of the
previous two, may be worth considering. In a hybridogenic system
there is no reason why both sexes cannot occur. Consider two
species with genomes AA and BB that hybridize and produce male
and female offspring AB. When the F_1's combine, if females
produce only A type eggs and males only B type sperm, but of two
types, X or Y bearing, a self-perpetuating allodiploid species
will be initiated. The mechanism is not unlike some of those
found in races of the evening primrose, Oenothera (88). With
each genome kept intact through successive generations and thousands of males and females producing them, the probability of
bringing together exceptional diploid gametes is greatly increased.
What evidence do we have that such a system is possible? First
of all, hybridogenic males do occur in fish. Although a
Poeciliopsis monacha genome combined with a genome of P. lucida
or P. occidentalis results in all female offspring, when it is
combined with a genome of P. latidens, only males are produced (66).
These are mostly sterile but at least one was fertile for a short
time after it matured. This F_1 P. monacha-latidens male mated
to a P. monacha female produced only monacha-like offspring.
None of the many highly contrasting morphological characters
labeling the paternal genome were transmitted through the sperm
(89). With the knowledge that hybridogenesis can occur in males
and that diploid gametes apparently are occasionally produced,
this pathway to tetraploidy seems viable.

Hybridogenesis, so far, appears to be a rare phenomenon; in
fishes it is known only in the genus Poeciliopsis. On the other
hand, among more than 3,000 fish hybrids known, fewer than a
halfdozen have been reared in a way that would have revealed it.
The mechanism would be especially difficult to spot among wild
hybrids represented by both sexes. Any hybrid swarm that is
reproducing but shows no evidence of intergradation toward either
parental species could be hybridogenic. Among fishes there are
many of these. The only other substantial example of hybridogenesis
in animals is in the European frogs of the Rana esculenta complex
(90). Here the reproductive system comes very close to fulfilling
all the criteria for the third possible pathway to tetraploidy.
R. esculenta is a hybrid between R. ridibunda and R. lessonae.
In part of its range, where it lives with R. lessonae, it transmits
its R. ridibunda genome to its eggs and obtains a new R. lessonae
genome in each generation. Where it lives with R. ridibunda, the
R. lessonae genome is retained and a new R. ridibunda is added.
R. esculenta populations consist of both males and females; when
they interbreed, they produce the R. esculenta phenotype (91).

Apparently females pass the R. ridibunda genome to their eggs, while males pass the R. lessonae genome to their sperm; union of the two restores the R. esculenta phenotype. Triploid forms also occur (92) but Dr. Bogert will provide the details on these remarkable animals.

In 1925, Muller (86) wrote an article entitled: "Why Polyploidy is Rarer in Animals than in Plants." One of the points he made, which continues to be perpetuated (2), is that the presence of four randomly segregating sex chromosomes in tetraploids would result in sexual imbalance and a high frequency of sterile intersexes. Based on what we now know of the early stages of polyploidy, chromosomes do not segregate randomly but are transmitted as intact genome units. The process of polyploidization apparently is gradual and involves elimination of redundancy through deletions, mutations, and the silencing of duplicated genes (4, 87). There is no reason why sex-determining genes or their regulator genes would not be subject to the same process. Hybridogenesis prevents the formation of ill-adapted gene combinations while the process is taking place.

ADAPTIVE VALUE OF POLYPLOIDY

Polyploidy is the one mode of speciation universally accepted as being sympatric; polyploids, in fact, could not arise other than in contact with their progenitors. This means, then, that to survive, polyploids must either be immediately adapted to an alternative niche or they must be better adapted then their progenitors, in which case, they are likely to displace them.

Uyeno and Smith (27) consider catastomids and the tetraploid carp to be especially well adapted, ranking them among the most ecologically labile fishes in North America. They cite such traits as large size, long life, fast growth rate, and ecological adaptability, and postulate that these qualities derive from the increase in number of genes, recombination, and especially heterozygosity. This view runs counter to that of Stebbins (1) who believes that in polyploids "the large amount of gene duplication dilutes the effects of new mutations and gene combinations to such an extent that polyploids have great difficulty evolving truly new adaptive gene complexes." Consequently, "the major trends of evolution are all represented by diploid species." This may be true in plants, but in fishes, catostomids, and salmonids clearly represent major trends in evolution. As for the capacity of polyploids to evolve, selection for commercially important traits such as fast growth, early age of reproduction, disease resistance, high temperature resistance, and increased egg production among carp (93) and salmonids (94), dramatically demonstrate that their genetic systems are highly malleable.

It is generally held that autopolyploidy is a rare phenomenon in the wild and that its evolutionary significance is minimal

compared to alloploidy. White (2) believes that:
  The positive adaptive effects of allopolyploidy may
  be ascribed essentially to their hybrid condition,
  i.e. to heterosis in the most general sense. In
  some cases allopolyploids may be adapted to a wider
  range of environment than their diploid progenitors,
  presumably because they carry genes of both.
     Although the heterosis view has been widely accepted, it is
in conflict with basic tenet of the species concept which holds
that the boundaries between species protect coadapted gene pools
from disruption and that hybrids are less fit than the parental
species that produced them. Much of what is called hybrid vigor
is a form of somatic vigor or exuberance which may have little
function in nature or it may derive from restoration of heterozygosity when inbred lines are crossed. Although it is apparent
that heterosis is involved in the success of polyploids, clear
documentation of their superior fitness to parental precursors is
difficult to obtain since it requires that all biotypes be measured
under the same conditions. Such tests are almost totally unavailable, even uncontrolled experiments are hard to find.
     In the U.S.S.R., the rate of growth and viability of the 3x
unisexual and 2x bisexual silver goldfish were evaluated (41).
Based on a small sample, no difference in growth rate was observed
between fingerlings. Two year old unisexuals, however, had a
faster and more uniform rate of growth but their viability (50%)
was lower than that of the bisexuals (90%+). The data are biased
by the fact that some test animals were raised with other species,
and some alone. Also, the gonads of the unisexuals were less
well developed than the bisexuals, so energy that would have gone
into reproduction could go to growth in the two year olds.
     In another study, involving laboratory synthesized allotriploid
flatfishes, growth again was no faster in the triploids than in
the parental species until sexual maturity was reached; then the
sterile triploids grew faster (82).
     The possibility of establishing whether or not heterosis
contributes to the success of wild allodiploid and allopolyploid
fishes would appear to exist only in Poeciliopsis and Poecilia,
wherein the parental species and their hybrid derivitives coexist.
From a series of studies (59, 62, 68, 69, 79, 89, 95) comparing
frequencies of abundance, pregnancy rates, and brood sizes, a
mountain of conflicting data and opinion has emerged which only
points to the fact that assessment of this issue is not as simple
as initially envisioned. The direction opinion now seems to be
heading is that relative abundance, pregnancy rate, and brood
sizes differ among the biotypes from one locality to the next and
from one time of year to the next. As an example of the range of
abundance that occurs, from five collections taken at the same
locality between 1940 and 1969, the relative abundance of P.
monacha-occidentalis to P. occidentalis favored the unisexuals 65
to 97% (68). Although the other parental species, P. monacha,

occurs in this river (Rio Mayo), it is restricted to a small
population in one of the tributaries (59). In spite of the great
success of P. monacha-occidentalis at this locality, at others its
relative abundance ranges from only 0-3%.

Regarding the question of whether or not being an allotriploid
provides any advantage over being an allodiploid, in Poecilia
from the Rio Soto la Marina (79), the triploids outnumbered the
diploids in 19 out of 21 collections for an overall advantage of
356 to 83 but in other river systems triploids were rare or
absent. For Poeciliopsis monacha-lucida vs. P. monacha-2 lucida
(89,95),   the 2x prevailed in 6 out of 8 collections for a total
advantage of 269 to 165. In practically all samples, P. monacha-
lucida out numbered its host species, P. lucida, whereas P.
monacha-2 lucida outnumbered it only about half the time. Brood
records from the laboratory over a period of 20 years (73,95)
show the 2x unisexual outproducing the 3x by more than two to
one; yet in nature this is less apparent, again varying considerably
from one collection to another.

Although these kinds of conflicting data do not resolve the
question of which biotype possesses the greatest fitness, what
does seem to emerge is that we are probably asking the wrong
question, at least as far as making field comparisons is concerned.
All of the biotypes are not competing for the same niche; and
although there may be some niche overlap, comparative measures of
success are not completely valid. Being able to occupy a broad
niche may be construed as heterosis; but, in part, success still
depends on how much of that niche is available.

Another major factor differentially influencing success of
unisexuals is the amount of clonal diversity that occurs from one
site to the next. Through the use of electrophoresis and tissue
graft analysis, it has been established that unisexual populations
of both Poecilia (97) and Poeciliopsis (65,66,98) are made up
of multiple clones. At any one locality they range in number
from 1 to 9; and, although it has not been quantified yet, those
sites with the greatest number of clones (in Poeciliopsis, at
least) have the greatest proportion of unisexuals relative to the
bisexual host species. Among clones of the same biotype, distinct
morphological and physiological differences have been identified,
involving such traits as genital pigment, dentition, size at
birth, maximum size attained, resistance to crowding, and to
temperature stress (62,73,99,100,102). That these kinds of
characters influence clonal successes and distribution was illustrated by two clones of Poeciliopsis-2 monacha-lucida which have
differences in dentition (100). By observing their habits it was
established that one clone feeds primarily on algae scraped from
rocks, the other on floating filamentous algae and detritus on
the bottom. The rock-scrapers were most abundant in head-water
arroyos where bedrock was abundant; the detritus-algae feeders
most abundant downstream in slow, sunbathed, manure-enriched

waters. In intermediate areas they both prospered, whereas in
extreme habitats, they virtually excluded each other.

The two clones of P. monacha-2 lucida illustrate how niche
breadth can be expanded by the addition of genetic variation.
Thus far, only three clones of this species have been identified
and only two of P. monacha-2 lucida; but in the two hybridogenic
forms in which clonal structure has been studied, there are no
fewer than 18 clones of P. monacha-lucida (65) and 19 P monacha-
occidentalis (99). The additional clonal diversity of the diploid
unisexuals over the triploids may account, at least in part, for
their greater abundance at most localities; this, plus the fact
that the hybridogens acquire a new locally adapted paternal
genome in each generation.

Given the complexity of community structures in Poecilia and
Poeciliopsis and the variety of temporal and special environments
available to influence the success of each biotype, the difficulty
of documenting heterosis in the field becomes obvious. In the
laboratory, however, some factors can be controlled a little
better and, although one cannot view heterosis as a whole, enough
of the parts may eventually be examined so its place in hybridization and polyploidy can be understood. From among a variety of
selective forces currently under examination, results from temperature stress experiments are now available (102). In the desert
streams where Poeciliopsis lives, temperatures fluctuate dramatically, both daily and seasonally; thus they are likely to be a
major selective force for these fishes. Resistance to heat and
cold stress was measured among many of the Poeciliopsis biotypes
discussed here. Poeciliopsis monacha-lucida was more resistant
to both heat and cold stress than either of its parental species,
P. monacha or P. lucida, and in terms of this trait, it is heterotic. Six clones of this unisexual were compared to each other;
some were more tolerant of cold and some more tolerant of heat.
One was more tolerant to both--it happens to be the most widespread clone of the 18 that have been identified from the Rio
Fuerte. Neither clone of P. monacha-2 lucida can be considered
heterotic for temperature stress. Although each was superior to
the parental species for one thermal trait, each was also inferior
for one. Between them, then, one was more resistant to heat and
one more resistant to cold, and in that sense, have adaptive
interclonal variation.

Once all of the information is in, the relationship of adaptation to the origin of polyploid species may run somewhat as
follows: When two species hybridize they produce many hybrid
offspring from a single mating, as well as the fact that more
than one mating is likely to occur. If the cross results in
unisexuality, many clones will be started, some will be broadly
adapted, some specifically adapted, and other maladapted.
Because of their reproductive process, any well adapted genotypes
they possess will not be disrupted by recombination but will be
multiplied and become widespread as clones made up of millions of

individuals. The step to triploidy, however rare it may be (apparently it is less common in <u>Poeciliposis</u> than <u>Poecilia</u>), is most likely to arise from an especially successful and abundant diploid clone. It may be a generalist but the probability seems greater that it will be a specialist. In either case, its long term survival will depend on a niche being available. Competition with parental species and among clones must be intense; but, once a clone is established, adaptation through the accumulation of favorable mutations, deletions, and the silencing of certain alleles can provide some fine adjustment. Advance to the tetraploid level, whether it is from a 2x or 3x unisexual, does not appear to be a high frequency event. Establishment of such a newcomer in a community of biotypes such as just described, would provide the ultimate example of "species packing."

THE SIGNIFICANCE OF POLYPLOIDY IN FISHES

The evolution of amphibians from fishes involved a substantial number of new adaptations of all of which had to be genetically coded for. Assuming that many of the loci in fish are already committed, mutations of new functions would be deleterious. The suggestion of Ohno and his colleagues (3), that numerous uncommitted loci made available by polyploidy can be redirected to code for new adaptations, provides a reasonable solution to the problem.

Another aspect of DNA is its quantitative relationship to specialization. When fishes are arranged in an array from the most generalized to the most specialized, the highest DNA values are found among generalized forms and the lowest among the specialized (7,18). Loss of parts, streamlining, and other alterations may leave certain loci without a function, if these are not redirected, they are likely to be lost, resulting in less DNA. Specialization in some groups of fishes and continuous loss of DNA presumable reaches the lowest allowable level beyond which additional adaptation cannot occur. Extinction rates may run high in such forms. Although fishes with generalized forms have high DNA levels, they apparently do not evolve much. One is faced with the dilemma that, if specialization leads to an adaptive breakthrough, evolution cannot capitalize on it. There will not be enough uncommitted DNA to code for the variety of new species usually associated with adaptive radiation. The most effective way out of this dilemma is by polyploidy.

LITERATURE CITED

1. Stebbins, G.L., 1977, "Process of Organic Evolution," ed. 3, Prentice-Hall, Englewood Cliffs, New Jersey.
2. White, M.J.D., 1978, "Modes of Speciation," W.H. Freeman, San Francisco.
3. Ohno, S., 1970, "Evolution by Gene Duplication," Springer-Verlag, New York.

4.   Ohno, S., 1974, "Animal Cytogenetics," Vol. 4, Chordata 1. Gerbrüder Borntraeger, Berlin.
5.   Schwartz, F.J., 1972, World Literature to Fish Hybrids with an Analysis by Family, Species and Hybrid. Gulf Coast Research Laboratory Museum, Ocean Springs, Mississippi.
6.   Ohno, S., Atkin, N.B., 1966, Comparative DNA values and chromosome complements of eight species of fishes. Chromosoma 18: 455-466.
7.   Hinegardner, R., 1968, Evolution of cellular DNA content in teleost fishes. Amer. Nat. 102: 517-523.
8.   Patterson, C., 1978, "Evolution," Cornell University Press, Ithaca, New York.
9.   Harrington, R.W., 1961, Oviparous hermaphroditic fish with interal self-fertilization. Science 134: 1749-1750.
10. Svärdson, G., 1945, Chromosome studies on Salmonidae. Report of the Institute of Freshwater Research. Drottningholm 23: 1-151.
11. Rees, H., 1964, The question of polyploidy in the Salmonidae. Chromosoma 15: 275-279.
12. Taylor, K.M., 1967, The chromosomes of some lower chordates. Chromosoma 21: 181-188.
13. Greenwood, P.H., Rosen, D.E., Weitzman, S.H., Myers, G.S., 1966, Phyletic studies of teleostean fishes, with a provisional classification of living forms. Bull. Amer. Mus. Nat. 131: 341-455.
14. Schultz, R.J., 1967, Gynogenesis and triploidy in the viviparous fish Poeciliopsis. Science 157: 1564-1567.
15. Chen, T.R., Ebeling, A.W., 1968, Karyological evidence of female heterogamety in the mosquitofish Gambusia affinis (Baird and Girad). Copeia 1968: 70-75.
16. Roberts, F.L., 1964, A chromosome study of twenty species of Centrarchidae. J. Morph. 115: 401-418.
17. Ohno, S., Wolf, V., Atkin, N.B., 1968, Evolution from fish to mammals by gene duplication. Hereditas 59: 169-187.
18. Hinegardner, R., Rosen, D.E., 1972, Cellular DNA content and the evolution of teleostean fishes. Amer. Nat. 106: 621-644.
19. Booke, H.E., 1968, Cytotaxonomic studies of the coregonine fishes of the Great Lakes, USA: DNA and karyotype analysis. J. Fish Res. Board Canada 25: 1667-1687.
20. Simon, R.C., 1963, Chromosome morphology and species evolution in the five North American species of Pacific salmon (Oncorhynchus). J. Morph. 112: 77-97.
21. Simon, R., Dollar, A., 1963, Cytological aspects of speciation in two North American teleosts, Salmo gairdneri and Salmo clarki lewisi. Canad. J. Genet. Cytol. 5: 43-49.
22. Viktorovsky, R.M., Chromosome sets of Coregonus peled and C. lavaretus baunti. Tsitologiya 6: 636-638.
23. Ohno, S., Muramoto, J., Klein, J., Atkin, N.B., 1969, Diploid-tetraploid relationship in clupeoid and salmonoid fish, pp. 139-147, in "Chromosomes Today," Vol. II, Darlington, C.D.,

Lewis, K.R. (eds.), Oliver and Boyd, Edinburgh.

24. Wolf, U., Engel, W., Faust, J., 1970, Zum Merchanismus der Diploidisierung in der Wirbeltierevolution: Koexistenz von tetrasomen disomen Genloci der Isozitrat-Dehydrogenasen bei der Regenbogenforelle (<u>Salmo irideus</u>). Humangenetik 9: 150-156.

25. Engel, W., Op't Hof, J., Wolf, U., 1970, Genduplikation durch polyploide Evolution: die Isoenzyme der Sorbitde-hydrogenese bei herings-und lacksartigen Fischen (Isospondyli). Humangenetik 9: 157-163.

26. Keyl, H.G., 1966, Increases of DNA in chromosomes, pp. 99-101, <u>in</u> "Chromosomes Today," Vol. I, Darlington, C.D., Lewis, K.R. (eds.), Oliver and Boyd, Edinburgh.

27 Uyeno, T., Smith, G.R., 1972, Tetraploid origin of the karyotype of catostomid fishes. Science 175: 644-646.

28. Romer, A.S., 1966, "Vertebrate Paleontyology," University of Chicago Press, Chicago.

29. Uyeno, T., Listed in Uyeno and Smith (Science 175: 644-646, 1972) as unpublished data.

30. Ohno, S., Muramoto, J., Christian, L., 1967, Diploid-tetra-ploid relationship among old world members of the fish family Cyprinidae. Chromosoma 23: 1-9.

31. Muramoto, J., Ohno, S., Atkin, N.B., 1968, On the diploid state of the fish order Ostariophysi. Chromosoma 24: 59-66.

32. Wolf, U., Ritter, H., Atkin, N.B., Ohno, S., 1969, Polyploidi-zation in the fish family Cyprinidae, order Cypriniformes. I. DNA-content and chromosome sets in various species of Cyprinidae. Humagenetik 7: 240-244.

33. Klose, J., Wolf, U., Hitzeroth, H., Riter, H., Ohno, S., 1969, Polyploidization in the fish family Cyprinidae, order Cypriniformes. II. Duplication of the gene loci coding for lactate dehydrogenase (E.c.: 1˙1˙1˙27) and 6-phosphogluconate dehydrogenase (E.c.: 1˙1˙1˙44) in various species of Cyprini-dae. Humagenetik 7: 245-250.

34. Quiroz-Gutierrez, A., Ohno, S., 1970, The evidence of gene duplication for S-form NADP-linked isocitrate dehydrogenase in carp and goldfish. Biochem. Genet. 4: 98-99.

35. Bender, K., Ohno, S., 1968, Duplication of the autosomally inherited 6-phosphogluconate dehydrogenase gene locus in tetraploid species of cyprinid fish. Biochem. Genet. 2: 101-107.

36. Kobayasi, H., Kawashima, Y., Takeuchi, N., 1970, Comparative chromosome studies in the genus <u>Carassius</u>, especially with a finding of polyploidy in the ginbuna. Jap. J. Ichthyol. 17: 153-160.

37. Kobayasi, H., 1971, A cytological study on gynogenesis of the triploid ginbuna (<u>Carassius auratus langsdorfii</u>). Zool. Mag. 80: 316-322.

38. Kobayasi, H., Hashida, M., 1977, Morphological and cytological studies in back-cross hybrids of F_1 fishes between the

kinbuna (Carassius auratus subsp.) and the crucian carp
(Carassius carassius). Jap. Women's Univ. J. (Home Economics)
Nol 24.
39. Kobaysi, H., 1977, Hybridization in Japanese funa, Carassius
auratus. Proc. 5th Japan-Soviet Joint Symp. Aquaculture.
Sept. 1976, Tokyo and Sapporo.
40. Liu, S., Sezaki, K., Hashimoto, K., Kobayasi, H., Nakamura,
M., 1968, Simplified techniques for determination of polyploidy
in ginbuna Carassius auratus langsdorfi. Bull. Jap. Soc.
Sci. Fisheries 44: 601-606.
41. Golavinskaya, K.A., Romashov, D.D., Cherfas, N.B., 1965, The
unisexual and bisexual forms of the silver goldfish (Carassius
auratus gibelio Block). Vopr. Iktiologii 5: 614-629.
42. Lieder, U., 1959, Über die Eientwicklung bei männchenlosen
Stämmen der Silberkarauche Carassius auratus gibelio (Block)
(Vertebrata, Pisces). Biol. Zbl. 78: 284-291.
43. Cherfas, N.B., 1966, Natural triploidy in females of the
unisexual form of silver carp [goldfish] (Carassius auratus
gibelio Block). Genetika 5: 16-24.
44. Kobayasi, H., 1976, Comparative study of karayotypes in the
small and large races of spinous loaches (Cobitus biwae).
Zool. Mag. 85: 84-87.
45. Sezaki, K., Kobayasi, H., 1978, Comparison of erythrocyte
size between diploid and tetraploid in spinois loach, Cobitis
biwae. Bull. Jap. Soc. Sci. Fisheries 44: 851-854.
46. Cimino, M.C., 1973, Karyotypes and erythrocyte sizes of some
diploid and triploid fishes of the genus Poeciliopsis. J.
Fish. Res. Board Canada 30: 1736-1737.
47. Swarup, H., 1959, Effect of triploidy on the body size,
general organization and cellular structure in Gasterosteus
(L.). J. Genetics 56: 143-155.
48. Purdom, C.E., 1973, Induced polyploidy in plaice (Pleuronectes
platessa) and its hybrid with the flounder (Platichythes
flesus). Heredity 29: 11-24.
49. Valenti, R.J., 1975, Induced polyploidy in Tilapia aurea
(Steindachner) by means of temperature shock treatment. J.
Fish. Biol. 7: 519-528.
50. Fankhauser, G., 1941, Cell size, organ and body size in
triploid newts (Triturus viridescens). J. Morph. 68: 161-177.
51. Nygren, A., Edlund, P., Hirsch, U., Aksgren, L., 1968,
Cytological studies in perch (Perca fluviatilis L.), pike
(Esox lucius L.), Pike-perch (Lucioperca lucioperca L.), and
ruff (Acerina cernua L.). Hereditas 59: 518-524.
52. Dingerkus, G., Howell, W.M., 1976, Karyotypic analysis and
evidence of tetraploidy in the North American paddlefish,
Polyodon spathula. Science 194: 842-844.
53. Ohno, S., Muramoto, J., Stenius, C., Christian, L., Kittrell,
W.A., 1969, Microchromosomes in holocephalian, chondrostean
and holostean fishes. Chromosoma 26: 35-40.

54. Miller, R.R., Schultz, R.J., 1959, All-female strains of the teleost fishes of the genus Poeciliopsis. Science 130: 1656-1657.

55. Schultz, R.J., 1966, Hybridization experiments with an all-female fish of the genus Poeciliopsis. Biol. Bull. 130: 415-429.

56. Schultz, R.J., 1969, Hybridization, unisexuality, and polyploidy in the teleost Poeciliopsis (Poeciliidae) and other vertebrates. Amer. Nat. 108: 605-619.

57. Vrijenhoek, R.C., 1972, Genetic relationships of unisexual-hybrid fishes to their progenitors using lactate dehydrogenase isozymes as gene markers (Poeciliopsis, Poeciliidae). Amer. Nat. 106: 754-766.

58. Vrijenhoek, R.C., Schultz, R.J., 1974, Evolution of a trihybrid unisexual fish (Poeciliopsis, Poeciliidae). Evolution 28: 306-319.

59. Moore, W.S., 1976, Components of fitness in the unisexual fish Poeciliopsis monacha-occidentalis. Evolution 30: 564-578.

60. Miller, R.R., 1960, Four new species of viviparous fishes, genus Poeciliopsis, from northwestern Mexico. Occasional Papers Mus. Zool., Univ. Michigan, No. 619. This publication lists one Rio Fuerte locality for P. monacha at Guirocoba; two others, one discovered by Miller at El Cajon is published under Vrijenhoek et al. 1978 and one discovered by J. Lanza is published under Bulger and Schultz 1979. The Rio Sinaloa site, discovered by Miller at Coronado, is unpublished.

61. Thibault, R.E., Schultz, R.J., 1978, Reproductive adaptations among viviparous fishes (Cyprinodontiformes: Poeciliidae). Evolution 32: 320-333.

62. Schultz, R.J., 1977, Evolution and ecology of unisexual fishes, pp. 277-331, in "Evolutionary Biology," Hecht, M.K., Steer, W.C., Wallace, B. (eds.), Vol. 10, Plenum, New York.

63. Cimino, M.C., 1972, Egg-production, polyploidization and evolution in a diploid all-female fish of the genus Poeciliopsis. Evolution 26: 294-306.

64. Schultz, R.J., 1961, Reproductive mechanisms of unisexual and bisexual strains of the viviparous fish Poeciliopsis. Evolution 15: 302-325.

65. Angus, R.A., Schultz, R.J., 1979, Clonal diversity in the unisexual fish Poeciliopsis monacha-lucida: a tissue graft analysis. Evolution 33: 27-40.

66. Schultz, R.J., 1973, Origin and synthesis of a unisexual fish, pp. 207-211, in "Genetics and Mutagenesis of Fish," Schröder, J.H. (ed.), Springer-Verlag, Berlin.

67. Schultz, R.J., 1961, Reproductive mechanism of unisexual and bisexual strains of the viviparous fish Poeciliopsis. 15: 302-325.

68. Moore, W.S., Miller, R.R., Schultz, R.J., 1970, Distribution adaptation and probable origin of an all-female form of Poeciliopsis (Pisces: Poeciliidae) in northwestern

Mexico. Evolution 24: 806–812.
69. Schultz, R.J., 1971, Special adaptive problems associated
     with unisexual fishes. Amer. Zool. 11: 351–360.
70. Schultz, R.J., 1973, Unisexual fish: laboratory synthesis of
     a "species." Science 179: 180–181.
71. Vrijenhoek, R.C., 1979, Factors affecting clonal diversity
     and coexistence. (in press).
72. Schultz, R.J., 1967, Gynogenesis and triploidy in the
     viviparous fish Poeciliopsis. Science 157: 1564–1567.
73. Schultz, R.J., (unpublished).
74. Cimino, M.C., 1974, The nuclear DNA content of diploid and
     triploid Poeciliopsis and other poeciliid fishes with reference
     to the evolution of unisexual forms. Chromosoma 47: 297–307.
75. Cimino, M.C., 1973, Meiosis in triploid all-female fish
     (Poeciliopsis, Poeciliidae). Science 175: 1484.
76. Hubbs, C.L., Hubbs, L.C., 1932, Apparent parthenogenesis in
     nature, in a form of fish of hybrid origin. Science 76:
     628–630.
77. Drewry, G.E., 1964, in "Interactions between a bisexual
     fish species and its gynogenetic sexual parasite," Bull.
     Texas Mem. Mus. No 8 Appendex 1, 67.
78. Balsano, J.S., Darnell, R.M., Abramoff, P., 1972, Electro-
     phoretic evidence of triploidy associated with populations
     of the gynogenetic teleost Poecilia formosa. Copeia 1972:
     292–297.
79. Rasch, E.M., Balsano, J.S., 1974, Biochemical and cytogenetic
     studies of Poecilia from eastern Mexico. II. Frequency,
     perpetuation, and probable origin of triploid genomes in
     females associated with Poecilia formosa. Rev. Biol. Trop.
     21: 351–381; and personal communication.
80. Rasch, E.M., Manaco, P.J., Balsano, J.S., 1978, Identification
     of a new form of triploid hybrid fish by DNA-feulgen cyto-
     photometry. J. Histochem. Cytochem. 26: 218 (abst.).
81. Tai, W., 1970, Multipolar meiosis in diploid crested wheat-
     grass, Agropyron cristatum. Amer. J. Bot. 57: 1160–1169.
82. Purdom, C.E., 1976, Genetic techniques in flatfish culture.
     J. Fish. Res. Board Canada 33: 1088–1099.
83. Stanley, J.G., Biggers, C.J., Schultz, D., 1976, Isozymes in
     androgenetic and gynogenetic white amur, gynogenetic carp,
     and carp-amur hybrids. J. Heredity 67: 129–134. (This
     article provides a good literature review on the subject of
     gynogenesis.)
84. Rasch, E.M., Darnell, R.M., Kallman, K.D., Abramoff. P.,
     1965, Cytophotometric evidence for triploidy in hybrids of
     the gynogenetic fish, Poecilia formosa. J. Exp. Zool. 160:
     155–170.
85. Schultz, R.J., Kallman, K.D., 1968, Triploid hybrids between
     the all-female teleost Poecilia formosa and Poecilia sphenops.
     Nature 219: 280–282.

86. Muller, H.J., 1925, Why polyploidy is rarer in animals than in plants. Amer. Nat. 59: 346-353.
87. Ferris, S.D., Whitt, G.S., 1977, Loss of duplicate gene expression after polyploidization. Nature 265: 258-260.
88. Cleland, R.E., 1936, Some aspects of the cytogenetics of Oenothera. Bot. Rev. 2: 316-318; Cleland, R.E., 1950, Studies on Oenothera cytogenetics and phylogeny. Indiana Univ. Publ., Sci. Ser. 16.
89. Schultz, R.J., Vrijenhoek, R.C., (unpublished).
90. Tunner, H., 1973, Das Albumin und andere Bluteiweisse bei Rana ridibunda Pallas, Rana lessonae Camerano, Rana esculenta Linné und daren Hybriden. A. Zool. Syst. Evol. Forschung 11: 219-233.
91. Uzzell, T., Berger, L., 1975, Electrophoretic phenotypes of Rana ridibunda, Rana lessonae, and their hybridogenetic associate, Rana esculenta. Proc. Acad. Nat. Sci. (Philadelphia) 127: 13-24.
92. Uzzell, T., Günther, R., Berger, L., 1977, Rana esculenta and Rana ridibunda: a leaky hybridogenetic system? Proc. Acad. Nat. Sci. (Philadelphia) 128: 147-171.
93. Moav, R., Brody, T., Hulata, G., 1978, Genetic improvement of wild fish populations. Science 201: 1090-1094.
94. Donaldson, L.R., Menasveta, D., 1961, Selective breeding of chinook salmon. Trans. Amer. Fish. Soc. 90: 160-164.
95. Thibault, R.E., 1978, Ecological and evolutionary relationships among diploid and triploid unisexual fishes associated with the bisexual species, Poeciliopsis lucida (Cyprinodontiformes: Poeciliidae). Evolution 32: 613-623.
96. Moore, W.S., 1976, Components of fitness in the unisexual fish Poeciliopsis monacha-occidnetalis. Evolution 30: 564-578.
97. Kallman, K.D., 1962, Population genetics of the gynogenetic telost, Mollienesia formosa (Girard). Evolution 64: 497-504; Kallman, D.K., 1962, Gynogenesis in the telost, Mollienesia formosa (Girard) (with discussion of the detection of parthenogenesis in vertebrates by tissue transplantation). J. Genetics 58: 7-21; Kallman, K.D., 1964, Homozygosity in a gynogenetic fish--Poecilia formosa. Genetics 50: 260-261; Darnell, R.M., Lamb, E., Abramoff, P., 1967, Matroclinous inheritance and clonal structure of a Mexican population of the gynogenetic fish, Poecilia formosa. Evolution 21: 168-173.
98. Moore, W.S., 1977, A histocompatability analysis of inheritance in the unisexual fish Poeciliopsis 2 monacha-lucida. Copeia 1977: 213-223; Vrijenhoek, R.C., Angus, R.A., Schultz, R.J., 1977, Variation and heterozygosity in sexual vs. clonally reproducing populations. Evolution 31: 767-781; Vrijenhoek, R.C., Angus, R.A., Schultz, R.J., 1978, Variation and clonal structure in a unisexual fish. Amer. Nat. 112: 41-45.
99. Angus, R.A., 1979, Geographical dispersal and clonal diversity in unisexual fish populations. Amer. Nat. (in press).

100. Vrijenhoek, R.C., 1978, Coexistence of clones in a hetero-
     geneous environment. Science 199: 549-552.
101. Keegan-Rogers, V., doctoral research in progress.
102. Bulger, A.J., Schultz, 1979, Heterosis and interclonal
     variation in thermal tolerance in unisexual fishes. Evolution
     33: (in press).

EVOLUTIONARY IMPLICATIONS OF POLYPLOIDY IN AMPHIBIANS AND REPTILES

James P. Bogart

Department of Zoology
University of Guelph
Guelph, Ontario

In plants, polyploidy is recognized to be a wide-spread phenomenon and of considerable practical and evolutionary importance, whereas polyploid animal species have been relegated for the most part, to insignificance in terms of their existence or evolutionary importance. Evolutionary and genetic authorities have adhered mostly to Mullers's 1925 (1) contention that sexual imbalance in polyploids would not permit bisexual polyploids to exist as natural entities in animals as they do in plants, which are capable of vegetative reproduction. Asexual polyploids are also condemned, in animals, by the commonly held, and mathematically "proven" (2) viewpoint that this method of reproduction reduces genetic recombination and is tantamount to phylogenetic suicide (3-5). It is evident, however, that an increasing number of polyploid amphibians and reptiles are being encountered in natural populations living in North America, South America, Europe, Asia, and Africa. To ignore their existence or to pass judgement on their evolutionary significance without adequate study is incomprehensible. In spite of the theoretical dogma surrounding animal polyploids, there is a growing bank of data which suggests that naturally occurring animal polyploids may play an interesting and significant role in population genetics and speciation.

In amphibians and reptiles, all the polyploid species are associated with diploid species. There are no distinctly polyploid families, genera, or even species groupings. Reptilian polyploids are all-female triploid lizards which are all thought to reproduce parthenogenetically. Amphibian polyploids are more diverse. Urodeles have demonstrated all-female triploid populations which supposedly reproduced gynogenetically and require sperm for egg activation from a related diploid bisexual species.

Anurans have bisexual, triploid, tetraploid, hexaploid, or octoploid populations or species. Those species or populations which
have been demonstrated to be polyploids are listed in Table 1.

Table 1. Amphibian and reptilian species and/or natural populations
          which are considered to be polyploid.[a]

Species with Classification	Reproductive Mode[b]	Diploid Chromosome No. (Ploidy)	Geographic Distribution (reference)
AMPHIBIA			
Anura			
Pipidae			
Xenopus			
ruwenzoriensis	B	108(6x)	Uganda (6,7)
X. vestitus	B	72(4x)	"
X. sp.	B	72(4x)	"
Leptodactylidae			
Ceratophrys			
dorsata	B	104(8x)	Brazil (8)
C. <<ornata>>	B	104(8x)	Argentina (9)
Odontophrynus			
<<americanus>>	B	44(4x)	Argentina & Brazil (10)
Pleurodema			
bibroni	B	44(4x)	Uruguay (11)
P. kriegi	B	44(4x)	Argentina (11)
Hylidae			
Hyla versicolor	B	48(4x)	e. North America (12)
Phyllomedusa			
<<burmeisteri>>	B	52(4x)	Brazil (13)
Bufonidae			
Bufo danatensis	B	44(4x)	Turkmen (14)
Bufo <<viridis>>	B	44(4x)	Kirghizia (15)
B. sp.D	B	40(4x)	Ethiopia (16)
Ranidae			
Dicroglossus			
<<occipitalis>>	B	52(4x)	Liberia (16)
Pxyicephalus			
<<delalandii>>	B	52(4x)	South Africa (16)
Rana <<esculenta>>	H	39(3x)	Europe (17.18)

Table 1. (continued)

Caudata			
Ambystomidae			
Ambystoma platineum	G	42(3x)	e. North America (19)
A. tremblayi	G	42(3x)	" (19)
A. texanum X laterale	P?G?	42(3x)	" (20)
REPTILIA			
Squamata			
Gekkonidae			
Gehyra variegata	P	63(3x)	Japan (21)
Hemidactylus garnotii	P	70(3x)	Indo-Pacific (22)
Agamidae			
Leiolepis triploida	P	54(3x)	Malaysia (21)
Teiidae			
Cnemidophorus exanguis	P	69(3x)	s.w. U.S. & n. Mexico (23)
C. flagellicaudas	P	69(3x)	s.w. U.S. (24)
C. opatae	P	69(3x)	n. Mexico (25)
C. sonorae	P	69(3x)	s.w. U.S. & n. Mexico (24)
C. tesselatus[a]	P	69(3x)	" (23)
C. uniparens	P	69(3x)	" (24)
C. velox	P	69(3x)	s.w. U.S. (23)

[a]Some species of frogs, indicated by << >> have been recognized to consist of diploid and polyploid populations as is Rana <<esculenta>> which is considered to be a hybrid "species." Cnemidophorus tesselatus also has recognized diploid (2n=46) clones which are parthenogenetic.

[b]Polyploid amphibians and reptiles differ with respect to their zygote production. Bisexual polyploids (B) have males and females which contribute equally to the zygote. Hybridogenetic (H) reproduction involves the elimination of one of the parental genomes in the F_1. All-female polyploids' eggs may initiate cleavage spontaneously and are considered to be parthenogenetic (P) or they may require stimulation from a male from some bisexual species and are considered to be gynogenetic (G).

Polyploid amphibians were recognized in some of the earliest chromosomal investigations under experimental conditions and even in natural populations. The early investigations are reviewed by Parmenter (26), Fankhauser (27), and Moore (28). Temperature shock has been used to induce triploidy in amphibians since the late 1930's (26) and pressure (29-32) is fairly commonly utilized in recent studies of polyploidy. The frequency of diploid eggs may be substantially increased using temperature shock or pressure, both of which have the effect of prohibiting the second polar body from being produced or escaping. Diploid eggs may develop gynogenetically if the sperm nucleus is not capable of fusing with the egg nucleus. This effect may be accomplished experimentally by using foreign or irradiated sperm (32-34). Certain percentages of eggs, even in control crosses not subjected to abnormal temperature or pressure, have been found to be diploid or tetraploid (35-38). Triploid progeny has been reported to be as high as 35% in control crosses using certain female Rana pipiens (37). A certain proportion of the progeny of many amphibian females might possible be polyploid since polyploid individuals have been encountered wherever large numbers of offspring have been examined. Finding polyploid populations or species may not be too surprising in the light of these experimental results and, indeed, finding polyploid individuals in natural populations may not be deemed a significant enough event to justify a detailed populational investigation. It is interesting, in retrospect, that the Hertwigs (39) discovered a naturally occurring triploid Rana <<esculenta>> as early as 1920. Because of the ease with which polyploidy may be experimentally induced in amphibians, the mechanism of polyploid production has been investigated in a number of species (28,30,33,35,36,40-46, and many others).

Experimentation in Anurans is simplified by the fact of external fertilization. Female Urodeles typically pick up a spermatophore with their cloacal lips and fertilization is internal, but artificial in vitro fertilization is still possible by using oviducal eggs or by squeezing the eggs from an uninseminated female (47-49). Similar types of manipulation are not possible in reptiles. Most of the information concerning meiotic behaviour has been obtained indirectly by examining progeny using a variety of techniques such as chromosome markers (30), compatible parents which have different chromosome numbers (35,36), or mutant genes (33,34,45). There is fairly general agreement concerning the female's responsibility for the production of polyploids when it is possible to determine responsibility. There is no direct evidence that polyploidy can be accomplished by polyspermy or unreduced sperm.

The Ambystoma Jeffersonianum Complex

As early as 1934, Clanton (50) described two forms of
Jefferson's salamander from Michigan. Salamanders of the "light
form" were all female and matings between "dark males" and light
females resulted in only females of the light form. In some
populations the ratio of females to males was as high as 50 to 1.
Bishop (51) recognized the "Clanton effect" (scewed sex ratio
with many more females than males) in New York. Jefferson's
salamanders in Indiana were analyzed by Minton (52) and he
concluded that Clanton's light all-female form represented interspecific hybrids involving two morphologically distinctive bisexual
species, Ambystoma jeffersonianum and A. laterale. Minton speculated that the hybridization was the result of secondary contact
of two populations which were originally divided, by the post-
Pleistocene eastward extension of the prairie Steppe, into a
northern (A. laterale) and a southern (A. jeffersonianum) species.
He also predicted that the ever-increasing proportion of females
to males could result in the extinction of populations which
relied on a steady migration of normal males in the contact zone.
Uzzell (19,53) uncovered the triploid nature of the all-female
hybrids and speculated that the hybrids represented two distinct
species. Uzzell (53) and Uzzell and Goldblatt (54) considered
the early (post-Pleistocene) hybridization of the diploid species
to have been an initial step for the evolution of the triploid
species and that the triploids each arose as a result of backcrosses involving the putative hybrid and A. laterale (to produce
A. tremblayi) or A. jeffersonianum (to produce A. platineum).
The triploid species so produced are all female and reproduce
gynogenetically so they must remain closely associated with the
original parental species which was involved in the backcross.
They exist as sexual parasites utilizing the sperm of normal
diploid males for the initiation of zygote development.
    Plasma proteins were examined by Uzzell and Goldblatt (54)
who found fixed heterozygosity and differential staining intensities at one plasma protein locus. This evidence supported the
hypothesis concerning the hybrid nature and expected genome
constitution in both of the triploids. Meiosis in one of the
triploids, A. tremblayi (55,56), appears to be preceded by a pre-
oögonial endomitosis so the eggs initiate meiosis in a hexaploid
state. Bivalents and occasional multivalent associations were
observed in first prophase. It is assumed that meiosis procedes
normally and results in the formation of triploid eggs.
    Recently, Downs (20) examined the Jeffersonianum complex in
Ohio, Indiana, and Michigan. He encountered some additional
complexities involving yet another species, Ambystoma texanum,
which is considered to be very distantly related to Jefferson's
complex species as well as to many other Ambystomatids (57).
Freytag (58) would even place A. texanum in a separate genus
(Linguelapsus). All-female diploid and triploid populations were

discovered by Downs (20) on the Bass Islands in Lake Erie. These
were interpreted to be hybrids between A. laterale and A. texanum
as evidenced by their intermediate morphological characteristics
and serum protein patterns. Diploid male and female A. texanum
were found on the middle Bass Island, but no Ambystoma males were
found on the north Island. Triploid females were determined to
have a genome which consists of two sets of A. texanum chromosomes
and one of A. laterale. Downs suggests that the all-female
diploids and triploids are parthenogenetic (at least on the north
Bass Island) and that A. texanum may interact with the Jefferson's
complex in other geographical areas where they occur in sympatry.
Downs found the diploid and triploid unisexuals to be heterozygous
for the same presumed locus studied by Uzzell and Goldblatt (54)
but also found electrophoretic heterozygotes in A. jeffersonianum
and A. texanum serum proteins. He suggests that we may be presently observing, with A. laterale and A. texanum a hybridization
event which is very similar to the original postulated hybridization which gave rise to A. tremblayi and A. platineum prior to
the time that the diploid, perhaps parthenogenetic, populations
were displaced by the allotriploids. Discovering mixed diploid-
triploid populations of Ambystoma is of extreme interest as it
parallels the situation observed in Cnemidophorus lizards and
frogs of the R. <<esculenta>> complex.

The Rana <<esculenta>> Complex

        In Europe and western Asia there exists another extremely
interesting group of related amphibian species which has been the
subject of considerable taxonomic confusion (Fig.1). This may
now be appreciated in the light of several recent studies which
have been summarized by Berger (17) and Dubois (59). The edible
frog, R. <<esculenta>>, has been determined to be a hybrid
<<species>> in numerous populations over much of its range and
is the product of crosses involving the lake frog, R. ridibunda
and the pool frog, R. lessonae. Populations have been studied
in Poland (17,60), Switzerland (61), Germany (62,63), Austria
(64,65), Denmark (66), and Sweden (67). There is considerable
variability in the sex ratios of R. <<esculenta>> in various
populations as well as the ratios of R. <<esculenta>> to the
"parental" species. R. <<esculenta>> is found in three different
associations. The most common association is with R. ridibunda
and by itself in so-called "pure" populations. The interaction
between the "parental" species and R. <<esculenta>> varies between
populations and this depends on their associations. Turner (64)
analysed a population consisting of male and female R. lessonae
and only female R. <<esculenta>>. He postulated a scheme by which
the eggs of R. <<esculenta>> females contain only the R. ridibunda
genome and R. <<esculenta>> is produced when these eggs are fertilized with R. lessonae sperm. This hybridogenetic reproduction
would be similar to the system described in unisexual poeciliid

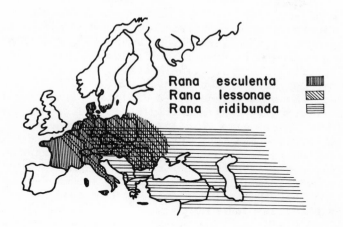

Fig. 1: Distribution of Rana ridibunda, R. lessonae, and
their hybrid, Rana esculenta, in Europe (modified from 59).

fish (68,69), but with the added complication of having, in
other populations, supposedly hybridogenetic male R. <<esculenta>>
(70). If R. <<esculenta>> is found with R. ridibunda, most of
the R. <<esculenta>> are males which transmit sperm containing
either a R. lessonae genome (2/3 of the time) or a R. ridibunda
genome (1/3 of the time) (17,70,71). "Pure" R. <<esculenta>>
populations contain both males and females (18,66,71) but as
many as 80% of the individuals (both male and female) are triploids
(18). Male triploids produce sperm of different sizes, and
considerable abnormalities have been observed in meiosis (72).
Crossing triploids results in offspring exhibiting all three
phenotypes (17). Clutches of R. <<esculenta>> eggs have occasionally been noted to include different size (73,74) and it is
assumed that triploid R. <<esculenta>> arise from fertilization
of diploid eggs produced by diploid R. <<esculenta>> (74).

Polyploid Reptiles

     Skewed sex ratios have been observed in a number of lizards
belonging to several families since the 1930's. In his review,
Cole (75) pointed out the existance of 26 all-female species of

lizards (from 6 families), as well as one all-female species of
snake. It is generally accepted (21,75-79) that the all-female
reptiles reproduce by parthenogenesis. Direct proof is available
for a few species which have been raised in isolation (76,79,80).
The absence of sperm in oviducts or cloacae of female unisexuals
which live in sympatry with sperm carring females of bisexual
species has been used as indirect evidence (81,82). Most of the
all-female unisexual lizards are believed to have arisen as the
result of hybridization involving bisexual species (76,83,84),
although some may have arisen spontaneously (75,85).

In addition to many recognized diploid parthenogenetic
species of lizards, several are triploid, as determined by chromosomal analysis (Table 1). Triploid lizards of the genus Cnemidophorus have received the most intensive investigation. Oögenesis
has been studied in only one triploid lizard, C. uniparens by
Cuellar (86), and it appears that meiosis is preceded by an
endomitotic event, as is the case with the salamander Ambystoma
tremblayi (55,56). However, meiosis in C. uniparens is soon
followed by cleavage and the embryo is fairly well developed at
the time of oviposition. The triploid unisexual Cnemidophorus
are all suspected to be the product of hybridization involving a
diploid unisexual parthenogenetic species and a normal bisexual
species (25,75). Chromosomes of C. sexlineatus group species are
not easily distinguished and it is not always easy to detect the
original parents involved in the allotriploid (25). It is generally assumed that triploidy is the result of a female diploid
parthenogenetic species which backcrossed to one or the other of
the original bisexual species. This produces an allotriploid
possessing a double complement of chromosome from some bisexual
species although the possibility exists that an allotriploid
could rarely have three separate genomes and may be referred to
three distinctive bisexual species (25). Normally unisexual
diploid parthenogenetic females may become inseminated with sperm
from a male of a bisexual species and this has resulted in the
occasional formation of triploids (76,87,88). Also, fertilization
of a normally parthenogenetic triploid female may sometimes
result in a tetraploid male (89) or female (76).

Cnemidophorus tesselatus is the only species of Cnemidophorus
which is recognized as having diploid and triploid all-female
populations (25). This species consists of allodiploids, modified
allodiploids, allotriploids, and modified allotriploids. The
diploid populations were formed by hybridization involving the
two bisexual species, C. tigris and C. septemvittatus, and the
triploid population involved a hybridization of the now all-female
allodiploid, C. tesselatus and C. sexlineatus (a third bisexual
species) (25). Parker and Selander (90) electrophoretically
examined diploid and triploid C. tesselatus. The triploid C.
tesselatus (identified electrophoretically) were all deemed to be
members of a single clone and the diploid parthenogenetic females

represented as many as 12 electrophoretically distinguishable clones. Clones of another allotriploid species, C. exsanguis, have been identified karyotypically (76).

Tetraploid, Hexaploid, Octoploid Frogs

In 1949, Wickbom (91) reviewed the available information and concluded that anuran chromosomes were very stable. Prior to 1959, most anuran species consistantly demonstrated chromosome numbers which confirmed this hypothesis, but in the examination of South American leptodactylid frogs, Saez and Brum's discovery (92,93) of 42 chromosomes in Odontophrynus americanus and up to 108 chromosomes in Ceratophrys ornata opposed such a generality. They also found some configurations in C. ornata which resembled multivalent associations. Saez and Brum did not attribute the elevated chromosome numbers to polyploidy but discussed chromosome number variability and "mixoploidy." In a subsequent study, Saez and Brum-Zorrilla (94) examined chromosomes from Uruguayan and Argentine populations and found O. americanus to have chromosome numbers of 42, 44 and 50 in different populations. Two other Odontophrynus species were found to have only 22 chromosomes. Rather than polyploidy, they considered O. americanus to be "a very polymorphic species." In the same year, M.L. Becak et al. (10) established that O. <<americanus>> in Brazil was a constant tetraploid. Additional studies in Argentina, Uruguay, and Brazil (8,9,95-98) clarified the polyploid nature of Odontophrynus <<americanus>> which has diploid and tetraploid populations in Argentina and Brazil. Barrio and Pistol de Rubel (95) examined 39 different populations in Argentina and Uruguay and found only diploids (2n=22) or tetraploids (2n=44). Individuals having 42 or 50 chromosomes were not found, nor were any diploid-tetraploid sympatric populations. There is no mention of the number of individuals sampled in either Saez and Brum-Zorilla's (94) study or that of Barrio and Pistol de Rubel (95). Ceratophrys <<ornata>> turned out to be an octoploid species with 104 chromosomes (9,96) as did C. dorsata in Brazil (8) but diploid (2n=26) populations of C. <<ornata>> are also found in Argentina (96,98).

The number of known bisexual polyploid species (or populations) has increased dramatically in the past few years: Hyla versicolor in North America (12); Pleurodema kreigi (11,98) in Argentina; Pleurodema bibroni (11) in Uruguay; Bufo <<kavirensis>> in Kirghizia (15); Xenopus ruwenzoriensis, X. vestitus, and X. sp. in Uganda (6,7); Dicroglossus [or Rana] <<occipitalis>>, Pyxicephalus [or Tomopterna or Rana] <<delalandii>>, and Bufo sp. D in Africa (16); Bufo danatensis in Turkmen (14) (Fig. 2-3). Many of the polyploid species have been found to have morphologically very similar diploid "cryptic species" (13,14,16,97,98). There is very little information concerning the population dynamics of many of the polyploid bisexual frog species (or populations) but, admittedly, most have only recently been discovered and some

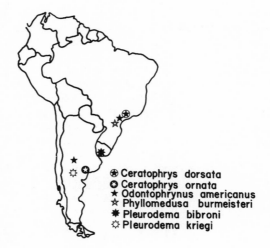

Fig. 2.   Localities in South America where polyploid anuran
species have been encountered.

occur in fairly remote regions.   Only <u>Hyla versicolor</u> has been
sufficiently studied to provide populational data which may be
relevant to bisexual polyploid frogs generally.   The diploid-
tetraploid cryptic species pair, <u>Hyla chrysoscelis</u> and <u>H</u>. versi-
<u>color</u> has received more attention than most as differences
between these species were recognized, not by morphology but by
acoustics, as early as 1958 by Blair (99), twelve years before <u>H</u>.
<u>versicolor</u> was determined to be a tetraploid.   In attempting to
explain the acoustical differences noted by Blair, Johnson (100)
analyzed calls from additional populations and produced viable
hybrids between "slow" and "fast-calling" populations.   Backcrosses
involving F_1 males only produced a few short-lived tadpoles which
justified specific designation for both call types.   The ranges
of the species have been outlined using pulse-rate analyses of
calling males (40,99,101-107).   Even though there appear to be
some minor differences in morphology in some areas (40,105) both

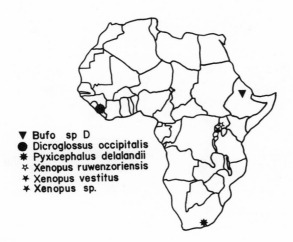

▼ Bufo sp D
● Dicroglossus occipitalis
✳ Pyxicephalus delalandii
✰ Xenopus ruwenzoriensis
✶ Xenopus vestitus
✴ Xenopus sp.

Fig. 3.   Localities in Africa where polyploid anuran species
have been encountered.

species are variable over their ranges and no over-all morphometric
analysis has been found to distinguish all members of either
species.
     Finding H. versicolor to be tetraploid and H. chrysoscelis
to be diploid (12,98) (see chromosomes, Fig. 4) helped to explain
the hybridization experiments of Johnson (100) in that the hybrids
would be triploids and, evidently, sterile. Also, chromosomal
information has assisted with the identification of females, which
do not vocalize, and in the establishment of more accurate ranges.
The distribution of both species is provided in Fig. 5, which
represents the compilation of data obtained from the previous acoustical studies, and information I have accumulated over the past six
years from chromosomes and nucleoli (108).   There is much more
overlap and apparent sympatry than has been indicated previously
(105,106), especially in the north. Viable triploid hybrids are
easily produced artificially, but only one "intermediate call"
which may be that of a hybrid (107), has ever been reported in
nature.   There are some indications that this cryptic species
pair may be a cryptic species complex involving three or even four

Hyla chrysoscelis and Hyla versicolor

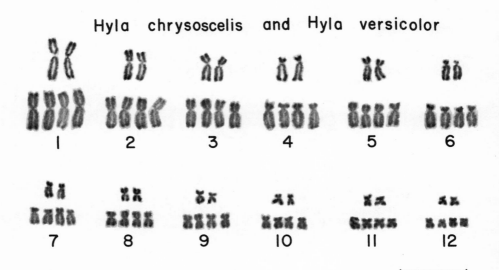

Fig. 4. Representative karyotypes of Hyla crysoscelis
(2n=24) and H. versicolor (2n=4x=48). H. chrysoscelis chromosomes
are above those of H. versicolor for each supposed homologous
set. Both specimens were males and came from a sympatric pond at
Lake Riviera Road and Highway 1, s.e. Manitoba. The scale is
20 μm.

species according to acoustical analyses (103,104,106), micro-
complement fixation (109), and electrophoresis (110).

DISCUSSION

     It is very likely that autopolyploids do arise from time to
time in natural populations as indicated by random sampling among
individuals in natural populations (27), the large number of
diploid eggs which some females seem to normally produce (35-37),
and the ease by which polyploidy can be experimentally induced.
The newly formed autopolyploid may be quite viable, but other
than any possible benefits of gene dosage, no unique combinations
of genes would be expected which would provide the individual
with a superior genotype, compared with normal diploids in a
natural population. As well as the physiological problems which
must be associated with increased cell size and an unbalanced

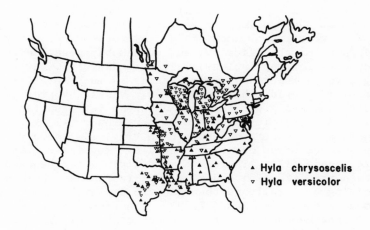

Fig. 5. Localities for tetraploid <u>Hyla</u> <u>versicolor</u> and diploid <u>Hyla</u> <u>chrysoscelis</u>.

genetic composition, gamete production could not procede in a normal fashion. Selection should be severe against autopolyploids living in competition with normally reproducing individuals having the same alleles. If, however, the original parents of a polyploid were genetically dissimilar, an allotriploid would have unique allelic combinations as well as maintaining a normal set of chromosomes from one parent.

Blair (see 111 for summary and references) has hybridized toads from all over the world. Chromosomal investigations from tadpoles produced from some of his several hundred cross combinations (35,36) demonstrated that polyploid tadpoles appear occasionally in control crosses, and in low frequencies if the parents are considered to be included in the same species group. The frequencies of polyploids increases substantially if the parents are from different species grouping and, in some crosses involving very distantly related species, only polyploids are found. It is not suggested that hybridization produces polyploids, since the number of polyploid individuals in any cross represents only a small fraction of the eggs which initially cleaved. Clearly, there is strong selection against certain diploid hybrids which

does not, in many cases, seem to affect the polyploids. Selection
would seem to operate against lethal genetic combinations, and
the addition of (a) maternal chromosome set(s) endows the hybrid
with viable gene combinations.

Although the crosses involving very divergent species of
Bufo demonstrated increased viability with polyploidy, there is
reason to doubt the applicability of this hypothesis to any of
the polyploid reptiles or amphibians. All of the presently known
polyploids have morphologically, and presumably genetically,
similar species (or populations) which are diploids. Hybridization
involving closely related diploid species is much more likely to
produce diploid hybrids than polyploids. Viable hybrids (presumably diploid) are produced when Ambystoma jeffersonianum is
crossed with A. laterale (53) or even A. texanum (47,49). Diploid
R. <<esculenta>> are more numerous than triploids and a R.
<<esculenta>> phenotype may be produced by crossing R. lessonae
with R. ridibunda (17). There are more diploid parthenogenetic
lizards than triploid (75) and triploid lizards have been produced
by hybridizing a normally parthenogenetic diploid female with a
male from a bisexual species (87,89). The formation of diploid
or triploid parthenogenetic or gynogenetic species by hybridization
has been proposed for many of the unisexual amphibians and reptiles
(20,25,54,89,112), as well as fish (68,69,113) and insects (114,115)
Initial hybrid advantage, if present, could be easily lost by
backcrossing and gene exchange with the parental species or
breeding among the hybrids. The obvious solution to these problems,
which has evolved independently in many groups of parthenogenetic
or gynogenetic animal species, is to maintain an independent gene
system meiotically.

Meiosis in polyploid females has been examined in only one
triploid salamander, Ambystoma tremblayi (55,56), and one triploid
lizard, Cnemidophorus uniparens (86). Observations, based on
numbers of chromosomes in first prophase, suggest that a premeiotic endomitosis produces a hexaploid oögonial cell which,
through meiotic reduction, results in triploid eggs. Most of the
synaptic complexes are bivalents but, of the twenty eggs from
three triploid females examined by MacGregor and Uzzell (56), two
quadrivalents were observed in one egg and one quadrivalent was
observed in each of two other eggs. They also found twice as
many chiasmata in the triploid as in the diploid eggs, but
assumed they involved pseudobivalents of sister chromosomes so
that any recombination would be meaningless genetically. In
spite of this limited information, the process of premeiotic
endomitosis has been widely disseminated as the mechanism for
maintaining somatic ploidy in virtually all parthenogenetic or
gynogenetic amphibians and reptiles (85,112,116). This same
mechanism is even speculated to occur in Rana <<esculenta>> for
the production of diploid eggs or sperm (70). In diploid R.
<<esculenta>> the genomes are apparently segregated such that the
R. ridibunda or R. lessonae genome ends up in the first polar

body, which is eliminated, and the remaining R. lessonae or R. ridibunda genome passes through a second meiotic equational division and remains intact in the female egg nucleus. This mechanism is termed "hybridogenesis" and has been likened to similar meiotic events postulated in some unisexual fish (68,69). Cytological documentation for these proposed meiotic events is not available, but they have been inferred based on numerous progeny which have resulted from several matings (17,65,70). Meiosis in male R. <<esculenta>> has revealed some multivalents and bridges (72), thus suggesting genetic recombination between non-sister homologues.

Observations of meiosis in tetraploid males often demonstrates quadrivalent associations involving the four supposedly homologous chromosomes (10,98,117). Meiosis in the octoploid Ceratophrys reveals bivalents, quadrivalents, hexavalents, and octovalents (8,92,96). However, only bivalents are usually found in both tetraploid Pleurodema species (11). The tetraploid species of Xenopus demonstrates bivalents, but multivalents were sometimes found in the hexaploid Xenopus (7). Tetraploid Dicroglossus occipitalis and Bufo sp. D have twice as many bivalents in the first metaphase of meiosis as do diploid Dicroglossus <<occipitalis>> and Bufo kerinyagae (a close relative of Bufo sp. D) and no multivalents were found in these two tetraploid species. Tetraploid Pyxicephalus <<delalandii>> did demonstrate some quadrivalents, but they may be considered "loose quadrivalents" for they either dissociate during prophase or metaphase, or are not formed in some cells (Fig. 6). Multivalent associations have generally been used as evidence for chromosomal homology such that if a polyploid demonstrates multivalents it is assumed to be an autopolyploid. Allopolyploids, on the other hand, would show few if any multivalents because the hybrid set of chromosomes would not be homologous. If this is true, multivalent associations could be used as evidence that some anuran polyploids were derived from hybridization involving genetically divergent parents (allopolyploidy), but others, which show multivalent associations evolved from a single species (autopolyploidy). Chromosome morphology has also been used to distinguish between autopolyploids and allopolyploids in triploid Cnemidophorus (76,118) and in the Pleurodema tetraploids which have some chromosomes which do not form a morphologically similar set of four for some of the groups (11,98). The Pleurodema species do not demonstrate multivalents. In the same context, it is interesting to note that the tetraploid Pyxicephalus <<delalandii>>, which does demonstrate some quadrivalent formation, has a karyotype in which 11 of the 13 chromosome sets of this species are easily grouped into 4 morphologically "homologous" chromosomes. This may be compared with only 5 of the 10 chromosome sets in Bufo sp. D and 8 of the 13 sets in Dicroglossus <<occipitalis>> (Fig. 7) which do not demonstrate quadrivalents (Fig. 6).

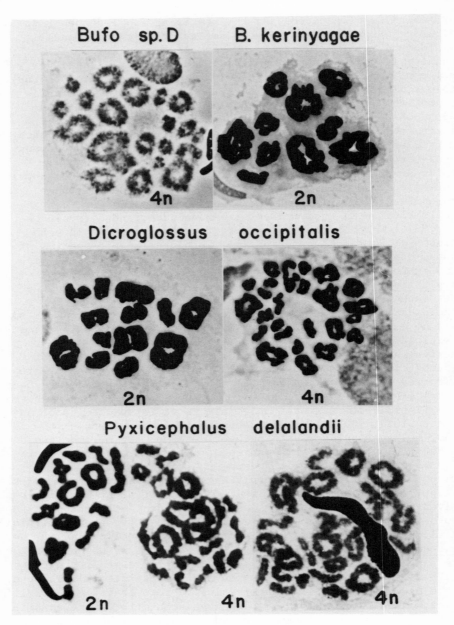

Fig. 6.   Meiotic metaphase I of diploid and tetraploid African bufonid and ranid cyptic species. Multivalents are not present in Bufo sp. D or the tetraploid Dicroglossus.   Some multivalents are demonstrated in some cells of the tetraploid Pyxicephalus (middle spread) but not other cells of the same male (right spread).

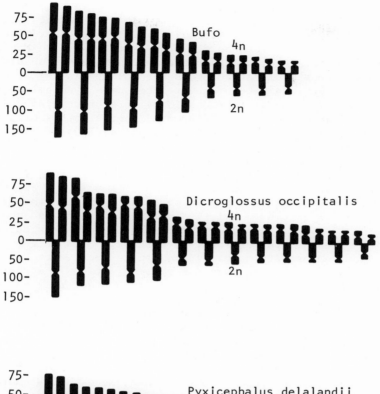

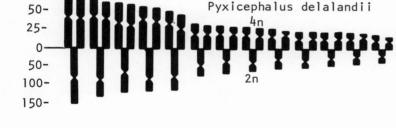

Fig. 7.   Idiograms of diploid and tetraploid African bufonid and ranid cryptic species.   The scale is the percent (X10) of the chromosome complement divided by 2.   If the haploid complement of the diploid species (below the axis) are compared with that of the tetraploid species (above the axis) it is evident that some chromosome sets of the tetraploid are not identical to the supposed homologous chromosome in the diploid.   This could be the result of allopolyploidy or chromosomal restructuring (diploidization) in the tetraploid.

It is possible, however, that mutational events would, over
time, alter the original genetic and chromosomal structure such
that homologies are lost. The multivalent association could,
perhaps, be a temporal indicator of polyploidy: recently evolved
autopolyploids would demonstrate multivalents but, over time,
fewer multivalent associations would be expected (98). Mancino
et al. (119) determined, using C-banded techniques which distinguished homologous from heterologous chromosomes in newts, that
chiasmata form between heterologous chromosomes even belonging to
the same specific genome (intra-haploid) in hybrids. Apparently,
synapsis in a hybrid may be so disrupted that pairings occur
between "re-duplicated" segments (sensu White (120)) which may
result in tri-, quadra-, hexa-, and octovalents even in a diploid!
This information clouds the issue concerning the use of multivalents to distinguish allo- from autopolyploids. But, if intra-
haploid associations do occur in hybrids of amphibians and reptiles,
we could be provided with a mechanism to help explain the segregation of parental genomes. Meiotic dysfunction, such as hybridogenesis, could evolve rapidly if intra-haploid synapses kept the
respective parental genomes intact. Perhaps, in those polyploids
which do not demonstrate multivalents, there are few or no re-
duplicated segments in the parental genome. It would appear that
the interpretation of multivalent association must rely on the
ability to distinguish truly homologous chromosomes.

Although functional retention of the second polar body in
meiosis accounts for the great majority of polyploid amphibians
under experimental conditions and may account for the formation
of diploid eggs in some parthenogenetic lizards (80), it is
probably not the mechanism currently used in polyploid amphibian
and reptile species or populations. Asher, Nace, and Richards
(33,121,122) mathematically demonstrated the consequences of
various meiotic mechanisms and concluded that homozygosity would
be attained rapidly in such a system even in a polyploid.
Homozygosity has not been encountered in any unisexual or polyploid
amphibian or reptile which has been examined electrophoretically
(20,54,90,110,123-128). Most of the electrophoretic studies have
demonstrated fixed heterozygosity and gene dosage which helps to
substantiate hybrid origin hypotheses for unisexual and polyploid
amphibians and reptiles. Heterozygosity could be maintained over
many more generations through a pre-meiotic endomitosis (116,122).
But, these same studies raise an additional problem, since Asher
and Nace (122) also determined that fixed heterozygosity could be
maintained over many generations only by very strong selection
and it is, therefore, surprising that heterozygous genotypes
referrable to original parental species would be encountered as
often as they are. For a heterozygous pattern to be maintained
from some Pleistocene event is extremely unlikely. Some of the
supposed fixed heterozygosity would best be interpreted as the
result of a relatively recent hybridization or to be more apparent

than real. Uzzell and Goldblatt (54) examined only one presumptive
gene locus in 22 individuals which consisted of eight Ambystoma
jeffersonianum, 18 A. laterale, 10 A platineum, and six A.
tremblayi. Their study has been used to claim fixed heterozygosity
and dosage effects which may be used to differentiate the two
diploid and two triploid species. Recently, Downs (20) demonstrated allelic variability for this, presumably, same locus in
the diploids, A. jeffersonianum and A. texanum. In Ontario
populations of the Ambystoma jeffersonianum complex there appears
to be a considerable amount of variability in the general proteins
and at more than a dozen enzymatic loci (unpublished). General
protein phenotypes (Fig. 8) represent some of the range of variability which has been encountered in Ontario. Certain of the
triploid specimens do demonstrate what might be considered fixed
heterozygosity and dosage as do some of the diploids. These
results may be more easily explained by assuming that there are
two, rather than one, loci (GP 3,4), and that certain alleles are
overlapping. The overlapping alleles have the same appearance as
the presumed dosage effects which were presented by Uzzell and
Goldblatt (54) and Downs (20). Increased variability in this
complex would be more consistant with the hypothesis of Asher and
Nace (122), who predict heterozygosity in polyploids over time.
Fixed heterozygosity would be apparent for a relatively short
time only if the parents were determined to be fixed homozygotes
for different alleles and would, if evidenced, provide documentation for a recent hybridization. If, on the other hand, polyploidy
did arise from some single event several hundred generations ago,
we would expect random mutation, any possible recombination, or
selection to have altered the gene frequencies such that a hybrid
origin would not easily be identifiable electrophoretically.

Few electrophoretic studies have actually been performed
using large numbers of amphibian or reptilian polyploid individuals
from several populations. Parker and Selander's (90) electrophoretic study of C. tesselatus involved 339 diploid and 67
triploid specimens as well as 69 C. tigris, 62 C. septemvittatus,
and 34 C. sexlineatus (which have been implicated in the evolution
of C. tesselatus). They found an extremely high level of heterozygosity (.714) in the triploid clone and a very high level
(.560) in the diploid clones. Mean heterozygosity for most
vertebrate species ranges from .04 to .1 (129-131). Uzzell
et al. (74) found no evidence of recombination in a examination
of the descendants of a single Rana <<esculenta>> female which
was heterozygous for four alleles. Other investigations, however,
do reveal possible introgression between Rana lessonae and R.
ridibunda through R. <<esculenta>>. Günther and Hähnel (125)
studied LDH patterns in 159 R. lessonae, 62 R. ridibunda, and 402
R. <<esculenta>> from eleven different populations in Germany.
They found 5.7% of the R. <<esculenta>> to be homozygous for the
R. lessonae allele or the R. ridibunda allele. Three R. lessonae
had a R. ridibunda allele while 12 R. ridibunda had a R. lessonae

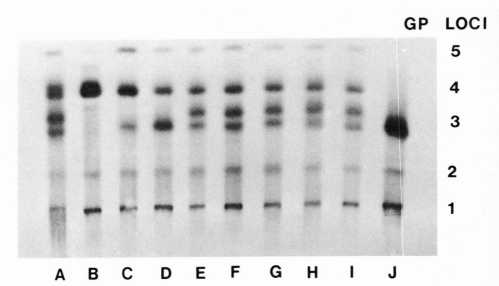

Fig. 8. Starch-gel electrophoretic patterns of serum proteins from members of the Ambystoma jeffersonianum complex in Ontario: triploid A. platineum (A,G,H,I); triploid A. tremblayi (C,D,E); A. laterale (B); A. jeffersonianum (J); and F is a triploid male. Loci 3 and 4 were examined by Uzzell and Goldblatt (54). They demonstrated fixed heterozygosity with dosage effects for the triploid female species. B,C,D, and J would appear similar to their figure for A. laterale, A. tremblayi, A. platineum, and A. jeffersonianum respectively. It appears that general protein loci 3,4, and 5 are polymorphic and have alleles which interact to produce the presumed dosage effect. It is not possible to use dosage as a species specific criterion in Ontario populations because of the evident variability in the triploid species. Variability among these loci was also demonstrated in Ohio (20).

allele. They concluded that gene flow had occurred between R. ridibunda and R. lessonae and that the R. ridibunda gene pool was less protected against R. lessonae genes than the R. lessonae pool was against those of R. ridibunda. Uzzell et al. (70) also indicated some slight gene flow between R. ridibunda and R. <<esculenta>>. Ralin and Selander (110) studied more than 300 specimens of Hyla versicolor and H. chrysoscelis electrophoretic- ally and determined that H. versicolor is much more variable than H. chrysoscelis and possesses more unique alleles.

Mechanisms for sex determination were originally postulated to be of paramount importance in the prevention of the formation of naturally occurring animal polyploids. Obviously, this obstacle has been independantly circumvented many times in animal populations. In the recognition of animal polyploids, it is now assumed that sex chromosomes are still in an initial state of differentiation for those groups which do demonstrate polyploidy (132). Of all the polyploids and possible ancestors in amphibians and reptiles, only Cnemidophorus tigris seems to have discernable sex chromosomes (133). Chromosomal evidence for female heterogamety in Xenopus laevis was presented by Weiler and Ohno (134) but these results were discredited by a more comprehensive chromosome study of normal and sex-reversed individuals of Xenopus laevis by Mikamo and Witschi (135). In Hyla arborea, Iriki (136) indicated that the male was chromosomally heterogametic, while Yosida (137) and Matsuda (138) claimed the female was heterogametic. Seto (139) did not find any difference in the male and female H. arborea karyotypes. Sex reversal experiments suggested that female toads (Bufo) and Ambystomatid salamanders are heterogametic (WZ) (140-142). In Rana, temperature shock treatments on eggs have produced all males (143) or all females (144) and the temperature during development may transform females into males (144). In some populations of Rana temporaria, females may change to males after having reached sexual maturity (146). Sex-reversal experiments indicate that the females of many species of Rana are homogametic (147). It is conceivable that selection can alter the frequencies of males and females in amphibians and reptiles in natural populations. Males are occasionally encountered in all-female populations but they may be selected against in the embryo, or they may be sterile (88). Females which produce males in all-female population would be selected against. Triploid R. <<esculenta>> may be male or female. Males contribute to the formation of R. <<esculenta>> in some diploid populations (with R. ridibunda) while females are more important for the continual production of R. <<esculenta>> in other populations (with R. lessonae). Tetraploids, hexaploids, and octoploids are bisexual and the mechanisms for maintaining sexual balance must have evolved independently several times. Perhaps genetic sexual balance is influenced by synaptic events in meiosis (98). Apparently, polyploids may be bisexual or all-female and this does not depend on the supposed heterogamety of either sex.

Evolutionary Considerations

Available information from presently known polyploids would suggest that most amphibian and reptilian polyploids arose through hybridization involving genetically divergent species or populations. The original hybrid produced would be genetically intermediate, probably diploid, and could survive in the same ecological situations as either parent (though not as successfully) but

could also survive in marginal or "average" habitats (more successfully). Selection would eliminate hybrids which engaged in large
amounts of genetic recombination with the parental species as
this would have the effect of strengthening isolating mechanisms
between the original parental populations. Those hybrids which
could maintain a hybrid advantage would survive over time and
this appears to have been accomplished by a meiotic mechanism in
which synapses between the original parental genomes is restricted.
Mancino et al.'s (119) discovery of intra-genome synapses in
hybrids is very significant and could provide a mechanism by
which original parental genomes could be segregated. Hybridogenesis could evolve under such a system and the particular
parental genome which would be maintained might be determined by
selection.   Genomes are selected differentially in populations of
Rana <<esculenta>> such that the R. lessonae chromosomes end up
in the majority of sperm cells if the female is R. ridibunda and
the R. ridibunda chromosomes usually are in the egg if the male
is R. lessonae. A pre-meiotic endomitosis could also circumvent
intergenomal synapses as sister homologous pair and any synapses
would be between these sister homogenetic chromosomes. Meiosis
would then procede fairly normally, and the eggs would be genetically and chromosomally identical to the female which produced
them. This mechanism has been proposed for parthenogenetic and
gynogenetic diploid and triploid species or populations. Most of
the information for amphibian and reptilian meiotic processes has
been obtained as inferrence from the analysis of the offspring
but it is assumed that the hybridogenetic mechanism in R.
<<esculenta>> is similar to that in poeciliid fish (68). All-
female diploid species may also have a premeiotic endomitosis as
suggested by Uzzell and Darevsky (112) for the Lacerta saxicola
comples, even though Darevsky (80) did not find the expected
altered number of chromosomes. Selection might operate to cull
out rapidly those individuals which were not capable of viable
solutions to reproduction, but there is some indication that
hybrids may, perhaps through the imbalance of chromosomes, be
able to achieve an endomitotic condition rapidly through the
process of hybridization. Hybrid Xenopus were produced by crossing
X. laevis and X. gilli (148, Kobel cited in 59) and females from
this cross produced two types of eggs (haploid and diploid). The
diploid eggs were the product of an endomitosis and bivalents
were formed between identical chromosomes. The diploid eggs were
fertilized using sperm of a third species (X. muelleri) and
produced trihybrid triploids. The triploid hybrids were viable
and the females produced triploid eggs by means of a premeiotic
endoduplication.

    Meiosis in triploid male R. <<esculenta>> appears to be
abherrant and there are various univalents, bivalents, multivalents, and bridges but there are also some normal-appearing
figures which, according to Günther (73) produce two size classes
of sperm. This can be referred to a haploid and a diploid

genetic constitution. The large (diploid) sperm cells are less common but may be involved in fertilization.

Objections which have been raised concerning parthenogenetic reproduction involving the reduction of genetic recombination and the subsequent accumulation of deleterious mutations (1,3-5) may not apply. It has been demonstrated that parthenogenetic species or populations are genetically variable (76,90) and do demonstrate enough recombination to counter the previous objections (33,121, 122). The parthenogenetic triploids or diploids have a greater reproductive potential than the bisexuals and it would seem that they would be able to disperse freely, colonize easily, and displace the original parental populations. Some parthenogenetic lizards which have not yet demonstrated a hybrid origin perhaps have displaced and eliminated one or both of their bisexual ancestors. In lizards, the mating behaviour may have some bearing on this problem. In many species (such as Cnemidophorus), males select females and may mate with anything that slightly resembles a conspecific female. This mating behaviour is important in the formation of hybrids and may also be important to confine the parthenogenetic females. Parthenogenetic females dispersing into the territories of a bisexual male would be inseminated. Experimental matings (76), planting females in natural populations containing bisexual males (87), and the sometimes finding of males in all-female populations, all demonstrate that this union produces triploids from diploid parthenogenetic females and tetraploids from triploid parthenogenetic females. Since there are no documented tetraploid parthenogenetic populations, it would seem that the tetraploid, having a balanced genetic system, may revert to random recombination. A tetraploid female may produce diploid eggs and a tetraploid male may produce diploid sperm. Assuming that the diploid gametes from the resulting tetraploids are viable, matings between the few rare tetraploids would be less common than backcrosses involving diploid bisexuals which would again produce triploids. So, the same rape-strategy in lizards which produces hybrid populations might also save parental populations.

Apparently, the gynogenetic triploid salamanders must depend on a bisexual male to initiate cleavage. If a parental bisexual male is not present in a population the triploids cannot survive, so the triploid females exist in a balance with the diploids. This situation if very difficult to comprehend for a number of reasons. It would appear that a diploid male who chose to mate with a triploid female could not contribute anything to future generations, and selection, operating at any level, would rapidly eliminate males which were not able to discriminate between members of their own species and the triploid parasites. Pre-mating isolating mechanisms, which are well developed in other salamander species, would be expected to evolve rapidly and this would eliminate the triploids. Also, in many populations, the triploids are much more successful than the diploids and ratios

of females to males may be as high as 50:1. One male would not
be able to provide enough spermatophores for 50 females and it
may be assumed that the ratio would be much higher if the males
were not a limiting factor in the production of triploid females
(Fig. 9). If, as has been suggested by several investigators

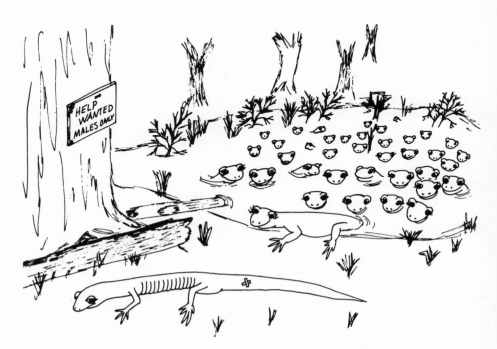

Fig. 9. Male salamanders in demand!

(20,53-55), some populations contain all female parthenogenetic
triploids or diploids, it would be expected that these clones
could easily eliminate the diploid bisexuals. The meiotic
mechanisms would be similar in the parthenogenetic and gynogenetic
females and the only difference would appear to be the mechanism
by which cleavage is initiated. The destiny of the sperm which
stimulates gynogenetic development in triploid Ambystoma has not
been investigated. In hybridization experiments, the sperm
nucleus unites with the egg nucleus unless the parents are
extremely genetically divergent such as in crosses between
families (34). Sperm has the capability of developing andro-
genetically even in cytoplasm of related species. Radiation is
usually employed to inactivate sperm nuclei for initiating
gynogenetic development. Most Ambystomatid hybridizations result

in normal zygote formation and not gynogenesis (47-49, 53,140). Parthenogenetic lizards may be inseminated and the sperm nucleus is incorporated. Occasional fusions would be expected to produce tetraploid offspring in the Ambystoma jeffersonianum complex but such individuals have not yet been encountered in this complex nor have mosaics, which might also be expected if the sperm may sometimes develop as a clone of haploid cells. A more reasonable hypothesis for the triploid Ambystoma would be the formation of diploid eggs so the sperm would be utilized to produce the triploids. This type of reproduction would satisfy most of the observations and provide a hybridogenetic mechanism similar to that believed to be operating in the Rana <<esculenta>> complex and poeciliid fish (68). Hybridization among A. jeffersonianum and A. laterale or A. laterale and A. texanum could produce a hybrid which, through a pre-meiotic endomitosis would produce diploid eggs. The egg could be fertilized by any available male of the complex producing triploids which would carry a full complement of genes from the sympatric diploid species, as well as a haploid set of chromosomes from one of the other species. The morphology of the triploid would be most similar to the sympatric species and this could explain the diploid bisexual - triploid unisexual pair associations. Triploid females could reject the male's haploid chromosomes by hybridogenesis and if an A. platineum dispersed into an A. laterale population, her fertilized eggs would result in the formation of A. tremblayi and account for the observed association in natural populations. Perhaps some percentage of the eggs or individuals are capable of parthenogenetic development either as diploid or, perhaps, as triploids. Parthenogenetic individuals could colonize easily and if diploid, could re-establish triploidy with other males. If the parthenogenetic female were triploid, the tadpoles would be expected to be tetraploid.

Unlike polyploid lizards and Ambystomatid salamanders in which the female cannot select an individual male, discrimination in anuran amphibians is a function of the female. Discrimination experiments amply demonstrate that females respond to conspecific vocalizations and may be essentially deaf to heterospecific males. Vocalization is considered to be the major isolating mechanism used by tetraploid Hyla versicolor and diploid H. chrysoscelis (103,104,106). In sympatry, females apparently discriminate very successfully. Perhaps this is the major reason that anurans demonstrate even-ploid polyploid bisexual populations, for even though tetraploid lizards of both sexes may be formed, there is no adequate mechanism to ensure that a tetraploid female will mate with a tetraploid male. The mechanisms for sound production and reception in anurans involve both the muscular system and the nervous system (149) and there is a possibility that increased cell size would alter male vocalization as well as the female's reception. The possibility also exists, however, that the demonstrated differences in vocalizations which have been found in <u>Hyla</u> <u>versicolor</u> and <u>H</u>. <u>chrysoscelis</u> or in diploid and tetraploid <u>Odontophrynus</u> <u>americanus</u> (98) were evolved subsequentially after polyploidization as a pre-mating isolating mechanism (Fig. 10).

Many anuran tetraploids have closely related diploid cryptic species or populations (13,14,16,96-98), and it may be assumed that the tetraploid arose from the similar diploid species. It

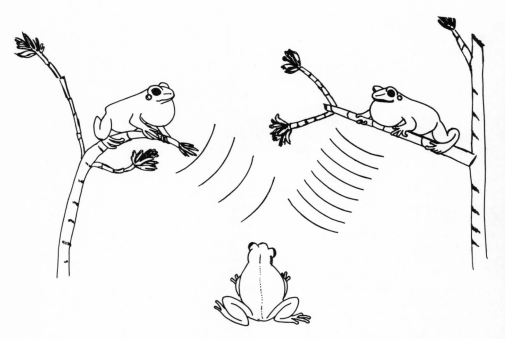

Fig. 10.   Discriminating female frogs!

is possible that a hybridization may have taken place which involved similar species or even genetically dissimilar populations of the same species. To be maintained, the hybrid would be expected to have a genotype which would be in some way advantageous. Present examination of tetraploids may not adequately provide the necessary information to outline their past history. Random recombination coupled with a larger possible number of alleles would, in a few generations, considerably alter the original ancestral genotype. Assuming a hybrid origin, successful tetraploids could eliminate one or both of the supposed parental populations. There is also the possibility that, if the tetraploid is an autopolyploid, it may eliminate diploids in certain parts of the former range resulting in partitioning of the

ancestral population into isolated groups. These isolates could
diverge genetically and speciate. Diploid eggs from a tetraploid
female may develop gynogenetically and produce diploid populations
derived from the tetraploid. I have tried various techniques
such as irradiated sperm, foreign sperm, and needle pricking to
induce gynogenetic development with Hyla versicolor eggs. The
very few diploids that do develop are never very viable and have
all died as tadpoles. I suspect that the large level of heterozygosity and possible mutant alleles in the tetraploid essentially
prohibits gynogenetic development. Also, if the tetraploid's
major advantage lies in its ability to carry a large variety of
alleles, the reduction in genetic variability which would be
necessary for the viability of a diploid gynogen would lead to
rare individuals which would be selected against.

In Kobel's (cited by Dubois (69)) experiments with Xenopus,
hybridization produced diploids which produced unreduced diploid
eggs. An additional hybridization involving the diploid eggs
produced triploids which also produced unreduced triploid eggs.
An additional hybridization or a backcross may produce a tetraploid. Triploid Rana <<esculenta>> apparently produce diploid
and haploid eggs or sperm (72,73). The possibility exists that
diploid eggs and sperm could unite and form a tetraploid although
this has yet to be demonstrated. I believe that if diploid and
haploid sperm are produced and are equally viable, the haploid
sperm would be more successful when competing for the same eggs.
I performed a simple experiment to justify my contention. Testes
were removed from diploid H. chrysoscelis and tetraploid H.
versicolor and minced together to form a sperm suspension which
consisted of haploid and diploid sperm. This suspension was used
to fertilize eggs of both H. versicolor and H. chyrsoscelis.
Sixty tadpoles were chromosomally sampled in each cross. All the
tadpoles from the H. versicolor eggs were triploid and all the
tadpoles from the H. chrysoscelis eggs were diploid. Obviously,
the haploid sperm were more successful. A small piece of testis
from each male was used for control crosses to ensure that each
male had viable sperm. Twenty control tadpoles from each female
were chromosomally examined and confirmed sperm viability. It
should be a simple matter to examine, chromosomally, the offspring
of triploid male and female R. <<esculenta>> to determine whether
the diploid sperm are capable of fertilizing diploid eggs.

The existing evidence for triploid lizards, salamanders, and
members of the Rana <<esculenta>> complex provides documentation
that triploids can arise by hybridization in natural populations
and that triploids are capable of producing triploid eggs.
Fertilization of the triploid eggs does produce tetraploids.
Because anuran tetraploid females are able to discriminate between
tetraploid and diploid males, tetraploid species are possible.
Higher levels of ploidy exist and may evolve from tetraploids.
Unreduced tetraploid eggs would be tetraploid and fertilization
by a diploid sperm would result in a hexaploid. Viable hexaploid

Hyla versicolor tadpoles are produced from time to time in control crosses (98). Even though this type of polyploidization could be termed autopolyploid, it would originate from a tetraploid which may be an allopolyploid and, thus, the hexaploid could be considered an autoallopolyploid. The octoploid species may have evolved from a tetraploid which produced completely unreduced eggs involving a tetention of the first polar body. These eggs would be octoploid and would have to develop gynogenetically. Octoploids could evolve from hexaploid unreduced eggs involving only the second polar body combined with diploid sperm from a tetraploid population. This mechanism would appear to be unlikely for it would involve tetraploid and hexaploid sympatric populations, although a situation such as this might be found when the hexaploid species is recently evolved. Retarded cleavage involving chromosomal division without cytokinesis in a tetraploid could also produce an octoploid, but this mechanism appears to be very rare even in experimental manipulations and would probably not initiate an interbreeding population of octoploids.

The evolutionary advantage of polyploidy in amphibians and reptiles would seem to rest in the ability to provide individuals with unique gene combinations. If selection can operate at the gene or chromosomal level, the gametes which are incorporated into the genome of a parthenogenetic diploid or triploid hybrid cannot be considered wasted. Rather, these genes can be clonally duplicated and, through genetic recombination, may eventually pass from one species into another such as has been evidence in the Rana <<esculenta>> complex (70,125). Similar introgression might be possible in the triploid lizards if males are produced which have viable sperm. Introgression might also be possible in the Ambystoma jeffersonianum complex. The genes which are passed would be expected to have been carefully screened by clonal selection and probably ideally suited to the existing environment. The polyploid triploid population may be likened to a gene bank account in which genes are deposited, accumulate rapidly in a new environment and, if they are withdrawn, can provide a distinct advantage to the individual receiving the new gene combination. Polyploid triploids may survive only under situations in which they maintain an advantage but then be displaced once the parental species have the genetic ability to live in the "hybrid" environment. Introgression might also be possible between diploid and tetraploid species through mismating, which produces, or recreates, triploids (14). Most tetraploids, however, and especially the higher even-ploid bisexual polyploids, have perhaps succeeded in escaping a situation which could lead to their demise. Genetic recombination and selection may enable the tetraploids, hexaploids, or octoploids to displace the diploid ancestors and even to speciate as polyploids in a normal fashion. Pleurodema bibroni and/or P. kriegi may have arisen from a tetraploid ancestor and Ceratophrys dorsata may have arisen from an octoploid ancestor (98). Over many generations, the polyploid nature of the genome duplications could be substantially altered as the species engage in diploidization. The fate of the tetraploid would be to become a diploid initially having an elevated number of chromosomes, additional loci, and a greater quantity of DNA. This process is assumed to have happened many times in vertebrate evolution (132,150), and contrary to previous speculations (151), may prove to be a significant aspect of speciation.

ACKNOWLEDGEMENT

I especially thank Doctors Cole, Ralin, and Selander for "preprints"; my graduate student, David Servage, for helpful suggestions and the use of electrophoretic information concerning the Ontario Ambystoma jeffersonianum complex; and my wife, Jo Ellen for assisting with the figures. Supported by grant No. A9866 from the National Research Council of Canada.

LITERATURE CITED

1. Muller, H.J., 1925, Why polyploidy is rarer in animals than in plants. Amer. Nat. 59: 346–353.
2. Kimura, M., Ohta, T., 1971, "Theoretical Aspects of Population Genetics," Princeton University Press, New Jersey. 219 pp.
3. Maynard Smith, J., 1971, What use is sex? J. Theor. Biol. 30: 319–335.
4. Maynard Smith, J., 1978, "The Evolution of Sex," Cambridge University Press, Cambridge, London. 222 pp.
5. Williams, G.C., 1975, "Sex and Evolution," Monographs in Population Biology. 8. Princeton University Press, New Jersey. 200 pp.
6. Fischberg, M., Kobel, H.R., 1978, Two new polyploid Xenopus species from western Uganda. Experientia 34: 1012–1014.
7. Tymowska, J., Fischberg, M., 1973, Chromosome complements of the genus Xenopus. Chromosoma 44: 335–342.
8. Becak, M.L., Becak, W., Rabello, M.N., 1967, Further studies on polyploid amphibians (Ceratophrydidae). I. Mitotic and meiotic aspects. Chromosoma 22: 192–201.
9. Bogart, J.P., 1967, Chromosomes of the South American amphibian family Ceratophridae with a reconsideration of the taxonomic status of Odontophrynus americanus. Canad. J. Genet. Cytol. 9: 531–542.
10. Becak, M.L., Becak, W., Rabello, M.N., 1966, Cytological evidence of constant tetraploidy in the bisexual South American frog Odontophrynus americanus. Chromosoma 19: 188–193.
11. Barrio, A., Rinaldi de Chiere, P., 1970, Estudios cito-genéticos sobre el genero Pleurodema y sus consecuencias evolutivas (Amphibia, Anura, Leptodactylidae). Physis 30: 309–319.

12. Wasserman, A.O., 1970, Polyploidy in the common tree toad, Hyla versicolor Le Conte. Science 167: 385-386.

13. Batistic, R.F., Soma, M., Becak, M.L, Becak, W., 1975, Further studies on polyploid Amphibians. A diploid population of Phyllomedusa burmeisteri. J. Heredity 66: 160-162.

14. Pisanetz, Ye.M., 1978, New polyploid species of Bufo danatensis Pisanetz, sp. nov., from the Turkmen SSR. SOPOV AKAD NAUK UKR RSP SER. B HEOL BIOL NAUKY (3): 277-282 (in Ukranian).

15. Mazik, E. Yu, Kadyrova, B.K., Toktosunov, A.T., 1976, Peculiarities of the karyotype of the green toad (Bufo viridis) of Kirghizia. Zool. ZH. 55: 1740-1742 (in Russian).

16. Bogart, J.P., Tandy, M., 1976, Polyploid amphibians: three more diploid-tetraploid cryptic species of frogs. Science 193: 334-335.

17. Berger, L., 1977, Systematics and hybridization in the Rana esculenta complex, pp. 367-388 in Taylor, D.H., Guttman, S.I. (eds.), "The Reproductive Biology of Amphibians," Plenum, New York and London.

18. Günther, R., 1975, Zum natürlichen Vorkommen und zur Morphologie triploider Teichfrösche, Rana <<esculenta>> L. in der DDR (Anura, Ranidae). Mitt. Zool. Mus. Berl. 51: 145-158.

19. Uzzell, T., 1963, Natural triploidy in salamanders related to Ambystoma jeffersonianum. Science 139: 113-115.

20. Downs, F.L., 1978, Unisexual Ambystoma from the Bass Islands of Lake Erie. Occas. Pap. Mus. Zool. Univ. Mich. 685: 1-36.

21. Hall, W.P., 1970, Three probable cases of parthenogenesis in lizards (Agamidae, Chameleontidae, Gekkonidae). Experientia 26: 1271-1273.

22. Kluge, A.G., Eckardt, M.J., 1969, Hemidactylus garnoti Dumeril and Bibron, a triploid all-female species of gekkonid lizard. Copeia 1969: 651-664.

23. Pennock, L.A., 1965, Triploidy in parthenogenetic species of the teiid lizard, genus Cnemidophorus. Science 149: 539-540.

24. Lowe, C.H., Wright, J., 1966, Chromosomes and karyotypes of cnemidophorine teiid lizards. Mamm. Chrom. Newsletter 22: 199-200.

25. Wright, J.W., Lowe, C.H., 1968, Weeds, polyploids, parthenogenesis, and the geographical and ecological distribution of all-female species of Cnemidophorus. Copeia 1968: 128-138.

26. Parmenter, C.L., 1933, Haploid, diploid, triploid, and tetraploid chromosome numbers and their origin in parthenogenetically developed larvae and frogs of Rana pipiens and Rana palustris. J. Exp. Zool. 66: 409-453.

27. Fankhauser, G., 1945, The effects of changes in chromosome numbers on amphibian development. Quart. Rev. Biol. 20: 20-78.

28. Moore, J.A., 1955, Abnormal combinations of nuclear and cytoplasmic systems in frogs and toads. Adv. Genet. 7: 139-182.

29. Dasgupta, S., 1962, Induction of triploidy by hydrostatic pressure. J. Exp. Zool. 151: 105-116.

30. Ferrier, V., Jaylet, A., 1978, Induction of triploidy in the newt Pleurodeles waltlii by heat shock or hydrostatic pressure. Interpretation of the different types of ploidy using a chromosomal marker. Chromosoma 69: 47-63.

31. Rugh, R., Marshland, D.A., 1943, The effect of hydrostatic pressure upon the early development of the frog's egg (Rana pipiens). I. Macroscopic observations. Proc. Amer. Phil. Soc. 86: 459-466.

32. Volpe, E.P., Dasgupta, S., 1962, Gynogenetic diploids of mutant leopard frogs. J. Exp. Zool. 151: 287-302.

33. Nace, G.W., Richards, C.M., Asher, J.H., Jr., 1970, Parthenogenesis and genetic variability. I. Linkage and inbreeding estimations in the frog, Rana pipiens. Genetics 66: 349-368.

34. Volpe, E.P., 1970, Chromosome mapping in the leopard frog. Genetics 64: 11-21.

35. Bogart, J.P., 1969, Chromosomal evidence for evolution in the genus Bufo. Ph.D. dissertation, Univ. of Texas at Austin. 217 pp.

36. Bogart, J.P., 1972, Karyotypes, pp. 171-195, in Blair, W.F. (ed.), "Evolution in the Genus Bufo," University of Texas Press, Austin.

37. Richards, C.M., Nace, G.W., 1977, The occurrence of diploid ova in Rana pipiens. J. Heredity 68: 307-312.

38. Wasserman, A.O., 1970, Chromosomal studies of the Pelobatidae (Salientia) and some instances of ploidy. Southwest. Nat. 15: 239-248.

39. Hertwig, G., Hertwig, P., 1920, Triploide Froschlarven. Arch. Mikr. Anat. 94: 34-54.

40. Jaslow, A.P., Vogt, C., 1977, Identification and distribution of Hyla versicolor and Hyla chrysoscelis in Wisconsin. Herpetologica 33: 201-205.

41. Kawamura, T., 1939, Artificial parthenogenesis in the frog. II. The sex of parthenogenetic frogs. J. Sci. Hiroshima Univ. Ser. B., Div. 1. 7: 39-86.

42. Kawamura, T., 1941, The sex of triploid frogs in Rana nigromaculata. Zool. Mag. (Tokyo) 53: 334-347.

43. Kawamura, T., 1952, Triploid hybrids of Rana japonica Günther female x Rana tempororia ornativentris Werner male. J. Sci. Hiroshima Univ. Ser. B., Div. 1, 12: 39-46.

44. Kawamura, T., Nishioka, M., 1977, Reproductive biology of Japanese anurans, pp. 103-139, in Taylor, D.H., Guttman, S.I. (eds.), "The Reproductive Biology of Amphibians," Plenum, New York and London.

45. Tompkins, R., 1978, Triploid and gynogenetic diploid Xenopus laevis. J. Exp. Zool. 203: 251-256.

46. Wright, D.A., Huang, C.P., Chuoke, B.D., 1976, Meiotic origin of triploidy in the frog detected by genetic analysis of enzyme polymorphisms. Genetics 84: 319-332.

47. Brandon, R.A., 1977, INterspecific hybridization among Mexican and United States salamanders of the genus Ambystoma under laboratory conditions. Herpetologica 33: 133-152.

48. Humphrey, R.R., 1962, Mexican axolotls, dark and mutant white strains: care of experimental animals. Bull. Philadelphia Herpetol. Soc. 19: 21-25.

49. Nelson, C.R., Humphrey, R.R., 1972, Artificial interspecific hybridization among Ambystoma. Herpetologica 28: 27-32.

50. Clanton, W., 1934, An unusual situation in the salamander Ambystoma jeffersonianum (Green). Occas. Pap. Mus. Zool. Univ. Mich. No. 290: 1-14.

51. Bishop, S.C., 1941, The salamanders of New York. Bull. N.Y. St. Mus. No. 324: 1-365.

52. Minton, S.A., Jr., 1954, Salamanders of the Ambystoma jeffersonianum complex in Indiana. Herpetologica 10: 173-179.

53. Uzzell, T., 1964, Relations of the diploid and triploid species of the Ambystoma jeffersonianum complex (Amphibia, Caudata). Copeia 1964: 257-300.

54. Uzzell, T.M.,Jr., Goldblatt, S.M., 1967, Serum proteins of salamanders of the Ambystoma jeffersonianum complex, and the origin of the triploid species of this group. Evolution 21: 345-354.

55. Cuellar, O., 1976, Cytology of meiosis in the triploid gynogenetic salamander Ambystoma tremblayi. Chromosoma 58: 355-364.

56. MacGregor, H.C., Uzzell, T.M., Jr., 1964, Gynogenesis in salamanders related to Ambystoma jeffersonianum. Science 143: 1043-1045.

57. Tihen, J.A., 1958, Comments on the osteology and phylogeny of ambystomatid salamanders. Bull. Florida State Mus. 3: 1-50.

58. Freytag, G.E., 1959, Zur Anatomie und Systematischen Stellung von Ambystoma schmidti Taylor 1938 und verwandten Arten. Vierteljahrsschr. Naturforsch. Ges. Zurich 104: 79-89.

59. Dubois, A., 1978, Les problémes de l'espéce chez les amphibiens anoures, pp. 161-284, in Bocquet, C., Génermont, Lamotte, M. (eds.), "Les Problémes de l'Espéce dans le Régne Animal II," Societé Zoologique de France.

60. Berger, L., 1968, Morphology of the F_1 generation of various crosses within Rana esculenta - complex. Acta Zool. Cracoviensia 13: 301-324.

61. Blankenhorn, H.J., Heusser, H., Vogel, P., 1971, Drei Phäno-typen von Grünfröschen aus dem Rana esculenta - Komplex in der Schweiz. Rev. Suisse Zool. 78: 1242-1247.

62. Günther, R., 1973, Über die verwandtschaftlichen Beziehungen zwischen den europäischen Grünfröschen und den Bastard-charakter von Rana esculenta L. Zool. Anz. 190: 250-285.

63. Günther, R., 1974, Neur Datenzur Verbreitung und Ökologie
    der Grünfrosche (Anura, Ranidae) in der DDR. Mitt. Zool.
    Mus. Berl. 50: 287-298.
64. Tunner, H.G., 1974, Die klonale Struktur einer Wasserfrosch-
    population. J. Zool. Syst. Evol.-Forsch. 12: 309-314.
65. Tunner, H.G., Dobrowsky, M.T., 1976, Zur morphologischen,
    serologischen und enzymologischen Differenzierung von Rana
    lessonae und der hybridogenetischen Rana esculenta aus dem
    Seewinkel und dem Neusiedlersee (Österreich, Burgenland).
    Zool. Anz. 197: 6-22.
66. Knudsen, K., Scheel, J.J., 1975, Contribution to the syste-
    matics of European green frogs. Bull. Soc. Zool. Fr. 100:
    677-679.
67. Ebendal, T., 1978, De gotfulla gröngrodorna. Fauna och
    flora 1: 9-22.
68. Cimino, M.C., 1971, Egg-production, polyploidization and
    evolution in a diploid all-female fish of the genus Poecilio-
    sis. Evolution 26: 294-306.
69. Schultz, R.J., 1969, Hybridization, unisexuality and poly-
    ploidy in the teleost Poeciliopsis (Poeciliidae) and other
    vertebrates. Amer. Nat. 103: 605-619.
70. Uzzell, T., Günther, R., Berger, L., 1977, Rana ridibunda
    and Rana esculenta: a leaky hybridogenetic system (Amphibia
    Salientia). Proc. Acad. Nat. Sci. Philadelphia 128: 147-171.
71. Uzzell, T., Berger, L., 1975, Electrophoretic phenotypes of
    Rana ridibunda, Rana lessonae and their hybridogenetic
    associate, Rana esculenta. Proc. Acad. Nat. Sci. Philadelphia
    127: 13-24.
72. Günther, R., 1975, Untersuchungen der meiose bei Männchen
    von Rana ridibunda Pall., Rana lessonae Cam. und der Bastard-
    form Rana <<esculenta>> L. (Anura). Biol. Zentrabbl. 94:
    277-294.
73. Günther, R., 1970, Der karyotyp von Rana ridibunda Pall. und
    das Vorkommen von Triploidie bei Rana esculenta L. (Anura,
    Amphibia). Biol. Zentralbl. 89: 327-342.
74. Uzzell, T., Berger, L., Günther, R., 1975, Diploid and
    triploid progeny from a diploid female of Rana esculenta
    (Amphibia Salientia). Proc. Acad. Nat. Sci. Philadelphia
    127: 81-91.
75. Cole, Ch.J., 1975, Evolution of parthenogenetic species of
    reptiles, pp. 340-355, in Reinboth, R. (ed.), "Intersexuality
    in the Animal Kingdom," Springer-Verlag, Berlin, Heidelberg
    and New york.
76. Cole, C.J., 1979, Chromosome inheritance in parthenogenetic
    lizards and evolution of allopolyploidy in reptiles. J.
    Heredity 70: 95-102.
77. Cuellar, O., 1974, On the origin of parthenogenesis in
    vertebrates; the cytogenetic factors. Amer. Nat. 108:
    625-648.

78. Maslin, T.P., 1971, Conclusive evidence of parthenogenesis in three species of Cnemidophorus (Teiidae). Copeia 1971: 156-158.

79. Maslin, T.P., 1971, Parthenogenesis in reptiles. Amer. Zool. 11: 361-380.

80. Darevsky, I.S., 1966, Natural parthenogenesis in a polymorphic group of Caucasian rock lizards related to Lacerta saxicola Eversmann. J. Ohio Herpet. Soc. 5: 115-152.

81. Cuellar, O., 1968, Additional evidence for true partheno-genesis in lizards of the genus Cnemidophorus. Herpetologica 24: 146-150.

82. Cuellar, O., Kluge, A.G., 1972, Natural parthenogenesis in the gekkonid lizard Lepidodactylus lugubris. J. Genetics 61: 14-26 + 2 pl.

83. Cole, C.J., 1978, Parthenogenetic lizards. Science 201: 1154-1155.

84. Wright, J.W., 1978, Parthenogenetic lizards. Science 201: 1152-1154.

85. Cuellar, O., 1977, Animal parthenogenesis. Science 197: 837-843.

86. Cuellar, O., 1971, Reproduction and the mechanism of meiotic restitution in the parthenogenetic lizard Cnemidophorus uniparens. J. Morph. 133: 139-165.

87. Darevsky, I.S., Danielyan, F.D., 1968, Diploid and triploid progeny arising from natural mating of parthenogenetic Lacerta armeniaca and L. unisexualis with bisexual L. saxicola valentini. J. Herpetology 2: 65-69.

88. Darevsky, I.S., Kupriyanova, L.A., Bakradze, M.A., 1978, Occasional males and intersexes in parthenogenetic species of Caucasian rock lizards (genus Lacerta). Copeia 1978: 201-207.

89. Lowe, C.H., Wright, J.W., Cole, C.J., Bezy, R.L., 1970, Natural hybridization between the teiid lizards Cnemidophorus sonorae (parthenogenetic) and Cnemidophorus tigris (bisexual). Syst. Zool. 19: 114-127.

90. Parker, E.D., Jr., Selander, R.K., 1976, The organization of genetic diversity in the parthenogenetic lizard Cnemidophorus tesselatus. Genetics 84: 791-805.

91. Wickbom, T., 1949, Further cytological studies on Anura and Urodela. Hereditas 35: 33-48.

92. Saez, F.A., Brum, N., 1959, Citogenetica de anfibios anuros de América del Sur. Los cromosomas de Odontophrynus americanus y Ceratophrys ornata. Anal. Fac. Med. Montevideo 44: 414-423.

93. Saez, F.A., Brum, N., 1960, Chromosomes of South American amphibians. Nature 185: 945.

94. Saez, F.A., Brum-Zorilla, N., 1966, Karyotype variation in some species of the genus Odontophrynus (Amphibia-Anura). Caryologia 19: 55-63.

95. Barrio, A., Pistol de Rubel, D., 1972, Encuesta cariotipica de poblaciones argentino-uruguayas de Odontophrynus americanus (Anura, Leptodactylidae) relacionada con otros rasquos taxonomicos. Physis 31: 281-291.

96. Barrio, A., Rinaldi de Chieri, P., 1970, Relaciones cario-sistematicas de los Ceratophryidae de la Argentina (Amphibia, Anura). Physis 30: 321-329.

97. Becak, M.L., Becak, W., Vizotto, L.D., 1970, A diploid population of the polyploid Amphibian Odontophrynus americanus and an artificial intraspecific triploid hybrid. Experientia 26: 545-546.

98. Bogart, J.P., Wasserman, A.O., 1972, Diploid-tetraploid cryptic species pairs: a possible clue to evolution by polyploidization in Anuran Amphibians. Cytogenetics 11: 7-24.

99. Blair, W.F., 1958, Mating call in the speciation of Anuran Amphibians. Amer. Nat. 92: 27-51.

100. Johnson, C., 1966, Species recognition in the Hyla versicolor complex. Texas J. Sci. 18: 361-364.

101. Bogart, J.P., Jaslow, A.P., 1979, Distribution and call parameters of Hyla chrysoscelis and Hyla versicolor in Michigan. Roy. Ontario Mus. Life Sci. Contr. 117: 1-13.

102. Brown, L.E., Brown, J.R., 1972, Mating calls and distri-butional records of treefrogs of the Hyla versicolor complex in Illinois. J. Herpetology 6: 233-234.

103. Gerhardt, H.C., 1974, Mating call differences between eastern and western populations of the treefrog, Hyla chrysoscelis. Copeia 1974: 534-536.

104. Gerhardt, H.C., 1978, Temperature coupling in the vocal communication system of the gray tree frog, Hyla versicolor. Science 199: 992-994.

105. Ralin, D.B., 1968, Ecological and reproductive differentiation in the cryptic species of the Hyla versicolor complex (Hylidae). Southwest. Nat. 13: 283-300.

106. Ralin, D.B., 1977, Evolutionary aspects of mating call variation in a diploid-tetraploid species complex of treefrogs (Anura). Evolution 31: 721-736.

107. Zweifel, R.G., 1970, Distribution and mating call of the treefrog, Hyla chrysoscelis at the northeastern edge of its range. Chesapeake Sci. 11: 94-97.

108. Cash, M.N., Bogart, J.P., 1978, Cytological differentiation of the diploid-tetraploid species pair of North American treefrogs (Amphibia, Anura, Hylidae). J. Herpetology 12: 555-558.

109. Maxson, L., Pepper, E., Maxson, R.D., 1977, Immunological resolution of a diploid-tetraploid species complex of tree frogs. Science 197: 1012-1013.

110. Ralin, D.B., Selander, R.K., 1979, Evolutionary genetics of diploid-tetraploid sibling species of treefrogs. (Anura: Hylidae). Evolution 33: 595-608.

111. Blair, W.F., 1972, Evidence from hybridization, pp. 196-232, in Blair, W.F. (ed.), "Evolution in the Genus Bufo," University of Texas Press, Austin.

112. Uzzell, T., Darvesky, I.S., 1975, Biochemical evidence for the hybrid origin of the parthenogenetic species of the Lacerta saxicola complex (Sauria:Lacertidae), with a discussion of some ecological and evolutionary implications. Copeia 1975: 204-222.

113. Abramoff, P., Darnell, R.M., Balsano, J.S., 1968, Electrophoretic demonstration of the hybrid origin of the gynogenetic telost Poecilia formosa. Amer. Nat. 102: 555-558.

114. Suomalainen, E., Saura, A., 1973, Genetic polymorphism and evolution in parthenogenetic animals. I. Polyploid curculionidae. Genetics 74: 489-508.

115. White, M.J.D., Contreras, N., Cheney, J., Webb, G.C., 1977, Cytogenetics of the parthenogenetic grasshopper Warramaba (formerly Moraba) virgo and its bisexual relatives. II. Hybridization studies. Chromosoma 61: 127-148.

116. Uzzell, T., 1970, Meiotic mechanisms of naturally occurring unisexual vertebrates. Amer. Nat. 104: 433-445.

117. Becak, M.L., Becak, W., 1970, Further studies on polyploid amphibians (Ceratophrydidae). III. Meiotic aspects of the interspecific triploid hybrid: Odontophrynus cultripes (2n=22) X O. americanus (4n=44). Chromosoma 31: 377-385.

118. Lowe, C.H., Wright, J.W., Cole, Ch.J., Bezy, R.L., 1970, Chromosomes and evolution of the species groups of Cnemidophorus (Reptilia, Teiidae). Syst. Zool. 19: 128-141.

119. Mancino, G.M., Ragghianti, M., Bucci-Innocenti, S., 1978, Experimantal hybridization within the genus Triturus (Urodela: Salamandridae) I. Spermatogenesis of F_1 hybrids, Triturus cristatus carnifex x T. vulgaris meridionalis. Chromosoma 69: 27-46.

120. White, M.J.D., 1961, The role of chromosomal translocation in urodele evolution and speciation in the light of work done on grasshoppers. Amer. Nat. 95: 315-321.

121. Asher, J.H.,Jr., 1970, Parthenogenesis and genetic variability. II. One-locus models for various diploid populations. Genetics 66: 369-391.

122. Asher, J.H.,Jr., Nace, G.W., 1971, Th genetic structure and evolutionary fate of parthenogenetic amphibian populations as determined by Markovian analysis. Amer. Zool. 11: 381-398.

123. Becak, W., Pueyo, M.T., 1970, Gene regulation in the polyploid Amphibian Odontophrynus americanus. Exp. Cell Res. 63: 448-451.

124. Ebendal, T., 1977, Karyotype and serum protein pattern in a Swedish population of Rana lessonae (Amphibia, Anura). Hereditas 85: 75-80.

125. Günther, R., Hähnel, S., 1976, Untersuchungen über den Genflusszwischen Rana ridibunda und Rana lessonae sowie die Rekombinationsrate bei der Bastardform Rana <<esculenta>> (Anura, Ranidae). Zool. Anz. 197: 23-28.

126. Neaves, W.B., 1969, Adenosine deaminase phenotypes among sexual and parthenogenetic lizards in the genus Cnemidophorus (Teiidae). J. Exp. Zool. 171: 175-184.

127. Neaves, W.B., Gerald, P.S., 1968, Lactate dehydrogenase isozymes in parthenogenetic teiid lizards (Cnemidophorus). Science 160: 1004-1005.

128. Neaves, W.B., Gerald, P.S., 1969, Gene dosage at the lactate dehydrogenase B locus in triploid and diploid teiid lizards. Science 164: 557-558.

129. Nevo, E., 1978, Genetic variation in natural populations: patterns and theory. Theor. Pop. Biol. 13: 121-177.

130. Powell, J.R., 1975, Protein variation in natural populations of animals, pp. 79-119, in Dobzhansky, T., Hecht, M.K., Steere, W.C. (eds.), "Evolutionary Biology" Vol. 8, Flenum, New York.

131. Selander, R.K., Johnson, W.E., 1973, Genetic variation among vertebrate species. Ann. Rev. Ecol. Syst. 4: 75-91.

132. Ohno, S., 1970, "Evolution by Gene Duplication." Springer-Verlag. New York, Heidelberg, Berlin. 160 pp.

133. Cole, Ch.J., Lowe, C.H., Wright, J.W., 1969, Sex chromosomes in Teiid Whiptail lizards (genus Chemidophorus). Amer. Mus. Novitates No. 2395: 1-14.

134. Weiler, C., Ohno, S., 1962, Cytological confirmations of female heterogamety in the African water frog (Xenopus laevis). Cytogenetics 1: 217-223.

135. Mikamo, A.E., Witschi, E., 1966, The mitotic chromosomes in Xenopus laevis (Daudin): normal, sex reversed and female WW. Cytogenetics 5: 1-19.

136. Iriki, S., 1930, Studies on amphibian chromosomes I. On the chromosomes of Hyla arborea japonica Guenther. Mem. Coll. Sci. Kyoto Imp. Univ. Ser. B. 5: 1-17.

137. Yosida, T.H., 1957, Sex chromosomes of the treefrog, Hyla arborea japonica. J. Fac. Sci. Hokkaido Univ. Ser. VI. Zool. 13: 352-358.

138. Matsuda, K., 1963, Culture technique with some amphibian tissues and a chromosome study of the tree frog Hyla arborea japonica. Zool. Mag. 72: 105-109.

139. Seto, T., 1964, The karyotype of Hyla arborea japonica with some remarks on heteromorphism of the sex chromosomes. J. Fac. Sci. Hokkaido Univ. Ser. VI Zool. 15: 366-373.

140. Humphrey, R.R., 1945, Sex determination in ambystomid salamanders: a study of the progeny of females experimentally converted into males. Amer. J. Anat. 76: 33-66.

141. Ponse, K., 1930, Le probléme du sexe et l'évolution de l'organe de Bidder du crapaud. Proc. 2nd Inter. Cong. Sex Res. Edinb. 202-210.

142. Ponse, K., 1941, La proportion sexuelle dans la descendance tissue des oeufs produits par l'organe de Bidder de crapauds femelles (Note préliminaire). Rev. Suisse Zool. 43: 541-544.

143. Kawamura, T., Tokunga, C., 1952, the sex of triploid frogs, Rana japonica Gunther. J. Sci. Hiroshima Univ. Ser. B. Div. 1, 13: 121-128.

144. Sato, M., 1952, The sex of triploid frogs, Rana limnocharis. J. Sci. Hiroshima Univ. Ser. B. Div. 1, 13: 155-161.

145. Witschi, E., 1927, Testis grafting in tadpoles of Rana temporaria L., and its bearing on the hormone theory of sex determination. J. Exp. Zool. 47: 269-294.

146. Witschi, E., 1928, Effect of high temperature on the gonads of frog larvae. Proc. Soc. Exp. Biol. Med. 25: 729-730.

147. Kawamura, T., Yokota, R., 1959, The offspring of sex-reversed females of Rana japonica Guenther. J. Sci. Koroshima Univ. Ser. B., Div. 1. 18: 31-38.

148. Muller, W.P., 1977, Diplotene chromosomes of Xenopus hybrid oocytes. Chromosoma 59: 273-282.

149. Martin, W.F., 1972, Evolution of vocalization in the genus Bufo, pp. 279-309, in Blair, W.F. (ed.), "Evolution in the Genus Bufo," University of Texas Press, Austin.

150. Bisbee, C.A., Baker, M.A., Wilson, A.C., Hadji-Azimi, I., Fischberg, M., 1976, Albumin phylogeny for clawed frogs (Xenopus). Science 195: 785-787.

151. Bush, G.L., 1975, Modes of animal speciation. Ann. Rev. Ecol. Syst. 6: 339-364.

POLYPLOIDY IN ANIMAL EVOLUTION: SUMMARY

Owen J. Sexton

Department of Biology
Washington University
St. Louis, MO 63130

The three papers making up this portion of the symposium
have made three important points. The first is that the study of
polyploidy in animals is alive and well. The dynamic aspect of
current research in this area, as exemplified by these papers,
has important consequences for workers in the study of polyploidy
in plants. I shall return to this point.
    Secondly, the role of polyploidy in the evolution of various
animal taxa is highly variable. Drs. Lokki and Saura have stressed
the notion that polyploidy is rare among the insects and that it
is always associated with parthenogenesis. They have documented
the verified cases of polyploidy among the orders of insects.
Dr. Schultz has summarized the data indicating the more central
role of polyploidy in the evolution of certain taxa of fishes.
Some of the more primitive fishes are tetraploids (e.g., Polyodon
spathula, an inhabitant of the larger streams and rivers of
Missouri and elsewhere in the Midwest). The primarily North
American family of fishes, the freshwater suckers (Catostomidae)
are tetraploids, while the majority of the species of the minnow
family (Cyprinidae), a group from which it is presumed that the
catostomids have diverged, is diploid. Dr. Bogart's position on
the importance of polyploidy in the evolution of amphibians and
reptiles, is, I think it safe to infer, that so few detailed
cytological studies have been made on populations of the species
of these two taxa that it is still to premature to generalize.
These findings, on the variability of the extent of polyploidy in
animal groups, mirror those reported by the participants in this
morning's session on Polyploidy in Plant Taxa. There were two
extreme cases of the role of polyploidy in major plant taxa
mentioned: Dr. Delevoryas stressed the probably insignificant
role of polyploidy in gymnosperms, while the Drs. Wagner indicated

379

the widespread nature of polyploidy in the pteridophytes. A
major lesson from both of today's sections is that a major cytological survey of the genomes of animal taxa might turn up higher
incidences of polyploidy than are now apparent.

The third contribution, shared by all three papers, was that
polyploid populations and species of animals are genetically much
more diverse than had been suspected. Furthermore, each paper
directly or indirectly, attacked the notion that parthenogenesis
and/or polyploidy were necessarily dead ends evolutionarily. The
first paper documented the genetic variation of several species
of insect, using techniques demonstrating both chromosomal and
enzymatic polymorphism. Drs. Lokki and Saura then discussed the
geographical distribution of various genotypes and showed that
certain genotypes are more frequently associated with specific
ecological associations (e.g., the distribution of the weevil,
Otiorhynchus scaber relative to phytogeographic zones). Dr.
Schultz demonstrated the existence of distinct clones within
unisexual populations of the poeciliid genera, Poeciliopsis and
Poecilia. Clones can be so specialized that they can diversify
trophically (e.g., rockscrappers versus detritus-algae feeders).
Dr. Bogart reviewed the data on heterozygosity in amphibians and
reptiles. That a significant proportion of this variation is
post-polyploid or post-parthenogentic may not be acceptable to
all.

Two aspects of this unsuspected amount of heterozygosity
should be stressed. Dr. Bogart emphasized the potential role of
parthenogenetic diploids or triploids, in the introgression of
adaptive complexes from one species to another. Dr. Schultz
reinforced the view of Ohno and his laboratory that one evolutionary role of polyploidy was to provide uncommitted loci for adaptive
radiation.

These three papers have stressed ecological phenomena more
than previous presentations did. Two ecological points should be
indicated as guidelines for future research. The first deals
with the fitness of polyploid versus diploid bisexual populations.
The inference was clear in all three papers that many polyploid
populations are superior to diploid ones in response to physiological stress. Several papers yesterday discussed the same
topic. Dr. Tal described his work with diploid and cholcicine-
induced autotetraploid tomatoes and demonstrated that the polyploids were less subject to water stress (i.e., had low transpiration rates, higher root pressure). Dr. Lewis reviewed similar
work by Prof. H. Mooney and his laboratory who had contrasted the
diploid and sterile triploids of Thalictrum alpinum. The polyploids exhibited a greater rate of photosynthesis, etc.

Such experimental findings reinforce the conclusions based
upon field observations that polyploids (particularly the neopolyploids discussed by Dr. Ehrendorfer) seem to exploit a different
set of resources than do the parental diploids. For example,
Drs. Lokki and Saura state, "...present evidence indicates that

polyploid insects are more efficient than their bisexual diploid ancestors in occupying whatever niche is available."

At this juncture I would like to suggest that such work comparing polyploids with their diploid ancestors is incomplete in the sense that only one side of an equation is present. The presented side stresses the physiological characteristics of the various populations. The missing side is a quantitative description of related aspects of the habitats, including estimates of the variances of the different parameters. The matching of the physiological characteristics of the populations to the habitat characteristics would provide a stage for the examination of the relative competitive abilities (including the "species packing" of biotypes described by Dr. Schultz) of diploid versus polyploid population. That is, do polyploids seem to occupy more extreme habitats than diploids because the former have eliminated the latter competitively, or are the polyploids exploiting resources not available to the diploids? Dr. Bogart's paper dealt with this concern.

The second ecological point deals with comparative demography. Mention has been made several times in this symposium of the relative fertility and/or fecundity of diploids versus polyploids. (Recall, however, that Dr. Bogart described the reproductive advantage which parthenogenetic populations can have.) Such information is critical to answer the question posed previously, that is, how do polyploids outcompete diploids? Given that polyploids often exhibit lower reproductive values, one wonders how they replace diploids. One inference is that polyploids must exhibit other aspects of fitness related to their resistance to stress. One such component of fitness would be expected to be survivorship. Hence, broad demographic analysis of the two types of populations would be instructive.

Finally, the two approaches outlined above can be used to place diploid-polyploid complexes into the connotation of the r-selection to K-selection spectrum. Such a fusion may well contribute to a furthering of our understanding of the genetic and ecological dynamics of diploid and polyploid populations.

PART IV

POLYPLOIDY IN AGRICULTURE

POLYPLOIDY AND DOMESTICATION:

THE ORIGIN AND SURVIVAL OF POLYPLOIDS IN CYTOTYPE MIXTURES

A.C. Zeven

Institute of Plant Breeding-I.v.P.
Agricultural University
Wageningen, The Netherlands

Mixtures of cytotypes occur in nature and are grown by man. Such mixtures are often cultivated as a landrace, i.e., the farmer does not pay any attention to the types he is growing, or, if he does, he only carries out a mild selection pressure. Of course, he is not aware of cytotypes. For example, farmers in Ethiopia grow a mixture of hexaploid bread wheat and tetraploid durum wheat. Owing to gene exchange both the cytotypes resemble each other (1), and therefore the crop is "sown as mixtures, grown as mixtures, reaped as mixtures, threshed and milled as mixtures, baked and brewed as mixtures" (1) and stored as mixtures.
The principal advantage of growing a mixture is yield stability. For farmers of less developed countries (and in earlier days in Europe, North America and elsewhere as well) a high yield stability is and was of vital importance and much more important than a high yield. Farmers prefer a yield of say about 80% every year to a yield of 120% for several years followed by one year with a crop failure. As there are no means of long storage and of large scale transport to import food from elsewhere, a crop failure in one year would starve the people. Hence yield stability is of utmost importance.
We must realize that within cytotypes several genotypes are present. The better the analyzing techniques like electrophoresis the more genotypes will be discovered. The many genotypes would bring about a polygenotype effect, for instance, to prevent the outbreak of an epidemic or severe damage by drought, etc. (I do not use the term multiline effect as this term can only be applied to a mixture of lines and is therefore restricted in its meaning.)
Studies of mixtures of cytotypes may indicate the fate of a polyploid after its spontaneous origin in a population with plants of a lower ploidy level. It may succumb because it can

not reproduce or, if it does reproduce, the seeds may not germinate because of allelopathic action of the seeds of the parental population, or because they are chromosomally or genetically ill-balanced. They may succumb also because of competition. Whatever the fate, many polyploids do survive because we find them and grow them.

Other examples of mixtures of cytotypes of wheat are available. The first is the almost extinct Zanduri wheat, which consisted of three cytotypes: <u>Triticum</u> <u>monococcum</u> L. (2n=2x, AA), <u>T</u>. <u>timopheevi</u> Zhuk. (2n=4x, AAB'B') and <u>T</u>. <u>zhukovskyi</u> Men. & Er. (2n=6x, AAAAB'B'). It should be mentioned that only one plant of the latter was found. Another mixture of <u>Triticum</u> species was Makha wheat, which consisted of <u>T</u>. <u>dicoccum</u> Schubl. (2n=4x=28, AABB), <u>T</u>. <u>macha</u> Dek. & Men. (2n=6x=42, AABBDD) and <u>T</u>. <u>paleocolchicum</u> Men. (2n=4x=28, AABB). In such mixtures interspecific hybrids may occur, but no analysis of these mixtures has been made.

Grass species often are made up of several cytotypes and these with other plant species are grown together to form a grass field. Beds with cultivars of hyacinths may be mixtures of cytotypes and so may be beds of Southwind lily (<u>Ornithogallum</u> <u>thyrsoides</u> Jacq.). The latter consists of diploids (2x=12), triploids, hexaploids, and aneuploids (2). Southwind lily material will be further investigated to find out whether there is any relation between number of chromosomes and phenotypic characteristics. Apparently, the multiplier does not know about his growing and trading a mixture of cytotypes.

SOME GENERAL CHARACTERS OF POLYPLOIDS

In general, polyploids have larger dimensions and a greater adaptability than diploids and therefore polyploids are attractive for cultivation. The larger sizes are not only of importance for production of food and forage, but also for bigger plant parts like flowers. The greater adaptability is attractive because polyploids can be grown in various environments. So natural polyploids have drawn the attention of man, who often has domesti-cated them. Polyploids originating from domesticated crops possibly have a still higher value as they combine the advantages of a polyploid with those of domestication. Several crops have developed a ploidy series like 2x, 3x, 4x, 5x and higher levels. Those with an odd number, the anorthoploids, are often sterile, while the orthoploids are often fertile. However, there are many exceptions. Furthermore, we find aneuploids and these are often sterile, too. The sterile plants can only be maintained if asexual propagation is possible. Levan (3) listed the conditions which lead to a successful autopolyploidization: (1) the number of chromosomes of the diploid should be suboptimal; (2) the chromosomes should not be too large; (3) the species should be a cross-fertilizer, because heterozygosity leads to a better

acceptance of the polyploidization and for breeding (and natural
selection) there are possibilities for selection; and (4)   the
plant should be grown especially for its vegetative parts,
because fertility is often low or absent.   Successful natural and
artificial autopolyploids meet these conditions, as for instance,
3x sugar beet, 4x ryegrass, 4x red clover, 4x alfalfa, many ornamentals, Gros Michel banana, 3x apple cultivars, and potato, if
this is not a segmental autotetraploid.   Condition four is less
important for the maintenance of allopolyploids as they are
often quite fertile.   Successful natural and artificial allopolyploids are durum wheat, bread wheat, tobacco, sugar cane, mustard,
swedes, oats, banana cultivars, tall fescue, cotton species, and
maybe Johnson grass (Sorghum halepense (L.) Pers.) if it is not
an autotetraploid.

But we must realize that for a newly arisen polyploid,
having no or little selective advantage as regards its parental
diploid(s), the probability of survival is very small.   It resembles
the fate of a newly arisen mutant allele in a population of self-
fertilizing individuals.   If the next generation derives from a
random sample of the sowing seed or other propagules, the probability of the polyploid being among the offspring is very small.
If it should be present, its frequency would still be very low
and the chance of its presence in the following generation would
again be very low.   Anyhow, it will be lost within a few generations.   I shall not discuss this subject here further.

A study of cytotype mixtures will help to understand the bi-
lateral effects of the cytotypes within a population and the way
a newly arisen polyploid succumbs or survives.   If it survives,
it may remain an admixture of the populations, apparently similar
to Triticum zhukovskyi in Zanduri wheat.   Or it may suppress its
parental species, which may have been the case with bread wheat
in emmer wheat.

Furthermore, a polyploid derived from a domesticated crop
may be better than a polyploid arisen from a wild plant.   So the
sequence domestication-polyploidization would be better for man
than the sequence polyploidization-domestication.   In the first
case man selected the polyploid from the population of cytotypes,
in the second it was done by nature.   Man must have applied
different selection criteria than nature.   I will come back to
this later.

Also of extreme importance is the loss or, at least, decrease
of the extent of self-incompatibility of a diploid becoming a
polyploid.   Hence, the plant changes from a cross-fertilizer into
a self-fertilizer.   Jain (4) has described what this means.   The
main point is probably the fact that a single polyploid plant is
able to reproduce by selfing.

EXAMPLES OF CYTOTYPE MIXTURES

I will discuss with the aid of examples various relationships between the polyploid and its parent or parents. More examples will be found in literature.

1. Spartina townsendii – a successful wild and planted allopolyploid

A case of successful ousting of a parent species by its allo-polyploid in nature is the replacement of Spartina maritima (Curt.) Fernald Roth. (2n=8x=26). This allopolyploid is a derivative of the American S. alternifolia Loisel (2n=10x=70) and the European S. maritima, originated on the south coast of Great Britain and first described in 1870. Around 1906 it occurred on the Atlantic coast of France and spread along the coast replacing S. maritima (5). At present the allopolyploid is actually planted for land reclamation, but no domesticated types are yet selected.

2. Festulolium loliaceum – successful but unimportant hybrids

Hybrids between perennial ryegrass (Lolium perenne L., 2n=2x=14, genome formula LpLp) (abridged to L plants) and meadow fescue (Festuca pratensis Huds., 2n=2x=14, FpFp) (abridged to F plants) and their backcross hybrids are found in the swards of several European countries. The F_1 hybrid (LF) has 2n=2x=14, while, depending on the backcross parent, the 3x backcross hybrids can be divided into festucoid (2n=3x=21, FFL) and loloid (2n=3x=21, FLL) hybrids (6). They apparently survive in a mixture of the parental species and other species that compose the sward. However, their survival is influenced by environment as observed by Wit (7) (Table 1).

Table 1. Percentage of 2x FL and 3x FFL and FLL hybrid plants in swards at two sites in the Netherlands (7).

Site	Genome formula			
	FL	FFL	FLL	No.
Wageningen	6	84	10	99
De Kaag	9	29	62	88

The Wageningen population occurred in the forelands of the River Rhine that are annually flooded and mainly hayed. The De Kaag

population occurred on a lake bank that is not flooded, but is
intensively grazed and hayed every second year. The great difference in frequencies of the two 3x hybrids is striking. How did
this come about? Whittington and Hill (8) found that when perennial ryegrass and meadow fescue plants were growing together
haying promoted the survival of meadow fescue plants; perhaps
this is the cause of the high frequency of the FFL plants in the
forelands of Wageningen. In an experiment, hybrids disappeared
quickly from a population of parents and hybrids, and when seedlings of meadow fescue and perennial ryegrass were growing together,
the population consisted of about 10,000 perennial ryegrass
plants and only 6 meadow fescue plants at the time of flowering
(9). Gymer and Whittington (10) further investigated the survival
of hybrids by studying the survival rate of one FL and 5 FFL
genotypes in cytotype mixtures. It appeared that under equal
conditions the crowding coefficients of the parents and the
hybrids were the same. An increase of soil fertility (by flooding)
and drought (during the summer) increased the crowding coefficients
of the hybrids as regards those of their parents. So, although
2x and 3x hybrids arise rarely (6), they are able to survive
owing to a higher crowding coefficient under sward conditions.
They are almost sterile and therefore they maintain themselves by
vegetative propagation.

3. Alfalfa - a successfully domesticated autotetraploid

Alfalfa (Medicago sativa L.) is an example of a successfully
domesticated autotetraploid (2n=4x=32), although a few diploids
are also known (11). The same is true for wild alfalfa, but I
did not find information on the occurrence of 2x and 4x plants in
nature. Do they grow isolated, mixed, or in a neighbouring but
pure population?
According to Bingham and Gillies (12), the progeny of 2x X
4x cross is 4x. If this can be extended to all 2x X 4x crosses,
it means that a newly originated 4x plant easily produces 4x
progenies. Furthermore, if in 4x alfalfa a natural dihaploid is
produced, it will be pollinated by neighbouring 4x plants producing
a 4x progeny. Other 2x plants growing close together in a 4x
population may fertilize each other producing 2x progenies.
These will suffer from deleterious and lethal genes in homozygous
condition and therefore will have a low fitness. In the long run
the 2x plants will probably disappear from the population but
apparently there are some factors that protect them from extinction.
Many comparisons between 2x and 4x varieties of a crop are
faulty because of the confounding of the genetic and ploidal
effects. Therefore, Dunbier et al. (13) made 2x and 4x populations
that were genetically similar. Differences of dry matter weight,
fresh weight of trifoliate leaves, and DNA contents of these

leaves were strongly influenced by ploidy level. G6PDA (glucose-6-phosphate dehydrogenase activity) was influenced by ploidy level and genotype. So in unrelated 2x and 4x material gene dosage (polyploidy) and genetic regulation play a role.

4. Helianthus multiflorus - a domesticated allotriploid

Somewhere in Europe, after the introduction of the parental species of sunflower (Helianthus annuus L., 2n=2x=34, and H. decapetalus L., 2n=4x=68), the sterile 3x hybrid, H. multiflorum (2n=3x=51), arose. Both parents came from North America. The chance that this hybrid species originated there is quite limited, because sunflower is not common in n.e. North America where H. decapetalus is found (14). Due to its introduction in Europe the geographical barrier was removed. After its origin, man must have selected this hybrid from the mixture of sunflower and hybrid plants for its beauty and maintained it asexually.

5. Red horse chestnut - a successful octoploid

The red horse chestnut (Aesculus x carnea Lois., 2n=8x=80) is an octoploid of the European common horse chestnut (A. hippocastanum L., 2n=4x=40) and the American A. pavia L. (2n=4x=40). As an ornamental it is grown in many countries, but its place of origin is not known. A backcross of this hybrid with the common horse chestnut resulted in the sterile 6x A. x plantierensis André (15). Both chance hybrids must have been found among the seedling plants of a common chestnut.
Apparently they survived the early stage before they were discovered by gardeners who protected them. It would be interesting to grow such a mixture again and to study the crowding coefficient of each cytotype.

6. Pyrethrum - domesticated diploids and triploids

Most varieties of the self-incompatible pyrethrum (Chrysanthemum cinerariaefolium Vis.) are 2x (2n=2x=18) clones. When these clones grow together among the progeny, 3x plants may be observed (16). Apparently, they originate easily, sometimes even 'at a high incidence.' In Yugoslavia wild plants are grown together and hence 3x plants may occur. However, Parlevliet (17), while collecting germplasm in Yugoslavia, did not find any plant with a typical 3x morphology. There may be two factors that cause the extinction of 3x seedling. Firstly, 3x plants develop slower than 2x plants, and they may succumb through competition with the wild flora. Secondly, 3x plants have a lower drought resistance than 2x plants. No studies have been carried out to measure the ability of 3x plants to compete with 2x plants.

7. European aspen – a naturally occurring 3x in 2x populations

Not much use is made of polyploidy in tree crops. In general, autotetraploids grow too slowly and therefore are of no use for wood production. But for ornamental trees the slow growth might be an attractive character, especially in those crops where a dwarf gene has not been found.

Triploids, however, grow faster than diploids and therefore they are very suitable for wood production. Triploids may originate in nature or can be made artificially. Thus a fast growing clone of the European aspen (Populus tremula L.) was found to be a triploid (2n=3x=57) (18). Additional 3x clones have been identified.

8. Hyacinths, tulips, and narcissi – their breeding history

The relationship between ploidy level and breeding of new cultivars of hyacinth (Hyacinthus orientalis L.) is quite extra-ordinary. As many old cultivars are still available it is possible to follow their breeding history and hence their increase in number of chromosomes with time (Table 2).

Table 2. Breeding history and ploidy level of cultivars of hyacinth (19), 2n=2x=16.

Period	Crosses	Ploidy level of cultivars
1560–1850	2x X 2x	2x
1700–1900	2x X 2x	3x
1800–1920	2x X 3x	2x to 3x
1850–1920	3x X 3x	2x to nearly 4x
1900–1950	3–nearly 4x X 3–nearly 4x	nearly 4x

So with time the number of chromosomes of the newly bred culti-vars increased. However, 4x cultivars were not registered although 4x seedlings have been observed. Apparently the 4x cytotype is less attractive, but no information is available. There is another peculiarity connected with the increase of chromosome number, viz., the increase of percentage of blue-flowered cultivars (Table 3).

As the chromosome number of the cultivars increased with time the frequency of blue-flowered cultivars also increased with time. Although no direct explanation can be given for this phenomenon there must be a relationship between number of chromosomes, blue-flower, and vigour as was already suggested by Hibberd in 1880 (from 19). It would be interesting to investigate this further,

Table 3. Number of cultivars and of blue-flowered cultivars as regards their chromosome number of hyacinth, 2n=2x=16.

2n=	Cultivars		% blue-flowered of total
	Total	Blue-flowered	
2x	31	5	16
17-23	6	1	17
3x	20	8	40
25-28	9	5	56
29-31	11	9	82

by growing a progeny of nearly 4x X nearly 4x and scoring the number of chromosomes, the vigour, and flower colour of the seedlings.

Most cultivars of tulip (Tulipa L.) are 2x, a few are 3x, and still less are 4x. The 3x may be derived from 2x X 2x crosses, one of the parents producing 2n gametes. Kroon and Van Eijk (20) found that some 2x cultivars (read genotypes) were inclined to produce 3x progenies and hence produced probably 2n female as well as 2n male gametes. The 4x cultivars are derived from 2x X 4x crosses. The latter were produced artificially. With time the frequencies of 3x and 4x cultivars increase as was shown for hyacinth by Darlington et al. (19). It should be remembered that several Tulipa species have been used and are still being used to breed new cultivars.

The initial breeding history of Trumpet narcissus (Narcissus pseudo-narcissus L., 2n=2x=14) and of the Poet narcissus (N. poeticus L., 2n=2x=14) indicate a course identical to that of hyacinth. Triploid cultivars of Trumpet narcissus were grown in 1860 and 4x cultivars in 1890. However, 3x wild Trumpet narcissi were found and they may have been included in the breeding population. For Poet narcissus the era in which the first 3x cultivars developed is not exactly known, but 4x cultivars were found in 1930 (21, 22). Tetraploidy is nearing the optimum chromosome number as no cultivar with a higher chromosome number has been registered, although plants with higher chromosome numbers have been observed. Thus Wylie (22) found a 2n=41 plant; it had small flowers and was less robust than 4x plants. Later the breeding course of narcissus developed differently from that of hyacinth due to the use of other Narcissus species.

9. Sweet potato – a successful autohexaploid

Sweet potato (Ipomoea batatas (L.) Lam.) is probably an autohexaploid (2n=6x=90), and as no wild hexaploids have been found –

Nishiyama's 'I. trifida' being a feral sweet potato (23) – it is
possible that the autopolyploidization took place during domestication. Nishiyama et al. (24) suggested that the parent is the 2x
I. leucantha Jacq. This latter species may be a hybrid of I.
lacunosa L. and I. trichocarpa (H.B.K.) G. Don (25). If so, I.
batatas is, depending on the genomic closeness of the parents, a
segmental autohexaploid. Man selected it for its high yield.

10. Potato – a successful autotetraploid

In South America several tuberous Solanum species related to our
potato (S. tuberosum L. group Tuberosum, 2n=4x=48) occur in the wild.
There are 2x, 3x, 4x and 6x races (n=12), while occasionally 2x, 3x,
and 5x hybrids are found. Most 2x species are self-incompatible,
whereas the 4x and 6x species are self-compatible. From some 2x
species cultivated (i.e., domesticated) 2x were developed. They are,
like their parents, self-incompatible. In our essay we refer to
them as phureja and stenotomum. Their domestication may have happened in Bolivia-Peru. After polyploidization the 4x andigena
potato developed. Whether it is an autotetraploid or a segmental
allotetraploid is irrelevant for what follows. The andigena is self-
compatible. Due to hybridization of andigena and stenotomum the 3x
S. x chaucha Juz. & Buk. arose. This hybrid is sterile.
In many areas of South America a potato crop is composed of 2x
and 4x plants with occasionally a few 3x hybrids. Jackson (26) was
the first to establish the frequencies of the various ploidy levels
in a potato field. He investigated two fields in southern Peru and
observed an abundance of 4x andigena plants (Table 4). In such

Table 4. Number of plant classified according to their ploidy
level in two potato fields in southern Peru (26), 2n=2x=24.

Field	2x	3x	4x	Nc	N
1	2	1	107	110	846
	(1.8%)	(0.9%)	(97.3%)		
2	10	5	311	326	326
	(3.1%)	(1.5%)	(95.4%)		

Nc = number of plants classified, N = total number of plants in the
field.

fields hybridization may occur with S. acaule Bitt. (2n=4x=48).
Hybridization with stenotomum results in the cultivated 3x hybrid S.
juzepczukii Buk. This hybrid crossed with andigena gives the cultivated S. x curtilobium Juz. & Buk. (2n=5x=60) (29).

From South America the potato was taken to Europe, Chile, Mexico
and elsewhere. We may assume that the first shipment of potato
existed of 2x, 3x, and 4x domesticated types, probably at the same
frequency as they are found today. But only the 4x type survived
in Europe, Chile, and Mexico. Why? First we will discuss the
transport of the potato to Europe. If the 2x phureja potato were
included, this cytotype would have disappeared during the voyage
owing to its lack of dormancy. Sprouted tubers must have occurred,
which would have been dead at arrival. We may assume that no
living phureja tuber reached Europe. Stenotomum and andigenum
reached Europe and among them some 3x cytotypes may have been
present. The first potato growing was done from true seed and
therefore 3x must have disappeared as this cytotype is sterile.
Stenotomum is self-incompatible, and fruit set and seed set depend
on the frequency of this cytotype. Due to the loss of phureja the
frequency of stenotomum must have been about 2% or less, i.e., 2
plants per 100. In the beginning of the potato growing in southern
Europe this plant was a curiosity and the chance that stenotomum
was present in a herb garden among the few 4x andigenum potato
plants would be extremely small. So one plant at most was present,
which could not fertilize itself. If pollen reached the stigmata
of a stenotomum plant, it must have been pollen from a 4x andigenum
plant. If this led to the development of a fruit and seeds, the
seeds then produced either sterile 3x plants or 4x andigenum-like
plants owing to 2n gametes from the 2x plant. So, any fertile
progeny of a 2x plant would be 4x. Furthermore, cross pollination
2x X 4x would have been restricted because of early flowering of
the 2x (28). Rowe (29) also found that 2x plants grown from true
seeds have a lower tuberization, and a smaller number of seed-size
tubers per plant than 4x plants grown from true seed (Table 5).

Table 5. Tuberization, number of tubers per plant, and average
tuber weight of 2x and 4x plants grown from true seeds (29).

Ploidy	Tuberization (%)	No. tubers/plant	Avg. tuber weight(g)
2x	80.6	9.9	13.8
4x	91.8	12.5	22.9

The lower tuberization could be a result of a stronger short day
sensitivity than andigenum. All these factors worked against the
survival of the 2x cytotype and it must have disappeared in a few

years after its introduction into southern Europe. When the
potato moved northward selection for daylength insensitivity
occurred.

In Chile and Mexico only 4x plants are grown and so, like in
Europe, 2x and 3x plants disappeared. I doubt that potato growing
in these countries started from true seed. If this were so, the
extinction of the 2x and 3x plants must have been due to 'drift'
or negative selection by man. However, on the Canary Isles a 3x
cultivar was present among the 10 primitive cultivars found (30).
It survived there for some 300 years.

In Mexico the 4x andigenum came into contact with S. demissum
Lindl. (2n=6x) resulting in the weedy 5x hybrid S. X edinense
Berthauld (31), but owing to the strong barrier between this
hybrid and andigenum (32) only a limited amount of demissum genes
apparently introgressed into the potato.

11. Bread wheat - a successful hexaploid

Bread wheat, Triticum aestivum (2n=6x=42, AABBDD), derives
from a hexaploid which must have originated where domesticated
emmer (Triticum dicoccum, 2n=4x, AABB) and a wild grass (Aegilops
squarrosa auct. non L., 2n=2x, DD) - its parental species - met.
From studies to be published elsewhere (33, 34), I came to the
conclusion that bread wheat was spread to n.w. Europe as an admixture of emmer. The mixture (including other plant species)
must have reached the Balkans in ca. 6000 BC and n.w. Europe ca.
4000 BC. Archeological finds show the presence of a few bread
wheat grains in emmer grains. But already in 3700 BC and also in
ca 2300 BC some almost pure bread wheat fields must have been
present (35). The cause of the demixing is not known, but apparently bread wheat could do so from the first bread wheat plant.

I have already referred to Zanduri and Makha wheat mixtures
and also to the bread wheat-durum mixtures of Ethiopia. Apparently
each component is capable of maintaining itself in the mixture.
Neither the genotype nor the ploidy level has an influence on
survival of the components or, if they have, their effects must
be oppositely directed and thereby neutralize each other. In an
artificial mixture of bread wheat and durum, the durum cultivar
was successful, for the more bread wheat cultivars were affected
by stem rust the quicker their frequency was reduced. In this
case the genetic effect, stem rust resistance/susceptibility,
played a major role, but a susceptible bread wheat variety,
escaping the disease due to its earliness, was still ousted by
the durum wheat (36).

12. Rye - a successful diploid but an unsuccessful tetraploid

Much research has been conducted with autotetraploid rye
with the hope of breeding a better rye crop than 2x rye. 4x and
2x rye types have been grown as a mixture to study competion.

However, when comparing a 2x population with a 4x one it should
be borne in mind that genetically these populations are not
identical, since the 4x population always derives from a limited
number of 2x plants. The 4x plants very likely do not represent
the total genetic information of the 2x population.

Levin (37) pointed out that in a cross-fertilizing population
of 2x and 4x plants the most frequent ploidy level will oust the
other ploidy level if the multiplication factors are the same.
This can easily be demonstrated by assuming one 4x plant in a 2x
population. This 4x plant will be pollinated by n pollen grains
from the 2x plants. The resulting 3x zygotes die in an early
stage. Hence the 4x ploidy level disappears from the population.
Identically one 2x plant in a 4x population will produce lethal
3x embryos and so 2x will also disappear from the population.

But in a 2x-4x mixture of rye the 2x will win as a result of
the bad seed yield of the 4x plants, even if the frequency of 2x
plants is low. As compared to 2x plants, 4x plants have a lower
culm number per plant limiting the number of seeds per plant.
Furthermore the seed set per ear of 4x plants is lower, reducing
the multiplication factor still more. Then, they are often
shorter, which means that they are shaded by neighbouring 2x
plants causing a reduction in seed set and seed weight. 4x
plants also produce aneuploids, which have a low seed set and do
not contribute to the maintenance of the 4x population. In
addition, there is certation resulting in a higher percentage of
the egg cells being fertilized by an n gamete than expected from
the n/2n pollen grain ratio. So 2x plants produce more 2x plants
and 4x plants less 4x plants than expected. Yet the 4x plants
have some advantages: the seeds have a higher weight which may
give the 4x seedlings a better start in the mixture, and their
better frost resistance is of advantage only in regions with a
severe winter. The disadvantage of a 4x plant will annul for a
great deal the advantages and therefore a 4x plant in a rye
population has no chance to survive unless it can protect itself
by isolation. Isolation by distance, but rye pollen grains carry
a long distance. Isolation from competition, but there are other
plants to compete with. Isolation from cross fertilization by
cleistogamy, but the observed tendency for self-fertilization is
facultative. Isolation by perenniality, like related species,
but this did not take place.

Hagberg and Ellerström (38) found however that a mixture of
2x:4x plants at a ratio of 0.32:0.68 was in balance. If the frequency of 4x plants was >0.68, then the 4x plants would oust the
2x plants. If the frequency of 2x plants was >0.32, then the 2x
would win. For breeding this is important as a 2x variety contaminated with 4x plants is 'self-cleaning,' and the same holds true
for a 4x variety contaminated with 2x plants.

However, in nature, 4x plants do not originate in great
numbers and certainly not at frequencies of >0.68. If they arise
it will be at a very low frequency and they have no chance of

producing a 4x offspring. Perhaps this is the reason that no 4x
rye variety has been found in nature.

13. Maize - unsuccessful as a tetraploid

In a mixture of 2x and auto-4x maize (Zea mays L.) the
survival rate of the 4x component is extremely low. This was
caused by the loss of 2n gametes due to certation (39) similar to
that described for rye. Even a mixture with an initial composition
of seed sown at 1(2x):9(4x) grown for two years produced a harvest
free of 4x seeds (39).

14. Rice and barley - artificial mixtures of 2x and 4x plants

I only know of two artificial mixtures of a diploid and its
autotetraploid. The first is rice, in which the autotetraploid
component was suppressed after a few generations (40). The
second is a mixture of barley and its autotetraploid component.
In this experiment the tetraploid component was also suppressed.
The main cause was the poor reproduction value of the latter,
viz., 2x=100% and 4x=ca.13% (40).

Triploid and aneuploid seeds set on wheat (2n=9x=63) and
barley plants infected by barley stripe mosaic virus (BSMV) (41-
43). If, for barley, such infected grains develop into plants
the progeny of these plants will consist of plants with 2n=14 to
39; 85% of them being 2n=14 to 19. Barley has apparently a high
tolerance for extra chromosomes. It is expected that in virus
free populations after a few generations the diploid plants will
dominate. The loss of chromosomes by an artificial autotetraploid
was also shown by Rykova (44) for flax. However, this loss was
not fast. In only 17 of the 70 tetraploid populations 2x plants
were found after 6 years of cultivation. The competition capacity
of these diploids as regards the 4x plants is not studied.

15. Perennial ryegrass - a successful artificial autotetraploid

Norrington-Davies and Harries (45) and Harries and Norrington-
Davies (46) studied mixtures of 2x and 4x cultivars of perennial
ryegrass (Lolium perenne L.). They observed that in these experimental mixtures the 4x component was in a competitive advantage
probably due to the higher seed weight. Furthermore, extracts of
4x seeds suppressed the germination of 2x seed more than extracts
of 2x seeds did with the germination of 4x seeds. However, care
should be taken with these data as only one 2x and one 4x variety
were used in the experiment. This must explain why in other
trials 4x plants were suppressed (see below).

In addition, environmental heterogeneity often plays a role
too as it often favours the minority component. However, in a 4x
population a 2x plant has a rather limited chance of surviving,

while a 4x plant in a 2x population will probably survive and
produce seed.

     It could be questioned why 4x plants did not originate in
nature or, if they did, why none have survived. Tetraploid
plants have been identified in seedlings, but at a very low
frequency, 0.7×10^{-6}. For seed production some 3.10^{6} seeds per
hectare are sown (47), so per hectare about two 4x plants may
occur. From mixtures of 2x and artificial 4x plants it has been
experienced that 4x plants have a low degree of persistence.
Hence in a grass field they are quickly suppressed by the 2x
plants.

     It must be borne in mind that in future the frequency of 4x
plants in perennial ryegrass populations might be much higher due
to the influx of 4x seeds from cultivated artificial 4x plants
(47).

     The artificial tetraploids are especially useful for produc-
tion grass type varieties. Thus in the Netherlands there are 18
varieties of the production grass type of L. perenne and of these
6 are 4x, while of the 17 varieties of the recreation grass type
none is 4x. These 4x varieties have no difficulty in maintaining
the 4x level. After initial high frequencies of aneuploid plants
an equilibrium is reached at a frequency of 6% (48). However, in
4x Italian ryegrass (Lolium multiflorum) this frequency is much
higher, viz., about 47% in advanced generations (49). If the
Japanese data are representative for the Dutch varieties apparently
no harm is done as 9 of 22 registered Italian and Westerwold
ryegrass varieties are 4x.

16. Sugar beet – anisoploid varieties as examples of a modern
     man–made cytotype mixture

     Autotriploid sugar beet and fodder beet (Beta vulgaris L.)
are grown in Europe because of the higher yield than 2x and
autotetraploid varieties. Triploid plants are sterile and therefore 3x seed has to be sown annually. This permits us to breed
3x F_1 hybrid varieties from inbred 2x and 4x lines. Before the
application of cytoplasmic male sterility it was not possible to
breed a purely 3x variety. A '3x variety' consisted of 2x, 3x,
and 4x plants, and the variety was named anisoploid variety. In
fact, it is an example of a modern man–made cytotype mixture.

     Such a mixture was bred by growing 2x and 4x plants together.
2x plants would produce many 2x plants and many 3x plants, while
4x plants would produce many 3x plants and many 4x plants. The
result would be about 50% 3x plants. Attempts have been made to
increase the 3x frequency and by screening anisoploid varieties
some varieties were found to possess a 3x frequency of 60-75%.
In Hungary it was even ruled that a registered variety should
have at least 60% 3x plants. However, Svab (50, 51) showed that
such high frequencies are the extremes of a normal distribution
with a mean of 50% and that if the rule was to become effective

each population had to be screened and a high percentage of the
good breeding material had to be discarded. This problem disappeared when male sterility was applied allowing the breeding of
purely 3x varieties.

17. Haploids – some are successful

Haploids, too, have been found in very low frequencies in
domesticated crops, but in general they are of no use. Due to
poor development, and hence low competing ability, and due to
generally occurring sterility they succumb in a population.
However, some haploids have reached the cultivar level like
'Gracilis' of Thuja plicata D. Don. This cultivar had been in
cultivation for some 70 years before Pohlheim (52) found in 1968
that it was a monohaploid (2n=x=11).
Similarly, the pelargonium cultivar Kleiner Liebling, already
grown since about 1925, is a monohaploid (2n=x=9) (53). Such
monohaploid cultivars could easily become a source of new cultivars
as any mutation (from dominant to recessive) would be constant,
as Pohlheim (52,54) indicated for Thuja.

SUGGESTIONS FOR FURTHER RESEARCH

The above examples show that the study of the relations
between domestication and polyploidy, and especially the origin
and survival of polyploids, is not intensive. Much needs to be
done. Therefore it might be helpful to give a few suggestions
for further research.
Our information about mixtures of cytotypes is quite limited.
We know that they exist in the wild, in the field and in the
garden. What kind of interactions occur? I have indicated that
autotetraploids have as a rule no or a low chance to survive in a
mixture with their diploid parents. Is this generally true? The
few studies on self-fertilizing crops show that autotetraploids
have a lower crowding coefficient than diploids. With cross-
fertilizing crops the advantage of n gametes over 2n gametes adds
to the disappearance of the 4x component, although this is not
true for alfalfa.
The increase of seed size as observed for 4x rye might give
the 4x plant a better advantage in the mixture. The lower seed
number of 4x plants is a disadvantage. This change from many
seeds with a low seed weight to less seeds with a higher seed
weight refers to a slight shift from r-selection in the direction
of K-selection. How important is this?
Apparently the 4x and 6x wheat plants in some Ethiopian
wheat fields grow 'happily' together. Their relation should be
investigated. This should also be done with that of the cytotypes
of Zanduri and Makha wheats (if these two are still available).
Additive data can be obtained from studying mixtures of natural
4x wheats and their 6x ABD-derivatives. However, in this study

it is impossible to separate the effects of the D genomes from
those of the D genes and their interactions with A and B genomes
or genes, respectively.

In general, we should know more about the population genetics,
or as I call it: mixture genetics (55) of mixtures of cross- and
self-fertilizing cytotypes. What is the fate of a newly arisen
polyploid? What is its fate when it has no or only a slight
selective advantage?

We have some information about the spread of 4x potato over
the world, but we do not know how the early introductions into
Europe appeared, because most potato material was wiped out there
by blight in the middle of the 19th century. If the old potato
cultivars of India (56) and southern Africa (57, 58) are derivatives of the old European potato an intensive research of this
material could shed some light on the first introductions into
Europe. Additional information could be obtained from the potato
on the Canary Isles which is derived from 17th century introductions (31).

A study of the loss of redundant gene expression (thus not
loci) after polyploidization should be intensified. For example,
data are available and are summarized by Garcia-Olmedo et al.
(59) for allohexaploid wheat. When more information becomes
available it might be possible to establish a relation between
percentages of loss and age of the polyploid. This relation will
be curvilinear as Garcia-Olmedo et al. (59) indicated that the
loss would be the highest soon after the origin of the polyploid.
In the first period there will be a selection against negative
heterotic interactions between homeoalleles and also against
disrupted dosage balance between functionally related genes.
Together with chromosomal imbalances these disadvantages would
result in a poor fertility and productivity (60) of the polyploid
and thus in its extinction.

What are the effects of a cross-fertilizing diploid becoming
a self-fertilizing autotetraploid? A cross-fertilizer maintains
its genetic variation by heterozygosity, while a self-fertilizer
does so by heterogeneity. A self-fertilizing autopolyploid
recently originated from a cross-fertilizing, i.e., heterozygotic
diploid, maintains its level of heterozygosity longer than a
self-fertilizing diploid.

I mentioned above whether or not the sequence of polyploidization followed by domestication would be different from the sequence
domestication followed by polyploidization, and if so, whether
the first is better than the second. All depends on the number
of parental plants becoming polyploid, the time since polyploidization has occurred, and the extent of hybridization with parental
and other species.

If a high number of parental plants become polyploid the
starter population will have a higher variation than if only a
few parental plants are involved. Furthermore, it is important
whether the polyploid is an auto- or an allopolyploid as the

latter has more than one parental species and the first only one.
Furthermore, a self-fertilizing autopolyploid will preserve its
genetic variation by heterozygosity better than a diploid.

Genetic variation may increase by mutations, their frequency
depending on the age of the polyploid and the presence of mutator
genes. The genetic variation may still further be increased by
hybridization, if the polyploid is not isolated from parental and
related species. This isolation could be genetic, chromosomal,
geographical, or temporal.

On the other hand, genetic variation may decrease owing to
stabilizing selection pressure and this may lead to genetic
poverty of a crop. Thus Dhaliwal (61) concluded that the genetic
variation of einkorn wheat (Triticum monococcum L.) was quite
small. He explained this by assuming that only a small population
of wild einkorn (T. boeoticum Boiss.) had been domesticated.
This could be true, but I believe that the intergenotypic competition resulted in the dominance of one or a few morphotypes may
give the present day einkorn population its quite uniform appearance. However, the genetic variation for neutral characteristics
might be still present. This assumption is supported by an
orientating study of an Austrian landrace of the alpine wheat
'Haunsberg'. The plants are morphologically quite alike, but
when ten grains were investigated for gliadin pattern, 8 patterns
were discovered. If more proteins had been investigated it is
quite likely that the plants with an identical gliadin pattern
would have been different for other proteins. Thus, like the
barley accessions (mostly improved varieties) investigated by
Allard and Kahler (62) with each having two or more genotypes, I
(33) postulated that this variation for gliadin composition has
existed for some 6000 years, i.e., 6000 generations, and that
apparently the genetic variation possibly had been maintained
mainly by the low yield of the landrace. Hence, a great part of
the harvest seed is used as sowing seed and so all or almost all
genetic variation is transferred to the next generation.

The spread of other polyploid crops and their cytotype
mixtures should be studied. Much is known about the spread of
various banana (Musa sp.) cytotypes (63), yet their distribution
over Africa and the Americas is not well known. The same studies
should be extended to crops like taro (Colocasia esculenta (L.)
Schott.) (64), sugar cane (Saccharum sp.) (65), and many others
possessing numerous cytotypes. Why did some cytotypes survive
when distributed? Such studies could shed light on the history
of the crops and also on the history of the peoples who grow them
as does my study (34) of the spread of the cytotypic mixture of
4x emmer and 6x bread wheat over Europe. Why did they demix?

The studies of the breeding history of hyacinth, tulip, and
daffodil should be continued. Why is the optimum number of
chromosomes of cultivars higher than that of the wild ancestors?
Why does a 4x hyacinth cultivar not exist while 4x seedlings have
been observed? Maybe since the study of Darlington et al. (19)

in 1951 such a cultivar has been bred. Why is there a positive correlation between high chromosome number and blue flower colour of hyacinth?

CONCLUSION

Much is known about the relation between polyploidy and domestication, but our knowledge of the interaction between cytotypes when grown together is still limited. The fact that this paper might be the first to summarize this subject for domesticated taxa could be an indication that this subject has not yet attracted much attention (see Lewis, p. 103, for wild species).

Studies of the evolution of polyploids, whether wild or domesticated, have started on a large scale and in the near future we shall hear more about them (59, 67-69, and others). These studies are being made possible by the wide introduction and application of (automated) apparatus for electrophoresis. The more data that are available the better our understanding will be of polyploids, wild and domesticated, as well as their mutual interference.

SUMMARY

The origin and survival of a polyploid in a mixture of this polyploid and its parent(s) is reviewed. With several examples a picture is drawn of the interference of cytotypes in a mixture of cytotypes.

Some natural polyploids, both wild and domesticated, are very successful. They, like bread wheat and banana, largely replaced their parents. The same is true for some artificial polyploids like autotriploid hybrid sugar beet in Europe and autotetraploid perennial ryegrass. But when grown together with their parents for several generations they will disappear from this mixture. Although in South America under primitive conditions, diploid, triploid, and tetraploid potatoes are grown, elsewhere only the tetraploids have survived. Various causes are presented to explain why the diploids and triploids succumbed.

Autotetraploids of maize, rye, barley, and rice cannot maintain themselves in diploid/tetraploid mixtures. The maintenance of diploid or tetraploid rye varieties is less difficult as both are "self-cleaning" with respect to the other.

Only two haploid cultivars exist but they can only maintain themselves with the help of man.

It is concluded that the survival chances of a polyploid after its origination is low. Firstly, under conditions of random sampling a rare type has a very small chance of occurring in the next generation. Furthermore, seedset of triploids and tetraploids is often low which limits their survival. In addition, in mixtures of cross-fertilizing diploid and autotetraploids the n gamete has an advantage over the 2n gamete. This limits the survival of the autotetraploids again.

It is concluded that our knowledge of the mutual interference of cytotypes in a cytotype mixture is quite limited. Much more research is needed and some proposals concerning this research are made.

LITERATURE CITED

1. Anderson, E., 1961, The analysis of variation in cultivated plants with special reference to introgression. Euphytica 10: 79–86.
2. Ramanna, M.S., personal communications, 1978/1979.
3. Levan, A., 1945, The present state of plant breeding by induction of polyploidy. Sveriges Utsädes-förenings Tidskrift 55: 109–143.
4. Jain, S.K., 1976, The evolution of inbreeding in plants. Ann. Rev. Ecol. Syst. 7: 469–475.
5. Huskins, C.L., 1930, The origin of Spartina townsendii. Genetica 12: 531–538.
6. Gymer, P.T., Whittington, 1973, Hybrids between Lolium perenne L. and Festuca pratensis Huds. 1. Crossing and incompatibility. New Phytol. 72: 411–424.
7. Wit, F., 1964, Natural and experimental hybrids of ryegrasses and meadow fescue. Euphytica 13: 294–304.
8. Whittington, W.J., Hill, J., 1961, Growth studies on natural hybrids between Lolium perenne and Festuca pratensis. J. Expl. Bot. 12: 330–340.
9. Gymer, P.T., Whittington, W.J., 1973, Hybrids between Lolium perenne and Festuca pratensis. 2. Comparative morphology. New Phytol. 72: 861–865.
10. Gymer, P.T., Whittington, W.J., 1976, Factors influencing the proportion of natural hybrids between Lolium perenne L. and Festuca pratensis Huds. in permanent pastures. J. Grassland Soc. 31: 165–169.
11. Bingham, E.T., Saunders, J.W., 1974, Chromosome manipulations in alfalfa: scaling the cultivated tetraploid to seven ploidy levels. Crop Sci. 14: 474–477.
12. Bingham, E.T., Gillies, C.B., 1971, Chromosome pairing, fertility, and crossing behavior of haploids of tetraploid alfalfa, Medicago sativa L. Canad. J. Genet. Cytol. 13: 195–202.
13. Dunbier, N.W., Eskew, D.L., Bingham, E.T., Schrader, L.E., 1975, Performance of genetically comparable diploid and tetraploid alfalfa: agronomic and physiological parameters. Crop Sci. 15: 211–214.
14. Heiser, Ch. B., Smith, D.M., 1960, The origin of Helianthus multiflorus. Amer. J. Bot. 47: 860–865.

15. Li., H.L., 1956, The story of the cultivated horse-
     chestnuts. Morris Arb. Bull. 7: 35-39.
16. Ottaro, W.C.M., 1977, The relationship between the ploidy
     level and certain morphological characteristics of
     Chrysanthemum cinerariaefolium Vis. Pyrethrum Post 14(1):
     10-11.
17. Parlevliet, J.E., 1979, Collecting pyrethrum in Yugoslavia
     for Kenya, pp. 91-96, in Zeven, A.C., van Harten, A.M.,
     (eds.), "Broadening the Genetic Base of Crops Proc. Conference,"
     and personal communication.
18. Müntzing, A., 1936, The chromosomes of a giant Populus
     tremula. Hereditas 21: 383-393.
19. Darlington, C.D., Hair, J.B., Hurcombe, R., 1951, The history
     of the garden Hyacinthus. Heredity 5: 233-252.
20. Kroon, G.H., van Eijk, J.P., 1977, Polyploidy in tulips
     (Tulipa L.); the occurrence of diploid gametes. Euphytica
     26: 63-66.
21. de Mol, W.E., 1923, The disappearance of the diploid and
     triploid Magnicoronatae narcissi from the larger cultures
     and the appearance in their place of tetraploid forms. Kon.
     Akad. Amsterdam. Proc. Sect. Sci. 25: 216-220.
22. Wylie, A.P., 1952, The history of the garden narcissi.
     Heredity 6: 137-156.
23. Austin, D.F., 1977, Hybrid polyploids in Ipomoea section
     Batatas. J. Heredity 68: 259-260.
24. Nishiyama, I., Miyazaki, T., Sakamoto, S., 1975, Evolutionary
     autoploidy in the sweet potato (Ipomoea batatas (L.) Lam.)
     and its progenitors. Euphytica 24: 197-208.
25. Austin, D.F., 1978, The Ipomoea batatas complex. I. Taxonomy.
     Bull. Torrey Bot. Club 105: 114-129.
26. Jackson, M.T., 1975, The evolutionary significance of the
     triploid cultivated potato, Solanum x chaucha Juz. & Buk.
     PhD thesis, University of Birmingham, 191 p. and appendices.
27. Hawkes, J.G., 1962, The origin of Solanum juzepczukii Buk.
     and S. cutilobum Juz. and Buk. Zeitschr. Pflanzenz.
     47: 1-14.
28. Rowe, P.R., 1967, Performance of diploid and vegetatively
     doubled clones of phureja-haploid tuberosum hybrids. Amer.
     Potato J. 44: 195-203.
29. Rowe, P.R., 1967, Performance and variability of diploid and
     tetraploid families. Amer. Potato J. 44: 263-271.
30. Zubeldia Lizarduy, A., Lopez Campos, G., Sanudo Pazaluelos,
     A., 1955, Estudio descripcion y classificacion de un grupo
     de variedades primitivas de patata cultivades en los Isles
     Canarias. Bol. Inst. Invest. Agron. Madrid 15: 287-325.
31. Ugent, D., 1967, Morphological variation in Solanum x edinense,
     a hybrid of the common potato. Evolution 21: 696-712.
32. Ugent, D., 1968, The potato in Mexico: geography and primi-
     tive culture. Econ. Bot. 22: 108-123.

33. Zeven, A.C., 1979, The prehistoric spread of bread wheat into Asia, pt. I: 103-107, Proc. 5th Inter. Wheat Genetics Symp., New Delhi.

34. Zeven, A.C. The spread of bread wheat over the Old World since the Neolithicum as indicated by their genotypes for hybrid necrosis (in preparation).

35. van Zeist, W., 1968, Prehistoric and early historic food plants in the Netherlands. Palaeohistoria (publ. 1970): 41-72.

36. Klages, K.H.W., 1936, Changes in the proportion of the components of seeded and harvested cereal mixtures in abnormal seasons. J. Amer. Soc. Agron. 28: 935-940.

37. Levin, D.A., 1975, Minority cytotype exclusion in local plant populations. Taxon 24: 35-43.

38. Hagberg, A., Ellerstrøm, S., 1959, The competition between diploid, tetraploid and aneuploid rye. Theoretical and practical aspects. Hereditas 45: 369-416.

39. Cavanah, J.A., Alexander, D.E., 1963, Survival of tetraploid maize in mixed 2n-4n plantings. Crop Sci. 3: 329-331.

40. Sakai, K.-I., 1955, Competition in plants and its relation to selection. Cold Spring Harbor Symp. Quant. Biology 20: 137-157.

41. Linde-Laursen, I., Siddiqui, K.A., 1974, Triploidy and aneuploidy in virus infected wheat, _Triticum_ _aestivum_. Hereditas 76: 152-154.

42. Sandfaer, J., 1979, Frequency of aneuploids in progenies of autotriploid barley, _Hordeum_ _vulgare_ L. Hereditas 90: 213-217.

43. Sanfaer, J., 1979, The influence of different strains of barley stripe mosaic virus on the frequency of triploids and aneuploids in barley. Phytopath. Zeitschrift (in press).

44. Rykova, R.P., 1977, (Depolyploidization in induced autotetraploid flax). Byull. Vses, Ord. Lenina no. 69:34-38. From Pl. Breeding Abstr. 48 (1978):10796.

45. Norrington-Davies, J., Harries, J.H., 1977, Competition studies in diploid and tetraploid varieties of _Lolium_ _perenne_. 1. The influence of density and proportion of sowing. J. Agric. Sci. Cambridge 88: 405-410.

46. Harries, J.H., Norrington-Davies, J., 1977, Competition studies in diploid and tetraploid varieties of _Lolium_ _perenne_. 2. The inhibition of germination. J. Agric. Sci. Cambridge 88: 411-415.

47. van Dijk, G.E., personal communication, March 1978.

48. Ahloowalia, B.S., 1971, Frequency, origin and survival of aneuploids in tetraploid ryegrass. Genetica 42: 129-138.

49. Nagata T., Okabe, T., 1978, Frequency of aneuploids in autotetraploid populations of Italian ryegrass _(Lolium_ _multiflorum_ Lam.). Jap. J. Breeding 28: 205-210.

50. Svab, J., 1966, Ueber die genetische Stabilität anisoploider Zuckerrübensorten. Zeitschr. Pflanzenz. 55: 241-259.

51. Svab, J., 1973, Population-genetical aspects of variety maintenance, pp. 89-93, Proc. First Meeting Section Biometrics in Plant Breeding of Eucarpia.

52. Pohlheim, F., 1968, Thuja gigantea gracilis Beissn. - ein Haplont unter den Gymnospermen. Biologische Rundschau 6: 84-86.

53. Daker, M.G., 1966, 'Kleiner Liebling', a haploid cultivar of Pelargonium, Nature 211: 549-550.

54. Pohlheim, 1972, Untersuchungen zur Sprossvariation der Cupressacea 4. Zur Auslese von Mutations-Chimaren und mutanten der Haploiden. Thuja gigantea gracilis. Arch. Zuchtungs-forsch. 2: 223-235.

55. Zeven, A.C., 1977, Domesticatie en evolutie van de cultuur-planten. Course, Institute of Plant Breeding, Agricultural University, Wageningen, 206 p. (mimeographed).

56. Swaminathan, M.S., 1958, The origin of early European potato-evidence from Indian varieties. Indian J. Genet. Pl. Breeding 18: 8-15.

57. van der Plank, J.E., 1946, Origin of the first European potatoes and their reaction to length of day. Nature 157: 503-505.

58. Brücher, H., 1966, Wildkartoffeln in Afrika. Zeitschr. Pflanzenz. 16: 147-163.

59. Garcia-Olmedo, F., Carbonera, P., Aragoncillo, C., Salcedo, G., 1978, Loss of redundant gene expression after polyploidization in plants. Experientia 34: 332-333.

60. Albuzio, A., Spettoli, P., Cacco, G., 1978, Changes in gene expression of diploid and autotetraploid status of Lycopersicon esculentum. Physiol. Pl. 44: 77-80.

61. Dhaliwal, G.C., 1977, Origin of Triticum monococcum. Wheat Information Service 44: 14-17.

62. Allard, R.W., Kahler, A.L., 1972, Patterns of molecular variation in plant populations. Proc. Sixth Berkeley Symp. on Mathematical Statistics and Probability 5: 237-254.

63. Simmonds, N.W., 1976, Sugarcanes, pp. 104-108, in Simmonds, N.W. (ed.), "Evolution of Crop Plants," Longman, London & New York.

64. Yen, D.E., Wheeler, J.M., 1968, Introduction of taro into the Pacific: the indications of the chromosome numbers. Ethnology 7: 259-267.

65. Plucknett, D.L., 1976, Edible aroids, pp. 10-12, in Simmonds, N.W. (ed.), "Evolution of Crop Plants," Longman, London & New York.

66. Simmonds, N.W., 1976, Bananas, pp. 211-215, in Simmonds, N.W. (ed.), "Evolution of Crop Plants," Longman, London & New York.

67. Barber, H.N., Driscoll, C.J., Long, P.M., Vickery, R.S., 1969, Gene similarity of the Triticinae and the study of segmental interchanges. Nature 221: 897-898.

68. Hart, G.E., Langston, P.J., 1977, Chromosomal location and
     evolution of isozyme structural genes in hexaploid wheat.
     Heredity 39: 263-277.
69. Adams, W.T., Allard, R.W., 1977, Effect of polyploid on
     phosphoglucose isomerase diversity in Festuca microstachys.
     Proc. Nat. Acad. Sci. USA 74: 1652-1656.

PROBLEMS OF ALLOPOLYPLOIDY IN TRITICALE

Arne Müntzing

Institute of Genetics
University of Lund
Lund, Sweden

Intergeneric allopolyploids combining genomes of bread wheat
(<u>Triticum</u> <u>aestivum</u>) and rye (<u>Secale</u> <u>cereale</u>) were first produced
by Rimpau (1). The true breeding strain which he had produced
attracted great attention and was regularly cultivated for a long
time in a plant breeding garden in Halle, Germany. According to
Tschermak (2), this strain had also been cultivated for more than
40 years in the garden of the Agricultural University of Vienna.

In 1935 the true breeding hybrid was cytologically examined
(3-5) and found to have 2n=56, i.e., the sum of the chromosome
numbers in bread wheat (2n=42) and rye (2n=14).

This information fitted results obtained five years earlier
at the Agricultural Experiment Station of Saratov in southeastern
Russia. During the period 1918 to 1934 the director of the
institute, G.K. Meister, and his associates, were active in the
field of wheat-rye hybridization. Besides large amounts of male-
sterile hybrids obtained by spontaneous crosses, hybrid derivatives
were later observed which were true breeding and fertile. Such
so-called balanced wheat-rye hybrids were suspected to be polyploid
as indicated by Tiumiakov (6) and Meister (7). Cytological
analysis of this material was carried out by Lewitsky and Benetzkaja (8-10) who made a careful study of mitosis and meiosis. They
observed that the somatic chromosome number was 56 in three
different families. Thus, the constant intermediate and fertile
rye-wheat hybrids were definitely amphiploids of hexaploid wheat
and rye.

For health reasons, Professor Müntzing was unable to attend
the Conference, but he kindly submitted his invitational paper
for publication. (Editor)

Investigations of the mode of meiosis in the pollen mother cells, as well as on the female side, revealed a frequent occurrence of irregularities caused by the presence of univalent chromosomes. The disturbed chromosome pairing could not be due to a lack of homology and must therefore be assumed to have other causes, either a general incompatibility between the parental chromosome sets or an antagonism between the female cytoplasm and the male chromosome set which represented another genus.

Lewitsky and Benetzkaja also discussed the mode of origin of the amphiploids and had to base their arguments on the fact that all the primary wheat-rye hybrids at Saratov were completely male-sterile. Under such circumstances they had to assume an apogamous development of F_1 ovules with a somatic number of chromosomes, and that the chromosome set was then doubled in the first division of the egg cell.

However, this complicated theory could soon be abandoned. In 1935 F_1 plants from crosses between Swedish varieties of bread wheat and rye were studied by the present writer. In this case the production of a new triticale strain was made possible by the spontaneous formation of small somatic sectors with a doubled chromosome number including anthers as well as ovules, or perhaps even quite local areas of chromosome doubling, leading to single dehiscing anthers, or parts of anthers, with unreduced pollen. Such an occurrence may, of course, easily be overlooked but probably represents a mechanism of general importance that had been at work also in the previous cases of spontaneous origin of octoploid types of triticale. Thus, the hypothesis of apogamous development followed by chromosome doubling became superfluous (5).

The name triticale was used for the first time by Lindschau and Oehler (3). This name had been proposed to them by Tschermak, one of the three rediscoverers of Mendel's laws. It is interesting that Tschermak used the denomination Triticale in a few papers but then changed his mind and proposed the name Secalotricum in analogy to previous cases of allopolyploidy. However, Secalotricum did not become accepted, and for a long time Triticale was used as a common name to designate all allopolyploids derived from crosses between wheat (genus Triticum) and rye (genus Secale).

Baum (11) suggested Triticosecale Wittmack as a Latin generic name, and this denomination has now been accepted. However, as a handy term triticale (with a small t and not in italics) is now in general use instead of the older Latin name Triticale (in italics and with a capital T).

Though Secalotricum was not accepted as a general denomination for allopolyploids between wheat and rye, it is now used as a specific name for those allopolyploids which are derived from F_1 hybrids between rye as the female parent and wheat as the male parent. Investigations of such material have led to various interesting results, including cytoplasmic effects (for literature references, see [12], pp. 12-13).

OCTOPLOID TRITICALE

In the 1930's cytogenetic studies and preliminary breeding work with octoploid triticale were carried out, especially in Germany and Sweden. After 1937, when chromosome doubling by colchicine treatment had been discovered, work with octoploid triticale was started in several other European countries. By and by the positive and negative agronomic characteristics of octoploid triticale became known (see 12-16).

As a rule octoploid triticales have good winter hardiness, grow well on light soils, and have early flowering and seed maturity. Other positive characters are large kernels with interesting biochemical properties. The protein content is higher than in the parent species and as a rule the baking properties are excellent.

Among the negative characters, partial sterility is especially disturbing, but this is in part compensated for by the large size of the kernels. The kernels are often shrivelled, which leads to lower values of test weight than in wheat. Octoploid triticale has also a tendency to sprout at harvest time if the weather is rainy. By breeding work, such characters as well as a tendency to lodging could be slowly improved, but in most countries strains of octoploid triticale are not yet sufficiently good to be released to farmers.

As reported by Müntzing (12) an interesting exception to this rule occurs in China. On the Yunnan-Kweichow plateau in southwestern China successful cultivation of octoploid triticale was started in 1973. Available data indicate that in this area, at high altitude and with bad soil, the triticale strains are clearly superior to wheat and rye. It was also stated that octoploid triticale had much more desirable properties than hexaploid triticale. Octoploid triticale is now also cultivated in the Ningshiahui region of northern China.

In recent years the earlier reports about the general occurrence of meiotic disturbances in octoploid triticale have been verified and supplemented by many workers especially Krolow (17-20), Tsuchiya (21), and Weimarck (22-24). Much of the discussion now concerns correlations between sterility, meiotic disturbances, and rate of aneuploidy. My co-worker, A. Weimarck, who has analysed triticale material cultivated at the Institute of Genetics in Lund, Sweden, has reached the following main conclusions: In bulk populations, as well as in progenies of euploid plants, recombined strains from hybrid populations are characterized by lower degrees of aneuploidy than primary strains. The recombined strains also have higher fertility and a more stable meiosis than the primary strains.

A close relationship was found between somatic chromosome number and fertility, the euploids clearly having higher fertility than the aneuploids. It should be observed, however, that no positive correlation was found by Weimarck between the degree of meiotic disturbances and sterility. Indirectly, however, meiotic irregularities tend to decrease the average fertility in the next generation by the production of a higher rate of aneuploids than plants with a more regular meiosis. On the other hand, especially in winter types of octoploid triticale, it is likely that a higher proportion of aneuploid than euploid seedlings are eliminated during the long period between sowing in the autumn and harvest the following summer. Such selection is especially obvious in Siberia. According to Khvostova and Shkutina (25), aneuploid plants appearing in the plots of octoploid triticale are less viable and perish during the harsh winter in the Irkutsk area.

Other kinds of elimination and selection in octoploid triticale have been revealed by Pieritz (26,27). In the first place he showed that there is a strict selection against aneuploidy among the male gametes in octoploid triticale, whereas all kinds of deviating chromosome constitutions are transmitted by the ovules. By improved technical methods, Pieritz also succeeded in distinguishing morphologically between wheat and rye chromosomes. Thanks to this distinction he could confirm other indirect evidence that in octoploid triticales the univalents occurring at meiosis are predominantly rye chromosomes. As pointed out by Müntzing (15), this is indicated by the fact that certain strains or hybrid populations with many univalents at meiosis have a more or less pronounced tendency to revert to hexaploid wheat.

Meiosis in octoploid triticale has not only been examined in primary strains and stable recombination products. Weimarck (24) studied meiosis in 9 F_1-combinations in comparison with meiosis in the parent strains. In all cases the frequency of univalents at first metaphase was higher in the F_1 hybrids than in the parents. This much larger material confirmed previous observations by Müntzing (14) and Bjurman (28) concerning two primary strains and their F_1 and F_2 hybrids. Hence, it seems to be a general phenomenon that in octoploid triticale parental strains have a more regular meiosis than hybrid plants from different cross combinations. This fact is also correlated with a significantly lower degree of fertility in the hybrids than in the homozygous parents.

HEXAPLOID TRITICALE

From Tentative Beginning to Global Distribution

It is possible that the interest in triticale as a potential new crop would have tapered off entirely if the efforts had been limited to octoploid material. However, this was successfully prevented by an enormous development of work with hexaploid triticales.

The first amphiploid between tetraploid wheat and rye was reported by Derzhavin (29). In this case it was a union of Triticum durum (2n=28) with the wild species Secale montanum (2n=14). Of more interest from the breeding point of view, was the amphiploid between Triticum durum and cultivated rye (Secale cereale) produced by O'Mara (30) and the combination of Triticum turgidum (2n=28) and rye made by Nakajima (31). A more concentrated effort of producing a broader and more variable material of hexaploid triticale was made in Spain by Sanchez-Monge and Tjio (32) and Sanchez-Monge (33,34). This work was primarily made to get triticales of good grain quality as a substitute for the mixture of wheat and rye that was rather widely cultivated in certain regions of Spain. Sanchez-Monge realized that it was not possible to obtain, directly, a hexaploid triticale with good properties, but believed that it would be possible to improve this material by recombination and selection.

This optimistic belief was convincingly demonstrated in Canada. The first organized effort to develop triticale as a commercial crop in North American was initiated by L.H. Shebeski at the University of Manitoba, Winnipeg. The starting material was the hexaploid durum X rye amphiploid produced by O'Mara (30). Several additional hexaploid triticales were developed from new crosses, and seeds of other existing wheat X rye amphiploids, both hexaploid and octoploid, were collected. Many of the best triticale lines from all sources were intercrossed in 1958. Important progress was made through the discovery of day length-insensitive early maturing types of triticale, and dwarf and semidwarf wheat lines which were used as a source of shorter and stronger straw in the triticales. These characteristics, as well as disease resistance and grain-quality improvement, showed that hexaploid triticale could fill the need for a feed crop for domestic animals.

By 1969 one cultivar, "Rosner," was licensed and became recognized as a new crop of commerce. Results from livestock feeding experiments, distilling and brewing tests, and also from experimental manufacture of breakfast cereals indicate that triticale has considerable potential as a cereal crop.

In 1964 N.E. Borlaug initiated triticale research in Mexico as a cooperative project between the University of Manitoba and CIMMYT (Centro Internacional de Mejoramiento de Maiz y Trigo). Funds were provided by the Rockefeller Foundation. The main objective was to develop a grain crop that would be competitive with other cereals, particularly in improving human nutrition in developing countries. During the first years this program was directed by Borlaug, but since 1968 F.J. Zillinsky is the leader of this very comprehensive and intensive work.

In 1969 CIMMYT initiated an international triticale testing program in which numerous countries around the world could cooperate. Each year about 50 different stations in more than 30 countries take part in this program. In this way valuable results

concerning yield and other agronomic characters are collected as
a guide for further work.

Different Kinds of Highbred Triticales

   Secondary Hexaploids and Octoploids. In the 1960's good
results from crosses between octoploid and hexaploid triticales
were reported by Pissarev (35) in the U.S.S.R., Kiss (36-39) in
Hungary, and Jenkins (40,41) in Canada and U.S.A. The new secondary hexaploids derived from these crosses were reported to be
clearly superior in several respects to the original hexaploid
parents.
   Theoretically it was difficult to understand why such crosses
between triticales with 56 and 42 chromosomes should give better
results than hybridization and selection within the hexaploid
group itself. For a very long time tetraploid species of wheat
were known to have the genome formula AABB and hexaploid species
AABBDD. However, thanks to Canadian research workers, it became
clear that the A and B genomes of tetraploid wheat are not identical with the A and B genomes in hexaploid wheat. Kerber (42)
succeeded to extract the AABB part of bread wheat and found that
these extracts were dwarf plants that differed in many ways from
tetraploid wheat species and that they were especially adapted to
cooperate with the D-genome derived from Aegilops squarrosa.
Later on, Kaltsikes et al. (43) carried out similar extraction.
   From such data it was evident that in hybrids between octoploid and hexaploid triticale there will be a comprehensive
genetic recombination between the A and B genomes derived from
tetraploid wheat and those derived from hexaploid wheat. This
recombination, when followed by selection, will lead to favourable
results. As indicated above, in the 1960's very good results
from crosses between octoploid and hexaploid triticales were
obtained by workers in the U.S.S.R., Hungary, Canada, and U.S.A.
Later on the production of such secondary hexaploid triticales,
as they are now called, has become one of the main standard
methods in breeding work with triticale.
   In work performed by the present writer (12,16,44) not only
improved secondary hexaploids have been obtained but also valuable
secondary octoploid triticales. To avoid chromosome elimination
in the latter case, the octoploid X hexaploid F_1 hybrids were
backcrossed reciprocally to octoploid strains.

   Cytoplasm. The superiority of secondary hexaploids is not
only due to favourable recombination of genes in the A and B
genomes contributed by tetraploid and hexaploid wheat species:
cytoplasmic factors are also involved. This was first suggested
by Sisodia and McGinnis (45) and conclusively proved by Larter
and Hsam (46) and Hsam and Larter (47). As a general conclusion
of these investigations, Hsam and Larter pointed out that evidently
the hexaploid wheat cytoplasm had been modified by the presence

of the D genome from <u>Aegilops squarrosa</u>, and that the production
and utilization of secondary triticales with the favourable
hexaploid wheat cytoplasm should form an integral part of a
triticale breeding program.

    <u>Triple Hybrids from Three-way Crosses</u>. Addition of the
genomes of two wheat species and rye was reported by Müntzing
(48). F_1 hybrids between the tetraploid wheat species <u>Triticum</u>
<u>turgidum</u> and rye were produced and found to be highly sterile.
However, unreduced ovules with 21 chromosomes were formed in the
F_1 and could be "picked up" by pollen grains from bread wheat
with the same chromosome number as the unreduced ovules.
    The "triple hybrids", carrying the genomes of three species
(Fig. 1), had very poor fertility, but some offspring could be
raised and they were studied for a few generations. This material
was then discarded since the production in this way of agronomically useful products seemed to be exluded.
    However, better results were later obtained by pollinating
F_1 hybrids from crosses between bread wheat and rye with pollen
from already existing octoploid triticales (14, pp. 410-421).
    This led to the production of new heterozygous strains of
octoploid triticale (Fig. 2), from which useful and stable octoploid triticales could later be selected. Research work of this
kind is still in progress, but now the primary hybrids between
bread wheat and rye are pollinated with hexaploid, instead of
octoploid, strains of triticale. This gives rise to triple
hybrids with 2n=49 from which, in later generations, new strains
of hexaploid triticale may be selected.
    Such work is carried out especially because A.F. Shulydin
(working in Charkov, U.S.S.R.) has obtained very good results
with this method. Some triticales, derived from triple hybrids
in Shulyndin's material, considerably surpassed bread wheat in
grain yield and amount of protein per hectar. The triple hybrid
derivatives also had the best winter hardiness. Some of them are
recommended for cereal production and other ones for forage or
green matter production (49,50).
    Another large group of triple hybrids from three-way crosses
has been produced at the Southwestern Great Plains Research
Center, Bushland, Texas (51). Numerous F_1 seed of male-sterile
wheat X rye and of F_1 seed of the three-way crosses of (male-
sterile wheat X rye F_1's) X hexaploid triticale were produced in
field crossing blocks. Among the F_3's of such three-way crosses
800 plants were selected. Their F_4 and F_5 progenies were found
to vary in height, maturity, fertility, grain yield, and seed
quality, and ranged from true winter to spring in growth habit.
Yield trials showed that most of the F_3 plant progenies equaled
or exceeded the yield and test weight of one or more the the
commercial triticale varieties used in Texas. The number of
promising lines selected from the 800 F_3 families suggest that

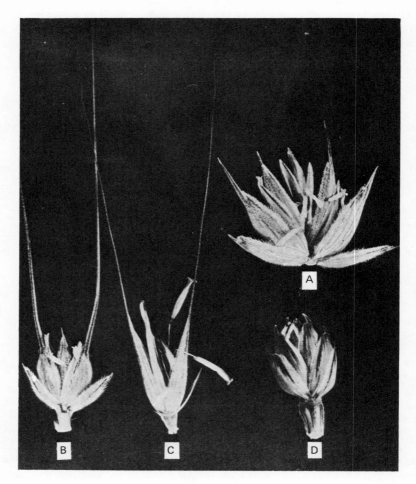

Fig. 1.   Spikelets of a triple hybrid (A) between <u>Triticum</u> <u>turgidum</u> (B), <u>Secale</u> <u>cereale</u> (C), and <u>Triticum</u> <u>aestivum</u> (D).

the vastly more diverse breeding material later produced in the same way at this station holds real promise for triticale improvement.   Such experiences are evidently quite similar to those made by Shulyndin in the Soviet Union as regards the value of three-way crosses for the production of outstanding new triticale strains.

<u>Substitutions</u>.   In breeding work with hexaploid triticales at CIMMYT, Mexico the so-called Armadillo strains have played an important role.   As reported (52,53), these strains were found to

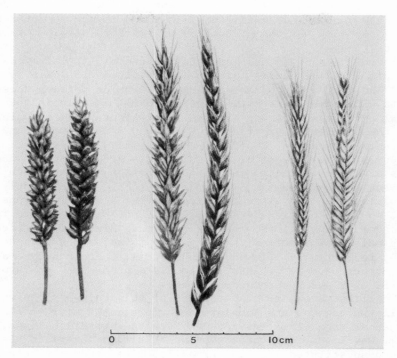

Fig. 2. Ears of a new triticale product (in the middle) in comparison with ears of the bread wheat parent (to the left) and the rye parent (to the right). The triticale ears are from two different I_2 plants derived from a new triticale heterozygote. This heterozygote (2n=56) arose from pollination of a primary wheat X rye hybrid (2n=28) with triticale pollen (In=28) (14).

have high fertility, improved test weight, better grain yield, insensitivity to day length, one gene for dwarfness, early maturity, and good nutritional quality. Investigations on the origin of the unusual characteristics of the Armadillo strains revealed that they must have been introduced by a spontaneous hybrid between hexaploid triticale and a Mexican bread wheat having a dwarfing gene.

On account of their outstanding properties the Armadillo strains were used extensively in crosses to other hexaploid triticales during the following generations. Selections with fertility approaching that of the Armadillo parent were obtained among the segregating populations. By 1970 practically all the material in the CIMMYT triticale program originated from crosses having Armadillo as a progenitor (54).

Positive results with triticales derived from artificial crosses between hexaploid triticale and bread wheat have been reported by several workers (40,55-58), and is now one of the standard methods for the production of improved strains of hexaploid triticale.

To understand why such crosses are useful, it is necessary to recall that the genome formula of hexaploid triticale is AABBRR and that of bread wheat AABBDD. Hybrids between these parents will have the constitutions AABBRD. At meiosis the typical chromosome pairing will be 14 bivalents + 14 univalents, where the bivalents comprise all the A and B chromosomes and the univalents represent 7 R and 7 D chromosomes.

During meiosis some of the univalents are eliminated and the others are transmitted to the next generation together with all the A and B chromosomes. Since the plants are predominantly selfpollinating, the ultimate effect, after a number of generations, would theoretically be a multitude of plants with different chromosome constitutions, ranging from pure hexaploid triticales to typical bread wheats with the genome formulas AABBRR and AABBDD, respectively. In addition to this, there could be a large number of more or less intermediate products with favourable mixtures of R and D chromosome pairs.

The first known representatives of this category, in which not all the genomes are complete but represent a mixture of chromosomes from different genomes, are the Armadillo lines. In 1973 it was found that chromosome pair 2D from hexaploid wheat had been substituted into the Armadillo line, thus replacing one pair of rye chromosomes (59). Evidence was also obtained that the complete A and B genomes were present. Shortly after this discovery, Gregory (60) reported other cases of crosses between hexaploid triticale and bread wheat in which D genome chromosomes had been substituted for rye chromosomes.

As previously mentioned the favourable properties of the Armadillo strains were rapidly utilized in the triticale program at CIMMYT, Mexico, and soon practically all the triticale strains involved in the breeding work were derived from crosses involving Armadillo lines as one of the parents. As it is now known that at least one of the rye chromosomes from the D genome, it is obvious that such substitutions must be widespread in the present CIMMYT material. That such is the case was shown by Merker (61), who studied the chromosome complements of 48 lines of hexaploid triticale and triticale X wheat intercross lines belonging to the CIMMYT breeding program. At that time the development of the Giemsa technique for staining chromosomes had opened new horizons for triticale cytogenetics. Thus it was possible to distinguish accurately between rye and wheat chromosomes during mitosis. According to Merker (62), rye chromosomes have telomeric and wheat chromosomes centromeric heterochromatin or no heterochromatin at all. Using such a technique, it was possible to determine with precision how many pairs of rye chromosomes that are present

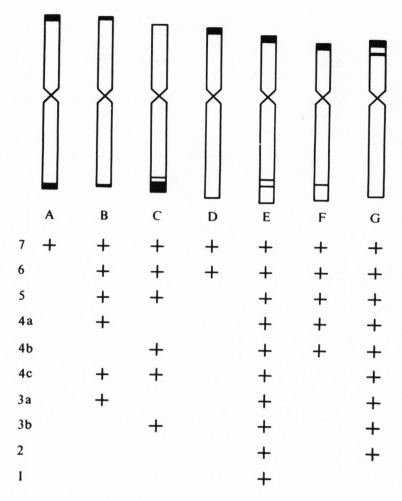

	A	B	C	D	E	F	G
7	+	+	+	+	+	+	+
6		+	+	+	+	+	+
5		+	+		+	+	+
4a		+			+	+	+
4b			+		+	+	+
4c		+	+		+		+
3a		+			+		+
3b			+		+		+
2					+		+
1					+		

Fig. 3.   Substitutions in hexaploid triticales.   Idiogram of the rye chromosomes and chromosome compositions of the investigated lines.   Black regions of the chromosomes represent heterochromatin. Letters A to G indicate the seven rye chromosomes.   Further explanation in the text (61).

in a triticale line and the identity of these chromosomes (61).
    The aim of Merker's investigation was to elucidate to what extent rye chromosomes in advanced lines from the CIMMYT program had been replaced by wheat chromosomes.   From the absence of a pair of rye chromosomes the presence of the homoeologous D genome chromosome pair could be detected.

The pattern of heterochromatic staining is indicated in Fig. 3. This represents the rye idiogram as found in the material investigated. The letters A to G indicate the seven rye chromosomes. Some variation exists but the idiogram represents the most frequent type of each chromosome. Black regions in the chromosomes represent heterochromatin. Fig. 3 shows the different types of rye chromosomes found to be present in the material investigated. A + sign indicates the presence of the rye chromosome in question; the absence of + indicates the absence of the rye chromosome in question and the presence of the homoeologous wheat chromosome of the D genome. The figures to the left indicate the 10 different chromosome constellations observed among the 48 lines examined.

Of these lines only four carried all the rye chromosomes whereas 44 lines represented more or less comprehensive substitutions. In the majority of these lines one, two, or three rye chromosome pairs had been replaced by the corresponding chromosomes in wheat genome D.

Merker's investigation also included studies of meiosis in three different F_1 combinations. The mode of chromosome pairing was in perfect harmony with the substitutions observed in somatic cells. If two lines differ in the identity of one pair of chromosomes, a minimum of two univalents are expected, and so on. This is exactly what was found in the analyzed F_1's. Thus these investigations clearly demonstrate that the results obtained should be interpreted as substitutions and not as loss of heterochromatin in the rye chromosomes.

In Merker's material there was a gross correlation between chromosome composition and the morphological appearance of the plants. On the whole the more wheaty types had fewer rye chromosomes. However, data were obtained which indicate that the specific triticale characters are mainly induced by genes in chromosomes 3R and 5R.

The substitutional polyploidy discussed by Merker (61,63) is probably one of the reasons for the superiority of triticales derived from crosses between typical triticale and bread wheat. A number of lines with one, two, or three pairs of D genome chromosomes substituting for rye chromosomes are advanced lines with agronomically important characters such as high yield, disease resistance, insensitivity to day length, and resistance to lodging. Thus, chromosome substitutions and the establishing of lines with mixed genomes seem to produce new chromosome combinations and genotypes of high agronomic potential. Most probably this is possible only in polyploid species where the other genomes have a buffering effect.

It should be observed, however, that preferential selection of wheat-rye substitutions does not occur only as a consequence of human selection, for natural selection may also play a role (64,65). This natural selection acts on chromosome size and/or DNA content. In a recent investigation (66) it was possible to ascertain which wheat-rye chromosome substitutions occur in hexaploid wheat X hexaploid triticale populations where no artificial selection pressure had been applied. Thus, the largest of the rye chromosomes (2R) was the first to be lost and was present only when all seven rye chromosome pairs were present. On the other hand, the smallest rye chromosome (1R) was present in all the plants.

Though substitutions now seem to be of great importance in triticale breeding it should be observed, however, that a surprisingly good alternative to complicated substitutions has recently appeared: In a few cases new hexaploid triticales have been produced which are entirely free from substitutions but nevertheless have quite good properties, including vigour and fertility. Two strains of this kind, Beagle and DRIRA, have been produced in the CIMMYT program and of the two, especially Beagle has behaved very well in the Swedish environment. It should be mentioned that these strains have the bread wheat cytoplasm and low amounts of heterochromatin which explains part of their good properties. Such data suggest that parallel to the research with substitutional triticales new triticales of more classical types should still be produced and tested.

As to the effects of heterochromatin further data were gathered by Merker (67). He observed variation in the heterochromatic pattern in an advanced strain of hexaploid triticale. In some plants the largest telomeric heterochromatic region was deleted. This made it possible to select isogenic lines with presence and absence of the heterochromatic region, as well as plants in which one homolog carried the region and the other one lacked it. The heterochromatic region in question is the largest one in the whole chromosome complement of this strain. Plants with this region absent have about one-third fewer univalents at first metaphase as compared to plants with the region present. In plants where one homolog carries the region and the other does not, this rye chromosome pair forms an open bivalent or two univalents in most of the pollen mother cells. In such plants, univalents of this rye chromosome pair constitute about one-third of the total number of univalents. These data experimentally verify Bennett's view (68) that heterochromatin plays a major role in meiotic pairing failure and cytological instability of triticale.

Analysis of progenies of selfed plants heterozygous for the presence of the heterochromatic region indicated a tendency to selection against the homolog carrying the region. This is in harmony with the fact that many advanced lines of triticale have a reduced quantity of heterochromatin as compared to rye. This is probably the result of an indirect selection for cytological stability.

CONCLUDING REMARKS

From another and more comprehensive report concerning results and problems of research with triticale (12), it is evident that such work is now carried out by numerous plant breeders and scientists, representing many different organizations and institutes throughout the world.

In the present paper some information has been given concerning the origin and properties of various kinds of triticale. At first research was mainly devoted to octoploids, but during the last 30 years the hexaploid triticales have dominated the scene. The primary types and their recombination products were soon followed by secondary triticales with good properties derived from crosses between octoploids and hexaploids. Triple hybrids, representing combinations between hexaploid and tetraploid wheat with diploid rye, were found to have useful properties and are produced in several countries. Then, less than decade ago, the substitutional triticales became known, showing that the individual chromosomes from various genomes, especially D and R, could be combined in many different ways with important results.

Though breeding work with triticale has to meet several difficult problems such as meiotic irregularity, partial sterility, aneuploidy, and seed shrivelling, several strains have been found to be good enough to be cultivated in practice. Various cultivars of triticale are now utilized in Hungary, Spain, Canada, United States, and China for different purposes (food, feed, forage).

From a theoretical point of view, triticale represents a good example of induced polyploidy, which in several respects deserves to be compared with spontaneous polyploids in nature.

LITERATURE CITED

1. Rimpau, W., 1891, Kreuzungsprodukte landwirtschaftlicher Kulturpflanzen.   Landwirtschaftl. Jahrb. 20: 335-371.
2. Tschermak-Seysenegg, E., 1936, Wirkliche, abgeleitete und fragliche Weizen-Roggen-Bastarde (Triticale-Formen), pp. 1-4, Vorläuf. Mitteil. Sitzung Mathem.-naturwiss. Klasse vom 29, Oktober 1936.   Akak. Wiss.schaft. Wien.
3. Lindschau, Oehler, E., 1935, Untersuchungen am konstant intermediären additive Rimpau'schen Weizen-Roggen-Bastard. Züchter 7: 228-233.
4. Müntzing, A., 1935, Berättelse över verksamheten vid Sveriges Utsädesförenings kromosomavdelning under tiden 1 Oktober 1931-30 September 1935. Sveriges Utsädesförenings Tidskr. 305-320 (in Swedish).
5. Müntzing, A., 1936, Über die Entstehungsweise 56-chromosomiger Weizen-Roggen-Bastarde. Züchter 8: 188-191.
6. Tiumiakov, N., 1928, Neue Erscheinungen, beobachtet an Roggen-Weizenhybriden des Zwischenstadiumtypus der Genera-

tionen F_2 und F_3, pp. 104-105, Verh. d. USSR Bot.-Kongr.

7. Meister, G.K., 1928, Das Problem der Speziesbastardierung, pp. 1049-1117, Z. Indukt. Abstamm.-Vererbungsl. Suppl. Bd. 2. Verh. 5 Inter. Kongr. Vererb.-Wissensch.

8. Lewitsky, G.A., Benetzkaja, G.K., 1929, Cytologische Untersuchung der konstant-intermediären Weizen-Roggen-Bastarden, pp. 197-198, Zusätzen zur Liste der Vorträge und Thesen des UDSSR-Kongresses f. Genet., Pflanz.- u. Tierzüchtg (in Russian).

9. Lewitsky, G.A., Benetzkaja, G.K., 1930, Cytological investigation of constant-intermediate rye-wheat hybrids, pp. 345-352, Proc. All-Union Congr. Genet. Sel., Leningrad 1929 (in Russian with English summary).

10. Lewitsky, G.A., Benetzkaja, G.K., 1931, Cytology of the wheat-rye amphidiploids, pp. 241-264, Bull. Appl. Bot. Genet. Plant Breed. (Leningrad) 27 (in Russian with English summary).

11. Baum, B.R., 1971, The taxonomic and cytogenetic implications of the problem of naming amphiploids of Triticum and Secale. Euphytica 20: 302-306.

12. Müntzing, A., 1979, Triticale. Results and Problems. Adv. Pl. Breeding 10: 1-103.

13. v. Berg, K.H., Oehler, E., 1938, Untersuchungen über die Cytogenetik amphidiploider Weizen-Roggen-Bastarde. Züchter 10: 226-238.

14. Müntzing, A., 1939, Studies on the properties and the ways of production of rye-wheat amphidiploids. Hereditas 25: 387-430.

15. Müntzing, A., 1957, Cytogenetic studies in rye-wheat (Triticale). Cytologia (Suppl.): 51-56.

16. Müntzing, A., 1972, Experiences from work with octoploid and hexaploid rye-wheat (Triticale). Biol. Zentralbl. 91: 69-80.

17. Krolow, K.D., 1962, Aneuploidie und Fertilität bei amphidiploiden Weizen-Roggen-Bastarden (Triticale). I. Aneuploidie und Selektion auf Fertilität bei oktoploiden Triticale-Formen. Z. Pflanzenzüchtg. 48: 177-196.

18. Krolow, K.D., 1963, Aneuploidie und Fertilität bei amphidiploiden Weizen-Roggen-Bastarden (Triticale). II. Aneuploidie-und Fertilitätsuntersuchungen an einer oktoploiden Triticale-Form mit starker Abregulierungstendenz. Z. Pflanzenzüchtg. 49: 210-242.

19. Krolow, K.D., 1969, Cytologische Untersuchungen an Kreuzungen zwischen 8x and 6x Triticale. I. Untersuchungen an den Eltern, an der F_1 und der F_2. Z. Pflanzenzüchtg. 62: 241-271

20. Krolow, K.D., 1969, Cytologische Untersuchungen an Kreuzungen zwischen 8x und 6x Triticale. II. Untersuchungen and F_2- (Meiosis), F_3- und F_4-Pflanzen. Z. Pflanzenzüchtg. 62: 311-342.

21. Tsuchiya, T., 1973, Frequency of euploids in different seed size classes of hexaploid triticale. Euphytica 22: 592-599.

22. Weimarck, A., 1973, Cytogenetic behaviour in octoploid
    Triticale. I. Meiosis, aneuploidy, and fertility. Hereditas
    74: 103-118.

23. Weimarck, A., 1974, Elimination of wheat and rye chromosomes
    in a strain of octoploid Triticale as revealed by Giemsa
    banding technique. Hereditas 77: 281-286.

24. Weimarck, A., 1975, Cytogenetic behaviour in octoploid
    Triticale. II. Meiosis with special reference to chiasma
    frequency and fertility in F_1 and parents. Hereditas 80:
    121-130.

25. Khvostova, V.V., Shkutina, F.M., 1975, The causes of low
    fertility in triticale, pp. 186-190, in "Triticale, Studies
    and Breeding," Proc. Inter. Symp. 1973, Leningrad.

26. Pieritz, W.J., 1966, Untersuchungen über die Ursachen der
    Aneuploidie bei amphidiploiden Weizen-Roggen-Bastarden und
    über die Funktionsfähigkeit ihrer männlichen und weiblichen
    Gameten. Z. Pflanzenzüchtg. 56: 27-69.

27. Pieritz, W.J., 1970, Elimination von Chromosomen in amphid-
    iploiden Weizen-Roggen-Bastarden (Triticale). Z. Pflanzen-
    züchtg. 64: 90-109.

28. Bjurman, B., 1958, Note on the frequency of the univalents
    in some strains of Triticale and their hybrids. Hereditas
    44: 189-192.

29. Derzhavin, A., 1938, Results of work on breeding perennial
    varities of wheat and rye. Izv. Acad. Nauk. USSR, Ser.
    Biol. 3: 663-665 (in Russian).

30. O'Mara, J.G., 1948, Fertility in allopolyploids. Rec.
    Genet. Soc. Amer. 17: 52.

31. Nakajima, G., 1950, Genetical and cytological studies in
    breeding of amphidiploid types between Triticum and Secale.
    I. The external characters and chromosomes of fertile F_1
    T. turgidum (n=14) X S cereale (n=7) and its F_2 progenies.
    Jap. J. Genet. 25: 139-148.

32. Sanchez-Monge, E., Tjio, J.H., 1954, Note on 42 chromosome
    Triticale. Caryologia Suppl. 2: 748.

33. Sanchez-Monge, E., 1956, Studies on 42-chromosome Triticale.
    I. The production of the amphidiploids. An. Aula Dei 4:
    191-207.

34. Sanchez-Monge, E., 1959, Hexaploid Triticale, pp. 181-194,
    Proc. 1st Inter. Wheat Genet. Symp., Winnipeg.

35. Pissarev, V., 1966, Different approaches in Triticale breed-
    ing. Proc. 2nd Inter. Wheat Genet. Symp. 1963, Lund, Sweden.
    Hereditas Suppl. 2: 279-290.

36. Kiss, A., 1966, Neue Richtung in der Triticale-Züchtung. Z.
    Pflanzenzüchtg. 55: 309-329.

37. Kiss, A., 1966, Kreuzungsversuche mit Triticale. Züchter
    36: 249-255.

38. Kiss, A., 1971, Origin of the preliminary released Hungarian
    varieties, Nos. 57 and 64. Wheat Inform. Serv. 32: 20-22.

39. Kiss, A., 1974, Triticale-breeding experiments in Eastern

Europe, pp. 41-50, in "Triticale," IDRC-024e. Proc. Inter. Symp. 1973, El Batan, Mexico.

40. Jenkins, B.C., 1969, History of the development of some presently promising hexaploid triticales. Wheat Inform. Serv. 28: 18-20.

41. Jenkins, B.C., 1974, Hexaploid triticale: past, present and future, pp. 56-61, in "Triticale," First Man-made Cereal. Proc. Inter. Symp. 1973, St. Louis, Publ. by Amer. Assoc. Cereal Chem.

42. Kerber, E.R., 1964, Wheat: reconstitution of the tetraploid component (AABB) of hexaploids. Science 143: 253-255.

43. Kaltsikes, P.J., Evans, L.E., Larter, E.N., 1969, Morphological and meiotic characteristics of the extracted AABB tetraploid component of three varieties of common wheat. Canad. J. Genet. Cytol. 11: 65-71.

44. Müntzing, A., 1975, Some results from cytogenetic studies and breeding work in triticale, pp. 70-75, in "Triticale, Studies and Breeding," Proc. Inter. Symp. 1973, Leningrad.

45. Sisodia, N.S., McGinnis, R.C., 1970, Importance of hexaploid wheat germ plasm in hexaploid triticale breeding. Crop Sci. 10: 161-162.

46. Larter, E.N., Hsam, S.L.K., 1973, Performance of hexaploid triticale as influenced by source of wheat cytoplasm, pp. 245-251, in Proc. 4th Inter. Wheat Genet. Symp. 1973, Agric. Exp. Sta., Columbia, Missouri.

47. Hsam, S.L.K., Larter, E.N., 1974, Influence of source of wheat cytoplasm on the synthesis and plant characteristics of hexaploid triticale. Canad. J. Genet. Cytol. 16: 333-340.

48. Müntzing, A., 1935, Triple hybrids between rye and two wheat species. Hereditas 20: 137-160.

49. Shulyndin, A.F., 1972, Wheat-rye allopolyploids (Triticale) and problems of immunity, quality, winter-hardiness and grain production. Genetica 8: 61-74.

50. Shulyndin, A.F., 1975, Genetical grounds of synthesis in various triticales and their improvement by breeding, pp. 53-69, in "Triticale, Studies and Breeding," Proc. Inter. Symp. 1973, Leningrad.

51. Porter, K.B., Tuleen, N.A., 1976, The performance, fertility, and cytology of progeny of male sterile wheat-rye F_1/triticale hybrids, in Proc. Inter. Triticale Symp. 1973, Lubbock, Texas, ICASALS Publ. 76-1: 73-78.

52. Zillinsky, F.J., Borlaug, N.E., 1971, Progress in developing triticale as an economic crop. CIMMYT Res. Bull. 17: 1-27.

53. Zillinsky, F.J., 1974, The development of triticale. Adv. Agron. 26: 315-348.

54. Zillinsky, F.J., 1974, The triticale improvement program at CIMMYT, pp. 81-85, in "Triticale," IDRC-024e, Proc. Inter. Symp. 1973, El Batan, Mexico.

55. Larter, E.N., Tsuchiya, T., Evans, L., 1968, Breeding and

cytology of triticale, pp. 213-221, in Proc. 3rd Inter.
Wheat Genet. Symp. 1968, Australian Acad. Sci., Canberra.

56. Jenkins, B.C., 1975, Hexaploid triticale: past present and
     future, pp. 26-30, in "Triticale, Studies and Breeding"
     Proc. Inter. Symp. 1973, Leningrad.

57. Popov, P., Tsvetkov, S., 1975, Development of winter primary
     and secondary hexaploid triticale (2n=42), pp. 151-157, in
     "Triticale, Studies and Breeding," Proc. Inter. Symp. 1973,
     Leningrad.

58. Kolev, D., 1975, Characteristics of Triticale (2n=58) AD-
     COC-3 and some of its hybrids, pp. 96-107, in "Triticale,
     Studies and Breeding," Proc. Inter. Symp. 1973, Leningrad.

59. Gustafson, J.P., Zillinsky, F.J., 1973, Identification of D-
     genome chromosomes from hexaploid wheat in a 42-chromosome
     triticale, pp. 225-232, in Proc. 4th Inter. Wheat Genet.
     Symp. 1973, Agric. Exp. Sta., Columbia, Missouri.

60. Gregory, R.S., 1974, Triticale research program in the
     United Kingdom, pp. 61-67, in "Triticale," IDRC-024e, Proc.
     Inter. Symp. 1973, El Batan, Mexico.

61. Merker, A. 1975, Chromosome composition of hexaploid triticale.
     Hereditas 80: 41-52.

62. Merker, A., 1973, A Giemsa technique for rapid identification
     of chromosomes in Triticale. Hereditas 75: 280-282.

63. Merker, A., 1976, Chromosome substitution, genetic recombin-
     ation and the breeding of triticale. Wheat Inform. Serv.
     41-42: 44-48.

64. Gustafson, J.P., Bennett, M.D., 1976, Preferential selection
     for wheat-rye substitutions in 42-chromosome triticale.
     Crop Sci. 16: 688-693.

65. Gustafson, J.P., 1976, The evolutionary development of
     triticale: the wheat-rye hybrid. Evol. Biol. 9: 107-135.

66. Gustafson, J.P., Zillinsky, F.J., 1978, Influences of natural
     selection on the chromosome complement of hexaploid triticale.
     Proc. 5th Inter. Wheat Genet. Symp., New Delhi (in press).

67. Merker, A., 1976, The cytogenetic effect of heterochromatin
     in hexaploid triticale. Hereditas 83: 215-222.

68. Bennett, M.D., 1974, Meiotic gametophytic, and early endosperm
     development in Triticale, pp. 137-148, in "Triticale," IDRC-
     024e, Proc. Inter. Symp. 1973, El Batan, Mexico.

USES OF WHEAT ANEUPLOIDS[1]

G. Kimber and E. R. Sears

Department of Agronomy, University of Missouri, and
Science and Education Administration of USDA
Columbia, MO   65201

The constructive use of aneuploids in any type of study
obviously depends on the availability, fertility, and viability
of an essentially complete series of aberrant types. In cultivated wheat (Triticum aestivum, 2n=6x=42) there are available
collections of aneuploids unequaled in any other organism. For
example, in the cultivar Chinese Spring, Sears (1) produced
complete sets of nullisomics, monosomics, trisomics, and tetrasomics, and Sears and Sears (2) have accumulated 41 of the 42
possible telocentrics. Furthermore, many combinations of these
aneuploids have been constructed for analyzing specific chromosomal, genetic, and evolutionary situations. Similar but less
complete sets of aneuploids in other cultivars have been derived
from the Chinese Spring material or have been produced independently. These developments have allowed the investigation of the
cytogenetics and evolution of T. aestivum with an elegance and
precision currently unattainable in few if any other higher
organisms. The ramifications of these investigations are seen
not only in the evolutionary and genetic framework so constructed,
but also in actual and potential practical manipulations now
available that allow a precise and often predictable genetic
control over introduced diversity in the species.

---

[1] Cooperative investigations of SEA, USDA, and the Agronomy
Department, University of Missouri. Journal Series No. 8361 of
the Missouri Agricultural Experiment Station.

GENETICS

Monosomics

Genes are located on chromosomes; it therefore follows
that the irregular distribution of a genetically marked monosomic
chromosome at meiosis will disturb the genetic segregation ratios
observed in euploids. It is this disturbance of segregation
ratios that allows genes to be assigned to specific chromosomes
of the set, and incidentally provides a most convincing demonstration of the fact that genes are indeed located on chromosomes.

In undertaking monosomic analysis in wheat, use is made of
the fact that the female transmission of gametes deficient for
the monosomic chromosome is approximately 75%. It is therefore
conventional to pollinate the monosomic series with the line or
variety being analyzed. Certation mitigates against the use of
monosomics as male parents. Hence, the univalent chromosome in
the hybrid progeny is, neglecting univalent shift, derived from
the male parent. The phenotype of the hemizygous progeny, if the
gene is recessive, or the disturbed segregation of the selfed
progeny clearly indicates the identity of the critical chromo-
some(s) involved. The more common segregation patterns are
listed in Table 1.

Monosomic analysis involves maintaining the 21 lines of the
tester series, recognizing their cytological makeup and checking
for the absence of univalent shift. This is a time-consuming
task that requires the skill of a cytologist. Consequently, the
use of monosomics in genetic analysis has not been as widespread
as would be anticipated from the potential and elegance of the
method. Monotelo- or monoisosomics can be used instead of monosomics to prevent univalent shift, but some of these are poorly
fertile. Double monotelosomics (20"+t'+t') may be more useful,
since they are of satisfactory fertility.

Some examples of the utilization of monosomic analysis for
locating genes that affect different attributes are (1) morphological characters (3-5); (2) lethality (6); (3) disease resistance (7-10); and (4) metric characters (11). Maan and Lucken
(12), using a modified monosomic analysis, were able to locate
genes that interact with the cytoplasm to produce male sterility.
By recording the association of nucleoli with the micronuclei
derived from the aberrant segregation of univalents at the preceding divisions, Crosby (13) was able to identify the location
of the nucleolar organizer regions with specific chromosomes.
Various workers (14-18 and others) have used other aneuploids,
often nullisomic-tetrasomics, in locating biochemical markers in
wheat.

Bielig and Driscoll (19,20) described the production of
monosomic alien substitution lines (MAS) in wheat as having 20
pairs of chromosomes from wheat and a univalent chromosome from
an alien species substituted for a pair of wheat homologs. In

Table 1. The anticipated segregation patterns in $\underline{T.\ aestivum}$ when a complete set of 21 monosomics of recessive phenotype is pollinated with euploids of differing genetic constitution.

No. of genes	Euploid inheritance	Euploid segregation	Monosomic F_1 segregation[1]	Selfed progeny of F_1 monosomics
1	Recessive[a]	3:1	20 lines all with dominant phenotype; 1 critical line with recessive phenotype	
1	Hemizygous ineffective	3:1	All 21 lines dominant phenotype	All 21 lines segregate 3:1; in critical line only disomics have recessive phenotype
1	Dominant	3:1	All 21 lines dominant phenotype	20 lines segregate dominant; 1 recessive; one 1 line all dominant to zero recessive[b]
2	Duplicate dominants	15:1	All 21 lines dominant	19 lines segregate 15 dominant : 1 recessive; two lines all dominant to zero recessive[b]
2	Complementary dominant	9:7	All 21 lines dominant phenotype	19 lines segregate 9:7; two lines segregate 3:1
3	Triplicate dominant	63:1	All 21 lines with dominant phenotype	18 lines segregate 63:1; three lines all dominant to zero recessive[b]

[a]In this case the monosomic would have to be dominant.

[b]Because of the infrequent recovery of nullisomics, occasional plants with the recessive phenotype will be recorded, less frequently in the case of duplicate dominants and even less frequently in the case of triplicate inheritance.

each case the alien chromosome carries a genetic marker allowing
its identification without recourse to cytology. The use of
these lines as the female parent in monosomic analyses or in the
production of intervarietal chromosome substitutions reduces the
amount of cytology necessary and simultaneously permits detection
of univalent shift by genetic means.

Morris (21) published a list of genes in wheat that had been
located on specific chromosomes, mainly by monosomic analysis,
and has updated the list each year in Wheat Newsletter.

Telocentric Mapping and Analysis

The chromosome complement of Triticum aestivum consists of
21 pairs of chromosomes, none of which has a terminal or subterminal centromere. Although this situation causes difficulty in
recognizing individual chromosomes by size and arm-ratio comparisons, it incidentally provides the background against which
misdivision products, particularly telocentrics, can easily be
recognized.

The fortunate karyotypic situation coupled with the fertility and stability of almost all lines containing one or more
telocentrics makes this type of material particularly valuable in
genetic analysis and in studies of evolution.

Sears (22) recognized that the presence or absence of a
telocentric chromosome can be used as a phenotypic character,
just as any other marker. It follows that because the segregation
of telocentrics (as any other chromosome) depends on which pole
the centromere moves to, the frequency of occurrence of a telocentric chromosome in a progeny segregating for genes on that
chromosome arm can be used as a means of mapping the distance
between the centromere and other linked loci.

The technique of Sears consists of crossing the euploid
marker stock with the appropriate ditelocentric stocks and then
using the F_1 as a male parent onto homozygous recessive euploid
females. The recombination value between the marked locus and
the centromere is derived in a conventional manner from the
proportion of parental (marked whole chromosomes or unmarked
telocentrics) and recombinant (marked telocentric or unmarked
whole chromosomes) types among the progeny. The original analysis
gave the B2, Srll, and Ki loci, respectively, 0.44, 45.1, and
51.3% recombination to the centromere on the long arm of chromosome
6B (22). Other workers have used this or modified techniques, to
locate other genes; e.g., Williams and Maan (23) have mapped
genes for disease resistance, and Law and Worland (11) summarized
the analysis of both quantitative and qualitative characters on
chromosome 7B of the cultivar Hope. McIntosh (24) lists linkage
of various loci in T. aestivum together with 31 examples of
linkage to the centromere.

The technique of telocentric mapping may also be applied to
alien chromosomes added to a wheat background when both the

appropriate telocentrics and marker stocks are available. Chang
et al. (25) in a preliminary analysis mapped the Hp (hairy ped-
uncle) gene of rye as more than 50 crossover units from the centromere
on the long arm of chromosome 5R. The labor and difficulties
associated with this type of analysis of alien chromosomes would
often make the experiment prohibitive in cost and time; however,
it does demonstrate the power of the technique, which allows the
centromere mapping of genes on chromosomes of diploid species
where the maintenance of aneuploids is often difficult or impossible.

    Gill and Kimber (26) also took advantage of the fact that
telocentric chromosomes can be unequivocally identified in somatic
cells when they constructed the Giemsa-banded karyotype of T.
aestivum. By examining only the banding pattern of the known
telocentrics it was possible to synthesize a definitive karyotype
involving 41 of the 42 chromosome arms. Following the production
of this karyotype it was possible to identify the characteristic
patterns of the three genomes and relate these to the putative
diploid progenitors. The A and D genomes could be well matched
to T. monococcum and T. tauschii, respectively, whereas the B
genome is totally different from any of the species previously
proposed as donors. Clearly, this now allows for the search of
the B-genome donor through examination of the karyotypes of other
diploids.

    Another use of telocentric aneuploids was made by Fu and
Sears (27), who demonstrated a 1:1 relationship between chiasmata
and crossing over. They recorded the chiasma frequency in a
heteromorphic bivalent consisting of a telocentric and a complete
chromosome. The telocentric and the corresponding arm of the
complete chromosome were heterozygous for genetic markers, and
the recombination of these characters was observed in the progeny.
Interestingly, the chiasma frequency at metaphase was lower than
would have been predicted from the recombination frequency.
However, the chiasma frequency at diakinesis did show a clear 1:1
correspondence. The lower frequency of chiasmata at metaphase
was attributed to terminalization prior to observation. Barlow
and Driscoll (personal communication) observed an even greater
discrepancy between crossing over and metaphase pairing of bivalents
that included a telocentric chromosome not completely homologous
with its mate.

    Because one of the important characteristics of a chromosome
arm is its length relative to that of the other arm of the same
chromosome, it is essential that an accurate method be available
for making this determination. Simply measuring the respective
telocentrics is not satisfactory, due to the great variation from
cell to cell. L. Sears (in 2) solved this problem by measuring
the telocentrics in cells of dimonotelosomic plants (containing
two telocentrics for one arm and one for the opposite arm).
Relatively few cells had to be measured to establish whether the

two telocentrics of nearest the same length were longer or shorter
than the third one.

Linde-Laursen and Larsen (28) used double monotelodisomics
to identify translocations in T. aestivum and thus achieved a
precise resolution unobtainable with monosomics alone.

Regulation of Chromosome Pairing

The regular bivalent formation in polyploids has classically
been ascribed to differential affinity. That is a preferental
synapsis of homologs to the exclusion of pairing between similar
(homoeologous) chromosomes from the constituent species of the
polyploid. The first clear recognition of the genetic control of
the cytological diploidization of polyploids came from studies of
aneuploid conditions in wheat and wheat hybrids (29,30) and
inferentially in other polyploid species (31).

In T. aestivum (and by circumstantial evidence in T. turgidum,
T. timopheevii, and T. zhukovskyi) the major gene regulating the
normal chromosome pairing pattern is located on the long arm of
chromosome 5B some 50 crossover units from the centromere
(32). When this Ph locus is present, even in the hemizygous
condition, chromosome pairing is restricted to homologous chromosomes. In aneuploid conditions (e.g., nullihaploid or hybrids
deficient for chromosome 5B) in which no homologous chromosomes
are present, the pairing of homoeologous chromosomes takes place
at a frequency considerably higher than when chromosome 5B is
present (30,33). In aneuploid situations in which homologous
chromosomes are present but chromosome 5B is absent (e.g., nullisomic 5B or nullisomic 5B tetrasomic 5D), both homologous and
homoeologous chromosomes often pair in very complex configurations
(30,34).

From studies of chromosome pairing in various aneuploids and
aneuploid hybrid situations at low, normal, and higher temperatures,
several workers have provided evidence for the action and interaction of loci on both the long and short arms of chromosomes of
homoeologous groups 3 and 5. Loci on both normal and supernumerary
chromosomes of alien species interact with loci on chromosomes of
T. aestivum (35-38).

From measurements of the distance between two telocentrics
in the same somatic cell (39,40), the effect of various aneuploid
conditions on the secondary association of chromosomes has been
determined.

The evidence concerning the regulation of chromosomal pairing
in wheat has been most recently reviewed by Sears (41).

Intervarietal Chromosome Substitution

Aneuploids have been employed extensively in analyzing
quantitative characters of cultivated varieties of wheat. The
basic manipulation is the construction, in a common background,

of sets of lines in each of which a single unrecombined chromosome is substituted from a donor variety. Thus the effects of single chromosomes, their interactions with an essentially uniform background, and the effects of recombination in single chromosomes may be studied (11). The production of substitution lines is essentially a matter of pollinating a series of monosomics by another variety and using the monosomics in F_1 and subsequent generations as males in backcrosses to the respective monosomics of the recipient variety. To avoid univalent shift, the latter monosomics are preferably monotelosomic, monoisosomic, or double monotelosomic.

BREEDING

Introduction of Alien Variation

It is axiomatic that in order to practice selection there must be variability. Equally, the greater the range of variability available, the greater the probability that a breeder will be able to locate and utilize desirable alleles in a breeding program. It is with the aim of increasing the available pool of genetic variability that cytogeneticists have attempted to introduce genetic material from alien, but related, species into wheat. Many cases involve the use of aneuploids.

The original introduction of alien variation into a wheat chromosome using aneuploids was the induced translocation of the Lr9 gene of chromosome 6^{Cu} onto chromosome 6B of T. aestivum cv. Chinese Spring by Sears $(42)_{Cu}$ A plant to which had been added the long arm of chromosome 6^{Cu} monoisosomically was irradiated just prior to meiosis. Euploid T. aestivum was pollinated with pollen from the irradiated plant, and plants with the Lr9 locus were recognized by disease testing. Cytological examination of these resistant progeny allowed the isolation of several trans-locations, one of which was eventually released as breeders' material and was appropriately named Transfer.

Following the production of Transfer several other introductions of alien genes have been produced by similar manipulation, others by modification of Sears' technique, and still others by utilizing both aneuploids and alleles that effect chromosome pairing in hybrids. It has further been recognized that the spontaneous introduction of whole alien chromosomes into wheat varieties has taken place and the substitution lines were only indentified and characterized subsequent to their release as cultivars.

Driscoll (43) devised a technique for introducing alien genetic material into wheat chromosomes which reduces the time-consuming cytological analyses of other techniques. The manipulation requires inducing translocations by irradiation of seed of lines in which an alien chromosome is added disomically to the normal wheat complement. The irradiated seed is grown and selfed.

In the next generation ear/row progenies are examined for the
segregation of the character being investigated. Segregation of
the trait usually occurs for two different and recognizable
reasons.

First, if the irradiated parent was an unrecognizable monosomic
addition, it should segregate so that approximately 75% of the
progeny does not show the desired trait. Second, if a translocation has been induced, then depending on the frequency of production, orientation, and segregation of the resultant quadrivalent,
a small proportion of progeny do not exhibit the phenotype being
investigated. It is from these families that the translocated
type may be recovered. The cultivar Transec was developed by
this technique (44).

A currently untested technique, which combines features of
both Sears' and Driscoll's techniques, was devised by Kimber
(45).

The first successful use of induced homoeologous chromosome
pairing in an aneuploid situation to transfer a character to
wheat was that of Riley et al. (46) who transferred resistance to
the yellow-rust fungus from T. comosum to T. aestivum. The
technique involved crossing a disomic addition of chromosome 2M
of T. comosum with a form of T. speltoides which, even in the
presence of chromosome 5B, allows homoeologous chromosome pairing
to take place. Compair, the cultivar that was eventually isolated,
includes a chromosome containing the segment of 2M that carries
the allele which conditions resistance, yet with enough chromosome
2D to allow the translocated chromosome to pair normally with
chromosome 2D.

Using lines in which Agropyron elongatum chromosomes were
substituted for wheat chromosomes 3D and 7D and wheat aneuploids
deficient for chromosome 5B, Sears (47) was able to recover
numerous 3D/Ag and 7D/Ag transfer chromosomes with the leaf-rust
resistance conditioned by two different Agropyron chromosomes.

Zeller (48) and Mettin et al. (49) described the identification
of wheat varieties already in cultivation that carried rye chromosome 1R substituted for wheat chromosome 1B or that had wheat-rye
translocated chromosomes. The varieties all originated from
material which had been derived from hybrids involving rye.

A similar process is seen to occur in hexaploid Triticale,
where some of the rye chromosomes can be replaced, usually by
chromosomes of the D genome of T. aestivum. Gustafson and Zillinsky
(50) identified wheat chromosome 2D spontaneously substituted for
2R (and possibly also 5D for 5R) in the hexaploid Triticale cv.
Armadillo. Evans (51) observed similar spontaneous chromosome
substitution in crosses between two artifically induced amphiploids.

When chromosomes are univalent they tend to misdivide at or
near the centromere during meiosis, with a frequency apparently
dependent on the species involved, the particular genotype, and
the chromosome concerned. The resultant telocentrics can, presumably for only a short period of time, reunite with each other

or with any other recently misdivided chromosome. Sears (52)
took advantage of this situation by producing plants that were
simultaneously monosomic for a genetically marked wheat chromosome
and a rye chromosome that also carried genetic markers. Plants
were derived containing chromosomes that had one arm of the rye
chromosome and one arm of the wheat chromosome joined by a common
centromere.

Hybrid Wheat

The commercial production of hybrid wheat is accomplished by
utilization of cytoplasms inducing male sterility and chromosomal
genetic restoration factors. Driscoll (53,54) devised a system,
using aneuploids, in which male sterility is induced by a recessive
gene (or deletion) on a wheat chromosome, and fertility is restored
by a corresponding epistatic gene on a homoeologous alien chromosome.

The system involves the production of three lines, designated
as X, Y, and Z, each of which is homozygous for the recessive
male-sterile locus and carries, respectively, 2, 1, and 0 doses
of the alien chromosome carrying the epistatic restoring factor.
The X line has 44 chromosomes, makes 22 bivalents, is male and
female fertile, and relatively true breeding. The Y line has 43
chromosomes, makes 21 bivalents and one univalent, is male- and
female-fertile, but produces two types of gametes, one with 21 wheat
chromosomes and the other with 21 wheat plus one alien. The 21-
chromosome pollen grains in the Y line do not contain the epistatic
restorer but are viable because the recessive male-sterile locus
acts on sporophytic tissue. Because line Y is hemizygous for the
epistatic restorer, it can produce both types of pollen. Only the
21-chromosome male gametes function because of certation effects
against the hyperploid pollen. The Z line has 42 chromosomes,
makes 21 bivalents, and is male sterile.

Following the initial production of small quantities of the Z
seed from selfed progenies of the Y line, part of the plants from
the Z seed are pollinated by pollen from the X line. The seed
produced is all Y type. The bulk of the Y line so produced is used
as male parent for the remainder of the Z plants. All the seed
produced in this cross is Z in type and can be used as the female
parent for hybrid production by crossing with any normal variety.
The hybrid seed so produced does not carry the alien chromosome, is
fertile, and is potentially a new hybrid variety.

Evolution

One of the early uses of wheat aneuploids in evolutionary
studies was in the assignment of chromosomes to the three genomes,
A,B, and D. Sears (55) was able to identify the D-genome monosomics
by crossing the monosomic set with the tetraploid T. turgidum. The
hybrids involving the A- and B-genome monosomics had 13 bivalents

and 8 univalents at first meiotic metaphase, whereas the hybrids involving the D-genome monosomics had 14 bivalents and 6 univalents. The A-genome monosomics were distinguished from the B-genome monosomics by similar analysis of hybrids involving a synthetic AADD allotetraploid (56).

Following the identification of the individual chromosomes, Sears (57) identified the homoeologous wheat chromosomes. By developing plants that were nullisomic for one wheat chromosome and simultaneously tetrasomic for another chromosome, he was able to observe the interaction of the chromosome dosages so produced. Two major classes were recognized as compensating and noncompensating. In the compensating class the phenotype and fertility were restored to relative normality, whereas the phenotype in the noncompensating class was even more aberrant than either the simple nullisomic or tetrasomic alone, and in many cases the noncompensating combinations were nonviable.

Of particular interest and great significance was the fact that the compensating combinations occurred in seven sets of three. That is, if the tetrasomy of one chromosome compensated for the nullisomy of the second, and the tetrasomy of the second compensated for the nullisomy of the third, then the tetrasomy of the third would compensate for nullisomy of the first. Furthermore, these three chromosomes would then not compensate for any of the remaining 18 in the set.

The compensating chromosomes were recognized as genetically similar and were called homoeologous. It was further recognized that in every homoeologous group there was one chromosome from each of the three genomes, A, B, and D.

The recognition of the genetical similarity of the homoeologous chromosomes by these aneuploid studies has considerable evolutionary significance in illustrating the divergence of the three genomes in T. aestivum from a common ancestor; yet it also shows how the individual chromosomes have changed mainly by mutation without obliterating their initial identity. As can be anticipated from this analysis and has been demonstrated by numerous workers, other species in the Triticinae have chromosomes which also presumably diverged from the same archetypical and common ancestor and are therefore also homoeologous to the wheat chromosomes.

The cytological equivalent of the genetic demonstration of homoeology was made by Riley and Kempanna (34), who induced translocations between chromosomes in the absence of chromosome 5B and then identified the translocation products by telocentric analysis. As all the translocations recovered involved homoeologous chromosomes, it is possible to conclude that only homoeologs are able to pair by deletion of chromosome 5B.

Riley and Chapman (58) determined the homoeologies of the arms of certain homoeologs through the use of telocentric chromosomes. They first crossed two ditelosomic lines together, producing F_1 plants with two heteromorphic bivalents. These were then pollinated by T. speltoides, whose genome suppresses the action of the gene Ph and thereby permits homoeologous pairing to occur. Offspring were selected that had both telocentrics. If these paired, they were homoeologous. If they did not pair with each other but occasionally with opposite arms of the same chromosome, they were non-homoeologous. L. Sears (in 2) used the same technique to confirm genetic data indicating homoeology of 4BL (the long arm of chromosome 4B) with 4DS and to establish the homoeology of 2BL with 2AS and 2DS.

The homoeology of alien chromosomes can be investigated, using aneuploids, by two methods: (1) their genetic compensating ability and (2) their cytological pairing ability when the regulation of pairing to strictly homologous chromosomes is relaxed.

The genetic analysis can be accomplished by attempting to substitute the alien chromosome for wheat chromosomes, when one alien chromosome will generally substitute for the chromosome of one homoeologous group only. Riley (59) substituted rye chromosome II of the variety King II for all three chromosomes of group 6, thereby demonstrating the homoeology of the alien chromosome to its wheat counterparts. Chromosome II of the King II addition set is now, of course, designated 6R. Similarly Sears (60) substituted a single rye chromosome (now designated 2R) for wheat chromosomes 2A, 2B, and 2D. The literature contains many references to other alien chromosome substitutions. However, rye chromosome 3R shows some homoeology with both group 3 and group 1 (61,62) and 5R substitutes for 4A in addition to group 5 chromosomes (63). One possible explanation for these apparent mismatches may be the presence of translocations between rye chromosomes, which make each of them partially homoeologous to two wheat groups.

Establishing the cytological relationships of single alien chromosomes to their wheat homoeologous groups generally involves hybridizing telocentric wheat aneuploids to an addition line and then inactivating the Ph locus on chromosome 5B, usually by hybridization with high-pairing forms of T. speltoides. Under these circumstances, the wheat telocentric chromosome will pair with the alien chromosome only when the telocentric is homoeologous to the alien. It is also necessary that the alien chromosome be identified cytologically either as a telocentric or from a subterminal centromere position. Johnson and Kimber (64) and Dvorak (35) demonstrated the cytological homology of Agropyron telocentric chromosomes by this technique, and Athwal and Kimber (65) showed that chromosome A of T. umbellulatum, recognizable as an extreme subterminal, was homoeologous to wheat group 6. By algebraic analysis, Riley and Chapman (58), also using wheat telocentrics, inferred the homoeology of the chromosome of T. speltoides that is similar to the chromosome of wheat group 5.

Kimber and Athwal (65), Kimber (66,67), and Gill and Kimber (26) questioned the relationships of T. speltoides to the B genome of T. aestivum. This reconsideration was stimulated by

the discovery of genotypes of T speltoides that did not suppress
the regulating activity of chromosome 5B (35,36). The chromosomes
of these strains did not pair with the chromosomes of the B
genome, contrary to expectation if T. speltoides were the source
of that genome.

Sallee and Kimber (68) recorded the pairing frequencies of
41 of the 42 telocentrics of T. aestivum and were able to show
that a chromosome arm paired with the same facility when it was
telocentric as when it was part of a bibrachial chromosome.
Kimber and Hulse (69) developed methods allowing the calculation
of numerical similarities between the A, B, and D genomes of T.
aestivum and genomes in related species on the basis of the
pairing of telocentric chromosomes in hybrids.

CONCLUSIONS

It was stated initially that the constructive use of aneuploids in any genetic study depends on the availability, fertility,
and viability of an essentially complete series of the aberrant
types. The examples of the use of aneuploids of T. aestivum
described in this paper, although obviously incomplete, indicate
the analytic power and conceptual elegance of aneuploid analysis.

The geneticist can place genes on specific and recognizable
chromosomes and map their position relative to the centromere.
The cytologist can investigate the pairing and segregation of
specific chromosomes recognizable by their centromere position,
and can relate behavior to chemical and physical treatments and
chiasma frequency to recombination. Individual chromosomes have
been stained by the Giemsa technique and are recognizable in
hybrids and aneuploids. The evolutionist has an unequaled range
of powerful tools available for phylogenetic investigations.
Finally, the breeder is now in the position where the appreciation
of his crop is both genetically diverse and detailed; moreover,
the use of aneuploids allows the introduction and utilization of
new, novel, and otherwise unobtainable variation.

SUMMARY

There is available in wheat a unique series of aneuploids
ranging from all 21 possible monosomics to complex types that are
simultaneously deficient for one chromosome and duplicate for
another. Furthermore, lines with chromosomes from related alien
species either added to or substituted for wheat chromosomes are
in common cytological use.

This contribution considers the use of this range of material
in studies designed to elucidate the evolutionary relationships
of the species, in investigations of the genetics of a polyploid
with cytological diploidization, and in potential breeding manipulations.

LITERATURE CITED

1. Sears, E.R., 1954, The aneuploids of common wheat. Missouri Agr. Exp. Sta. Res. Bull. 572: 59.
2. Sears, E.R., Sears, L.M.S., 1978, The telocentric chromosomes of common wheat, 1: 389-407, Proc. 5th Inter. Wheat Genet. Symp., New Delhi.
3. Sears, E.R., 1947, The sphaerococcum gene in wheat. Genetics 32: 102-103.
4. Unrau, J., 1950, The use of monosomics and nullisomics in cytogenetic studies of common wheat. Sci. Agric. 30: 66-89.
5. Driscoll, C.J., Jensen, N.F., 1964, Chromosomes associated with waxlessness, awnedness and time of maturity of common wheat. Canad. J. Genet. Cytol. 6: 324-333.
6. Tsunewaki, K., 1960, Monosomic and conventional analysis in common wheat. III. Lethality. Jap. J. Genet. 35: 71-75.
7. Sears, E.R., Rodenhiser, H.A. 1948, Nullisomic analysis of stemrust resistance in Triticum vulgare var. Timstein. Genetics 33: 123-124.
8. Heyne, E.G., Livers, R.W., 1953, Monosomic analysis of leaf rust reaction, awnedness, winter injury and seed color in Pawnee wheat. Agronomy J. 45: 54-58.
9. Macer, R.C.F., 1966, The formal and monosomic genetic analysis of stripe rust resistance in wheat. Proc. 2nd Inter. Wheat Genet. Symp., Lund, Hereditas (Suppl.) 2: 127-142.
10. McIntosh, R.A., Baker, E.P., 1968, A linkage map for chromosome 2D, pp. 305-309, Proc. 3rd Inter. Wheat Genet. Symp., Australian Acad. Sci., Canberra.
11. Law, C.N., Worland, A.J., 1972, Aneuploidy in wheat and its uses in genetic analysis, pp. 25-65, Ann. Rep. Plant Breed. Inst., Cambridge.
12. Maan, S.S., Lucken, K.A., 1966, Development and use of an aneuploid set of male sterile Chinese Spring wheat in Triticum timopheevii Zhuk. cytoplasm. Canad. J. Genet. Cytol. 8: 398-403.
13. Crosby, A.R., 1957, Nucleolar activity of lagging chromosomes in wheat. Amer. J. Bot. 44: 813-822.
14. Shepherd, K.W., 1968, Chromosomal control of endosperm proteins in wheat and rye, pp. 86-96, Proc. 3rd Inter. Wheat Genet. Symp., Australian Acad. Sci., Canberra.
15. Waines, J.G., 1973, Chromosomal location of genes controlling endosperm protein production in Triticum aestivum cv. Chinese Spring, pp. 873-877, Proc. 4th Inter. Wheat Genet. Symp., Columbia, Missouri.
16. May, C.E., Vickery, R.S., Driscoll, C.J., 1973, Gene control in hexaploid wheat, pp. 843-849, Proc. 4th Inter. Wheat Genet. Symp., Columbia, Missouri.
17. Hart, G.E., 1970, Evidence for triplicate genes for alcohol dehydrogenase in hexaploid wheat. Proc. Nat. Acad. Sci. USA 66: 1136-1141.

18. Hart, G.E., 1979, Genetical and chromosomal relationships among the wheats and relatives. Stadler Genet. Symp. 11, in press.

19. Bielig, L.M., Driscoll, C.J., 1971, Production of alien substitution lines in Triticum aestivum. Canad. J. Genet. Cytol. 13: 429-436.

20. Bielig, L.M., Driscoll, C.J., 1973, Release of a series of MAS lines, pp. 147-150, Proc. 4th Inter. Wheat Genet. Symp., Columbia, Missouri.

21. Morris, R., 1959, Location of genes for wheat characters by chromosomes. Wheat Newsl. 6: 2-16.

22. Sears, E.R., 1966, Chromosome mapping with the aid of telocentrics. Proc. 2nd Inter. Wheat Genet. Symp. Hereditas (Suppl.) 2: 370-380.

23. Williams, N.D., Maan, S.S., 1973, Telosomic mapping of genes for resistance to stem rust of wheat, pp. 765-770, Proc. 4th Inter. Wheat Genet. Symp., Columbia, Missouri.

24. McIntosh, R.A., 1973, A catalogue of gene symbols for wheat, pp. 893-937, Proc. 4th Inter. Wheat Genet. Symp., Columbia, Missouri. (Supplemented yearly in Wheat Newsletter.)

25. Chang, T.D., Kimber, G., Sears, E.R., 1973, Genetic analysis of rye chromosomes added to wheat, pp. 151-153, Proc. 4th Inter. Wheat Genet. Symp., Columbia, Missouri.

26. Gill, B.S., Kimber, G., 1974, Giemsa C-banding and the evolution of wheat. Proc. Nat. Acad. Sci. USA 71: 4086-4090.

27. Fu, T.K., Sears, E.R., 1973, The relationship between chiasmata and crossing over in Triticum aestivum. Genetics 75: 231-246.

28. Linde-Laursen, I., Larsen, J., 1974, The use of double-monotelodisomics to identify translocations in Triticum aestivum. Hereditas 78: 245-250.

29. Okamoto, M., 1957, Asynaptic effect of chromosome V. Wheat Inf. Serv. 5: 6-7.

30. Riley, R., Chapman, V., 1958, Genetic control of the cytologically diploid behaviour of hexaploid wheat. Nature 182: 713-715.

31. Kimber, G., 1961, Basis of the diploid-like meiotic behaviour of polyploid cotton. Nature 191: 98-100.

32. Wall, A.M., Riley, R., Gale, M.D., 1971, The position of a locus on chromosome 5B of Triticum aestivum affecting homoeologous meiotic pairing. Genet. Res. Cambridge 18: 329-339.

33. Mello-Sampayo, T., Canas, A.P., 1973, Suppressors of meiotic chromosome pairing in common wheat, pp. 709-713, Proc. 4th Inter. Wheat Genet. Symp, Columbia, Missouri.

34. Riley, R., Kempanna, C., 1963, The homoeologous nature of the nonhomologous meiotic pairing in Triticum aestivum deficient for chromosome V (5B). Heredity 18: 287-306.

35. Dvorak, J., 1972, Genetic variability in Aegilops speltoides affecting homoeologous pairing in wheat. Canad J. Genet. Cytol. 14: 371-380.

36. Kimber, G., Athwal, R.S., 1972, A reassessment of the course of evolution in wheat. Proc. Nat. Acad. Sci. USA 69: 912-915.
37. Dover, G.A., 1973, The genetics and interactions of "A" and "B" chromosomes controlling meiotic chromosome pairing in the Triticinae, pp. 653-666, Proc. 4th Inter. Wheat Genet. Symp., Columbia, Missouri.
38. Rubenstein, J.M., Kimber, G., 1976, The genetical relationships of the systems regulating chromosome pairing in hybrids and aneuploids of hexaploid wheat. Cereal Res. Commun. 4: 263-272.
39. Feldman, M., Mello-Sampayo, T., Sears, E.R., 1966, Somatic association in Triticum aestivum. Proc. Nat. Acad. Sci. USA 56: 1192-1199.
40. Avivi, L., Feldman, M., 1973, Mechanism of non-random chromosome placement in common wheat, pp. 627-633, Proc. 4th Inter. Wheat Genet. Symp., Columbia, Missouri.
41. Sears, E.R., 1976, Genetic control of chromosome pairing in wheat. Ann. Rev. Genet. 10:31-51.
42. Sears, E.R., 1956, The transfer of leaf-rust resistance from Aegilops umbellulata to wheat. Brookhaven Symp. Biol. 9: 1-22.
43. Driscoll, C.J., 1963, A genetic method for detecting induced intergeneric transfers of rust resistance. Proc. 2nd Inter. Wheat Genet. Symp., Lund, Hereditas (Suppl.) 2: 460-461.
44. Driscoll, C.J., Anderson, L.M., 1967, Cytogenetic studies of Transec--a wheat-rye translocation line. Canad. J. Genet. Cytol. 9: 375-380.
45. Kimber, G., 1971, The design of a method, using ionising radiation, for the introduction of alien variation into wheat. Indian J. Genet. Plant Breed. 31: 580-584.
46. Riley, R., Chapman, V., Johnson, R., 1968, The incorporation of alien disease resistance in wheat by genetic interference with the regulation of meiotic chromosome synapsis. Genet. Res. 12: 199-219.
47. Sears, E.R., 1973, Agropyron-wheat transfers induced by homoeologous pairing, pp. 191-199, Proc. 4th Inter. Wheat Genet. Symp., Columbia, Missouri.
48. Zeller, F.J., 1973, 1B/1R wheat-rye chromosome substitutions and translocations, pp. 209-221, Proc. 4th Inter. Wheat Genet. Symp., Columbia, Missouri.
49. Mettin, D., Blüthner, W.D., Schlegel, G., 1973, Additional evidence on spontaneous 1B/1R wheat-rye substitutions and translocations, pp. 179-184, Proc. 4th Inter. Wheat Genet. Symp., Columbia, Missouri.
50. Gustafson, J.P., Zillinsky, F.J., 1973, Identification of D-genome chromosomes from hexaploid wheat in a 42-chromosome Triticale, pp. 225-231, Proc. 4th Inter. Wheat Genet. Symp., Columbia, Missouri.

51. Evans, L.E., 1964, Genome construction within the Triticinae.
    I. The synthesis of hexaploids (2n=42) having chromosomes
    of Agropyron and Aegilops in addition to the A and B genomes
    of Triticum durum. Canad. J. Genet. Cytol. 6: 19-28.
52. Sears, E.R., 1972, Chromosome engineering in wheat. Stadler
    Symp. 4: 23-38, Columbia, Missouri.
53. Driscoll, C.J., 1972, XYZ system of producing hybrid wheat.
    Crop. Sci. 12: 516-517.
54. Driscoll, C.J., 1973, A chromosomal male-sterility system of
    producing hybrid wheat, pp. 669-674, Proc. 4th Inter. Wheat
    Genet. Symp., Columbia, Missouri.
55. Sears, E.R., 1944, Cytogenetic studies with polyploid species
    of wheat. II. Additional chromosomal aberrations in Triticum
    vulgare. Genetics 29: 232-246.
56. Okamoto, M., 1962, Identification of the chromosomes of
    common wheat belonging to the A and B genomes. Canad. J.
    Genet. Cytol. 4: 31-37.
57. Sears, E.R., 1966, Nullisomic-tetrasomic combinations in
    hexaploid wheat, pp. 29-45, in "Chromosome Manipulations and
    Plant Genetics," Riley, R., Lewis, K.R. (eds.), Oliver & Boyd,
    London.
58. Riley, R., Chapman, V., 1966, Estimates of the homoeology of
    wheat chromosomes by measurements of differential affinity
    at meiosis, pp. 46-58, in "Chromosome Manipulations and
    Plant Genetics," R. Riley, K. R. Lewis (eds.), Oliver & Boyd,
    London.
59. Riley, R., 1965, Cytogenetics and plant breeding. Genetics
    Today. Proc. XI Inter. Congr. Genet. 3: 681-688.
60. Sears, E.R., 1968, Relationships of chromosomes 2A, 2B, and
    2D with their rye homoeologue, pp. 53-61, Proc. 3rd Inter.
    Wheat Genet. Symp., Australian Acad. Sci., Canberra.
61. Gupta, P.K., 1969, Studies on transmission of rye substitution
    gametes in common wheat. Indian J. Genet. Plant Breed. 29:
    163-172.
62. Lee, Y.H., Larter, E.N., Evans, L.E., 1969, Homoeologous
    relationship of rye chromosome VI with two homoeologous
    groups from wheat. Canad. J. Genet. Cytol. 11: 803-809.
63. Zeller, F.J., Baier, A.C., 1973, Substitution des Weizen-
    chromosomenpaares 4A durch das Roggenchromosomenpaar 5R in
    den Weihenstephaner Weizenstamm W70a86 (Blaukorn). Z.
    Pflanzenzüchtg. 70: 1-10.
64. Johnson, R., Kimber, G., 1967, Homoeologous pairing of a
    chromosome from Agropyron elongatum with those of Triticum
    aestivum and Aegilops speltoides. Genet. Res. Cambridge 10:
    63-71.
65. Athwal, R.S., Kimber, G., 1972, The pairing of an alien
    chromosome with homoeologous chromosomes of wheat. Canad.
    J. Genet. Cytol. 14: 325-333.

66. Kimber, G., 1973, The relationships of the S-genome diploids to polyploid wheats, pp. 81-85, Proc. 4th Inter. Wheat Genet. Symp., Columbia, Missouri.
67. Kimber, G., 1973, A reassessment of the origin of the polyploid wheats. Genetics 78: 487-492.
68. Sallee, P.J., Kimber, G., 1978, An analysis of the pairing of wheat telocentric chromosomes. Proc. 5th Inter. Wheat Symp., New Delhi (in press).
69. Kimber, G., Hulse, M.M., 1978, The analysis of chromosome pairing in hybrids and the evolution of wheat. Proc. 5th Inter. Wheat Symp., India (in press).

SOME APPLICATIONS AND MISAPPLICATIONS OF INDUCED POLYPLOIDY TO PLANT BREEDING

Douglas R. Dewey

U.S. Department of Agriculture, SEA-AR
Utah State University
Logan, Utah 84322

Plant breeders are eternal optimists, always searching for and expecting significant breakthroughs in plateaus of yield, quality, or adaptation. These breakthroughs have been achieved in some crops, notably maize (Zea mays) and grain sorghum (Sorghum bicolor) (1); but they have been elusive in others, particularly forage crops, in which conventional breeding methods have usually produced disappointing results (2,3). With the 1937 discovery of the "colchicine technique" for inducing polyploidy, breeders seized upon this then-unconventional technique as a means of penetrating yield barriers. Since 1937, breeders, using polyploid methods on many crops, have gone through repeated cycles of high expectations followed by low realizations. The foremost lesson to be learned from the breeders' 40-year experience ("struggle" may be a better word) with induced polyploidy is that it is not a panacea for plant improvement. Nevertheless, as a forage breeder-cytogeneticist, I still look on the intelligent manipulation of polyploidy as one of the most, if not the most, promising means of improving yields of certain crop plants, particularly the perennial forages.

Induced polyploidy can be used in three basic ways by plant breeders: 1) to elevate the chromosome number of a species (induced autoploidy), 2) to elevate the chromosome number of a species-hybrid (induced alloploidy = amphiploidy), and 3) to serve as a genetic bridge between ploidy levels or between species. The intent of breeding induced autoploids is to capitalize on the direct consequences of chromosome duplication, i.e., larger cells and plant parts. Amphiploidy is used to restore fertility to sterile species-hybrids and, ultimately, to synthesize new species or resynthesize existing species. In addition to their direct uses, induced autoploidy and amphiploidy may be used to facilitate

445

genetic transfer between taxa, thus serving as agents of introgression.

From the onset of polyploid breeding, it has been apparent
that different types of crop plants respond differently to induced
polyploidy. Original ploidy level, genome structure, mode of
reproduction, perenniality, and the plant part for which the crop
is grown all have a bearing on breeding success or failure. The
plant breeder must match the characteristics of his plant material
to the specific application of induced polyploidy that maximizes
his opportunities for success. The breeder should carefully
weigh the relative merits of polyploid breeding vs. conventional
breeding and commit his resources to the program that offers the
greatest potential for his material and needs. Often a program
using both conventional and polyploid breeding methods will be
appropriate.

The intent of this paper is to consider some successful and
unsuccessful applications of induced polyploidy to plant breeding
and thereby provide guidelines that can lead to more effective
use of artificial polyploidy by plant breeders.

HISTORICAL PERSPECTIVES

In a benchmark paper written 23 years ago, Ledyard Stebbins
(4) assessed the status and future of "Artificial Polyploidy as
a Tool in Plant Breeding." In comparing Stebbins' 1956 outlook
with the realities in 1979, little has changed in the realm of
polyploid breeding in almost a quarter of a century. With a few
relatively minor modifications, Stebbins' assessment is as
applicable now as it was then. Now as in 1956, induced autoploidy
has a greater impact on agriculture than does amphiploidy, although
I sense the balance is changing. As examples of successful or
potentially successful artificial autoploids, Stebbins cited
sugarbeets (Beta vulgaris), red clover (Trifolium pratense),
alsike clover (Trifolium hybridum), rye (Secale cereale), grapes
(Vitis spp.), watermelons (Citrullus lanatus), and various ornamentals.

How have those potentially valuable induced autoploids fared
in the past 23 years? None has lived up to expectations. At
first glance, polyploid sugarbeets would appear to be the genuine
success story of polyploid breeding. By 1970, with impetus given
by cytoplasmic male-sterility, most ot the European sugarbeet
acreage was devoted to triploids or anisoploids. However, the
mass shift to the use of triploids was made without clear evidence
of their superiority over genetically equivalent diploids (5).
In more recent years, the trend in Europe has been to return to
diploid varieties and that trend may continue (6). Polyploid
sugarbeets have never been used extensively in North America.

Some contend that "breeders might have produced far better varieties if they had confined their attention to diploid material" (7).

Tetraploid red clover has been only semi-successful, and it is grown to some extent in Europe (8). The tetraploids have never gained acceptance in North America because of the poor performance of unadapted European-bred strains (personal communication, N.L. Taylor). Were it not for the yet unsolved problems of low seed production, tetraploid red clover might replace the diploid in many agricultural areas. In spite of its well-documented superiority over the diploid in the United Kingdom, tetraploid red clover accounts for less than 20% of the production (8). Absence of economic incentives to produce tetraploid seed is largely responsible for the limited use of polyploid red clover.

Although alsike clover responds quite favorably to chromosome doubling and its seed set poses no serious problem, the tetraploids have never achieved wide usage. European-derived tetraploids have performed poorly in North America (personal communication, C.E. Townsend). Being of minor agricultural importance, alsike clover probably does not warrant the time and expense associated with a polyploid breeding program, at least in most areas of the world.

Tetraploid rye is frequently cited in plant-breeding texts as the single example of a cereal crop that has benefited directly from chromosome doubling. The current importance of tetraploid rye is difficult to assess because most of it is grown in East European countries, particularly the U.S.S.R., and acreage figures cannot be easily obtained. Nevertheless, frequent reference to tetraploid rye in recent Plant Breeding Abstracts suggests that it has considerable agricultural importance both as a grain crop and as a forage crop. 'Tetra Petkus' rye was grown on a limited scale in the U.S. and Canada in the 1950's, but it or other tetraploid varieties are not now important as a grain crop in North America. The tetraploids are finding minor usage as forage or green-manure crops in the U.S. (personal communication, L.W. Briggle).

In the 1950's, induced autoploidy was considered to be an important method of improving grapes because of the increased fruit size of the tetraploids. Yet today not a single tetraploid, either natural or induced, has become commercially important, primarily because of their erratic bearing (9).

Brief commercial interest was shown in seedless triploid watermelons (10), but now they are grown only as a gourmet specialty item and contribute only in a minor way to the melon industry. Inquiries sent to 12 floriculturists across the U.S. uncovered no appreciable use of autoploidy in flowers, although tetraploid snapdragons (Antirrhinum majus) and zinnias (Zinnia elegans) were mentioned as being of minor importance.

The two most promising amphiploids cited by Stebbins (4) were Triticum-Agropyron, perennial wheat, and Triticum-Secale, triticale. Even as early as 1956, it was apparent that little hope existed in developing a perennial wheat that would be competitive with annual wheat for either yield or quality. Although most breeders have given up on perennial wheat, Soviet breeders, led by Academician N.V. Tsitsin, are continuing their efforts to develop both a perennial wheat and a forage wheat. Tsitsin (11) recently reconfirmed his goal "to develop perennial wheat varieties of commerical value." Although he recognizes that this goal has not been reached, he is confident that "the solution of this problem is not far distant." A forage-wheat variety, 'After-growing-38,' has been released from Tsitsin's program, but its economic value has yet to be determined.

After 40 to 45 years of breeding effort in several countries, triticale is still on the threshold of becoming an important cereal crop. Although triticale is grown commercially in parts of North America, Europe, and Asia, it still must be considered as a minor cereal crop. Nevertheless, the future prospects for triticale are promising. As little as 10 years ago, Canadian triticales yielded only half as much as adapted wheat varieties (12). The most recently released triticale variety, 'Welsh,' yields as well as the best wheat varieties and 16% more than the only previously released Canadian variety, 'Rosner' (13). Progress of this magnitude indicates that triticale is rapidly approaching the status of a major cereal crop.

Now as in 1956, induced polyploidy has its greatest and most varied plant-breeding application as a vehicle of genetic transfer. The transfer of disease resistance from a wild species to its cultivated relative via induced polyploidy has become a relatively common practice in many crops, and it is now almost a standard procedure in tobacco (Nicotiana tabacum) breeding (14). Many other crops including wheat (Triticum aestivum), oats (Avena sativa), potatoes (Solanum tuberosum), and cotton (Gossypium hirsutum) have been beneficiaries of genes for disease or insect resistance from their non-cultivated relatives. Even quantitatively inherited traits such as fiber quality in cotton (15) and forage quality in grasses (16) have been transferred with the aid of induced polyploidy.

In 1956, some felt that Stebbins' appraisal of the potential of polyploid breeding was unduly pessimistic, but time has demonstrated that he was, if anything, overly optimistic. Generally speaking, induced autoloidy has fallen short of the 1956 expectations; the outcome is still pending on the breeding contributions of amphiploidy; and induced polyploidy as a genetic bridge has performed more or less as expected.

The less-than-spectacular plant-breeding progress that has been achieved through induced polyploidy should not be construed to mean that polyploid breeding should be abandoned or even diminished. Rather, it means that breeders must be increasingly discriminating in the choice of crops and breeding situations in which to use induced polyploidy. More attention must be given to the biological and economic factors that promote successful polyploid breeding and then a program must be fashioned that will work in harmony with those success factors.

CURRENT TRENDS

Failure of polyploid breeding to reach its projected potential has not deterred research and breeding with induced polyploids. A computer-aided search of the Commonwealth Agricultural Bureaux (C.A.B.) data base, which consolidates listings from 28 abstracting services, uncovered from January 1972 to January 1979 about 500 publications keyed to the word "polyploid(y)" in conjunction with "induced" or "colchicine." Although the publication data are far from precise and must be interpreted cautiously, they serve as an index of research and breeding activity relating to induced polyploids. Many important publications were undoubtedly over-looked because the search failed to indentify them with the key index words that I had chosen. Although the summary data in Tables 1 and 2 are incomplete with respect to numbers of publications, the relative proportions of publications in the various categories are probably quite accurate.

Table 1. Estimated research activity (by country) on induced polyploidy, in terms of number of publications obtained from the C.A.B. data-base from January 1972 to January 1979.

Country	Research Publications	
	No.	% of total
USSR	175	38.0
India	75	16.3
United States	43	9.4
United Kingdom	26	5.6
Japan	17	3.7
Poland	10	2.2
Bulgaria	10	2.2
Czechoslovakia	10	2.2
Netherlands	9	2.0
Canada	9	2.0
Belgium	8	1.7
Sweden	8	1.7
France	8	1.7
West Germany	7	1.5
24 other countries	45	9.8
Total	460	100.0

Research on induced polyploidy is being conducted in at least 38 countries, but more than half of it is concentrated in two, the U.S.S.R. and India (Table 1). Historically, Soviet plant breeders and geneticists have had a great interest in wide hybridization and induced polyploidy dating back to G.D. Karpechenko's synthesis of Raphanobrassica in 1928. This interest continues to flourish under the strong influence of 80 year-old N.V. Tsitsin, probably the world's foremost advocate of wide crossing and induced polyploidy. The scope of the Soviet effort is indicated by the 600 participants, representing more than 60 institutions, attending a symposium on "Wide Hybridization in Plants and Animals" in Moscow in 1958 (17). The number of publications coming from the Soviet Union in recent years suggest that their efforts in wide crossing and induced polyploidy have not diminished.

The considerable scientific effort being devoted to induced polyploidy in India may come as a surprise to some. However, India has traditionally produced an abundance of capable cytogeneticists. Furthermore, good quality cytogenetic research can be accomplished with a moderate investment in laboratory space, equipment, and supplies, meaning that a nation need not be particularly affluent to support this type of research. Much of the Indian effort seems to be directed toward observing the effects of induced polyploidy rather than toward breeding applications. This emphasis is probably responsible for their large number of publications.

As a group, the West European countries accounted for about 14% of the publications on induced polyploidy, followed by the U.S. and Canada with a combined 11%. European plant breeders have always used induced polyploids much more extensively than

Table 2. Estimated research activity (by crop class and type of polyploidy) on induced polyploidy, in terms of number of publications listed by the C.A.B. data-base from January 1972 to January 1979.

Crop class	Type of induced polyploidy		
	Autoploidy	Amphiploidy	Total
Root and vegetable crops	86	20	106
Grain crops	36	27	63
Forage grasses	23	27	50
Forage legumes	35	5	40
Small fruits and berries	23	15	38
Fruit trees	30	6	36
Non-fruit trees	32	4	36
Seed legumes	22	5	27
All other	68	30	98
Total	355	139	494

have North American plant breeders. Polyploids of sugarbeets,
red clover, rye, ryegrass (Lolium spp.), and various Brassica
species are important to European agriculture, but those polyploids
have had little impact on North American agriculture. The
reasons for the different attitudes in Europe and North America
toward the agricultural merits of polyploids are not readily
apparent. Presumably if one breeding method is decidely superior
to another, economics will dictate its adoption.

Much more research is being done with induced autoploids
than with amphiploids. About 70% of the publications appeared to
deal with autoploidy and only 30% with amphiploidy (Table 2).
The emphasis on autoploidy over amphiploidy can be attributed, at
least in part, to the easier acquisition of autoploids and to the
greater economic benefits currently accruing from autoploids.
Amphiploidy requires the accumulation of species-hybrids, whereas
induced autoploidy is practiced on already-existing species. As
long as autoploids continue to give the greater economic returns,
one can reasonably expect that they will attract more research-
breeding attention.

Research on induced polyploidy is being conducted on a vast
array of plant species from more than 150 genera. The most
widely studied genera include Beta (beets), Solanum (potatoes),
Trifolium (clover), Ribes (currants and gooseberries), Gossypium
(cotton), Cucumis (melons and cucumbers), Nicotiana (tobacco),
and Morus (mulberry). The type and quantity of polyploidy
research differs widely in different groups of crop plants (Table
2). Root and vegetable crops, which generally respond well to
chromosome doubling, are the object of a great deal of breeding
and research involving induced autoploidy. Over half of the
research in this crop-group is devoted to two crops, sugarbeets,
and potatoes. The work with sugarbeets involves autoploidy
exclusively, whereas autoploidy and amphiploidy are being used
almost equally in potatoes.

Although autoploidy has been of little immediate benefit to
the grain crops, except possibly rye, more than half of the
publications on polyploidy in grain crops still deal with autoploidy. Most of the autoploidy research is being conducted in
barley (Hordeum vulgare), rye, and buckwheat (Fagopyrum esculentum);
whereas amphiploidy papers usually involve bigeneric combinations
such as Triticum-Aegilops, Triticum-Elymus, Triticum-Agropyron,
Triticum-Hordeum and some trigeneric combinations, Triticum-
Secale-Agropyron.

The forage grasses are the only crops where amphiploids
appear to be as important as induced autoploids. The large
amount of research on the Lolium-Festuca hybrid complex accounts
for much of the current emphasis on amphiploidy. In contrast to
the grasses, amphiploidy is playing only a minor role in the
forage and seed legumes. About half of all work on induced
polyploidy in forage legumes is with red clover, and all of the
red clover effort involves autoploidy.

Trees, with their extended life cycles, are not very well
adapted to amphiploid breeding, which usually requires repeated
hybridization and selection. Consequently, the research on
polyploidy in trees is concentrated on autoploidy. Among non-
fruit trees, the genus Populus (poplar) is receiving the most
attention. Species of Morus (mulberry), Malus (apple), and
Prunus (apricot, plum) are the fruit trees most commonly subjected
to induced polyploidy.

Because of their shorter life cycles, the small fruits and
berries are better adapted to improvement through amphiploidy
than are the trees. Amphiploidy accounts for about 40% of the
polyploidy research being conducted on small fruits. Ribes
(gooseberry, currant) and Fragaria (strawberry) are the genera
attracting the most attention from small-fruit breeders and
geneticists who are working with induced polyploidy.

A significant amount of polyploidy research is being conducted
on species in two genera, Nicotiana and Gossypium, included in
the "all other" category in Table 2. All but one of the 14
Nicotiana publications dealt with amphiploidy, as did 12 of the
15 Gossypium publications.

CONDITIONS AFFECTING SUCCESS IN POLYPLOID BREEDING

The two more or less universal effects of chromosome doubling
are increased cell size and decreased fertility (18). Consequently,
crops that benefit most from increased cell size and suffer least
from reduced fertility are inherently predisposed to benefit from
polyploid breeding. Polyploid breeding success obviously comes
easier in crops that mesh well with the natural tendencies of
induced polyploidy than in crops that are sensitive to the adverse
consequences of induced polyploidy.

Very early in the history of polyploid breeding, Levan (19)
concluded that crops most amenable to improvement through chromosome doubling should 1) have a low chromosome number, 2) be
harvested primarily for their vegetative parts, and 3) be cross-
pollinating. Two other conditions, the perennial habit and
vegetative reproduction, have a bearing on the success of polyploid
breeding by reducing a crop's dependence on seed production.
Finally, the length of time required to cycle a sexual generation
is very important to polyploid breeding programs, which are
unavoidably longer-term than are conventional programs. Success
in either type of program is closely associated with the number
of generations and the size of populations that can be screened.

Of the three conditions listed by Levan as favoring polyploid
breeding, I place the greatest importance on low chromosome
number. Most species have an optimum chromosome number or ploidy
level beyond which additional chromosomes turn to the detriment
of the plant. Most crops have already achieved their optimum
ploidy level and a further increase serves no useful purpose.

Few crop plants are successful beyond the hexaploid level. None of the important grain crops, root crops, or fiber crops exceed this level. As a group, the forage grasses probably contain the greatest number of species with octoploid or higher chromosome numbers, but even they represent only a small part of the total. Exceptions to the hexaploid-or-less rule in crop plants include strawberries (Fragaria X annanassa) and smooth bromegrass (Bromus inermis), both of which are octoploid (2n=56).

Amphiploids whose chromosome number is increased beyond the hexaploid level often lose chromosomes or full genomes in later generations. The octoploid amphiploid (2n=56) of Lolium multiflorum (annual ryegrass) X Festuca arundinacea (tall fescue) is unstable, and the advanced-generation progenies drift toward hexaploidy where they become stabilized (16). Decaploid amphiploids (2n=70) of Phalaris tuberosa (bulbous canarygrass) X Phalaris arundinacea (reed canarygrass) stabilized at 2n=56 after eight generations (20). Triticum-Agropyron amphiploids ranging from 2n=70 to 84 become stabilized at 2n=56 (21). The early work with triticale involved octoploids (2n=56), but the most successful recent breeding work is being done with hexaploids (2n=42) (12). In each of the above cases and in many others, the lower ploidy levels are the most stable and desirable from a breeding standpoint. The implications of the ploidy level data should be readily apparent to plant breeders. Rarely, if ever, will an advantage be realized by doubling the chromosome number of a sexual species or a species-hybrid if it is already at the tetraploid level.

It has become almost axiomatic that polyploid breeding has its greatest opportunities in crops that are grown primarily for their vegetative parts. The reasoning is obvious; such crops benefit from one universal consequence of induced polyploidy, larger plant parts, and suffer least from the other, reduced fertility. The large amount of research and breeding being conducted on polyploidy in root and vegetable crops and forage crops (Table 2) suggests that many breeders subscribe to that reasoning.

Although reduced fertility is not as devastating to a root or forage crop as it is to a cereal crop, good seed production is essential to all crops that are commercially propagated by seed. The poor seed production of induced tetraploid red clover is largely responsible for the limited use of that crop (8). Seed production becomes less important in long-lived perennials than in short-lived perennials, biennials, or annuals; but breeders of induced polyploids cannot afford to ignore fertility in any sexually reproduced crop. Only when a crop can be propagated vegetatively on a commercial scale does seed production become relatively unimportant to the breeder.

The existence of two highly successful allopolyploid cereal crops, wheat and oats, demonstrates that amphiploidy and high seed production are not necessarily incompatible. Fertility and seed production of triticale and tetraploid rye have steadily increased, but only after intense selection over many generations.

The rationale underlying Levan's (19) third condition favoring success in polyploid breeding, the cross-pollinating habit, is that numerous genetic combinations must come together before the most favorable gene combination and balance is achieved. Cross-pollination fosters free-mixing of genes in a breeding population, whereas self-pollination restricts genetic mixing. A corollary condition to unrestricted genetic mixing is the inclusion of a large number of diverse genotypes in the original breeding population prior to chromosome doubling. A broad genetic base is a prerequisite of any successful breeding program, conventional or polyploid, but it is more difficult to achieve in a polyploid program. Inadequate variation in the original breeding population has undoubtedly contributed to the failure of many polyploid breeding programs.

Breeding experience seems to support Levan's cross-pollinating rule, at least with respect to induced autoploidy. The most successful induced autoploid crops -- ryegrass, red clover, sugarbeets -- are naturally cross-pollinating. Furthermore, most naturally occurring autoploid species -- alfalfa (Medicago sativa), orchardgrass (Dactylis glomerata), crested wheatgrass (Agropyron cristatum), timothy (Phleum pratense) -- are also cross-pollinating. Induced or natural autoploidy has been of little consequence in self-pollinating crops. The potato, a self-fertilizing autoploid, is an exception to this rule, but vegetative reproduction makes the type of sexual reproduction of less consequence.

The cross-pollinating habit appears to be less essential in the breeding of amphiploids than in autoploids. Some of our most successful crops -- wheat, oats, cotton, and tobacco -- are self-fertilizing allopolyploids. Amphiploid triticale is likewise self-fertilizing. Cross-pollination provides for free genetic mixing, whereas self-pollination facilitates the fixing of desirable gene combinations. Consequently, the advantages and disadvantages of allogamy vs. autogamy may offset one another. Gustafson (12) observed in triticale that: "It appears that hybridization...coupled with predominantly self-pollination furnishes hexaploid triticale with an efficient genetic system for the rapid evolution of a species. On one side, inter- and intra-specific connections...provide an easily available source of genetic and chromosome variation. On the other side, self-pollination causes the immediate fixing of gene or chromosomal combinations for natural or artificial selection." Whether breeding self- or cross-pollinating autoploids or amphiploids, the over-riding consideration should be the building of large and genetically diverse segregating populations. Such populations may be easier to construct in cross-pollinating polyploids, but the desired segregates are easier to fix in self-pollinating polyploids.

Simple economics may outweigh all of the biological considerations in determining whether a polyploid breeding program is brought to a successful conclusion. Because of their economic potential, breeding programs of amphiploid cereal crops such as perennial wheat or triticale have survived even though they run counter to several of the biological conditions that favor success. On the other hand, support for polyploid breeding programs may be difficult to obtain in economically less important species even though they might be biologically suited to polyploid breeding.

Polyploid breeding programs must compete with conventional breeding programs for financial support. If the conventional programs have been successful and have not appreciably exhausted the existing germplasm resources, there is little justification to invoke the more expensive, long-term, and uncertain induced-polyploid breeding methods. Lack of significant progress in many of the forage crops through traditional plant-breeding methods may be the single-most important factor justifying the expanded use of polyploid breeding in these crops. When conventional breeding approaches fail to produce desired results, breeders naturally look to unconventional methods, particularly wide hybridization and induced polyploidy.

BREEDING OPPORTUNITIES AND STRATEGIES

Induced Autoploidy

The amount of research and breeding effort that has been expended on induced autoploids is highly disproportionate to their relative importance in nature. Less than 10% of the natural polyploid species are autoploids, yet considerably more than half of the polyploid research and breeding effort has been concentrated on that class of polyploids. In the future, less emphasis should probably be placed on breeding induced autoploids. All major crops, most minor crops, and many non crops have already had their chromosome complements doubled; and few have benefited from it even after long-term breeding and selection. Further indiscriminant chromosome doubling without a specific purpose or breeding objective cannot be justified.

In recent correspondence (January–April 1979) with breeders of various crops in several countries regarding their experience with induced polyploidy, I failed to locate a single plant breeder who was enthusiastic about using induced autoploids per se. Some typical responses were: "We have not found any practical use for autotetraploids per se" in tobacco. "We used polyploidy extensively (in various forages) in the 1960's...However since then we have made little use of this method and consider our 'era of colchicine' to be virtually over." "After considerable hope and very disappointing results, the trend is now toward lesser experimentation on induced tetraploids in the viticultural research stations." "In my opinion the value of induced tetraploidy for breeding red clover...is not very high." In sugarbeets "the trend seems to be toward diminished utilization of triploids and greater concentration on breeding and development of diploid hybrids." "The trend is away from tetraploids [buckwheat] and I have thrown out all of my experimental autotetraploids." "I don't believe auto-polyploidy would be of any use in cotton improvement." "In recent years, polyploid breeding in Japan is not as active as previously. Generally speaking, the synthesized polyploid forms are not promising." These responses may not represent the attitudes of all breeders who have worked with autoploids, but they do reflect a general consensus that autoploid breeding is at a low ebb and may decline even further.

Increased breeding emphasis on induced autoploidy may be justified in at least one group of crops, the perennial forages. The fact that most naturally occurring autoploids are perennial forages -- alfalfa, orchardgrass, crested wheatgrass, Hordeum bulbosum, and Hordeum violaceum -- suggests that they would be adaptable to induced polyploid breeding. Furthermore, many of the perennial forages meet all of Levan's (19) conditions for success in a polyploid breeding program.

Although red clover has been the object of considerable polyploid breeding without producing varieties that have wide acceptance, additional breeding emphasis appears to be warranted. Tetraploid red clover appears to have almost everything in its favor except seed production. Everywhere that the tetraploid has been grown, it has produced considerably less seed than comparable diploids. Poor seed yields result from a combination of fewer seed heads, a flower structure that discourages pollination by bees, and meiotic irregularity. The success or failure of tetra-ploid red clover hinges to a large extent on the ability of breeders to alleviate these shortcomings. New germplasm sources must be doubled and merged with existing tetraploid populations to broaden the genetic base from which to select for fertility.

Induced tetraploids of annual ryegrass (Lolium multiflorum) and perennial ryegrass (Lolium perenne) have been bred in several European countries since the early 1960's. In a recent summary comparison of diploid vs. tetraploid varieties from several countries van Bogaert (22) showed that the tetraploids averaged 8 to 18% higher green-matter yields, but the dry-matter yields of the two groups were almost identical. Although dry matter production was not increased, the tetraploids had advantages in other aspects including 1) increased disease resistance, 2)higher palatablity, 3) more non structural carbohydrates, 4) less crude fiber, and 5) higher digestibility. In contrast to red clover, seed yields of the ryegrass tetraploids are adequate, producing more seed than diploids on a weight basis but less in terms of seed numbers. Although tetraploid ryegrasses may not exceed the diploids in forage yield, their superior quality factors may lead to expanded use. More than 40 varieties of tetraploid ryegrass have been released by six European countries (22). Although

tetraploid ryegrass is not being bred in North America, some
European varieties are now being marketed on this continent.

Induced autoploidy appears to offer an excellent opportunity
to improve the productivity of the perennial diploid grasses of
the Triticeae tribe. At least four Triticeae grasses -- Agropyron
cristatum (crested wheatgrass), Agropyron spicatum (bluebunch
wheatgrass), Hordeum violaceum, and Hordeum bulbosum (bulbous
barley) -- form naturally occurring diploid-autoploid series (23-
26). In every instance, the tetraploid is more robust and
productive and has larger seed than the diploid. Increased seed
size is particularly important to the establishment of small-
seeded grass species that are used to revegetate harsh arid range
sites. Two of these species complexes, Agropyron cristatum and
Hordeum violaceum, have diploid (2n=14), tetraploid (2n=28), and
hexaploid (2n=42) races; and no agronomic advantage is associated
with the hexaploid over the tetraploid. Consequently, grass
breeders should probably confine themselves to the synthesis of
autotetraploids.

Doubling the diploids of the Agropyron spicatum complex
should be especially appealing to grass breeders. This species
is one of the most widespread and important range grasses in the
western U.S. It contains the common genome found in all North
American wheatgrasses (27). The diploid race is the most prevalent,
with the larger and more productive tetraploids being confined to
the Pacific Northwest. Chromosome doubling of diploid strains
and ecotypes from all regions of the western U.S. should provide
a unique and valuable germplasm pool. Agropyron spicatum has
closely related diploid counterparts in the Middle East and
Central Asia -- A. libanoticum, A. stipifolium, and A. ferganense
(28). These species, all of which are useful range forage
grasses, should likewise be raised to the tetraploid level for
breeding purposes.

Another unique opportunity to use induced polyploidy in the
perennial Triticeae grasses is with diploid Elymus junceus (Russian
wildrye). No naturally occurring tetraploid races of Russian
wildrye are known. This species, the only diploid in the genus
Elymus, has come into wide usage in the U.S. and U.S.S.R. to
revegetate arid rangeland. It would find even much wider use
were it not for its poor seedling vigor. If chromosome doubling
did nothing more than improve the stand establishment characteristics of Russian wildrye by increasing seed size, it would be
a significant advance. One collection of Russian wildrye was
doubled about 10 years ago (A.E. Slinkard, unpublished), and it
does indeed have larger seed, about 80% heavier than the diploid.
Breeders have treated this induced tetraploid more or less as a
novelty; however, a concentrated effort has been recently initiated
at Logan to double the chromosome complement of a wide range of
the best diploid strains.

The ploidy situation in the perennial bromegrasses (Bromus
group Bromopsis) makes them amenable to polyploid breeding even

though most are already at the tetraploid level. The agronomically important strains of <u>Bromus inermis</u> (smooth bromegrass) are octoploid (2n=56). Nevertheless, this species and several of its closest relatives also contain chromosome races with 2n=28,42, and 70 (29). The tetraploids are the most likely group to respond favorably to chromosome doubling. Unfortunately, the tetraploid races are relatively uncommon and unavailable to breeders. An effort should be made to obtain additional collections of the tetraploids, which are reportedly quite common in northern Kazakhstan, U.S.S.R. (personal communication, V. Inosemtsev).

     Induced autoploidy probably has limited direct application to the improvement of alfalfa, orchardgrass, and crested wheatgrass, whose agriculturally important strains are already at the tetraploid level. Each of the three species-complexes consist of a natural autoploid series from diploid to tetraploid to hexaploid (23,30,31). Artificially doubled diploids are usually not competitive with the natural autotetraploids; nevertheless, the doubled diploids can be used to expand the germplasm pool of the tetraploids. This application will be discussed under the heading of "Induced Polyploids as a Genetic Bridge."

Induced Alloploidy

     It seems paradoxical that man has had his least success in manipulating polyploidy in the very area that nature has had its greatest success, i.e., in the synthesis of alloploid species. Many crop species (wheat, cotton, oats, tobacco, and many forage grasses) and numerous wild species are alloploids; but with a few possible exceptions, man has failed in his efforts to produce important crop plants through induced amphiploidy per se. Reasons for the breeder's inability to duplicate nature's feats in synthesizing species include: 1) choice of crops that do not lend themsleves to improvement in this fashion, 2) inadequate genetic variation in the initial breeding populations, 3) early abandonment of breeding programs because of lack of immediate success, and 4) failure to work at the lower ploidy levels.

     The most concentrated efforts to synthesize agronomically important amphiploids have been with the cereals. This emphasis may be justified in view of their economic importance; however, in the cereals, breeders have chosen one of the most difficult groups of plants to improve through amphiploid breeding. For the most part, these crops are self-fertilizing annuals that are grown for their seed. Their complete orientation toward seed production make the cultivated cereals highly vulnerable to even low levels of sterility, which is a certain consequence of amphiploidy. The 40- to 45-year breeding efforts to produce commercially acceptable triticales or perennial wheats are testimonials to the difficulty of synthesizing new cereal species.

Breeding an amphiploid cereal crop will almost certainly span
several generations of breeders from its inception until it
yields a new economically competitive species.

Securing adequate populations of genetically diverse interspecific or intergeneric F_1 hybrids and their amphiploid derivatives
is often so expensive and time consuming that the breeder is
forced to operate from a very narrow genetic base, and his chances
of success decline accordingly. The ease of obtaining F_1 hybrids
varies widely, but in every instance a considerable investment is
required to build a sizeable F_1 hybrid populaton from which to
launch an amphiploid breeding program. Unfortunately, ease of
crossing between taxa is usually negatively correlated with the
success of their amphiploid hybrid. Although there are exceptions
to the observation by Clausen, Keck, and Heisey (32) that the
most successful amphiploids come from hybrids between the more
distantly related taxa, the concept is generally valid. Never--
theless, the breeder in his quest for a superior amphiploid
should recognize that some hybrids can be too wide. Intertribal
hybrids and amphiploids such as those between wheat and oats (33)
have not proven to be important from an agronomic standpoint. The
interaction of genetic systems of species from different tribes
are likely to result in genic and genomic imbalances and dis-
harmonies that prevent their hybrids and amphiploids from reaching
even the capabilities of the parent species. Consequently, plant
breeders probably should not at present concern themselves with
hybrids between members of different tribes.

Because of impatience on the part of a breeder or his employer,
a genuinely worthy breeding program may be abandoned before its
potential has been determined and exploited. Tsitsin (personal
communication) insists that breeders must carry amphiploid hybrids
at least 10 generations to obtain a realistic measure of their
potential. Many amphiploid breeding programs are abandoned far
short of this minimum. In an annual cereal crop, 10 generations
can be advanced and evaluated in as few as 5 years. Perennial
crops, of course, require much more time to turn over each generation and to evaluate it. The short generation time is one great
advantage that the annual cereals have over the perennials in an
amphiploid breeding program.

I consider the use of low-chromosome-number species, preferably
diploids, to be the key element to successful breeding of amphiploids. Love (34) had the same philosophy and attributed the
poor performance of most amphiploids to the failure of the breeders
to work with diploid species. The desirability of synthesizing
amphiploids with lower chromosome numbers can be illustrated in
the cytogenetic program with the perennial grasses of the Triticeae
tribe (Agropyron, Elymus, Sitanion, Hordeum) at Logan. This
tribe contains about 200 perennial species worldwide, and their
chromosome numbers range from 2n=14 to 84. Roughly 10% of the
species are diploids, 65% are tetraploids, 20% are hexaploids,
and the remaining 5% are octoploids or higher. The fact that

two-thirds of the species are tetraploids immediately suggests
that the greatest opportunities for species synthesis lie in the
production of tetraploid amphiploids. Of the 50 different amphiploids that have been produced at Logan, only 1 is tetraploid
(2n=28), 15 are hexaploid (2n=42), 32 are octoploid (2n=56), and
2 are decaploid (2n=84). This array of ploidy levels, which was
developed for purposes in addition to breeding, is vastly different
from that of the natural species.

   Our early breeding experience with these amphiploids,
especially at the higher ploidy levels, has been consistently
disappointing. Although fertility was restored to satisfactory
levels in the initial amphiploid generation, C_0, it declined in
subsequent generations. This decline was much more rapid in the
octoploids than in the hexaploids (1) (Fig. 1). In one amphiploid

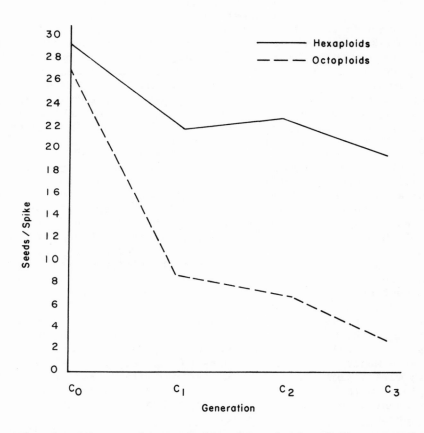

   Fig. 1. Mean seed set of five hexaploid and four octoploid
perennial Triticeae amphiploids in each of four generations after
chromosome doubling (35).

population, <u>Elymus canadensis</u>-<u>Agropyron subsecundum</u>, fertility dropped continuously through six generations and by the C_5 generation it was only one-tenth as fertile as the C_0 (36). Not only did the generation means decline in all octoploids, but the range in genetic variability decreased also.

Prospects of stabilizing fertile amphiploids at the hexaploid level are much brighter. Although mean seed set tended to decline in advanced generations, the decline was moderate. More important, the range in seed set remained as high in the C_3 as in the C_1 generation. In fact, individual C_3 plants in some populations were more fertile than the most fertile C_1 plants. Variation of this scope gives the breeder ample opportunity to maintain or even increase the fertility level in subsequent generations.

In addition to the devastating decline in fertility, the octoploid perennial Triticeae amphiploids sustained a substantial loss in vegetative vigor from the F_1 to C_0 generation. The <u>E. canadensis</u>-<u>A. subsecundum</u> C_0 amphiploid yielded only one-third as much as its genetically equivalent F_1 (36). Even in subsequent generations, yields of the amphiploids were no more than half as much as those of the F_1's. Yield losses from the F_1 to C_0 in other octoploids were, with a few exceptions, similar to those sustained by the <u>E. canadensis</u>-<u>A. subsecundum</u> amphiploid. The hexaploid amphiploids suffered little or no loss in vigor when compared to their F_1 counterparts.

The combination of reduced fertility and reduced vegetative vigor in the 56-chromosome amphiploids has caused us to abandon all efforts to synthesize octoploid Triticeae grasses and to concentrate on the hexaploids and tetraploids. Although hybrids between the diploid species are difficult to make, the extra effort to obtain them is probably justified. Inasmuch as crossing is easier among tetraploids, our first goal is to double all available diploids and then hybridize the induced tetraploids to produce allotetraploids.

Our unsatisfactory experience in producing high-ploidy-level amphiploids has been similar to that reported by McWilliam (20) in <u>Phalaris</u>. After eight cycles of selection in a 70-chromosome amphiploid population derived from a hybrid between <u>P</u>. <u>tuberosa</u> (2n=28) and <u>P</u>. <u>arundinacea</u> (2n=42), fertility remained low and agronomic characters were inferior to those of the F_1. He concluded that 2n=70 was probably above the optimum chromosome level of the species and that a fertile 70-chromosome amphiploid with desirable forage characters could not be obtained.

The importance of working at the lowest possible ploidy level is further demonstrated in the <u>Lolium</u>-<u>Festuca</u> complex, a group of species that range from 2n=14 to 2n=70. Wide hybridization and induced polyploidy has been practiced more extensively in these grasses than in any other forage crop. It is notable that the only stable, fertile, and agronomically important amphiploids have come from diploid parents, <u>Lolium</u> <u>perenne</u> and <u>Lolium</u>

multiflorum. At least three commercially acceptable varieties of
this amphiploid hybrid are now in use in Great Britain and in
Europe (37).

Sterility problems in many amphiploids, particularly those
with a high chromosome number, are associated with homoeologous
chromosome pairing, resulting in genetically unbalanced gametes.
Suppression of homoeologous pairing and promotion of exclusive
bivalent pairing would substantially reduce the sterility and
cytological instability that plague most newly formed amphiploids.
Great strides have been made in wheat in the understanding of the
genetic control of homoeologous pairing and how to manipulate it
(38). A genetic effect on homoeologous pairing has also been
recognized in other species, including tall fescue (39); however,
recognition of an effect and controlling it are quite different
matters. Although the control of homoeologous pairing would be a
significant advance in the synthesis of stable and fertile amphiploids, its use in all but a few species is in the distant future.
In the meantime, simple selection for fertility and monitoring of
chromosome number are probably as effective and simple as any
other means of stabilizing amphiploids.

I am convinced that synthesis and breeding of amphiploids is
on the threshold of an era of expansion. Breeding of autoploids
has probably peaked and will decline, but the potential of amphiploids remains largely unexploited. The immediate future of
amphiploid breeding depends somewhat on the ability of triticale
or perennial wheat to become established as major crops. Unqua-
lified success in either of these amphiploids, but most likely
triticale, would stimulate renewed interest in synthesizing
amphiploids not only in the cereals but in all crops. Regardless
of the outcome of triticale, breeders and cytogeneticists should
continue to synthesize new amphiploids, while recognizing that
indiscriminant synthesis of amphiploids is no longer appropriate.
If breeders are intent on capitalizing on the potential of amphiploidy, they should select those crops that are best adapted
(biologically or economically) to amphiploid breeding, work at
the lowest possible ploidy level, generate large and genetically
diverse populations, and be prepared to invest a lifetime on the
project.

Induced Polyploidy as a Genetic Bridge

The conditions that effect the success or failure of induced
polyploids per se are not so important when the polyploids are
used as a genetic bridge. The polyploids in this circumstance
simply serve as vehicles for gene transfer and are not evaluated
as end products themselves. Because the restrictions on polyploids
as genetic bridges are so few, their usage in this capacity has
been varied and widespread.

The agronomic benefits to be derived from induced polyploidy
per se are often unpredictable. On the other hand, induced

polyploidy as a bridge is more likely to be used in a breeding situation whose outcome can be predicted from the beginning, for example, the transfer of a specific gene or gene-block from one species to another. Induced autoploidy plays an important bridging role in two ways: 1) as a means of facilitating gene flow between chromosome races within an autoploid species or species-complex and 2) by enhancing the crossability of two species.

In the diploid-autoploid species complexes of alfalfa, orchardgrass, and crested wheatgrass the tetraploids are the predominant cultivated forms. However, the diploids of each species contain certain characteristics that would be advantageous to the tetraploids. Crested wheatgrass serves as a good example of the use of induced autoploidy to facilitate gene flow across ploidy barriers. Gene flow between diploid and polyploid crested wheatgrasses is virtually nonexistent because of barriers to crossing and almost complete hybrid sterility (40). The small amount of genetic exchange that occurs between diploids and polyploids is unidirectional, from diploid to polyploid (41). Doubling the chromosome number of diploid crested wheatgrass overcomes the crossing barriers, results in fertile interploid hybrids, and makes gene flow bidirectional (42,43). Now the genetic resources of all crested wheatgrasses, regardless of ploidy level, are available to breeders for improving the agronomically important tetraploids or for transferring traits from the genetically variable tetraploid taxa to the highly uniform diploids.

Alfalfa breeders and cytogeneticists have provided a model in the effective use of an autoploid series that could well be followed by those working with cytologically analogous crops. With the aid of induced autoploidy, unreduced gametes, and interploidy hybridization, a complete autoploid series from 1x to 8x has been built in the Medicago sativa-falcata complex (44). This series gives the breeder great versatility for moving genes between ploidy levels; and it provides a powerful tool to study evolutionary processes, inheritance patterns, gene action, and morphological, cytological, and physiological effects of polyploidy. Similar ploidy series should be generated in all autoploid species.

Doubling the chromosome number of a diploid often increases its capability to hybridize with other species, particularly if both are diploids. I have repeatedly attempted to hybridize diploid Agropyron cristatum with diploid Agropyron spicatum but without success. Only when autotetraploid races of one or both species were used was the cross successful. Similarly, I have been unable to hybridize diploid A. spicatum or diploid A. stipifolium with hexaploid A. repens, but crossing occurred readily when the autotetraploid races were used. Similar results from a wide range of crop plants -- Medicago (45), Trifolium (46), Fragaria (47), Nicotiana (14), Solanum (48), and Lamium (49), -- leave little doubt of the enhancing effect of induced autoploidy on interspecific or intergeneric crossability.

Amphiploidy has found its widest and possibly most important application as a means of effecting genetic transfer between species (controlled introgression). The necessity of using amphiploidy as a genetic bridge increases in direct proportion to the sterility of the F_1 hybrid. It offers the only opportunity of moving genes between species whose F_1 hybrids are totally sterile, but its use is not restricted to situations of complete F_1 sterility. Backcross progeny of partially fertile F_1's may themselves be sterile, whereas backcrosses of the amphiploid may be fertile because of the buffering effect of additional chromosomes. However, induced amphiploidy may only complicate genetic transfer if the F_1 hybrid has reasonable fertility.

The outcome of controlled introgression may range from transfer of whole genomes to movement of single genes from one species to another. Ordinarily the goal is to transfer the desired gene(s) with as little extraneous genetic material as possible, because additional genetic material almost always carries undesirable effects with it. Sears' (50) transfer of leaf rust (Puccinia triticina) resistance from Aegilops umbellulata to bread wheat (Triticum aestivum) via an amphiploid of T. dicoccoides X A. umbellulata is the classical model of integrated use of wide hybridization, amphiploidy, irradiation, and conventional backcrossing and selection procedures to insert a small chromosome segment from one species into another.

Cauderson's (21) description of stepwise transfer of a genome, a chromosome, and a gene from perennial intermediate wheatgrass (Agropyron intermedium) to annual wheat illustrates the effects of various stages of introgression. Through a series of backcrosses and selection, a stable octoploid (2n=56) strain was obtained that contained the full chromosome complement of wheat (2n=42) and 14 of the 42 chromosomes of intermediate wheatgrass. Although fertile and stable, the "partial amphiploid" was agronomically unacceptable; yet it was resistant to three wheat rusts. Further backcrossing and selection resulted in 44-chromosome strains with the full wheat complement plus a pair of intermediate wheatgrass chromosomes. As the amount of wheatgrass genetic material was reduced from a full genome to one chromosome, the agronomic qualities of the strains improved. Finally, through suppression of homoeologous pairing, it was possible to transfer the genes for rust resistance from the Agropyron chromosomes to the Triticum chromosomes, resulting in an agronomically acceptable wheat with rust resistance.

The cytogeneticists' recently discovered ability to "turn on" or "turn off" genetic exchange between certain species through control of homoeologous pairing will undoubtedly stimulate activity in controlled introgression, much of which will involve amphiploids at one stage or another. Unfortunately, control of homoeologous pairing has been explored in depth only in Triticum, and its manipulation has become possible only after 20 years of intensive cytogenetic investigations in numerous laboratories. If breeders of other crops expect to benefit from the use of genetic control of chromosome pairing, they must first pay the price (hopefully on a reduced scale) that wheat cytogeneticists and breeders have paid, i.e., many years devoted to the accumulation of basic cytogenetic information and acquisition of genetic stocks.

With a few exceptions, breeders of other crops cannot expect to obtain cytogenetic support comparable to that given to wheat. Nevertheless, considerable progress in gene transfer has been and will continue to be made without the sophisticated and sometimes complex procedures used in wheat. Mechanisms of interspecific gene transfer in cotton are at least one step down in elegance from those currently used by wheat cytogeneticists, yet the practical results in cotton have probably exceeded those in wheat. The triple hybrids (TH) of cotton, which involve the induced amphiploid of Gossypium aboreum X G. thurberi crossed to G. hirsutum, have been used widely in cotton breeding programs to improve fiber strength of upland cotton(15). Other agronomically important characteristics transferred from wild diploid cottons to tetraploid cultivated cotton, often via hexaploid amphiploids, include resistance to several insects, plant smoothness, the nectariless trait, and cytoplasmic male sterility (51).

Breeding procedures are even less refined in the forage crops than in wheat or cotton, yet significant progress has been achieved through introgression via amphiploidy in some forages. The superior quality of 14-chromosome annual ryegrass was incorporated into 42-chromosome tall fescue through their 56-chromosome amphiploids. The amphiploids were crossed as males to their F_1 counterparts, somehow resulting in 56-chromosome progeny, which in later generations dropped to 2n=42, the same as that in tall fescue (16). After extensive evaluation, a 42-chromosome synthetic variety, 'Kenhy,' was released primarily on the basis of its improved quality (52). Although the exact machanism by which the genetic transfer took place is obscure, the end results were agronomically significant. The development of Kenhy poses quite a contrast to the methods and consequences of introgression in wheat. Cauderon (53), in summarizing controlled introgression between Triticum and Agropyron, conceded that the derivatives obtained to date do not represent an important improvement in wheat. She concluded with the statement, "We do not know where we must go [to make important improvements], but we know how to get there." The breeders of Kenhy knew where to go and they got there, but they didn't know exactly how they got there.

Introgression via induced polyploidy will undoubtedly increase in its importance to plant breeders as more efficient means of effecting gene transfer are devised through basic cytogenetic research. Breeders can then look more and more to related taxa in their search for additional genetic variation. Wheat breeders for example can look forward to making greater use of genes from the perennial grasses of the Triticeae tribe. By its very nature, introgression cannot usually be expected to lead to major break-

throughs in the yield barrier in a single jump, rather it can add
new genes or gene complexes to the breeder's genetic portfolio,
which in time can have a significant impact on the adaptation and
productivity of a crop.

SUMMARY

The performance of induced polyploids as agricultural crops
has consistently fallen short of expectations. Artificial autoploids once thought to have considerable agricultural merit --
sugarbeets, rye, red clover, alsike clover, grapes, watermelons,
and ornamentals-- are being grown less today than they were 10 to
15 years ago. The two most publicized amphiploids, Triticum-
Secale (triticale) and Triticum-Agropyron (perennial wheat) have
yet to become important agricultural crops, although triticale is
rapidly approaching the status of a major crop. Induced polyploidy is finding its most varied application as a vehicle of
controlled introgression between taxa through the transfer of
genes, gene-complexes, whole chromosomes, and partial genomes.
In spite of modest agricultural successes, research and
breeding work on induced polyploids is still very popular. More
than 50% of about 500 recent publications on induced polyploidy
originated from two countries, the U.S.S.R. and India. European
plant breeders are showing much more interest in artificial
polyploids than are North American plant breeders. About 70% of
the recent research and breeding appears to be conducted on
autoploidy and only 30% on amphiploidy.
Plant breeding success comes more readily in crops that
benefit most or suffer least from the two universal effects of
induced polyploidy, increased cell size and reduced fertility.
Crops most amenable to polyploid breeding should have a low
chromosome number and be harvested primarily for their vegetative
parts. Other biological factors that have a bearing on a crop's
predisposition to polyploid breeding include mode of reproduction
(self pollinating, cross pollinating, or asexual), length of
reproductive cycle, and perennial vs. annual growth habit.
Economic factors may override all other factors in determining
whether to pursue polyploid breeding. As a group, the forages
are probably best adapted to polyploid breeding and the cereals
are among the least adapted. Yet, the economic importance of the
cereals has led to a concentrated and prolonged polyploidy breeding
effort that is nearing success.
Induced autoploids have a doubtful future in agriculture.
Many breeders who have worked with artificial polyploids have
become disillusioned with them and are returning to traditional
breeding methods. Induced autoploidy has its greatest breeding
application in the perennial forages, which contain several of
the world's important natural autoploid species including alfalfa,
orchardgrass, and crested wheatgrass.

Although induced amphiploidy has not yet had a significant impact on agriculture, it holds greater promise than does autoploidy. Alloploidy is a much more common phenomenon in nature than is autoploidy, and the opportunities of synthesizing agriculturally important crops via amphiploidy are good if the breeder 1) chooses crops that lend themselves to polyploid breeding, 2) works at the lowest possible ploidy level, 3) generates large and genetically diverse breeding populations, and 4) is prepared to invest a professional lifetime to the project.

Conditions affecting the agricultural success or failure of artificial polyploids per se become relatively unimportant when they are used as a genetic bridge. Induced autoploidy plays an important bridging role by facilitating gene flow between chromosome races within a species-complex and by enhancing the crossability of two species. Amphiploidy offers the only opportunity for introgression between species if their F_1 hybrids are totally sterile. As a bridge, amphiploidy has been used most frequently in transferring simply inherited disease resistance from wild to cultivated species; however, complex quality traits have also been transferred between species. Introgression via induced polyploidy will undoubtedly increase in importance as cytogeneticists devise more efficient means of genetic transfer, e.g., control of homoeologous pairing. Controlled introgression cannot usually be expected to lead to single large junps in yield, but it can add new genes and gene-complexes to the breeder's germplasm pool, which in time can have a major cumulative effect on the adaptation and productivity of a crop.

LITERATURE CITED

1. National Plant Genetics Resources Board, 1979, Plant genetic resources: conservation and use. Unnumbered publication, 20 pp. U.S. Govt. Printing Office. Washington D.C.
2. Hanson, A.A., 1972, Breeding of grasses, pp. 36-52, in Younger, V.B., McKell, C.M. (eds.), "The Biology and Utilization of Grasses," Academic Press, New York.
3. van Bogaert, G., 1977, Scope for improving the yield of grasses and legumes by breeding and selection, pp. 29-35, in Gilsenan, B. (ed.), "Proc. Inter. Meeting on Animal Production from Temperate Grassland," Dublin.
4. Stebbins, G.L., 1956, Artificial polyploidy as a tool in plant breeding, pp. 37-52, in "Genetics in Plant Breeding," Brookhaven Symposia in Biology No. 9. Brookhaven National Laboratory, Upton, New York.
5. Hecker, R.J., Strafford, R.E., Helmerick, R.H., Maag, G.W., 1970, Comparison of the same sugarbeet F_1 hybrids as diploids, triploids, and tetraploids. Amer. Soc. Sugarbeet Tech. 16: 106-116.

6.   Hornsey, K.G., 1974, The exploitation of polyploidy in
     sugarbeet breeding. J. Agric. Sci. Camb. 84: 543–557.
7.   Hornsey, K.G., 1970, The future for polyploids. Br. Sugar-
     beet Rev. 38: 163–170.
8.   Frame, J., 1976, The potential of tetraploid red clover and
     its role in the United Kingdom. J. Br. Grassland Soc. 31:
     139–152.
9.   Einset, J., Pratt, C., 1975, Grapes, pp. 130–153, in
     Janick, J., Moore, J.N. (eds.), "Advances in Fruit Breeding,"
     Purdue University Press, West Lafayette, Indiana.
10. Yamashita, K., Kihara, H., Nishiyama, I., Matsumara, S.,
     Matsumoto, K., 1957, Polyploidy breeding in Japan. Proc.
     Inter. Genetics Symp. 1956: 341–346.
11. Tsitsin, N.V., 1975, Organization of new species and forms
     of plants. Address to the Twelfth International Botanical
     Congress. Leningrad, 23 pp.
12. Gustafson, J.P., 1976, The evolutionary development of
     triticale: The wheat-rye hybrid. Evol. Biol. 9: 107–135.
13. Larter, E.N., Gustafson, J.P., Zillinsky, F.J., 1978, Welsh
     triticale. Canad. J. Plant Sci. 58: 879–880.
14. Chaplin, J.F., Mann, T.J., 1961, Interspecific hybridization,
     gene transfer, and chromosomal substitution in Nicotiana.
     North Carolina State College Tech. Bull. 145. 31 pp.
15. Culp, T.W., Harrell, D.C., 1973, Breeding methods for improv-
     ing yield and fiber quality of upland cotton (Gossypium
     hirsutum L.). Crop Sci. 13: 686–689.
16. Webster, G.T., Buckner, R.C., 1971, Cytology and agronomic
     performance of Lolium–Festuca hybrid derivatives. Crop Sci.
     11: 109–112.
17. Tsitsin, N.V. (ed.), 1960, "Wide Hybridization in Plants,"
     Israel Program for Scientific Publications, Jerusalem, 364 pp.
18. Eigsti, O.J., Dustin, A.P., 1955, "Colchicine in Agriculture,
     Medicine, Biology, and Chemistry," Iowa State College Press,
     Ames, 470 pp.
19. Levan, A., 1945, Polyploidiförädlingens nuravande läge.
     Sverges Utsädesför. Tidskr. 55: 109–143.
20. McWilliam, J.R., 1974, Interspecific hybridization in Phalaris,
     pp. 243–249, Proc. XII Inter. Grassland Congress.
21. Cauderon, Y., 1977, Alloploidy, pp. 131–143, "Interspecific
     Hybridization in Plant Breeding," Proc. 8th Eucarpia Congress,
     Madrid.
22. van Bogaert, G., 1975, A comparison between colchicine
     induced tetraploid and diploid cultivars of Lolium species,
     pp. 61–78, in Nuesch, B. (ed.), "Ploidy in Fodder Crops,"
     Eucarpia Report, Zurich, Switzerland.
23. Asay, K.H, Dewey, D.R., 1979, Bridging ploidy differences in
     crested wheatgrass. Crop Sci. 19: 519–523.
24. Dewey, D.R., 1965, Morphology, cytology, and fertility of
     synthetic hybrids of Agropyron spicatum X Agropyron dasystach-
     yum-riparium. Bot. Gaz. 126: 269–275.

25. Dewey, D.R., 1979, The Hordeum violaceum complex of Iran. Amer J. Bot. 66: 166-172.

26. Rajhathy, T., Morrison, J.W., Symko, S., 1963, Interspecific and intergeneric hybrids in Hordeum, pp. 194-212, in "Barley Genetics I," Proc. 1st Inter. Barley Genet. Symp., Wageningen.

27. Stebbins, G.L., Snyder, L.A., 1956, Artificial and natural hybrids in the Gramineae, tribe Hordeae. IX. Hybrids between western and eastern North American species. Amer. J. Bot. 43: 305-312.

28. Dewey, D.R., 1975, Genome relations of diploid Agropyron libanoticum with diploid and autotetraploid Agropyron stipifolium. Bot. Gaz. 136: 116-121.

29. Carnahan, H.L., Hill, H.D., 1961, Cytology and genetics of forage grasses. Bot. Rev. 27: 1-162.

30. Jones, K., 1962, Chromosomal status, gene exchange, and evolution in Dactylis. 2. The chromosomal analysis of diploid, tetraploid, and hexaploid species and hybrids. Genetica 32: 272-295.

31. Lesins, K., Singh, S.M., Baysal, I., Sadasaviah, R.S., 1975, An attempt to breed hexaploid alfalfa (Medicago spp.). Z. Pflanzenzüchtg. 75: 192-204.

32. Clausen, J., Keck, D.D., Hiesey, W.M., 1945, Experimental studies on the nature of species. II. Plant evolution through amphiploidy and autoploidy, with examples from the Madiinae. Carnegie Inst. Washington, Publ. No. 564. 174pp.

33. Kruse, A., 1969, Intergeneric hybrids between Triticum aestivum L. (v. Koga II, 2n=42) and Avena sativa L. (v. Stal. 2n=42) with pseudogamous seed formation. Kgl. Vet.-og Landbohjsk. Arsskr. 1969: 188-200.

34. Love, R.M., 1972, Selection and breeding of grasses for forage and other uses, pp. 66-73, in Younger, V.B., McKell, C.M. (eds.), "The Biology and Utilization of Grasses," Academic Press, New York.

35. Asay, K.H., Dewey, D.R., 1976, Fertility of 17 colchicine-induced perennial Triticeae amphiploids through four generations. Crop Sci. 16: 508-513.

36. Dewey, D.R., 1977, Morphology, cytology, and fertility of F_1 and induced-amphiploid hybrids of Elymus canadensis X Agropyron subsecundum. Crop Sci. 17: 106-111.

37. Welsh Plant Breeding Station Annual Report., 1977, Aberystwyth varieties currently in agriculture. pp. 242-249.

38. Riley, R., 1974, Cytogenetics of chromosome pairing in wheat. Genetics 78: 193-203.

39. Jauhar, P.P., 1975, Genetic control of diploid-like meiosis in hexaploid tall fescue. Nature 25: 595-597.

40. Knowles, R.P., 1955, A study of variability in crested wheatgrass. Canad. J. Bot. 33: 534-546.

41. Dewey, D.R., 1971, Reproduction in crested wheatgrass triploids. Crop Sci. 11: 575-580.

42. Dewey, D.R., 1977, A method of transferring genes from tetraploid to diploid crested wheatgrass. Crop Sci. 17: 803–805.

43. Dewey, D.R., Pendse, P.C., 1968, Hybrids between *Agropyron desertorum* and induced-tetraploid *Agropyron cristatum*. Crop Sci. 8: 607–611.

44. Bingham, E.T., Saunders, J.W., 1974, Chromosome manipulations in alfalfa. Scaling the cultivated tetraploid to seven ploidy levels. Crop Sci. 14: 474–477.

45. Lesins, K., 1972, Interspecific crosses involving alfalfa. VII. *Medicago sativa* X *M. rhodopea*. Canad. J. Genet. Cytol. 14: 221–226.

46. Quesenberry, K.H., Taylor, N.L., 1978, Interspecific hybridization in *Trifolium* L. Section *Trifolium* Zoh. III. Partially fertile hybrids of *T. sarviense* Hazsl. X 4x *T. alpestre* L. Crop Sci. 18: 551–556.

47. Ellis, J.R., 1962, *Fragaria-Potentilla* intergeneric hybridization and evolution in *Fragaria*. Proc. Linn. Soc. London 173: 99–106.

48. Livermore, J.R., Johnson, E.E., 1940, The effect of chromosome doubling on the crossability of *Solanum chacoense*, *S. jamsii*, and *S. bulbocastarum* with *S. tuberosum*. Amer. Potato J. 17: 170.

49. Bernstrom, P., 1953, Increased crossability in *Lamium* after chromosome doubling. Hereditas 39: 241– 246.

50. Sears, E.R., 1956, The transfer of leaf-rust resistance from *Aegilops umbellulata* to wheat, pp. 1–22, *in* "Genetics in Plant Breeding," Brookhaven Symposia in Biology No. 9, Brookhaven National Laboratory, Upton, New York.

51. Meyer, V., 1974, Interspecific cotton breeding. Econ. Bot. 28: 56–60.

52. Buckner, R.C., Burrus, P.B., Bush, L.P., 1977, Registration of Kenhy tall fescue. Crop Sci. 17: 672–673.

53. Cauderon, Y., 1979, Use of *Agropyron* species for wheat improvement, pp. 129–139, "Proc. Conf. Broadening Genetic Base of Crops," Wageningen.

MAXIMIZING HETEROZYGOSITY IN AUTOPOLYPLOIDS

E. T. Bingham

Department of Agronomy
University of Wisconsin
Madison, WI 53706

Polyploidy appears dependent on heterozygosity! The largest group of polyploids, the allopolyploids (disomic polyploids), have fixed heterozygosity in the two or more divergent genomes they possess (e.g., wheat, oats, cotton, tobacco, etc.). Hexaploid wheat, for example, although self-pollinated and basically homozygous at loci in each of its three genomes, has internal hybridity among loci with similar function in its three genomes. Disomic polyploids thus are able to capitalize on the merits of both the self- and cross-fertilizing systems (1).

The autopolyploids (polysomic polyploids) insure their heterozygosity through cross-pollination (e.g., alfalfa, birdsfoot trefoil, potato, and many grasses). We can find no example in crop plants of a successful polysomic polyploid species which is self-pollinated. Evidently the polysomic condition can not tolerate the homozygosity associated with self-pollination. The biochemical and physiological advantages of heterozygosity must be an important component of polyploid vigor (2).

Polysomic polyploids are represented by segregating and heterogeneous populations where maximum heterosis may be expressed by a few elite individuals in the population but not by the population per se. (Apomixis can preserve and perpetuate the elite polyploid individuals but will not be reviewed here.) In our seed reproduced polysomic polyploids we can maximize the frequency of elite genotypes, but at present we cannot fix such genotypes in cultivated populations. As will be illustrated in this paper, maximum heterozygosity and heterosis does not occur in the F_1 or single cross generation when parents are inbred (as it does in diploids or disomics) but occurs in the segregating double cross or an even later generation. Under polysomic polyploid conditions, the more inbred the parents, the lower the

performance of the F_1 (3,4). Thus it is more difficult to capitalize on advantages of hybrid vigor in seed reproduced polysomics
than it is in seed reproduced diploids, disomic polyploids, or in
asexually reproduced crops.

The thrust of this paper will be to review evidence that
maximum heterozygosity is important and to show how knowledge of
the genetic structure of polysomic polyploids can be coupled with
modified breeding methods to maximize the frequency of elite
individuals in cultivars. Additionally, a potential now exists
for using genetic control of the meiotic process in diploids of
cultivated polyploids to sexually produce elite tetraploid hybrids
from diploid hybrid parents.

COMPLEXITY OF POLYSOMIC HETEROZYGOSITY

Heterosis in disomic species is rather straightforward
genetically, although the biochemistry of heterosis is still not
fully understood. There is only one form of heterozygosity at a
disomic locus and only one interaction product, e.g., that between
A and a.

In polysomics the familiar terms nulliplex, simplex, duplex,
triplex, and quadruplex, used to describe the number of times a
dominant allele is represented at a tetraploid locus, are an
extension of diploid theory and based on a two allele model (Fig.
1). Here again there can be only one heterozygous interaction
product, i.e., that between A and a. These familiar terms are

Classical terminology – two alleles

Nulliplex	a a a a
Simplex	A a a a
Duplex	A A a a
Triplex	A A A a
Quadruplex	A A A A

Terminology for multiple alleles

Mono-allelic	nulliplex or quadruplex	$a_i a_i a_i a_i$
Di-allelic	simplex or triplex	$a_i a_j a_j a_j$
Di-allelic	duplex	$a_i a_i a_j a_j$
Tri-allelic		$a_i a_i a_j a_k$
Tetra-allelic		$a_i a_j a_k a_l$

Fig. 1. Terminology for genetic structure of loci in
polysomic polyploids.

not adequate, however, to describe any polysomic locus possessing more than two alleles. In the case of multiple alleles in a polysomic tetraploid for example, the terms mono-allelic, di-allelic, tri-allelic and tetra-allelic (Fig. 1) appear appropriate. A tetra-allelic locus would exhibit maximum heterozygosity and would have six first order dominance interactions of alleles taken two at a time ($a_i a_j$, $a_i a_k$, $a_i a_l$, $a_j a_k$, $a_j a_l$, $a_l a_k$) as well as potential second and third order interactions for a total of eleven allelic interactions. Only the tetraploid case will be considered here; polysomic hexaploids and above would be an extension of the tetraploid.

Another important point in the discussions to follow is that an allele cannot be distinguished from a chromosome segment (Fig. 2). The chromosome segment could contain linked genes, and as can be seen in situation II (Fig. 2), homologous segments from diverse parents could each contain a favorable non-allelic dominant which in terms of desirability would be equivalent to the situation with multiple alleles.

I **Multiple alleles at a locus**

$$a_i a_j a_k a_l \; > \; a_i a_j a_k a_k \; > \; a_i a_j a_j a_j \; > \; a_i a_i a_i a_i$$

II **Linkage blocks - two alleles per locus**

A a a a		A a a a		A a a a		A A A A
b B b b	>	b B b b	>	b B B B	>	b b b b
c c C c		c c C C		c c c c		c c c c
d d d D		d d d d		d d d d		d d d d

III **Linkage blocks -- mono-, di-, and multi-allelic loci**

M M M M[a]		M M M M		M M M M		M M M M
A a a a		A a a a		A a a a		A A A A
b B b b	>	b B b b	>	b B B B	>	b b b b
$c_i c_j c_k c_l$		$c_i c_j c_k c_k$		$c_i c_j c_j c_j$		$c_i c_i c_i c_i$
$d_i d_j d_k d_l$		$d_i d_j d_k d_k$		$d_i d_j d_j d_j$		$d_i d_i d_i d_i$

Fig. 2. Genetic constitution and order of desirability under I: Hypothesis of multiple alleles; II: Hypothesis of genetic linkage blocks; and III: Combination of I & II.

[a] M = mono-allelic locus for a monomorphic trait such as leaf shape.

Situation III (Fig. 2) I feel is the most realistic. In this case the linked chromosome segments contain mono-allelic

loci for monomorphic traits, and loci with two to several alleles
for polymorphic traits. Such segments are likely involved in
alfalfa since frequently there is only one chiasma per bivalent
and rod bivalents are common (5). This in fact may well be the
mechanism for bivalent pairing in alfalfa; multiple chiasmata
necessary for quadrivalents are infrequent and quadrivalents
average fewer than one per cell even in raw autotetraploids (6).

RESEARCH ON MAXIMUM HETEROZYGOSITY

Theoretical and practical research on heterosis in polysomic
polyploids is comparatively recent. Carnahan suggested in 1960
that heterosis was more complicated than in diploids in that four
different alleles at a locus were needed for maximum heterozygosity
(7). Shortly thereafter, Demarly published theoretical models
and practical results with alfalfa supporting the importance of
tetra-allelism (or four different chromosome segments) in heterosis
(8).

Inbreeding research on polysomic polyploids is also pertinent
since inbreeding depression is the opposite of heterosis. Since
the approach to homozygosity upon inbreeding is much slower in
polysomic polyploids than in diploids, less inbreeding depression
would also be expected. This has not been the case, however, in
natural polysomic polyploid species. Inbreeding depression was
greater in alfalfa (9-11) and wheat grass (12) than would be
predicted on the basis of the coefficient of inbreeding in a two
allele model. This is indirect evidence for the existence of
multiple alleles. Busbice and Wilsie (9) suggested that the
rapid inbreeding depression was similar to the theoretical rate
at which first order interactions were lost from tri- and tetra-
allelic loci.

In potato, vigor and tuber yield data from two studies
(13,14) can be used to compare heterozygous (di-allelic duplex)
autotetraploids (derived by doubling diploid hybrids) with heterozygous (di-, tri-, and tetra-allelic) tetraploids produced by
intermating the di-allelic duplex parents. The di-allelic duplex
clones were lower yielding than comparable diploids, whereas the
potentially tri- and tetra-allelic hybrids were higher yielding
than comparable diploids. This suggests that genetic interactions
involving more than the two alleles in the di-allelic duplex
state were important determinants of vigor.

Among the several natural diploids which have been doubled
(see Dewey, p.445) maize and rye have been used in research which
bears directly on the concept of maximum heterozygosis. In
maize, Randolph found that tetraploids produced by direct doubling
of inbred diploid lines were weak and essentially sterile (15,16).
In contrast, tetraploids produced by doubling diploids from open-
pollinated varieties and hybrid stocks were vigorous and fertile.
In fact, tetraploids derived from heterozygous stocks were 70-90%

fertile and as vigorous or more vigorous than the parent stocks.
These relationships were also observed in a study using some of
Randolph's stocks in an autotetraploid linkage analysis (17).
Tetraploids derived from diploid inbreds would be largely mono-
allelic whereas those from hybrids would be largely di-allelic
duplex.

In rye, which like maize is naturally a cross-pollinated
diploid species, it was also difficult to establish inbred autotetraploids by doubling diploid inbreds (18). Of 29 diploid
inbred lines treated with colchicine, 13 tetraploids were obtained
of which only 7 lines survived the first season in the tetraploid
state and only 6 were vigorous enough to use in research.

A finding in Randolph's work (15) supports the notion that
polyploids are more dependent on heterozygosity than are diploids.
Maternal haploids (diploids) which occurred spontaneously in his
tetraploids were completely fertile whether they were from fertile
or sterile tetraploids! As discussed by Randolph, the sterility
in the tetraploids cannot be entirely due to meiotic irregularities
associated with multivalents; highly fertile and highly sterile
tetraploid maize had essentially the same synaptic behavior at
meiosis and chromosome number relations in their gametes. Also
there are examples of autotetraploids with small chromosomes and
bivalent synapsis that are quite sterile (6).

Inbreeding depression in autotetraploid maize essentially
paralleled the decrease in heterozygosity in independent studies,
and could be explained on the basis of a standard inbreeding
coefficient (16,19,20). Similarly in autotetraploid rye inbreeding
depression was parallel with the rate of reduction of heterozygosity (18). Isogenic diploid and tetraploid rye was compared
and, as expected, tetraploids displayed less inbreeding depression.

These inbreeding results from autotetraploids of naturally
diploid species are in marked contrast to inbreeding results with
naturally polysomic species. In alfalfa and wheat grass, for
example, vigor and fertility declined much faster than the theoretical rate of reduction in heterozygosity. If the greater than
predicted inbreeding depression is due to loss of first order
interactions from tri- and tetra-allelic loci (9), then these
multiple allelic interactions are more important in natural
polysomic polyploids than in recent autotetraploids.

Mac Key (1) described how, during the evolutionary history
of an outbreeding polysomic species, a precise genetic balance is
achieved for quantitative and qualitative traits in terms of both
dosage relationships and allelic interactions. Natural polysomic
polyploids evidently have evolved mechanisms to exploit all the
heterotic interactions not possible in disomic inheritance.

In order to test critically the hypothesis that maximum
heterozygosity (the highest frequency of tetra-allelic loci which
can be achieved through normal sexual reproduction) is required
for maximum heterosis at the population level, it is necessary to
start with parents having defined genotypic structure. Also it

is necessary to produce from these parents, populations possessing
the same genes and gene frequencies and which differ only in the
relative proportions of genotypic structures they contain.

These requirements were satisfied in an elegant study by
Lundqvist (18) using isogenic diploid and tetraploid inbreds of
rye. Inbreds were diallel mated to produce F_1 and F_1 x F_1
hybrids. Tetraploid F_1 hybrids (expected to be largely di-allelic
duplex as were Randolph's double diploid hybrids of maize) were
much more vigorous than their inbred parents (mono-allelic).
Heterosis was apparent in the F_1's at both diploid and tetraploid
levels. The F_1 x F_1 matings were a powerful tool in demostrating
the difference between disomic and polysomic heterosis and showed
that F_1 x F_1 mating lead to "progressive heterosis" in the tetraploids. At the diploid level F_1 progeny were about equal or
superior to F_1 x F_1 progeny, but at the tetraploid level F_1 x F_1
progeny involving four different inbred parents exceeded the
performance of the F_1 often by as much as the F_1 exceeded the
inbred tetraploid parents. Thus tetraploid heterosis progressed
from F_1 to F_1 x F_1 in autotetraploid rye, and in a similar study in
autotetraploid maize (19). The realized heterosis (F_1 x F_1 > F_1 >
Parents) corresponds to the theoretical changes in the
potential number of alleles at a locus (Table 1). The genetic
structure of loci in the progeny of F_1 x F_1 mating could potentially
be nearly 89% tri- and tetra-allelic.

In alfalfa, so called progressive heterosis of double crosses
over single crosses has also been observed where partial inbreds
(S_1 to S_4) obtained by conventional selfing were used as parents
(4,8). These results support the theoretical expectations under
the maximum heterozygosity model, although the genotypic structures
were not defined in the partial inbred parents. The difficulty
in obtaining parents with defined genotypic structures in alfalfa
and other natural polysomic polyploids was thoroughly discussed by
Dunbier (21). It has not been possible to begin with complete
inbreds since inbreeding depression is so great in natural polysomic species. Furthermore, the completely heterozygous or
tetra-allelic state cannot be assumed as a starting point because,
as Dunbier noted, there is a small probability of drawing tetra-
allelic parents from random mating populations (Table 1).

The approach we took to produce autotetraploid parents with
a defined genotypic structure in alfalfa required several steps:
1) natural tetraploids were scaled down to diploids using haploidy
(22), 2) diploid hybrids ($a_i a_j$, etc.) were produced, and 3)
diploid hybrids were doubled by colchicine treatment to obtain
defined di-allelic duplex ($a_i a_i a_j a_j$) autotetraploid parents (23).

Chromosome doubling has an inbreeding effect on the resulting
autotetraploid which has been interpreted by some workers as
being equivalent to 3.8 generations of conventional selfing
(6,24,25) and by others as 2.2 generations of selfing (21,26).
As will be seen in data to follow, the di-allelic duplex condition

Table 1. Theoretical genetic structure of polysomic tetraploid generations; calculated under assumptions that frequency of different alleles per locus was equal and that single and double crosses were made by mating unrelated parents.

Generation	Parents Produced by Doubling	
	Inbreds (e.g., $a_i a_i$; $a_j a_j$; etc.)	F_1 hybrids (e.g., $a_i a_j$; $a_k a_1$; etc.)
Parents	100% mono-allelic	100% di-allelic duplex
Single cross (F_1)	100% di-allelic duplex	11.1% di-allelic duplex 44.4% tri-allelic 44.4% tetra-allelic
Double cross ($F_1 \times F_1$)	11.1% di-allelic 44.4% tri-allelic 44.4% tetra-allelic	1.2% di-allelic 19.8% tri-allelic 79.0% tetra-allelic
Random mating equilibrium[a]	1.6 mono-allelic 18.7 di-allelic simplex, triplex 14.1 di-allelic duplex 56.2 tri-allelic 9.4 tetra-allelic	

[a] From Dunbier (21), based on equal frequencies of four alleles.

in alfalfa is definitely a partially inbred condition with inbreeding depression equivalent to between 2 and 3 generations of selfing.

It is important to note that in the experiments to follow, we used more diverse parents and more exacting pollination control (hand crosses and emasculation) than often possible in practical breeding. In a recent alfalfa study eight cultivated diploid hybrids were doubled to obtain eight di-allelic duplex autotetraploid parents (4xCD) which were mated to produce four unrelated single cross (SC) and two unrelated double cross (DC) experimentals. Clonal propagules were used so that original diploids and 4xCD materials could be compared with plants in SC and DC generations. Cuttings were made from shoots of 2x and 4xCD parent clones and from a sample of four genotypes in each SC

and DC. The study was based on 6 propagules per entry per plot
spaced 0.8 x 0.8 m and replicated four times.

The 4xCD parents (P) yielded slightly but not significantly
less than the diploids from which they were derived (Table 2).
As in the rye study, there was progressive heterosis with the SC
producing twice as much herbage as the 4xCD parents and the DC
yielding one-third more than the SC. The ranking was clearly
DC > SC > P, and differences were significant (p=0.05).

Over the past six years, three separate experiments also
have been completed comparing SC and DC generations using plants
established from seed and in seeded plots. These independent
experiments have involved 20 unrelated 4xCD parents. Results for
fertility relationships and herbage yield in percent of DC are
summarized in Table 3. The 4xCD clones are essentially self-
sterile, low in cross-fertility, and yield only half as much
herbage as the DC in spite of the fact that they are di-allelic
duplex heterozygotes for polymorphic loci. Clearly, the di-
allelic level of heterozygosity is not sufficient for full fertility or vegetative vigor. Heterosis for both seed and herbage
yield was pronounced and progressed once again from the SC to DC.
Seed yield increased from SC to DC generation consistently about
35%, and herbage has increased 7-20% depending on materials.

Table 2. Herbage yield in gram fresh weight per plant
(gfw/plt) of 2x and 4x parents (P) and hybrids (SC & DC); and a
unique family from 2x parents (H and G) which include a 4x hybrid
from chromosome doubling (HG2 4x) and from 2n gametes (HxG 4x).

Entry	Ploidy	Herbage yield		
	level	Cut 1	Cut 2	Mean
		- - - - - gfw/plt.[a] - - - - - -		
P ($\bar{x}$ of 8)	2x	193	255	224
SC ($\bar{x}$ of 4)	2x	205	230	218
P ($\bar{x}$ of 8)	4x	148	237	193
SC ($\bar{x}$ of 4)	4x	217	540	379
DC ($\bar{x}$ of 2)	4x	315	684	500
H	2x	80	108	94
G	2x	167	230	199
HG2	2x	162	234	198
HG2	4x	174	306	240
HxG	4x	214	630	422

[a] gfw/plt = grams fresh weight per plant.

Table 3. Fertility and herbage yield relationships among 4xCD partial inbreds, SC, and DC hybrids (summarized from Dunbier and Bingham (23), and Bingham, unpublished).

Entry	Fertility (% of DC)		Herbage (% of DC)
	Selfed	Crossed	
4xCD	0	35	50[a]
SC	50-60	65	80-93[b]
DC	100	100	100[b]
two generations beyond DC		85-95	

[a] Extrapolated from clonal studies.
[b] Based on plants from seed and seeded plots.

The 4xCD, SC, and DC generations have the same alleles and allelic frequencies, but different genotypic structures of the alleles at respective loci in individuals in different generations. Consistent ranking of DC> SC> 4xCD correlates with the theoretical increase in the frequency of tetra-allelic loci and supports the hypothesis that maximum heterozygosity maximizes heterosis. Thus, there is strong evidence for both the existence of multiple allelic series (or blocks of linked loci with favorable alleles) and the importance of the tri- and tetra-allelic conditions in influencing plant performance. Moreover, the difference in performance of the SC and DC populations suggests that the tetra-allelic condition is the most important especially for fertility (23). The sum of tri- and tetra-allelic loci is not greatly different in the SC and DC populations (88.9 and 98.8%, respectively); however, the proportion of tetra-allelic loci is quite different (44.4 and 79%, respectively).

In autotetraploid genetic theory it has been demonstrated that with a two allele model in crosses between duplex parents, the SC has a higher proportion of both heterozygous loci and loci that contain at least on dominant allele than the DC population (27). The SC should therefore be superior in a two allele situation. The increase from the SC to the DC in the alfalfa research clearly indicates that a two allele model is not adequate and supports the maximum heterozygosity concept.

BREEDING METHODS TO MAXIMIZE HETEROZYGOSITY

In developing cultivars of seed reproduced polysomics such as alfalfa, birdsfoot trefoil, and many grasses, there is often

several generations of selection in a given population for a
desired trait such as diesease resistance prior to selection of
superior parents from the population. The cultivar is then
synthesized by intermating the selected parents (Syn. 1) and
increasing the seed to commercial levels by successive generations
of synthesis (e.g., Syn 2, 3, and 4). The resulting cultivar is
often approaching equilibrium in terms of allelic structure of
loci. Unfortunately, the peak frequency of tri- and tetra-
allelic has long past when equilibrium is reached (4, 23). Thus
the synthetic method of cultivar development usually does not
capitalize on potential maximum heterozygosity.

Populations with the same allelic frequencies can have
different allelic structures at a locus as a result of the way
they were developed (23). For example, if four unrelated duplex
clones A, B, C, and D are to be used as parents, and if they are
random mated until equilibrium is achieved, the genotypic structure
will be mono-allelic 0.19%, di-allelic simplex or triplex 5.47%,
di-allelic duplex 4.10%, tri-allelic 49.22%, and tetra-allelic
41.02%. If, however, they are mated AXB and CXD and they ABXCD
then the resultant population will have 1.2% di-allelic duplex,
19.8% tri-allelic, and 79.0% tetra-allelic loci. Thus, to the
extent that tetra-allelic loci are important in plant vigor, the
double cross should be superior to the equilibrium population.

Double cross hybrid production in alfalfa (11,28) was
proposed long before we were aware of the advantages it offered
in maximizing hybrid vigor. However, only two out of more than
100 alfalfa cultivars are known to be double crosses. These were
made without pollination control and are a mixture of chance
double crosses and single cross sibs. Until recently, alfalfa
lacked a pollination control mechanism to produce exacting single
and double cross hybrids. Suitable cytoplasmic male sterility is
now available, but it is difficult to produce commercial quantities
of hybrid seed on male-steriles because of limited cross-
pollination by bees. The best pollinating bees, the pollen
collectors, prefer to visit the pollen-parents and not the male-
sterile seed-parents. Hence, exacting double cross hybrids from
controlled pollination are not yet economical.

A modified and practical approach we are using in cultivar
synthesis involves concurrent selection for required disease
resistance and agronomic traits in four or more diverse populations
(A, B, C, and D) instead of one (23). The four populations
are then synthesized in a two step process, 1) AXB and CXD
(termed SC or Syn. 1) and 2) ABXCD (DC or Syn. 2), where seed
of parent populations is blended and grown in isolation. The DC
is a mixture of chance double crosses as well as single cross
sibs. The hypothesis is that chance double crosses are better
than relying on equilibrium populations. In the practical work
thus far, DC or Syn 2 populations have yielded 5 to 15% more
herbage than the parent populations. Thus as much as 15% gain in
yield has been obtained by a slight modification of the cultivar

synthesis method. Synthesis of a cultivar for field testing from
di-allelic duplex parents obtained by doubling diploid hybrids is
underway, but it is two years away from testing. This approach
is considerably more difficult and significant gains will be
required to justify its use in practical breeding.

It is our observation that knowledge of the existence and
importance of multiple allelic interaction in polysomic polyploids
is prompting some breeders to modify cultivar synthesis to take
advantage of maximum heterozygosity. Two such practical modifications are greater diversity of parents and production of commercial
Syn. 2 seed.

UNIQUE METHODS TO MAXIMIZE HETEROZYGOSITY

Two alternatives to normal sexual reproduction exist which
could uniquely fix heterozygosity at or near the maximum in the
first hybrid product in polysomic polyploids: 1) somatic fusion
of hybrid diploid cells, and 2) hybridization of gametes with the
unreduced chromosome number (2n gametes) from diploid hybrids.
These methods are particularly well suited for polysomic tetraploid
crops (e.g., potato) where diploids are available (e.g., via
haploidy) and where the commerical product is asexually reproduced
(e.g., tubers). Somatic hybridization appears to have potential
use, and 2n gametes are already in use.

In somatic cell fusion, donor protoplasts from different
diploid hybrids within the same species complex (e.g., $a_i a_j$ and
$a_k a_l$) could be fused and regenerated to produce hybrid tetraploids
($a_i a_j a_k a_l$). All the genetic variation of donor diploids would be
transmitted to hybrid tetraploid--a fete not possible in the
normal sexual process. At this time, however, there is no known
example of somatic fusion being used for this purpose.

2n gametes have a similar potential for maximizing heterozygosity when they are produced by restitution of the first meiotic
division or an equivalent process. Importantly, 2n gametes occur
naturally at a low frequency in many plant species (29) and
simple genetic control for their production has been identified
in diploid derivatives of potato (30) and alfalfa (31).

Genetic theory and application of 2n gametes is well documented in potato (30,32-34). In brief, of the several mechnanisms
by which 2n gametes may be produced (not including some types
associated with apomictic seed production), first division restitution (FDR) and FDR-type 2n gametes are preferable in breeding
to maximize heterozygosity. This is because they transmit all of
the heterozygosity from the centromere to the first crossover,
and half of that beyond the first crossover. If there is a
second crossover, the heterozygosity transmitted is: 100% from
centromere to first crossover, 50% between first and second
crossover, and 75% beyond second crossover. In species such as
potato and alfalfa, where there is often only one chiasma per

bivalent, probably at least 80% of the heterozygosity in the
diploid may be transmitted via FDR 2n gametes.

Normal microsporogenesis and FDR-type 2n microspore formation
resulting from parallel spindles at metaphase II (MII) are dia-
gramed in Fig. 3. Parallel spindles at M II of microsporogenesis
in diploid alfalfa (Fig. 4) positions T II nuclei in one plane
(Fig. 5). This conditions one division furrow through the parallel
spindles (instead of two furrows in different planes in the
normal case) which produces a dyad of 2n microspores (Fig. 6).
As seen in Fig. 4, normal and parallel spindles occur in adjacent
meiocytes in the same anther. This results in both normal (n)
and 2n pollen (Fig. 7) produced by the same plant. This permits
the plant to be used as a parent in crosses with diploids or
tetraploids. Importantly, diploids producing n and 2n pollen
have full fertility in both 2x-2x and 4x-2x crosses in potato
(34) and in alfalfa (35).

Genetic consequences of parallel spindles are equivalent to
FDR (Fig. 3). The mechanism insures that alleles on sister
chromatids linked to the centromere reside in different TII nuclei.
Division across the parallel spindles insures that maternal and
paternal centromeres and their linked chromatids reside in the
same 2n microspore, thus restoring much of the heterozygosity
present in the MI nucleus. Second division restitution (34) has
opposite genetic consequences and alleles on sister chromatids
linked to the centromere reside in the same gamete resulting in
much homozygosity.

Superiority of FDR-type 2n gametes in potato over normal n
and SDR 2n gametes was manifested in both the gametophyte (pollen
vigor) (36) and sporophyte (tuber yields) (33). Tuber yields of
certain tetraploid hybrids of tetraploid x diploid FDR 2n gamete
producers outyielded not only the mid-parent but the best tetraploid cultivars (33). The unusually high mean performance was
interpreted as a manifestation of FDR 2n pollen to pass onto its
progeny the already heterotic diploid genotype in a largely
intact array.

Genetically mediated FDR 2n gamete formation in alfalfa (31,
37) was identified in cultivated alfalfa at the diploid level
which was developed from cultivated tetraploids over the past ten
years by haploidy and breeding (35). To test the value of such
2n gametes in alfalfa, tetraploid hybrids were produced 1) by FDR
2n gametes (2n=2x=16) from diploid clone 'W31' ($a_i a_j$) and 2) by
normal n gametes (n=2x=16) from autotetraploid clone '4xW31'
($a_i a_i a_j a_j$) obtained by colchicine doubling. Both were crossed
onto a standard tetraploid male sterile tester. Both parents
possessed the same genes, and their functional gametes in the
cross had the same chromosome number; however, the level of
heterozygosity in the gametes was different. The exact heterozygosity of the FDR 2n gametes cannot be specified, but could
be as much as 80%; that of the n gametes of 4xW31 cannot exceed
67%. Forage yields of respective hybrids in seeded rows and as

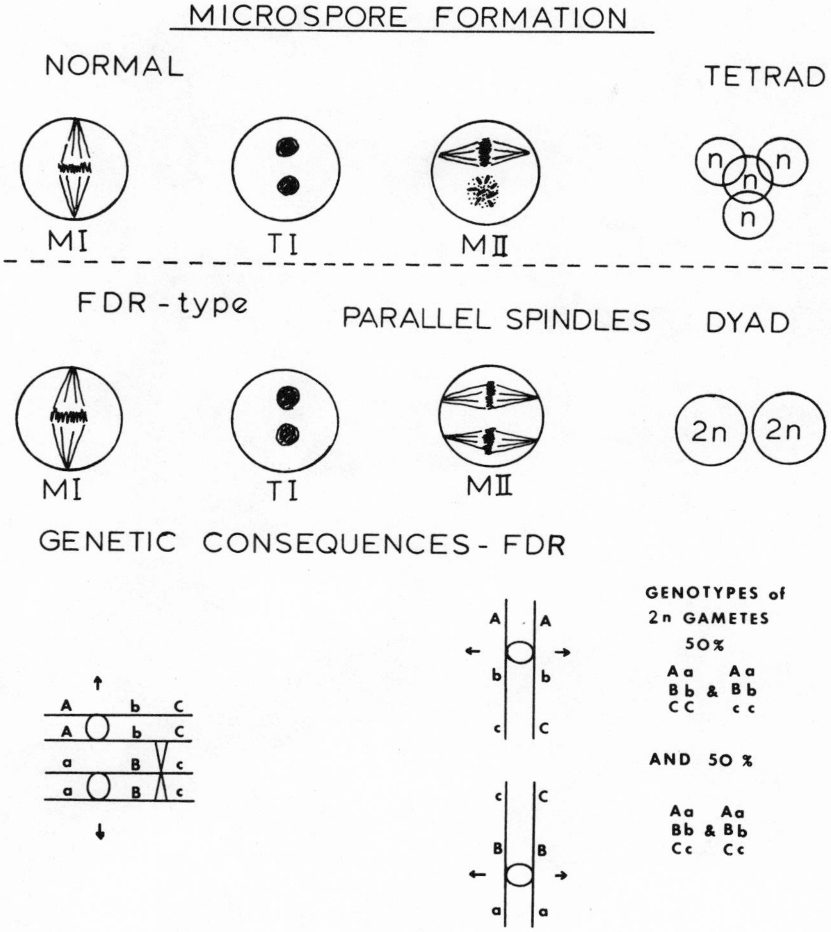

Fig. 3. Diagram of normal mircroscope formation, FDR-type resulting from parallel spindles at metaphase II (MII), and genetic consequences of FDR-type gamete formation.

spaced plants over a two-year cutting period were consistently greater (some cuttings significantly greater at P=0.05%) in the case of hybrids from 4x tester x FDR 2n gametes. Thus FDR 2n gametes, which theoretically could transmit more heterozygosity than normal gametes, produced offspring with greater hybrid vigor.

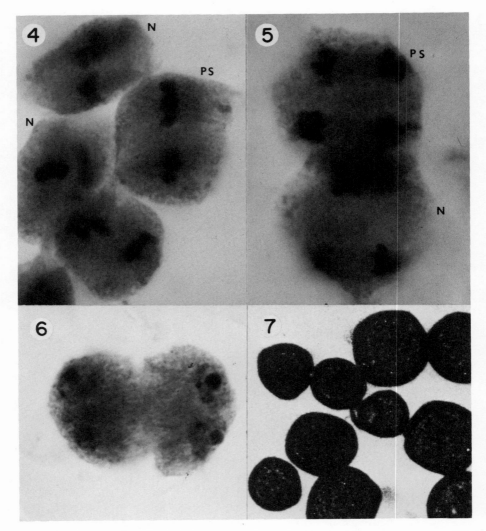

Fig. 4-7 Photomicrographs of normal (N) and parallel spindles
(PS) in alfalfa at metaphase II (Fig. 4) and at telaphase II
(Fig. 5). Formation of a dyad resulting from parallel spindles
(Fig. 6); and mature n and 2n pollen of alfalfa (Fig. 7).

Diploid hybrids (a_ia_j) producing 2n gametes presently can be
used as pollen parents in 4x-2x crosses to produce tetraploid
hybrids which are at least as heterozygous as the double cross
hybrids previously discussed. We are experimenting with this

approach, but ideally the 4x seed parent should be a male-sterile single cross hybrid, and as previously discussed, it has thus far been difficult to obtain economic levels of seed production on male-steriles.

The ultimate use of 2n gametes in maximizing heterozygosity would be the union of FDR-type 2n eggs and FDR-type 2n pollen from hybrid diploid parents. An example of union of two 2n gametes to produce a sexual polyploid is entry HXG 4x (Table 2). It was obtained along with diploid hybrid HG2 in a cross of diploid clones H and G. The 2n pollen was FDR-type, but the status of the 2n egg was not known. Diploid HG2 was doubled to obtain HG2 4x. Thus, it was possible to make a sibling comparison of an autotetraploid from chromosome doubling (di-allelic duplex) with a sexually produced autotetraploid (potentially tetra-allelic at many loci). Heterosis was great in the more heterozygous hybrid HxG 4x; it yielded nearly twice as much herbage as HG2 4x in the clonal study.

A few diploids which produce 2n eggs at a high frequency (good seedset in 2x-4x matings) have been identified and used in matings with diploids which produce 2n pollen. Thus far, these diploid x diploid matings have produced about 25% tetraploid and 75% diploid progeny (triploid embryos are also produced but generally abort due to endosperm failure). This frequency of tetraploid hybrids would not be adequate for commercial purposes in a seed reproduced tetraploid such as alfalfa. However, this frequency would be more than adequate in an asexually reproduced tetraploid such as potato, where the elite hybrid could be selected and propagated asexually.

IMPLICATIONS ON CHROMOSOME DOUBLING

Doubling the chromosome number of a diploid, even a diploid hybrid ($a_i a_j$) results in half of the chromosomes in the autotetraploid being strictly alike by descent ($a_i a_i a_j a_j$). Such autotetraploids are partial inbreds on the basis of theoretical and practical research on maximum heterozygosity and they are not expected to be as vigorous as the progeny of the next two sexual generations. Hence the potential yield of a new autotetraploid cannot be immediately evaluated.

Research reviewed suggests that the most productive autotetraploid will be obtained by doubling a sufficient number of diverse diploid hybrids to insure allelic diversity in the breeding population. Further, it will be necessary to synthesize the autotetraploid cultivar using a SC and DC sequence or synthetic equivalent and market seed of the generation with maximum hybrid vigor. This will generally be the DC or second synthetic generation if di-allelic duplex autotetraploid parents are used.

Alternatively, maximum hybrid vigor can be achieved by somatic fusion and in the first hybrid product of FDR-type 2n gametes from diploid hybrids. These approaches are equally well-suited for maximizing hybrid vigor in auto- or allotetraploids and are currently practical for asexually reproduced crops where a vegetative organ is the commercial product. The 2n gamete approach also holds potential for seed reproduced tetraploid crops where diploid representatives of the cultivated tetraploid are available, and genetic control is established for FDR-type production of 2n eggs and 2n pollen.

SUMMARY AND CONCLUSIONS

1. Heterozygosity is an important component of both allo-polyploids (disomic polyploids) which have internal hybridity, and autopolyploids (polysomic polyploids) which are cross-pollinated.

2. Heterozygosity is more complicated in polysomic polyploids than in diploids or disomic polyploids due to the multiplicity of heterozygous states possible at a locus: di-allelic simplex, duplex and triplex, and tri- and tetra-allelic.

3. In tetraploid alfalfa using di-allelic duplex ($a_i a_i a_j a_j$) parents (P) to make single crosses (SC) and double crosses (DC) the frequency of maximally heterozygous tetra-allelic loci ($a_i a_j a_k a_l$) in each generation was P (0%), SC (44%), and DC (79%). The theoretical order of desirability (DC > SC > P) based on frequency of tetra-allelic loci was the same as the level of heterosis for seed and herbage yield in several studies.

4. Research on heterosis reviewed in autotetraploid maize, rye, potato, and alfalfa was all consistent with the theory of maximum heterozygosity. This provided evidence for both the existence of multiple alleles (indistinguishable from blocks of linked genes) and the importance of tetra-allelism.

5. Whereas maximum heterozygosity (heterosis) is achieved in F_1 hybrids of diploids (or disomic polyploids), it is progressive in polysomics and requires two to three successive hybridizations to maximize using inbred parents and normal sexual processes.

6. Breeding implications are that methods of producing cultivars should attempt to maximize heterozygosity in the generation used for commercial production. This will usually be the double cross or second synthetic generation.

7. Somatic fusion and 2n gametes are unique methods of maximizing heterozygosity. Somatic hybridization of cells from divergent diploid hybrids would maximize heterozygosity and should be practical in asexually reproduced species. The 2n gamete method is very practical and applicable to several species where the cultivated form is tetraploid and diploids are available.

8. Knowledge of the importance of maximum heterozygosity and breeding methods to exploit it, should underpin production of new autopolyploids by somatic doubling or sexual polyploidy.

LITERATURE CITED

1.   Mac Key, J., 1970, Significance of mating systems for chromo-
     somes and gametes in polyploids. Hereditas 66: 165-176.
2.   Roose, M.L., Gottlieb, L.D., 1976, Genetic and biochemical
     consequences of polyploidy in Tragopogon. Evolution 30: 818-
     830.
3.   Dessureaux, L., Gallais, A., 1969, Inbreeding and heterosis
     in autotetraploid alfalfa I. Canad. J. Genet. Cytol. 11:
     706-715.
4.   Gallais, A., Guy, P., Lenoble, M., 1970, Models for varieties
     in cross-fertilised forage plants. pp. 254-259, Proc. 11th
     Inter. Grassl. Congress.
5.   Stanford, E.H., Clement, W.M.,Jr., Bingham, E.T., 1972,
     Cytology and evolution of the Medicago sativa - falcata
     complex, pp. 123-141, in Hanson, C.H. (ed.), "Alfalfa Science
     and Technology," Amer. Soc. Agron. Monograph 15.
6.   Obajimi, A.O., Bingham, E.T., 1973, Inbreeding cultivated
     alfalfa in one tetraploid-haploid-tetraploid cycle: Effects
     on morphology, fertility, and cytology. Crop Sci. 13: 36-39.
7.   Carnahan, H.L., 1960, Some theoretical considerations of
     the consequences of multiple alleles in relation to inbreeding
     and testing procedures in autopolyploids, pp. 19-22, in
     Rept. 17th Nat. Alfalfa Improv. Conference.
8.   Demarly, Y., 1963, Genetique des tetraploids et amelioration
     des plantes. Ann. Amelio. Plant. 13: 307-400.
9.   Busbice, T.H., Wilsie, C.P., 1966, Inbreeding depression and
     heterosis in autotetraploids with application to Medicago
     sativa L. Euphytica 15: 52-67.
10. Panella, A., Lorenzetti, F. 1966, Selfing and selection in
     alfalfa breeding programmes. Euphytica 15: 248-257.
11. Tysdal, H.M., Kiesselbach, T.A., Westover, H.L., 1942,
     Alfalfa breeding. Res. Bull. Nebr. Agric. Exp. Sta. 124.
     46 p.
12. Dewey, D.R., 1966, Inbreeding depression in diploid, tetra-
     ploid and hexaploid crested wheatgrass. Crop Sci. 6: 144-
     147.
13. Rowe, P.R., 1967, Performance of diploid and vegetatively
     doubled clones of Phureja-haploid tuberosum hybrids. Amer.
     Potato J. 44: 195-203.
14. Rowe, P.R., 1967, Performance and variability of diploid
     and tetraploid potato families. Amer. Potato J. 44: 263-271.
15. Randolph, L.F., 1941, An evaluation of induced polyploids
     as a method of breeding crop plants. Amer. Nat. 75: 347-363.
16. Randolph, L.F., 1942, Influence of heterozygosis on fertility
     and vigour in autotetraploid maize. Genetics 27: 163.
17. Bingham, E.T., Burnham, C.R., Gates, C.E., 1968, Double and
     single backcross linkage estimates in autotetraploid maize.
     Genetics 59: 399-410.

18. Lundqvist, A., 1966, Heterosis and inbreeding depression in autotetraploid rye. Hereditas 56: 317-366.

19. Levings, C.S., III, Dudley, J.W., Alexander, D.E., 1967, Inbreeding and crossing autotetraploid maize. Crop Sci. 7: 72-73.

20. Rice, J.S., Dudley, J.W., 1974, Gene effects responsible for inbreeding depression in autotetraploid maize. Crop Sci. 14: 390-393.

21. Dunbier, M.W., 1974, The use of haploid-derived autotetraploids to study maximum heterozygosity in alfalfa. Ph.D. thesis, University of Wisconsin.

22. Bingham, E.T., 1971, Isolation of haploids of tetraploid alfalfa. Crop Sci. 11: 433-435.

23. Dunbier, M.W., Bingham, E.T., 1975, Maximum heterozygosity in alfalfa: Results using haploid-derived autotetraploids. Crop Sci. 15: 527-531.

24. Clement, W.M. Jr., Lehman, W.F., 1962, Fertility and cytological studies of a dihaploid plant of alfalfa, Medicago sativa L. Crop Sci. 2: 451-453.

25. Hougas, R.W., Peloquin, S.J., 1958, The potential of potato haploids in breeding and genetic research. Amer. Potato J. 35: 701-707.

26. Mendoza, H.A., Haynes, F.L., 1974, Genetic basis of yield in the autotetraploid potato. Theor. Appl. Genet. 45: 21-25.

27. Dudley, J.W., 1964, A genetic evaluation of methods of utilizing heterozygosis and dominance in autotetraploids. Crop Sci. 4: 410-413.

28. Bolton, J.L. 1948. A study of combining ability of alfalfa in relation to certain methods of selection. Sci. Agric. 28: 97-126.

29. Harlan, J.R., deWet, J.M.J., 1975, On Ö Winge and a prayer: the origins of polyploidy. Bot. Rev. 41: 361-390.

30. Mok, D.W.S., Peloquin, S.J., 1975, The inheritance of three mechanisms of diplandroid (2n pollen) formation in diploid potatoes. Heredity 35: 295-302.

31. McCoy, T.J., Bingham, E.T., 1979, Inheritance of 2n gametes in cultivated alfalfa at the diploid level. (In preparation)

32. Mendiburu, A.O., Peloquin, S.J., Mok, D.W.S., 1974, Potato breeding with haploids and 2n gametes, pp. 249-258, in Kasha, K.J. (ed.), Proc. 1st Inter. Symp., "Haploids in Higher Plants," University of Guelph, Guelph, Ontario.

33. Mendiburu, A.O., Peloquin, S.J., 1977, The significance of 2n gametes in potato breeding. Theor. Appl. Genet. 49: 53-61.

34. Mok, D.W.S., Peloquin, S.J., 1975, Three mechanisms of 2n pollen formation in diploid potatoes. Canad. J. Genet. Cytol. 17: 217-255.

35. Bingham, E.T., McCoy, T.J., 1979, Cultivated alfalfa at the diploid level: origin, reproductive stability, and yield of seed and forage. Crop Sci. 19: 97-100.

36. Simon, P.W., Peloquin, S.J., 1976, Pollen vigor as a function
     of mode of 2n gamete formation in potatoes. Heredity 67:
     204-208.
37. Vorsa, N., Bingham, E.T., 1979, Cytology of 2n pollen forma-
     tion in diploid alfalfa. (Submitted Canad. J. Genet. Cytol.)

POLYPLOIDY AND AGRICULTURE: SUMMARY

Keith A. Walker

Monsanto Agricultural Products Co.
St. Louis, MO   63166

As an outsider to this field with modest understanding of
polyploidy and its implications to agriculture, there is little
that I can add to the discussion. The contributions which compose
this session on the relevance of polyploidy to agriculture have
provided a wealth of information on a broad array of subjects
ranging from the relation between polyploidy and plant domestication to the very elegant uses of a unique series of aneuploids in
wheat. There have been several striking conclusions and observations made by the various contributors some of which deserve
special notice.
     First among these is the emerging implication that the
formation of 2n gametes (unreduced gametes) may be substantially
responsible for the appearance of polyploid plant species or
races. This has been discussed elsewhere in this volume, but its
special relevance to domesticated species such as alfalfa,
potato, and tulip was underscored by Doctors Zeven and Bingham.
Apart from the mechanism of polyploidization, Dr. Zeven reviewed
the means where by polyploids would be maintained or lost from a
population of mixed cytotypes. With the exception of a few
examples of the cultivation as land races of a mixture of cytotypes such as with the Zanduri and Maka wheats and cytotype
mixtures of potato in South America, Dr. Zeven pointed out that
in most instances the autopolyploids can not maintain themselves
in cultivated mixtures with the counterpart diploids. A few
exceptions to this rule exist, such as sugar beet and sweet
potato, but these polyploid cytotypes have been maintained or
developed by the direct intervention of man. He pointed out the
need for additional research to establish whether or not the
sequence of polyploidization followed by domestication would be

different or better than the sequence of domestication followed
by polyploidization.

In a second major point of emphasis, Dr. Dewey reviewed the
contributions of polyploid breeding to the improvement or development of new crop species. He stated that, "The performance of
induced polyploids as agricultural crops has consistantly fallen
short of expectations." While identifying a number of difficulties
limiting the performance of induced polyploids, Dr. Dewey underscored as a major problem the failure to obtain adequate genetic
diversity in the breeding populations because of the constraints
of time and expense. The resultant effect has been reduced vigor
and fertility in the polyploid deviatives of the breeding populations. Dr. Müntzing has cogently documented in his review of
triticale that developing a truly successful polyploid crop may
be a long-term process. While much of the future of triticale as
a major crop may still lay ahead, the collective experiences of
those who have labored to improve its quality substantiates the
concerns raised by Dr. Dewey regarding the impact of plant vigor
and fertility on the usefulness of any particular polyploid. Dr.
Müntzing identified the important role that the triple hybrids
representing the combination of hexaploid and tetraploid wheat
and diploid rye played in obtaining hexaploid triticales with
desirable properties.

Perhaps the most persuasive argument that heterogygosity is
an important component to the successful development of both
allopolyploids and autopolyploids was offered by Dr. Bingham.
Based upon data which he had obtained in alfalfa, Dr. Bingham
concluded that the existence of multiple allelic series, supported
by strong circumstantial evidence, and maximizing the tri- and
tetra-allelic condition most favorably influence plant performance.
I found Dr. Bingham's discussion of possible methods to maximize
heterozygosity, with particular reference to alfalfa, very exciting.
The production of maximally heterozygous tetraploids by the
fertilization of gametes with the unreduced chromosome number
obtained from heterozygous diploids was a method of particular
interest. To capitalize on this method Dr. Bingham stressed the
need to have available exploitable systems for 2n gamete formation
in the target species and well characterized divergent individuals
at the lower ploidy level.

Has the idea on the use of unreduced gametes in polyploid
breeding brought us full circle? The emergence of polyploid
production in natural populations via the mechanism of unreduced
gametes as well as their potential for use in the synthesis of
maximally productive polyploids are exciting observations.
However, the question remains as to whether or not the observations
suggest a possible route to the development of successful agronomic
polyploid crops on a wider scale.

PART V

POLYPLOIDY: FUTURE PROSPECTS

POLYPLOIDY IN PLANTS:

UNSOLVED PROBLEMS AND PROSPECTS

G. Ledyard Stebbins

Department of Genetics
University of California
Davis, CA 95616

The papers that have been presented at the present synposium provide in themselves ample evidence that problems connected with polyploidy are of prime importance for understanding the evolution not only of most plants, but also of many groups of animals. Although chromosome doubling as a tool for plant breeders has become much reduced in importance during recent years, its revival may become practical as more becomes known and understood about the reasons why this process has been of great importance for the origin of species in nature (1).

First and foremost, neither evolutionists nor plant breeders will understand their problems completely if they pay too much attention to the process of chromosome doubling itself. This quantitative change in chromosome number and nuclear DNA content is only one of a series of complex processes that must take place for polyploidy to be successful in nature. Hybridization that produces genetic and/or chromosomal heterozygosity, mutation at the polyploid level, inactivation or elimination of duplicate gene loci, and gene-controlled regularization of chromosome pairing: all of these changes are as important for successful polyploid evolution as is doubling or trebling the chromosome number. The cytogeneticist, taxonomist, and plant breeder must always distinguish between polyploidy as an individual process and polyploid evolution as a complex series of processes. The present review deals with polyploid evolution in its entirety. In it, I pose and attempt to answer six questions of major importance.

1. TO WHAT EXTENT IS POLYPLOIDY REVERSIBLE?

Several years ago, Raven and Thompson (2) suggested that the common belief of cytogeneticists in the irreversibility of polyploid evolution might be erroneous. They pointed out that in many instances eggs of tetraploids, containing the reduced or diploid chromosome number, may develop parthenogenetically, giving rise to polyhaploid plants that have the diploid chromosome number. They failed to point out, however, that the majority of such polyhaploids, if they are produced from well-established tetraploids, are weak, sterile, or both. Later, deWet (3) showed that a polyhaploid derived from autotetraploid Dichanthium annulatum was fully viable and fertile if its tetraploid parent belonged to populations from India, but weak and sterile if derived from tetraploid populations of the same species native to the Mediterranean region. In a later publication (4), he referred to viable, fertile polyhaploids derived from two octoploid species, Bromus inermis and Parthenium argentatum. He then suggested that polyhaploids can be successful if they differ little genetically from the original diploid races that gave rise to autotetraploids. Their evolutionary importance, in his opinion, is that they make possible renewed evolutionary activity at the diploid level, long after the parental diploids have become extinct.

deWet's hypothesis shows how important is the distinction between polyploidy as a process and polyploid evolution. The distributional pattern of the genus Dichanthium as a whole indicates that D. annulatum tetraploids arose in India. Evolution even within this single species, that gave rise to its tetraploid Mediterranean ecotypes, was an irreversible series of processes that rendered impossible successful reversion to diploidy: the situation is exactly parallel to the distinction between individual mutations, that are reversible, and continuing evolution, that becomes increasingly improbable as the succession of carefully integrated processes becomes more and more complex (5).

At the level of genera, therefore, polyploid phylogeny can still be regarded as usually unidirectional, from lower to higher levels. Isolated diploid populations are likely to be derived from neighboring tetraploids by polyhaploidy only if the latter can be shown by genetic analysis to be unaltered autotetraploid strains. The diploids are much more likely to be relictual disjuncts that have evolved from other diploid species.

2. WHAT FACTOR OR FACTORS ARE RESPONSIBLE FOR THE SUCCESS OF POLYPLOIDS IN NATURE?

The recent experiences of plant scientists with natural and artificial polyploids has brought to the forefront a striking paradox. Although polyploids have been highly successful in nature, and include the majority of perennial weeds that thrive in association with man-made disturbance, newly synthesized

artificial polyploids have almost all failed to become valuable
crop or forage plants. Why have humans been unable to duplicate
the successful polyploid evolution that has been so ubiquitous in
nature?

Two of the plant breeders speaking at this symposium, Dewey
(1) and Bingham (6) have suggested an answer. Autotetraploids
are consistently less successful than their diploid progenitors
if such progenitors are a single viable and successful diploid
individual or population. Even moderate success of tetraploids
can be achieved only if their populations have a broad base of
genetic diversity and heterozygosity. This diversity is best
acquired by hybridization between different but related tetraploids,
followed by genetic recombination at the tetraploid level and
natural selection of the best adapted recombinants.

The failure of autotetraploid populations having a narrow,
restricted base of variability to succeed under natural conditions
is well illustrated by my own efforts to produce artificial
autotetraploids of various species of grasses and to establish
them under semi-natural conditions. During the early 1940's, I
produced autotetraploids of several species in the genera Elymus,
Stipa, Phalaris and Ehrharta, and planted them on grassy hillsides
back of the campus of the University of California, Berkeley.
The only species that succeeded at all was Ehrharta erecta,
native to South Africa. It is a broad leaved shade loving perennial, that produces great quantities of seeds. Since it is
normally self-fertilizing, it probably has a lower amount of
heterozygosity than have most outcrossed species of grasses,
although no quantitative analyses have been made. An autotetraploid produced by the colchicine method of somatic doubling
proved to be highly fertile, and was planted in a number of sites
on the Berkeley campus and in the hills behind it, as well as in
Carmel, near Monterey. In many of these sites the diploid controls
that were planted beside the tetraploids have succeeded very
well, and have spread for some distance beyond the original sites
of planting (7). On the other hand, the artificial tetraploid
failed completely in nearly every locality. In only one planting,
made on a steep, hillside in deep shade of live oaks (Quercus
agrifolia) did it out perform its diploid progenitor for a few
years. Even in this locality, however, the diploid controls have
during the past fifteen years become far more numerous than the
autotetraploids. While tetraploids have maintained themselves in
one of the original habitats, and in sites a few meters away from
the original seeding, where they are in deep shade and on steep,
well drained slopes, the diploids have spread more than a hundred
meters from the original site, and have occupied a variety of
habitats, including those characterized by deep shade and good
drainage. Polyploidy has enabled Ehrharta erecta to occupy a
habitat in which the diploid was less successful. Nevertheless,
once the tetraploids were established, they showed none of the

aggressiveness that is characteristic of naturally evolving tetraploid populations of grasses.

How could an adaptively inferior, ecologically restricted population like that of autotetraploid Ehrharta erecta become converted into an aggressive broadly adaptive autotetraploid like those of Dichanthium annulatum, Dactylis glomerata and many other species of grasses? Spontaneous chromosomal rearrangements cannot have been the basic cause, since artificial hybridizations between different tetraploid races of these species, that occupy different geographic regions, have revealed few or no chromosomal differences between them from their bottleneck of adaptive inferiority, particularly since the presence of three unmutated genes allelic to every one that has undergone a mutation would greatly reduce its effects.

We are left with hybridization as the only method by means of which a raw autotetraploid might escape from its bottleneck of adaptive inferiority. The hypothesis that hybridization is the major auxiliary process that contributes to the success of polyploids is in complete agreement with the experience of plant breeders, as mentioned above. It also agrees with the conclusions of an ecological physiologist, Moshe Tal, who in this symposium has stated (8) that the success of autotetraploids may be due to "balanced hybridity". At the level of gene loci, this balancing or buffering effect is due chiefly to the complex nature of tetrasomic inheritance, that automatically increases greatly the number of different kinds of alleles that can be present at any one locus. At the level of the expression of phenotypic characteristics, the effects of this buffering are twofold. In the first place, it partly stabilizes intermediate conditions with respect to quantitative characteristics that are determined by genes at many different loci: multiple factor or "polygenic" inheritance (9). Second, it can to some extent buffer any condition of heterozygote superiority or hybrid vigor that might result from crossing two genotypes having good combining ability.

To a taxonomists, who is accustomed to thinking of hybridization as crossing between two taxonomically recognized species, the concept of a hybrid autotetraploid has apparently been difficult to grasp. The opinion that I have often expressed in previous publications, that most if not all successful polyploids are of a hybrid nature, has been interpreted to mean that I regard allopolyploids as much more common than autopolyploids. The confusion is easily resolved on the basis of two considerations. First, a hybrid autopolyploid is a genotype that is derived from doubling the chromosome number of a hybrid between two parents that are alike in chromosome structure and segmental arrangement, but differ with respect to allelic genes that confer upon them different adaptive properties. If one should double the chromosome number of a hybrid corn, one would still have a hybrid genotype, but it would be unquestionably an autotetraploid. Second, the dichotomy

between autotetraploids and allotetraploids has been over-emphasized
and misinterpreted by many taxonomists. As originally defined
(10), autotetraploids are tetraploids derived from two chromosomally similar and genetically compatible genomes, while allopolyploids are derived from two genomes that are chromosomally
differentiated and genetically incompatible.

Many taxonomists, presumably to attain greater simplicity,
have perverted these definitions so that they regard as autopolyploids all polyploids that fall within the morphological
range of the aggregates that they regard as species, and as
allopolyploids those that fall morphologically between the species
that they recognize. This nomenclature is often combined with
rejection of the biological species concept, and adoption of the
older philosophy that a species is any entity that a competant
taxonomist, familiar with the group, chooses to call a species,
or is, in his or her opinion "a potentially satisfying mental
organization," as has been suggested by Cronquist (11). If this
kind of philosophy and reasoning were to be transferred to the
classification of polyploids, and the recent redefinition of
auto- and allopolyploidy on a taxonomic basis were to be retained,
an autopolyploid or allopolyploid could be recognized on the
basis of subjective judgments made largely because of morphological
similarities and differences. This is redefining a basically
cytogenetic concept to the point that it becomes an ultimate
absurdity.

The best solution to this dilemma would be to abandon completely the terms auto- and allopolyploid, particularly in taxonomic
treatments that are not well supported by cytogenetic data. One
could substitute the more neutral terms "intraspecific" and
"interspecific polyploids" or tetraploid, hexaploid, etc. cytotypes
(see Lewis, p.103). The term chromosomal races is inappropriate,
since it implies that the polyploid is an autopolyploid in the
original, cytogenetic meaning of the term.

If one follows the classifications generally accepted by
taxonomists, the terms auto- and allopolyploid are by no means
synonymous with intra- and interspecific polyploid. Two kinds of
exceptions can be recognized: polyploids derived from hybrids
between sibling species, and those that are derived from hybrids
between taxonomically recognized species that are nevertheless
genetically compatible with each other. An example of the former
would be a tetraploid derived from a hybrid between two of the
sibling species that are taxonomically recognized as Elymus
glaucus (12). An autotetraploid derived from an interspecific
hybrid could be produced by doubling the chromosome number of a
hybrid between Mimulus cardinalis and M. lewisii, two species
that are morphologically and ecologically separated by a large
gap, but are nevertheless similar in chromosomal organization and
form fully fertile hybrids (13).

The rejection of autopolyploid and allopolyploid as a valid
dichotomy for taxonomic classification is supported further by

the fact that conditions intermediate between the two genotypes
as originally recognized are now known to be so common that they
form the modal condition for natural polyploids. This fact has
often been pointed out in the more recent literature, and has
been recognized by deWet in the present symposium (14).

The terms auto- and allopolyploid are, nevertheless, very
useful if employed only according to their original cytogenetic
meaning. This is because the way in which polyploidy stabilizes
or buffers the hybrid condition differs greatly depending upon
whether the original hybrid contains two sets of completely
homologous and structurally similar chromosomes, or whether it
contains parental sets that are completely non-homologous, i.e.,
strongly differentiated structurally; or homoeologous, i.e.,
partly differentiated with respect to segmental rearrangements.
As has already been discussed, buffering of a cytogenetic autopolyploid is based entirely upon altered segregation of alleles
at individual gene loci. In a typical allopolyploid, derived
from parents having non-homologous chromosomes, the hybrid condition
is stabilized by the lack of pairing between chromosomes belonging
to the different parental species. In the intermediate condition,
known as segmental allopolyploidy, both genic buffering and
chromosomal stabilization via autosyndetic pairing can contribute
to perpetuation of the hybrid condition. If the parental chromosomes are relatively strongly differentiated from each other,
preferential pairing of homologues derived from the same parent
will occur frequently or regularly, and will bring about the same
kind of chromosomal stabilization that is characteristic of
typical allopolyploids. If the homeologous chromosomes belonging
to the different parents resemble each other more closely, the
raw segmental allopolyploid is likely to break down in later
generations and give rise to weak and sterile offspring, as was
reported by Wagner and Wagner (15) for certain hybrid polyploids
of ferns, and was found by Stebbins and Vaarama (16) in a polyploid
derived from Elymus glaucus X Sitanion jubatum. Segmental allopolyploids can be rescued from this kind of degeneration by the
incorporation of genes or gene complexes that reinforce preferential pairing, acting like the 5B chromosomal complex in wheat
(17). This kind of gene complex is probably widespread, although
it cannot be recognized unless a species has been intensively
analysed from the cytogenetic point of view, as has Triticum
aestivum.

How does the hypothesis that polyploidy becomes adaptive
chiefly in association with hybridization agree with recent
observations on polyploid complexes, particularly those involving
autopolyploidy? I have already presented many years ago several
examples of polyploid complexes based partly or entirely upon
autopolyploidy that are, nevertheless, derived from several
morphologically and ecologically distinct ancestral diploid
populations (9,18). More recently discussed examples are the
complexes of Betula papyrifera (19-22), Arabis hirsuta (23),

Ranunculus eschscholtzii (24), Montia perfoliata (25), and the genus Spergularia (26). Particular attention must be given to two examples, Galax aphylla and Epilobium angustifolium-latifolium.

The autotetraploid of Galax aphylla, a species belonging to a monotypic genus that is confined to the Applachian region of the eastern United States, was first reported by Baldwin (27) as more common than its parental diploid. On the basis of his information, I regarded it (18) as a typical autopolyploid of non-hybrid origin, derived from a single diploid ecotype. The species has now been studied in detail by Nesan (28), who has obtained scores of chromosome counts, representing the entire geographic range of the species. These show that tetraploid populations are actually far less numerous and widespread than are diploids, and are, in fact almost completely surrounded by them. These populations need to be more carefully studied, particularly with respect to differences in genes coding for isozymes, and with respect to ranges of ecological tolerance. It is entirely possible that autotetraploid Galax aphylla has arisen several times, and that the present array of tetraploid populations is the result of hybridizations between tetraploids and diploids having different ranges of ecological tolerance.

The second example that deserves attention consists of two related species, Epilobium (Chamaenerion) angustifolium and E. latifolium. Mosquin and Small (29,30) have maintained that each of these two species contains a diploid and tetraploid "race;" that the two autotetraploids have arisen independently of each other, and that hybridization between the two species, while it has admittedly occurred, has had no significant effect upon their evolution.

Two statements that they make indicate that this example needs to be more carefully analyzed, particularly with respect to ecology and cytogenetics. First, they state that everywhere, E. latifolium grows only in soils that are continuously moist, and imply that E. latifolium is more mesic than is E. angustifolium. In California, where E. latifolium occurs locally, but forms large populations, neither of these statements is correct. The populations of E. latifolium are found on loose talus or scree, that in the long periods of summer drought characteristic of the Sierra Nevada become completely dried out for several centimeters below ground level. The habitat is considerably more xeric than is that of E. angustifolium, which in the Sierra Nevada grows chiefly in coniferous forests and the margins of wet meadows. So far as I am aware, chromosome numbers of the Sierra Nevada populations of E. latifolium have not yet been obtained, but according to the map presented by Mosquin and Small, diploid populations are to be expected in this region. On the other hand, most of the ecological observations on E. latifolium appear to have been made by Mosquin and Small in regions where the populations are tetraploid.

A second comment made by these authors is that although
hybrids are known between diploid E. angustifolium and diploid E.
latifolium, the hybrids are not significant because they are
sterile. The authors do not state directly whether these hybrids
are themselves diploid or tetraploid, but the implication is that
they are diploid. If so, their sterility means nothing, since a
tetraploid derived from them would most probably be fertile, as
are most tetraploids derived from sterile diploid hybrids.
Bøcher (31) has reported the frequent occurrence of sterile
triploid hybrids in Greenland between diploid E. angustifolium
and tetraploid E. latifolium. Since these plants are long-lived
perennials, even a high degree of sterility might still permit
the formation of a few seeds after back crossing between the
triploid hybrid and tetraploid E. latifolium. Hence the occasional
introgression of genes from one to another of these two species
is not altogether ruled out. This example needs to be studied
much more carefully before it can be held up as an example of
autopolyploidy uninfluenced by hybridization.

3.   HOW DOES POLYPLOIDY AFFECT DISTRIBUTION PATTERNS?

The early research on polyploidy in relation to the distribution of species led to a number of hypotheses relating the
phenomenon to changes in ecological tolerance, particularly the
belief that polyploids are more tolerant of cold and drought than
their diploid relatives. More recent research has failed to
confirm these hypotheses (9). In the present symposium, Ehrendorfer
(32) has explained why this is so. The calculations that led to
the hypotheses failed to distinguish between polyploid series
within a genus and species belonging to genera that in their
entirety are of ancient polyploid origin. They also, for the
most part, failed to recognize that the incidence of polyploidy
is higher in perennial herbs than in annuals, so that floras
containing different proportions of these growth forms cannot be
compared.

Ehrendorfer showed in addition that the most meaningful
comparisons are between diploids and polyploids that are related
to each other, and that they must take into account the plant
associations to which the different cytotypes belong. He showed
that when these factors are properly evaluated, diploids can be
shown to be more common in the stable habitats of permanent or
climax communities, while polyploids are often found in labile or
successional biota. This newer, more critical and ecologically
oriented approach to the study of the distribution of polyploids
needs much more attention from botanists in various parts of the
world. It is the kind of synthetic approach that is essential
for solving basic problems connected with polyploidy or with any
other phase of evolution.

4. WHAT HAS BEEN THE FREQUENCY AND EVOLUTIONARY IMPORTANCE OF
    PALEOPOLYPLOIDY, THE ANCIENT STABILIZATION OF CHROMOSOME
    NUMBERS AT POLYPLOID LEVELS FROM WHICH SECONDARY POLYPLOID
    SERIES HAVE ARISEN?

The questions just discussed deal with the role of polyploidy
in the origins of modern floras, of species, and of population
systems within species. Other speakers in this symposium have
reviewed aspects of the problem of polyploidy in connection with
the origin of higher categories, such as genera and families.
Wagner and Wagner (15) have provided strong evidence to indicate
that nearly all genera of homosporous pteridophytes have basic
numbers that are tetraploid, hexaploid, or at higher levels
relative to the original numbers x=9, 10, and 11, although they
show that recent attempts to identify specific genomes purporting
to be x=6 are not in agreement with careful analyses of the same
groups. By contrast, Crosby (33) has shown that in bryophytes
not only are intrageneric polyploid series relatively uncommon
and confined to a few groups of mosses, but also the basic chromosome numbers of most or all genera belonging to this phylum or
series of phyla are such that paleopolyploidy can be assumed to
be absent. The same is true of fungi, as discussed by Maniotis
(34). High chromosome numbers reported for some algae, as reviewed
by Nichols (35), suggest that when they become better known
cytologically, paleopolyploidy may be found among them. In his
review of polyploidy in fishes, Schultz (36) has produced new
evidence to support previous claims that the entire family Salmonidae, containing the salmon, trout, and whitefish, as well as the
sucker family, Catastomidae, are both of polyploid origin.

I should like to amplify the discussion of paleopolyploidy
in angiosperms presented by Goldblatt (37). He supported previous
suggestions that several major families of monocotyledons have
basic numbers of x=14 or higher, suggesting paleopolyploid origin.
He also mentioned examples among dicotyledons, including both
relatively "primitive" or archaic families such as Magnoliaceae
(x=19) and more specialized, presumably recent, families such as
Bignoniaceae (x=20).

Since no modern woody genera are known that could possibly be
interpreted as ancestors of the above mentioned families, and
since woody families having basic numbers of x=7,8, or 9 (Annonaceae, Dilleniaceae, Dipterocarpaceae) are end products of special
evolutionary lines, one can only assume that the direct ancestors
of so-called "primitive" angiosperm families such as Magnoliaceae,
Winteraceae, and Illiciaceae are extinct. As I have already
stated (38), these families must be regarded as archaic rather
than primitive or ancestral.

One consequence of this situation is that among many higher
categories of vascular plants--classes, orders, and families--
genera that are the least specialized morphologically have the
highest basic chromosome numbers. Evolution by polyploidy appears

to have gone in a direction contrary to evolutionary specialization
of morphological characteristics. Several examples of this
inverse correlation can be mentioned. One of them is the Lycopsida,
discussed by Wagner and Wagner (15). The homosporous genus
Lycopodium (sensu lato) has consistently higher chromosome numbers
than the heterosporous genera Selaginella and Isoetes. Within
Lycopodium, the highest numbers (n=132,136) are found in species
placed by some authors in the genus Huperzia (L. selago, L.
lucidulum) and characterized by minimal specialization of their
reproductive structures. Species of the "genus" Diphariastum (L.
complanatum), that has far more highly specialized leaves and
reproductive structures, have the relatively low basic number
x=23. Among heterosporous Lycopsida, Selaginella species have
consistently n=9 or n=10, while a common basic number in Isoetes
is x=11.

    A similar correlation exists among true ferns. The fern
genus with the highest basic number, x=126, is Ophioglossum,
having the less specialized eusporangiate morphology. The lowest
number, x=11, is found in Hymenophyllum, a specialized offshoot
of the leptosporangiate group.

    Among angiosperms, the same situation prevails. The Annon-
aceae, having x=7,8, and 9, are with respect to woody anatomy,
perianth, and pollen grain structure definitely more specialized
than Magnoliaceae (x=19) or Degeneriaceae (x=12). In another
order, the Malvales, the relatively unspecialized woody Bombacaceae
have x=28 and x=44, while among the specialized herbaceous Malvaceae
basic numbers of x=5 (Sphaeralcea) and x=7 (Lavatera) are not
uncommon. In several different families, including the archaic
Winteraceae as well as the recent, highly specialized Asteraceae
and Poaceae, relatively unspecialized genera have chromosome
numbers that can be interpreted as multiples of those found in a
larger number of genera that are more specialized morphologically.
Some of these are listed in Table 1. For five of these seven
examples, information concerning relative degrees of specialization
has been obtained from publications of monographers, the references
for which are listed in the table. The two others, Winteraceae
and Liliaceae, require special mention. Among the Winteraceae,
only two basic numbers exist, x=43 and x=13. The genera having
the least specialized floral structure (Drimys sensu stricto,
Pseudowintera), have x=43. The number x=13 exists only in Tasmannia
(Drimys sect. Tasmannia), which has highly reduced unisexual
flowers that contain only a single carpel. Among the Liliaceae
the least specialized flowers are found in genera like Tofieldia
(x=15), that have flowers with perianth parts all alike, lack
specialized nectar glands, and with carpels that are nearly free
from each other and form an unspecialized septally dehiscent
capsule. Genera having x=7,8, or 9 include some that are relatively
unspecialized, such as Uvularia, but are still more specialized
than Tofieldia, as well as highly specialized genera like Allium
and the Brodiaea complex that are placed by many authors in a

Table 1. Families of angiosperms in which morphologically unspecialized genera are paleo-polyploids, while more specialized unrelated genera have lower chromosome numbers.[a]

Family	Genera or tribes and basic (x) chromosome numbers	
	Less specialized	More specialized
Asteraceae (40)	Heliantheae: 16,17,18,19	Cichorieae: 4,5,6,7,8,9
Brassicaceae (41)	Stanleya: 12 ; Thelypodium: 14	Arabis,etc.: 8,7; Arabidopsis: 5
Hydrophyllaceae (42)	Wigandia: 19	Nemophila: 9
Liliaceae	Tofieldia: 15	Trillium: 5; Scilla: 5,6,7
Poaceae (43)	Bambuseae, Arundinae: 12	Schismus: 6; Zingeria: 4,2
Polemoniaceae (44)	Cantua: 27; Cobaea: 26	Gilia: 9; Phlox: 7
Winteraceae	Drimys: 43	Tasmannia: 13

[a]Chromosomal data from (39); morphological data from references listed after the family name, or explained in the text.

different family. The lowest chromosome number found in the
Liliacean or Lilialean complex is x=5 that occurs in relatively
specialized genera such as <u>Trillium</u> and <u>Scilla</u>.

These correlations can be interpreted in two different ways.
One is to assume that the higher chromosome numbers were original
for the group, and that the lower numbers were derived by stepwise
aneuploid reduction in basic number. In most of the families
listed in Table 1, this interpretation is rendered highly improbable
by the absence of intermediate numbers. The alternate interpretation, that of paleopolyploidy, is more probable for two reasons.
First, the higher numbers are often multiples or combinations of
numbers frequently found in other genera of the family. For
instance, x=17,18, and 19 in the Heliantheae could easily have
been derived from the common numbers of Asteraceae, x=8,9, and
10. The number x=15 in <u>Tofieldia</u> could be derived from x=7
and/or x=8, both of which are common in the Liliaceae. The
numbers x=12 and x=24 (from x=6) in Poaceae, as well as x=26 and
x=27 (from x=8 and 9) in Polemoniaceae, are likewise easily
interpreted in this fashion. Second, as mentioned earlier in this
review, the buffering effect of polyploidy, that reduces the
effect on populations of individual mutations, would naturally
reduce greatly the rate of evolution due to gene changes, and so
would tend to preserve morphologically archaic genotypes.

The inverse correlation between polyploidy and morphological
specialization that is evident at the level of families, orders,
and classes contrasts strikingly with the situation that exists
within many genera, particularly those that belong to relatively
recent, actively evolving families. Table 2 lists 11 representative
examples, in which polyploidy is absent from the least specialized
and present in some of the more specialized species groups of the
genus. For five of them, the greater morphological specialization
that exists among the polyploid series is documented by references
cited in the table. For the remainder, the arguments are as
follows. Among the perennial species of <u>Helianthus</u>, the highest
and best known polyploid is the hexaploid <u>H</u>. <u>tuberosus</u>, characterized by specialized vegetative reproduction by means of tubers.
In <u>Hieracium</u>, the greatest morphological specialization exists in
the subgenus <u>Pilosella</u>, in which the floral scapes are elongate
and nearly or quite leafless, and which reproduce vegetatively by
means of specialized stolons. Most of these species are both
polyploid and apomictic (18). The great majority of species
belonging to <u>Hypochoeris</u> are diploids having gametic numbers n=4
and n=5. Polyploid (2n=16) exists, however, in <u>H</u>. <u>stenocephala</u> a
specialized cushion plant of the high Andes. In <u>Lactuca</u>, the
most widespread polyploids are specialized New World species such
as <u>L</u>. <u>canadensis</u> (n=17), that are clearly related to less specialized Old World species having n=8 and n=9. In <u>Mimulus</u>, the best
known polyploids are in the section <u>Simiolus</u> (47) which contains
both perennials and annuals, and with respect to both growth
habit and floral structure appears to be more specialized than

Table 2.   Genera belonging to advanced herbaceous families in which polyploids are among the most specialized morphologically of their genera.

Antennaria (Asteraceae, Inuleae, 38)
Crepis (Asteraceae, Cichorieae, 4)
Helianthus (Asteraceae, Heliantheae)
Hieracium (Asteraceae, Cichorieae)
Hypochaeris (Asteraceae, Cichorieae)
Lactuca (Asteraceae, Cichorieae)
Mimulus (Scrophulariaceae)
Paeonia (Paeoniaceae, 4)
Penstemon (Scrophulariaceae)
Phacelia (Hydrophyllaceae)
Solanum (Solanaceae)

---

strictly diploid sections such as the M. cardinalis complex and section Diplacus.   In Penstemon, nearly all species are diploid, but tetraploids, hexaploids, and octoploids are found in the section Saccantherae, characterized by the specialized structure of its anthers.   In Phacelia, the series Magellanicae, which forms a typical polyploid complex (48), possesses a gynoecium containing a reduced number of ovules, more specialized than that found in other perennial species, such as P. bolanderi and P. ramosissima. The great majority of the species of the large genus Solanum are diploids, but tetraploids and hexaploids are found in the specialized tuber-bearing group, as well as in the section Morella, that includes annuals having highly reduced flowers and inflorescences, as well as weedy tendencies.

Why should the correlation between polyploidy and morphological specialization among genera of a family often be the reverse of that found among species of a genus?   The only logical explanation must of necessity be based at least in part upon the fact that families are older, sometimes much older, than many of their modern genera.   During the course of evolution of a family, polyploids that, when first formed, are among the most morphologically specialized representatives of their family, later become no more specialized than the majority of diploid genera and species in the family, and finally become its least specialized members.

Two factors could account for this change; differential rates of evolution and extinction.   If a species acquires a high degree of specialization, and subsequently evolves very slowly, its relative degree of specialization, compared to other species in the family or genus, can change from most specialized to intermediate because newly evolved species have become even more specialized. It has been bypassed by more progressive lines of evolution. Then, if its more primitive ancestors become extinct, its position among the surviving species can change from intermediate to most primitive.

Such a change in phylogenetic position can be expected for polyploids. After they have been formed, they will evolve more slowly than their diploid relatives, for reasons that have already been discussed. Given hundreds of thousands of generations and exposure to a variety of new environmental challenges, one would expect that some of the diploid genera of a family would evolve new and more highly specialized morphological types, that would at least in part replace the less specialized diploids that, in the early stages of evolution of the family, gave rise to unspecialized polyploids.

Somewhat harder to explain is the postulate that relatively unspecialized diploids would have been more likely to become extinct than their morphologically comparable polyploid derivatives. Two factors could account for this differential extinction: the wide range of ecological tolerance possessed by the most successful polyploid species, and establishment in more stable plant communities. The fact that many polyploids have far wider ranges of geographic distribution than their diploid ancestors, and also occupy a wider range of ecological habitats is well known and has often been discussed (9,18). Given this difference, one would expect that as climates change and new species evolve during geological epochs and eras, the polyploids would have a greater chance of preserving at least some of their ecotypes than would the related diploids.

More important, however, is the fact that probably because of their greater vigor and competitive ability, the most successful polyploids can evolve ecotypes capable of invading and persisting in stable, climax associations from which their diploid ancestors were excluded because of their lower competitiveness. As I have already pointed out, and has been reaffirmed by Ehrendorfer (32) on the basis of far more complete evidence, polyploids usually become established in pioneer communities, or at least in early stages of succession. Establishment in such associations depends more upon reproductive success than upon vegetative vigor. The species composing them are subject to r-type selection (49). On the other hand, paleopolyploid woody genera such as Magnolia, Platanus, Alnus, Populus, Juglans, Carya, and Fraxinus, as well as herbaceous Compositae such as perennial species of Helianthus, Rudbeckia, and Adenocaulon, are entirely or at least partly established in stable climax communities, that have changed little for millions of years (50). The preservation of paleopolyploids, therefore, is apparently the result of a shift from dependence upon r-type selection to emphasis upon K-type selection for vegetative vigor. The intermediate step in this shift would naturally be a polyploid species having a wide range of ecotypes, some of which emphasize reproduction and the ability to colonize easily new pioneer habitats, while other ecotypes of the same species possess the vegetative vigor that enables them to compete successfully with or to coexist as subdominants with the dominant species of climax communities. The latter are usually, if not always, K-type strategists.

Polyploids having the necessary wide range of ecotypes, and therefore capable of making the transition, can be recognized in a number of temperate floras. Good examples are tetraploids of the Betula papyrifera complex, tetraploid species of Salix such as S. lasiandra, the stump sprouting Californian species of Arctostaphylos belonging to the complex of A. glandulosa-A. tomentosa, and among herbaceous species the complexes of Ranunculus californicus-occidentalis, Fragaria virginica-chiloensis, Achillea millefolium, Aster cordifolius-macrophyllus, Festuca ovina-rubra, Dactylis glomerata, Panicum virgatum, and Andropogon scoparius. The following succession of stages, therefore, can be postulated as capable of converting newly established r-selected polyploids that still exist sympatrically or parapatrically with their diploid ancestors, into paleopolyploid genera, adapted to climax habitats and a K-type adaptive strategy, and without existing diploid ancestors.

(1) Origin of polyploidy in association with hybridization either between species or between differently adapted races of the same diploid species.

(2) Establishment of the polyploid in a pioneer habitat.

(3) Expansion of the geographic range, and ecological tolerance of the polyploid species, via mutation, genetic and chromosomal recombination, hybridization, and introgression involving additional diploid species.

(4) Evolution of polyploid ecotypes having a K-type reproductive strategy, and adapted to subclimax or climax associations.

(5) Evolution at the diploid level of new species having greater morphological specializations.

(6) Extinction of the original diploid ancestors, as well as the polyploids that resemble them, because of climatic changes plus unfavorable competition with newly evolved diploids and still more recent polyploid derivatives, leaving the K-adapted derivatives of the original polyploids without close relatives.

(7) Speciation at the K-adapted polyploid level, giving rise to paleopolyploid genera that are descended from one or a few K-adapted polyploid ecotypes.

If paleopolyploid genera have evolved in this fashion, then careful analyses of several different polyploid complexes with this succession in mind should enable plant evolutionists to identify various stages of the succession. In my opinion, analytical and synthetic studies of this kind can be among the most fruitful approaches to bridging the gap between evolution at the level of races and species and the origin of higher categories.

The next question that comes to mind is: to what extent is this succession supported by paleobotanical evidence, and during

what geological periods did it occur?   Direct paleobotanical
evidence can never be obtained, since chromosome numbers of
extinct species cannot be determined.   Indirect evidence might,
however, be obtained from comparing sizes of cells of which the
walls have been preserved.   In this fashion, Miki and Hikita (51)
showed that the Metasequoia and Sequoia that flourished in Japan
during the Pliocene Epoch probably had, respectively, the somatic
numbers 2n=22 and 2n=66, as do their modern counterparts.   If the
present hypothesis is correct, then pollen having characteristics
of a modern paleopolyploid family such as Magnoliaceae, Platanaceae,
Salicaceae, or Oleaceae-Oleoideae should appear in the record
first as grains smaller than the modern ones, then as a mixture
of small and large grains.   Finally, the more recent strata,
the pollen grains should all have ranges in size comparable to
those of modern species.   Collaboration between paleobotanists
and cytogeneticists on problems such as this one should lead to
highly informative results.

The transition from r-type neopolyploid races to K-type
paleopolyploid genera has probably taken place, successively in
different groups, during much of the time during which angiosperms
have been dominant elements of the flora, from the middle of the
Cretaceous to the latter half of the Tertiary Period.   Leaves
resembling those of the modern paleopolyploid genera Trochodendron,
Tetracentron, and Cercidiphyllum, but much smaller in size, are
known from Siberian fossil deposits of early to mid-Cretaceous
age (55).   Perhaps these were borne by diploid ancestors of the
modern paleopolyploid relicts. Somewhat younger are leaf fossils
assigned to the Platanaceae (52,53) and possibly belonging to
diploid ancestors of the modern paleopolyploid genus Platanus
(x=21).   Most of the modern families of woody angiosperms have
become recognizable by the end of the Cretaceous Period (53), so
that the middle and latter part of this period would be the most
fruitful geologic age for detecting transitions of the type
postulated.

On the other hand, many of the paleopolyploid herbaceous
genera must be much younger.   Opinions differ as to the age of
the family Asteraceae (Compositae), but an early Tertiary (Eocene
or Oligocene) origin is the most likely (54).   If this is so,
then the most probable time for the origin of paleopolyploid
genera of this family, such as Helianthus, Rudbeckia, Wyethia,
and Adenocaulon is mid-Tertiary.   Other genera of Asteraceae,
such as Anaphalis, Antennaria, and Leontodon in the tribe Inuleae
have basic numbers x=14 and x=13, derived by polyploidy from the
basic number x=7 found in the neighboring genera Gnaphalium and
Helichrysum.   These genera must have acquired their secondary
polyploid status comparatively recently during the Miocene or
Pliocene epochs.   If they are to be classified as paleopolyploids,
then the succession of events postulated above can be regarded as
an ongoing process, and intensive research on modern genera,

tribes, and families might be expected to reveal various stages of the succession.

5. WHAT ARE THE EVOLUTIONARY CONNECTIONS BETWEEN POLYPLOIDY AND PARTHENOGENESIS OR APOMIXIS?

The high correlation between polyploidy and asexual production of zygotes and embryos, i.e., parthenogenesis or apomixis, has long been known (9,18). In the present symposium, the topic has not been reviewed with respect to plants, but all three of the participating zoologists have reported a similar correlation in insects (55) (Coleoptera: Curculionidae; Lepidoptera, genus Solenobia), fishes (36), and reptiles (56) (Lacertilia: Gekkonidae, Agamidae, Teidae). Moreover, all of them have commented on the high degree of genetic heterozygosity found in the polyploid apomicts, a condition that was recognized long ago in apomictic plants (Hieracium, 57). The question that comes immediately to mind is: are polyploidy and heterozygosity direct causes of apomictic reproduction, or are they merely conditions that favor the occurrence, establishment, and later success of apomicts?

The information presented in this symposium and elsewhere strongly favors the latter hypothesis. In plants, highly hetero-zygous and sterile hybrids have been discovered between diploid sexual species of Antennaria that are closely related to polyploid apomicts (58). In no case have these hybrids produced seed by apomixis. Moreover, the correlation diploidy-sexuality: polyploidy-apomix is far from perfect. Diploid apomicts have long been known in the Potentilla argentea complex (59), and in genera such as Citrus, Opuntia, Garcinia, and others (18). The genera Poa, Rubus, Antennaria, and others contain some polyploids that are obligate apomicts, some that are strictly sexual, and still others that are facultative apomicts, producing some viable seeds via the sexual process and others by apomixis. Recent research on Antennaria parlinii (60) has shown that all three of these conditions can exist among different individuals of the same interbreeding population system.

Among animals, Lokki and Saura (55) reported in this symposium that parthenogenesis is occasionally found in the diploid, sexual ancestors of triploid and tetraploid weevils (Curculionidae), and the genus Solenobia. In lizards, Bogart (56) has reported that sexual polyploids are frequent in the same genera that contain the triploid parthenogenesis or apomixis in either plants or animals. What, then, is the basis for the observed, widespread correlations between these three phenomena?

With respect to parthenogenesis and polyploidy, an interesting difference exists between plants and animals that may provide a clue to answering this question. As was stated above, in several plant genera sexual polyploids exist side by side with related apomicts having the same chromosome number. Since sexual polyploids

are far more common in plants than are apomicts, there is good
reason for believing that among angiosperms sexual polyploidy
precedes apomixis. This hypothesis is strengthened by the fact
that in Antennaria parlinii (60), and possibly other species of
that genus, sexual polyploids occupy older habitats than their
apomictic relatives. The latter are particularly common in the
glaciated regions of eastern North America, and in man-made
habitats such as roadsides and degraded pastures.

In animals, however, the reverse may be true. Numerous
examples of apomixis (called by him thelytoky) are reviewed by
White (61). The majority of those animals include diploid as
well as polyploid cytotypes, and in some insects, such as cave
crickets and the genus Warramaba (Orthoptera), Lonchoptera (Diptera),
scale insects (Coccidae, Hemiptera), and some genera belonging to
other classes, polyploidy is absent.

This difference between animals and flowering plants might
be explained by the difference in reproductive cycle between the
two kinds of organisms. In animals, meiosis takes place in the
mature oöcyte, and is followed immediately by fertilization. In
them, therefore, successful parthenogenesis requires only two
kinds of changes, both of them affecting a single kind of cell,
the oöcyte. Meiosis must be eliminated or circumvented, and the
oöcyte must be made capable of development without the stimulus
of the sperm. In angiosperms, however, the intercalation of a
gametophytic stage between meiosis and fertilization, plus the
formation and nutritive function of a triploid endosperm renders
the shift far more complex. Meiosis must be eliminated at an
early stage in development of the ovule, or the haploid embryo
sac must be replaced by a diploid gametophyte derived from a
somatic cell by means of apospory. The egg cell, which must be
altered physiologically so that it can develop without the stimulus
of the male nucleus, functions at a completely different developmental stage, and therefore under a completely different internal
environment than that of the megaspore mother cell in which
meiosis may become inhibited.

Moreover, the successful development of endosperm and embryo
in angiosperms depends upon a particular proportional relationship
between chromosome numbers of embryo sac, embryo, and endosperm,
that becomes altered in apomicts that form functional embryo
sacs. In a normal diploid this relationship is: embryo sac, n;
embryo, 2n; endosperm, 3n. In apomicts such as Antennaria, the
polar nuclei of the diploid embryo sac fuse as they do in haploid
embryo sacs of diploid species, so that the chromosome number of
the endosperm is twice that of the zygote and embryo. The relationship between embryo sac, embryo, and endosperm that in the
sexual cycle is n:2n:3n becomes in the apomictic cycle 2n:2n:4n.

There is ample evidence from the results of artificial
hybridization between sexual diploids and their autoploid derivatives to show that alterations of these chromosome number
relationships, unless compensated for in some way by changes in gene

dosage, will cause breakdown of embryo development (62). In
diploid X tetraploid crosses, the numerical relationship is
1:3:4. The result is rapid development of both endosperm and
embryo, but early breakdown of endosperm results in the failure
of the embryo to complete development unless it is extracted and
raised in artificial culture media. In tetraploid X diploid
crosses the numerical relationship is 2n:3n:5n, and development
is much retarded. The embryo may sometimes complete development,
but viable seed is rarely produced.

     Obviously, therefore, a harmoniously successful apomictic
cycle that includes embryo sac formation can be evolved only via
three different kinds of changes in regulatory mechanisms controlling gene action. These changes must differ from each other both
in the kind of regulation involved, and in the developmental
stage at which the regulation takes place. In sexually reproducing
angiosperms, therefore, polyploidy may aid in the origin and
establishment of apomixis by doubling or trebling the number of
gene loci at which favorable mutations might take place, while
hybridization not only increases the number of different kinds of
alleles that are present and might interact favorably with each
other, but it also reduces the number of alleles present as
duplicates that would minimize the effects of many mutations.

     Further evidence favoring this hypothesis comes from the
presence in genera such as Citrus and Garcinia of a different
kind of apomictic cycle that bypasses the megaspores, embryo sac,
and egg cell. This is the condition of adventitious embryony in
which the embryo develops directly from a somatic cell of the
nucellus or ovular integument (18). Particularly in interspecific
hybrids, in which abnormal meiosis usually renders gametophytic
haploid tissue weak or inviable, this kind of apomictic cycle can
evolve via a much simpler change in regulatory mechanisms, that
affect only the somatic cell or cells that are induced to form
embryos. One might expect to find in such plants both the diploid
chromosome number and polyembryony, and this is actually found in
the genera mentioned.

     In angiosperms, therefore, polyploidy aids in the success of
apomixis by increasing the size of the gene pool, while hybridization increases its diversity, and therefore renders more probable
the establishment of gene combinations coding for the necessary
shifts in the reproductive cycle. The evidence from animals,
however, suggests additional ways in which these processes aid in
the success of apomicts. The increased cell size found in polyploids may make them larger and more vigorous, provided that
their inherent tendency toward a slower tempo of the mitotic
cycle is counteracted by alterations of gene action. In both
animals and plants, some products of interspecific hybridization
may be vigorous and highly adaptive in particular environments,
but sexually sterile, as Schultz pointed out (36). As shown
originally by Darlington (63) and reaffirmed by White (61),
apomixis is in these examples an escape from sterility. This may

well be its most common and only adaptive advantages in animals.
In plants, however, the situation is more complex. This is
evident from the fact that in <u>Antennaria</u> and probably other
genera apomixis has evolved within species that are both polyploid
and sexually fertile. In such species, apomixis may be advantageous
chiefly because it aids in spreading the species by long distance
dispersal. If the sexual genotypes are dioecious or
self-incompatible, double colonization of new areas is necessary,
a condition that reduces greatly the possibility for successful
long distance dispersal. Apomixis can overcome this obstacle.

6.   WHAT ROLE, IF ANY, DID INTRAPSECIFIC OR INTRAGENERIC POLY-
      PLOID SEQUENCES PLAY IN THE ORIGIN OF DIPLOID LIFE CYCLES?

        In all probability, the earliest eukaryotes had life cycles
that were basically haploid, like those of many modern flagellates,
such as <u>Chlamydomonas</u>. Meiosis occurred as the first cellular
divisions after zygote formation, and somatic mitoses involving
an entire diploid set of chromosomes did not take place (64).
Protists having this kind of life cycle gave rise later to others
having a diploid life cycle, with meiosis being delayed until
just before fertilization, and to various kinds of algae and
archegoniates having isomorphic alternation of generations.
        If this phylogeny of life cycles is correct, the question
arises: What would have been the adaptive advantages that would
have enabled natural selection to favor the changes postulated?
Since animals have exclusively diploid life cycles, and in vascular
plants as well as complex algae such as the larger brown algae
the shift toward greater importance of the diploid generation has
been predominant, we can conclude that the diploid state is a
necessary precondition for the evolution of large, complex organisms. This is probably because diploid populations can enrich
their gene pools by harboring in the heterozygous conditions
large numbers of recessive mutations, thereby greatly facilitating
the formation of complex new gene combinations. This reasoning,
however, does not help us to understand how the diploid condition
could have arisen in the first place. The mutations that would
be most effective in bringing about the shift from haploidy to
diploidy would be those that would inhibit attractions between
homologous chromosomes, and so permit each chromosome to pass
through the mitotic cycle independently of the other chromosomes
on the spindle. These mutations may well have been similar to
those responsible for inhibiting association of partly homologous
chromosomes in wheat (17). There is no difficulty, therefore,
with the postulate that mutations of this kind could have arisen
in primitive eukaryotes. The difficult question is: What would
have been the adaptive value of these mutations that would have

favored their spread through populations of relatively simple
unicellular organisms?

A reasonable answer to this question can be deduced from the
effects of polyploidy in modern plants. If union of gametes
belonging to two genetically different haploid organisms should
produce a zygote that contained a heterozygous gene combination
promoting hybrid vigor, and contained also genes inhibiting
homologous association of chromosomes, that zygote would produce
rapidly a population of vigorous, highly competitive offspring.
Consequently, conditions favoring the origin of diploid life
cycles would be similar to those that favor the evolution of
polyploid series in modern organisms. As has been stated earlier
in this review, the ability to colonize pioneer habitats is one
of these conditions.

Two facts about the cytology of protists and green algae
favor this hypothesis. First, many protists have very high
chromosome numbers, some evidence suggests that genomes may be
present in duplicate. The enormously high chromosome number,
ca.1600, has been reported for the Radiolarian, Aulacantha
scolymantha, (65), and even the familiar Amoeba proteus has been
reported as having 500-600 chromosomes (66). The origin of such
high numbers by stepwise, aneuploid increase in chromosome number
is almost impossible to imagine. At least some doubling of
entire genomes must have been involved. Moreover, Nichols has
called our attention to the fact that in Euglena an anomalous
kind of nuclear fragmentation, not involving mitosis or meiosis,
can lead to viable cells having a chromosome number considerably
lower than the usual one, 86 (35). This would not be expected
unless normal cells of Euglena contain a high proportion of
duplicated gene loci. Sudden increases in chromosome number,
resembling polyploidy, may have been of general occurrence in
primitive unicellular eukaryotes. The more frequent was their
occurrence, the greater would have been the probability that,
occasionally, they would have incorporated genes inhibiting the
association of homologous chromosomes, and bringing about the
regular persistence of the diploid condition.

A second significant fact is that although polyploid series
are uncommon in algae, they are nevertheless present. Nichols
mentioned the genus Cladophora, and other examples are reviewed
by Godward (67). More careful study of these examples, particularly
from the ecological point of view, would be highly desirable.
Are young polyploid series in algae associated with the invasion
of ephemeral, pioneer habitats? Turning to the fungi, the remarks
of Maniotis made in this symposium (34) are highly relevant. The
water mold Allomyces and its relatives are unique among the fungi
in two ways. They alone possess both polyploid series as well as
isomorphic alternation of generations. Is this coexistence
purely a matter of chance, or does it result from the probability
that, as postulated in this section, environmental conditions

that favor polyploid series also favor the origin of life cycles
that include a diploid generation?

The discussion in this section has raised more questions
than it has provided answers. Its principal purpose has been to
suggest that unicellular eukaryotes and relatively simple algae
need to be studied much more carefully by biologists who are well
acquainted with modern cytogenetic techniques and phenomena, and
who can also study these forms in their natural ecological environments. In my opinion, evolutionary studies of a synthetic nature
on these organisms will prove to be the most fruitful approach to
understanding the most critical stages in the evolution of eukaryotic organisms.

CONCLUSIONS AND SUMMARY

The six questions that form the framework of this review can
be answered, at least tentatively, as follows. Polyploid evolution
includes much more than the mere doubling of chromosome numbers.
It must be studied in a synthetic fashion, using many different
avenues of approach. While the doubling itself is readily reversible, continuing evolution at polyploid levels quickly reduces
the probability that such reversals to diploidy will be successful.
Most polyploid series observed in nature represent unidirectional
evolution from lower to higher levels. The ecology of polyploid
series cannot be studied on the basis of statistical summaries of
entire floras, but must be built up from careful analyses of
particular series, supplemented by intimate knowledge of the
associations in which the plants live. When the problem is
approached in this fashion, correlations between polyploid and
occupation of pioneer, disturbed habitats become evident. Polyploidy often increases the size of organs, and less often the
size of entire plants. Its most significant effect, however, is
the buffering or balancing effect upon heterozygosity for both
gene combinations and entire chromosomes or chromosome segments.
This effect is evident in both auto- and allopolyploids. As
taxonomic categories, auto- and allopolyploids are often misinterpreted, and are so difficult to define that their use is as often
a hindrance as a help to understanding polyploid phylogeny.
Furthermore, most natural polyploids are now known to have characteristics that place them in positions intermediate between the
two categories.

Secondary polyploidy or paleopolyploidy is a common phenomenon
in vascular plants. It probably has come about via a complex
succession of events, of which the most important was the spread
of a series of interbreeding polyploid populations that included
some having an r-type of adaptive strategy, others having a
strategy of the K-type, and still others having intermediate
strategies. In this way the shift from the r-type strategy that

is characteristic of newly formed polyploids to the K-type strategy that characterizes paleopolyploid genera could have come about.

In a few groups of both plants and animals, polyploidy and hybridization are associated with reversion to asexuality, that is variously designated as parthenogenesis, apomixis, or thelytoky. In plants, both hybridization and polyploidy may precede the establishment of apomixis, while in most animal groups hybridization and parthenogenesis or thelytoky usually precede the formation of polyploids. This difference is probably due to the fact that establishment of apomictic life cycles requires many more complex genetic changes in plants than in animals, and is therefore aided by the richer gene pools that may be present in polyploids. In both animals and plants, the most valuable advantage of apomixis is preservation of highly adaptive and heterozygous gene combinations.

Finally, careful research on polyploid phenomena in unicellular eukaryotes and algae may provide greater insight into the factors responsible for the origin of chromosomal life cycles that are basic properties of both higher plants and animals.

LITERATURE CITED

1. Dewey, D.R., 1980, Some applications and misapplications of induced polyploidy to plant breeding. This volume, p. 445.
2. Raven, P.H., Thompson, H.J., 1964, Haploidy and angiosperm evolution. Amer. Nat. 68: 251-252.
3. deWet, J.M.J., 1968, Diploid-tetraploid-haploid cycles and the origin of variability in Dichanthium agamospecies. Evolution 22: 394-397.
4. deWet, J.M.J., 1971, Reversible tetraploidy as an evolutionary mechanism. Evolution 25: 545-548.
5. Simpson, G.G., 1953, "The Major Features of Evolution," Columbia University Press, New York.
6. Bingham, E.T., 1980, Maximizing heterozygosity in autotetra-ploids. This volume, p. 471.
7. Stebbins, G.L., 1949, The evolutionary significance of natural and artificial polyploids in the family Gramineae. Proc. 8th Inter. Congr. Genet, Hereditas, Suppl. Vol.: 461-485.
8. Tal, M., 1980, Physiology of Polyploids. This volume, p. 61.
9. Stebbins, G.L., 1971, "Chromosomal Evolution in Higher Plants," Edward Arnold, London.
10. Kihara, H., Ono, T., 1926, Chromosomenzahlen und systematische Gruppierung der Rumex-Arten. Zeitschr. Zellforsch. 4: 475-481.
11. Cronquist, A., 1978, Once again: what is a species?, pp. 3-20, in "Biosystematics in Agriculture," Beltsville Symp. Agr. Reg. 2, Allenheld, Osmuth & Co., Montclair, NJ.

12. Snyder, L.A., 1951, Cytology of inter-strain hybrids and the
     probable origin of variability in Elymus glaucus. Amer. J.
     Bot. 38: 195-202.
13. Hiesey, W.M., Nobs, M.A., Bjorkman, O., 1971, Experimental
     studies on the nature of species V. Biosystematics, Genetics,
     and physiological ecology of the Erythranthe section of the
     genus Mimulus. Carnegie Inst. Wash. Publ. 628, Washington,
     D.C.
14. deWet, J.M.J., 1980, Origins of Polyploids. This volume, p. 3.
15. Wagner, W.H., Jr., Wagner, F.S., 1980, Polyploid pteridophytes.
     This volume, p. 199.
16. Stebbins, G.L., Vaarama, A., 1954, Artificial and natural
     hybrids in the Gramineae, Tribe Hordeae. VII. Hybrids and
     allopolyploids between Elymus glaucus and Sitanion jubatum.
     Genetics 39: 379-395.
17. Riley, R., Chapman, V., 1958, Genetic control of the cyto-
     logically diploid behavior of hexaploid wheat. Nature 182:
     713-715.
18. Stebbins, G.L., 1950, "Variation and Evolution in Plants,"
     Columbia University Press, New York.
19. Brittain, W.H., Grant, W.F., 1965, Observations on Canadian
     birch (Betula) collections at the Morgan Arboretum. I. B.
     papyrifera in eastern Canada. Canad. Field-Nat. 79: 189-
     197.
20. Brittain, W.H., Grant, W.F., 1965, Observations on Canadian
     birch (Betula) collections at the Morgan Arboretum. II. B.
     papyrifera var. cordifolia. Canad. Field-Nat. 79: 253-257.
21. Brittain, W.H., Grant, W.F., 1967, Observations on Canadian
     birch (Betula) collections at the Morgan Arboretum. V. B.
     papyrifera and B. cordifolia from eastern Canada. Canad.
     Field-Nat. 81: 251-262.
22. Brittain, W.H., Grant, W.F., 1969, Observations on Canadian
     birch (Betula) collections at the Morgan Arboretum. VIII.
     Betula from Grant Manan Island, New Brunswick. Canad.
     Field-Nat. 83: 361-383.
23. Titz, W., 1972, Evolution of the Arabis hirsuta group in
     Central Europe. Taxon 21: 121-128.
24. Fisher, F., Rowley, J.A., Marchant, C., 1973, The biogeography
     of the western snow-patch Ranunculi of North America. C.R.
     Soc. Biogeogr. 438: 32-43.
25. Miller, J.M., 1979, Phenotypic variation in diploid and
     tetraploid populations of Claytonia perfoliata s.l.
     (Portulacaceae). Syst. Bot. (in press).
26. Ratter, J.R., 1976, Cytogenetic studies in Spergularia IX.
     Summary and Conclusions. Notes Roy. Bot. Gard. (Edinburgh)
     34: 411-428.
27. Baldwin, J.T., Jr., 1941, Galax: the genus and its chromosomes.
     J. Heredity 32: 249-254.
28. Nesan, G., unpublished data.

29. Small. E., 1968, The systematics of autotetraploidy in Epilobium latifolium (Onagraceae). Brittonia 20: 169–181.

30. Mosquin, T., Small. E., 1971, An example of parallel evolution in Epilobium (Onagraceae). Evolution 25: 678–682.

31. Bøcher, T.W., 1962, A cytological and morphological study of the species hybrid Chamaenerion angustifolium x C. latifolium. Bot. Tidsskr. 58: 1–34.

32. Ehrendorfer, F., 1980, Polyploidy and distribution. This volume, p. 45.

33. Crosby, M.R., 1980, Polyploidy in bryophytes. This volume, p. 193.

34. Maniotis, J., 1980, Polyploidy in fungi. This volume, p. 163.

35. Nichols, H.W., 1980, Polyploidy in algae. This volume, p. 151.

36. Schultz, R.J., 1980, Role of polyploidy in the evolution of fishes. This volume, p. 313.

37. Goldblatt, P., 1980, Polyploidy in angiosperms: monocotyledons. This volume, p. 219.

38. Stebbins, G.L., 1974, "Flowering Plants: Evolution above the Species Level," Harvard University Press, Cambridge, MA.

39. Fedorov, A.N. (ed.), 1969, "Chromosome Numbers of Flowering Plants," Acad. Sci. USSR Komarov Bot. Inst., Leningrad.

40. Cronquist, A., 1955, Phylogeny and taxomony of the Compositae. Amer. Midl. Nat. 53: 478–511.

41. Al-Shebaz, I.A., 1973, The biosystematics of the genus Thelypodium. Contr. Gray Herb. Harvard Univ. 204: 3–148.

42. Constance, L., 1963, Chromosome number and classification in Hydrophyllaceae. Brittonia 15: 273–285.

43. Stebbins, G.L., 1980, Major trends of evolution in the Gramineae and their possible significance (in press).

44. Grant V., 1969, "Natural History of the Phlox Family," M. Nijhoff, The Hague.

45. Babcock, E.B., 1947, "The Genus Crepis," Univ. Calif. Publ. Bot., Vols. 21,22.

46. Stebbins, G.L., 1939, Notes on the systematic relationships of the Old World species and of some horticultural forms of the genus Paeonia. Univ. Calif. Publ. Bot. 19: 245–266.

47. Vickery, R.K., Jr., Eldridge, F.A., II, McArthur, E.D., 1976, Cytogenetic patterns of evolutionary divergence in the Mimulus glabratus complex. Amer. Midl. Nat. 95: 377–389.

48. Heckard, L.R., 1960, Taxonomic studies in the Phacelia magellanica--polyploid complex with special reference to the California members. Univ. Calif. Publ. Bot. 32: 1–126.

49. MacArthur, R.H., Wilson, E.O., 1967, "The Theory of Island Geography," Princeton Univ. Press, Princeton, NJ, p. 149; Pianka, E., 1978, "Evolutionary Ecology," 2nd ed., p. 122.

50. Axelrod, D.I., 1976, History of the coniferous forests, California and Nevada. Univ. Calif. Publ. Bot. 70: 1–62.

51. Miki, S., Hikita, S., 1951, Probable chromosome number of fossil Sequoia and Metasequoia found in Japan. Science 113: 3–4.

52. Takhtajan, A. (ed.), 1974, "Fossil Flowering Plants of the USSR," Vol. 1. "Nauk" Publ., Leningrad.

53. Hickey, L.J., Doyle, J.A., 1977, Early Cretaceous fossil evidence for angiosperm evolution. Bot. Rev. 43: 3-104.

54. Raven, P., Axelrod, D.I., 1977, Origin and relationships of the California flora. Univ. Calif. Publ. Bot. 72: 1-134.

55. Lokki, J., Saura, A., 1980, Polyploidy in insect evolution. This volume, p. 277.

56. Bogart, J.P., 1980, Evolutionary implications of polyploidy in amphibians and reptiles. This volume, p. 341.

57. Ostenfeld, C.H., 1910, Further studies on the apogamy and hybridization of the Hieracia. Zeitschr. Ind. Abst. Verebungsl. 3: 241-285.

58. Stebbins, G.L., 1932, Cytology of Antennaria. I. Normal species. Bot. Gaz. 94: 134-151.

59. Müntzing, A., Müntzing, G., 1941, Some new results concerning apomixis, sexuality and polymorphism in Potentilla. Bot. Not. (Lund): 237-278.

60. Stebbins, G.L., Bayer, R., unpublished data.

61. White, M.J.D., 1978, "Modes of Speciation," W.H. Freeman, San Francisco.

62. Stebbins, G.L., 1958, The inviability, sterility and weakness of interspecific hybrids. Adv. Genetics 9: 147-215.

63. Darlington, C.D., 1939, "The Evolution of Genetic Systems," Cambridge Univ. Press, Cambridge.

64. Stebbins, G.L., 1960, The comparative evolution of genetic systems, pp. 197-226, in Tax, S. (ed.), "Evolution after Darwin," 1, University of Chicago Press, Chicago.

65. Grell, K.G., 1953, Die Chromosomen von Aulacantha scolymantha. Haeckel. Arch. Protistenk. 99: 1-54.

66. MacKinnon, D.L., Hawes, R.S.D., 1961, "An Introduction to the Study of Protozoa," Clarendon Press, Oxford.

67. Godward, M.B.E. (ed.), 1966, "The Chromosomes of the Algae," St. Martin's Press, New York.

POLYPLOIDY, PLANTS, AND ELECTROPHORESIS

Bruce Carr and George Johnson

Department of Biology
Washington University
St. Louis, MO 63130

In the last fifteen years the ability to characterize levels of genetic variation in animals using electrophoresis has produced a revolution of knowledge and interest. Similar studies in plants have lagged behind. A review of animal studies (1) lists 129 species (ten systems criterion), while a parallel review of plant studies (2) lists only 61 species, few of them investigated in comparable detail. The reasons for this disparity are partly technical and partly concern the different approach that plant biologists have utilized in their electrophoretic research. This paper attempts to document some of the present technical limitations and conceptual opportunities offered to plant biologists by electrophoresis.

The technical problems associated with electrophoresis can be divided into three categories: extraction, resolution, and assaying.

PRINCIPLE ISSUES

1. Getting It Out Alive. Perhaps the primary problem in applying electrophoresis to plant biology is the difficulty often experienced in obtaining active extracts from plant tissue. Either no activity is obtained, or "smeared" patterns are obtained, lacking resolution. Overcoming these difficulties has to date proven to be an individual enterprise, with different plant species requiring quite different approaches. No uniform set of experimental criteria are applied to diagnosing optimal extraction conditions for different plants species, despite the obvious utility of such an approach in addressing new electrophoretically "naive" species.

        The extraction problem has been approached in two ways. The
most popular method is to survey existing extraction techniques,
and to hope. In assessing the potential difficulties presented
by a new species, Robert Crawford of the University of St. Andrews
has suggested that a reasonable test of whether extraction will
be easy is whether or not you can eat it. A second and by far
superior alternative is to address the conditions which interfere
with the extraction of enzymes. In this regard, phenolase activity
in plant extracts has received a great deal of attention. Kelly
and Adams (3) have published an extraction method which utilizes
eight compounds specifically aimed at circumventing the problems
created by the phenolase enzyme complex (Table 1). Three methods
of dealing with phenolase inactivation of enzymatic activity in
crude extracts are recognized: (1) remove the phenolic substrates;
(2) inhibit the phenolase activity; and (3) remove the quinone
products, which usually derive from phenols, either by reconversion
to phenols or by condensing to an inactive form (4). In this
case a direct and considered chemical approach to the problem of
extraction was successful in producing active extracts from

Table 1. Plant enzyme extraction buffer.

Component	Function
0.1 M Tris-maleate buffer, pH 7	pH stabilization
0.2 M Na tetraborate	binds o-diphenols, substrate competitor
0.25 Na ascorbate	reduces quinones, phenols
0.02M Na meta-bisulfite	phenolase condensation to a non-reactive phenolase OH-sulfite compound
0.02M Na diethyldithiocarbomate	competes with phenolase for copper ions; thiol condenses quinones
0.01M germanium dioxide	binds o-diphenols, and so acts as a substrate competitor
10% DMSO	freeze stabilization
PVP (soluble)	binds phenolics
BuOH	removes phenolics from extracts
Et_2O	removes phenolics from extracts

Juniperus needles. Within the last year in our lab, extraction techniques have been developed for Distichlis and Gaura which permitted analysis on high resolution acrylamide gels (5; Carr, in preparation). Thus we can hope that our understanding of extraction-related problems of plant enzymes may be nearing a point where such a directed biochemical analysis of extraction difficulties provides a viable alternative to blind luck.

2. Sorting It All Out. Resolution problems are at least equal to those presented by extraction. Indeed resolution varies among the electrophoretic techniques available. Starch gels separate proteins on the basis of major net change differences. Polyacrylamide can be polymerized into gels of a range of pore sizes and thereby permit detection of variation in protein size and shape, as well as charge. However, the increased resolution of this approach is achieved only at a significant increase in experimental effort (especially extraction). Which technique is more appropriate will depend upon the nature of the investigation.

Much of the present difficulty in electrophoretic resolution is a direct result of using experimental protocols derived principally from Drosophila studies, protocols which were never designed to optimize resolution. Indeed, a good case could be made that these studies arrived through trial and error at a set of conditions which MINIMIZE resolution:

(a). Gel pore size. To maximize band sharpness, polyacrylamide gels of approximately 5-7% have been employed. We now know that electrophoretic mobility is determined by an interaction of both protein shape and change, and that at intermediate pore sizes of 5-7% these contributions often cancel (6). The result is that under these conditions many quite different proteins migrate similarly in electrophoresis, and cannot be resolved.

(b) Buffer pH. Most electrophoresis is carried out at alkaline pH, usually pH 8.5 or 9.0. At these pH levels, the two acidic residues (ASP, GLU) and two basic residues (LSY, ARG) are fully ionized. However, the pK of HIS is 7.7 and at pH values above 8.0 HIS is largely unionized. Thus at pH values commonly used, amino acid substitutions involving HIS produce no net change in charge. The result is that electrophoresis at pH 9.0 often fails to reveal variants which are detected by parallel analysis at pH 7 (7,8).

(c). Temperature. Most electrophoresis is performed in refrigerated cold boxes at 5°C, or under ice to produce similar temperatures. Protein shape is particularly sensitive to temperature, however, and because shape influences electrophoretic behavior, the temperature of the analysis may importantly affect resolution. Many proteins migrating identically at 5° migrate quite differently at higher temperature values (9).

(d). Buffer ion. Particularly in starch gel electrophoresis, different buffer recipes are commonly employed
for different enzymes to obtain optimal resolution. From
the variable resolution, it is obvious that the various
counterion differentially affect resolution. Rarely is the
effect dealt with explicitly, however, although counterion
radius appears as a discrete term in the diffusion constant
which lies at the heart of electrophoretic rate equations
(10).
The bottom line is that better isolation may be available
simply by more thorough investigation of what is presently known
about protein structure and how it interacts with experimental
conditions. To optimize resolution, plant workers would do well
to avoid the conditions of minimal resolution commonly employed
in insect work (T = 7%, pH 8.5, temp. = 5°C), and instead test
empirically a range of conditions. One may either design a pair-
wise arbitrary comparison protocol (T = 5% vs. 9%; pH 7.0 vs. 9.0
temp. = 0° vs 5°). (See for example the approach advocated by
Singh et al. (7), or carry out more detailed analysis to determine
more specific conditions of optimal resolution (10)).

3. <u>What Shall We Look At</u>? The selection of which enzyme
loci to examine by electrophoresis is often arbitrary, in both
animal and plant studies, the choice being largely dictated by
availability of convenient assays. Divorced from practical
concerns, one should like to select loci to suit the problem at
hand. There are at least four discrete and very different
problems addressed with electrophoresis by plant and animal
population biologists.
(a). Electrophoretic variants have proved very useful
as genetic markers. Electrophoretic variants often provide
a useful means of identifying genetic lines: many <u>crop lines</u>
differing primarily by quantitative characters are conveniently identified by "isozyme" markers. Many tissue culture
lines may not be differentiated in any other way. The
incidence of electrophoretic variation may also provide a
<u>useful index of the degree of inbreeding</u> (11). Perhaps,
most importantly, electrophoresis provides a ready means of
dealing with the population identity of plants for distinguishing spatially or temporarily contiguous populations,
identifying hybrid zones, and investigating identity.
(b). Phylogeny and Systematics. Because electrophoresis
produces discrete variants, it is widely employed in systematic
studies. The fundamental limitation of all such applications
is that <u>similar mobility on a gel does not necessarily imply
identity</u>. Thus it is primarily for closely-related groups
at the race or sibling species level that phylogenic comparisons are practical. More distantly-related groups are
usually characterized in terms of "genetic distance" (12), a
parameter which indexes genic similarity in terms of "isozyme"

similarity, with the difficulty that the index depends
critically upon the ability to demonstrate with electrophoresis
that pairs of proteins are identical (13).

   (c). Indexing Diversity. Much of the use of electrophoresis in population genetics is focused on attempts to
characterize the levels of genic variation in populations,
as reflected in protein variations. Such attempts are
primarily limited by resolution. As resolution has improved,
higher levels of variation have been reported (7).

   (d). Characterizing Specific Adaptations. Because
electrophoretically detected variant enzymes often differ
significantly in their functional properties, they provide
an avenue for investigating specific adaptations. Again it
is critical that all functionally different variants be
resolved from one another.

The choice of enzyme loci which may be most profitably
examined by electrophoresis depends upon which of these questions
is being addressed. The first two questions are really the same,
and do not depend upon the identity of the loci being examined.
The third question, however, presents a real sampling problem.
For the present, diversity studies require the broadest possible
selection of different enzymes, in order that the protein sample
adequately index the genome. The bias created by the particular
enzyme assays which are available is critical in this regard.
The fourth question, by contrast, requires the careful choice of
specific enzymes known to affect a particular physiological
process, omitting no enzyme which has an important influence.

POLYPLOID INVESTIGATIONS

   How do the foregoing considerations apply to the investigation of polyploidy per se? At this level the inclusion of polyploidy actually multiplies the problems outlined above.

   1. How do you find a variant? An added technical problem
encountered in applying electrophoresis to polyploids is that
variant proteins will often be present in very low concentrations
relative to the predominant form from which they are being resolved.
Diploids with one copy of a variant (genotype ab) produce 1:1
concentration ratios when heteromultimers are not found. If
heteromultimeric forms are formed, concentrations ratios are
1a:1b for monomers, 1aa:2ab:1bb for dimers, and 1aaa:3aaab:
4aabb:3abbb:1bbbb for tetramers. In tetraploids with one copy of
a variant (genotype abbb) the rare variant is present in lower
relative concentrations. If no heteromultimers are formed,
ratios of 1a:3b for monomers, 1aa:9bb for dimers, or 1aaa:81bbbb
for tetramers are obtained. If heteromultimers are found, the a-
containing variants relative concentration is reduced even further
(tetramers 1aaa:12aaab:54aabb:108abbb: 81bbbb - or 1/256 aaaa and
12/256 aaab). An increase in ploidy level or in number of protein

subunits magnifies this effect and protein classes may go unde-
tected.

There is no simple way to avoid these problems of differential
concentration of gene products in polyploids. This suggests that
electrophoretic techniques are not going to be very useful for
the study of polyploids in cases where successful detection of
all variants is critical (the third and fourth classes of question
listed above), unless careful attention is paid to resolution.
Where latitude exists in choice of enzymes, the two conflicting
effects of heterogeneity and resolution must be reconciled.
Enzymes which produce heterologous multimers (such as ab dimer)
produce multiple band classes and a potentially greater variability
on the gel. This advantage is dependent upon resolution and
concentration affects which limit detectability of some rare
classes. Concentrations effects can be minimized by selecting
enzymes with low subunit number.

2. Tracking ploidy. If the intensity of enzyme staining on
electrophoretic gels accurately reflects gene dosage, one might
in principle hope to be able to deduce ploidy level from the
number and relative intensities of gel bands, especially where
numerous enzymes of known subunit structure are available for
analysis. Unfortunately, the commonly employed stains rarely
follow Beer's law. Nor are the problems of accurately characterizing the densities of faint bands easily surmounted. In
addition, dosage estimates based on staining intensity require
that regulation of gene expression in polyploids and their diploid
progenerators be proportional.

3. Alternative approaches. An essential experimental
question for anyone proposing to employ electrophoresis in the
study of polyploids is: "Are other techniques liable to be more
useful?" For all but the fourth class of question discussed
above, direct study of DNA diversity using restriction endonucleases may well prove a far superior approach. Problems of
gene dosage are largely avoided, and the techniques are no more
difficult to master and carry out. Using restriction endonucleases to characterize DNA sequence diversity has the added
virtue that it deals directly with DNA, which after all, is the
intended focus of all but the fourth class of question.

WHERE ARE WE NOW (TECHNICALLY)?

In the widespread employment of electrophoresis in plant
biology, several areas of difficulty are apparent. We list five.

1. Magic incantations. No general protocols are widely
accepted for systematically determining optimal extraction procedures. A new investigator has no reasonable guide to direct
him, and even the most seasoned investigators often adopt widely
divergent approaches.

2. <u>Starch gels</u>. High resolution electrophoretic techniques have only recently been publicized, and they usually involve a significant increase in experimental effort. Most work is still carried out on starch gels, which lack optimal resolution.

3. <u>Drosophila enzymes</u>. To a large degree, the enzyme assays first adopted by <u>Drosophila</u> population geneticists remain the focus of electrophoretic studies of plants. Little work has been done on photosynthetic carbon fixation or any of the other physiological processes peculiarly important to plant biology.

4. <u>Gene dosage</u>. In most work gels are not scanned with a densitometer, so that relative band intensity data are rarely available; an added complication is the complexity contributed by polyploidy.

5. <u>Alternative approaches</u>. Restriction endonucleases have been only recently introduced. At least for chloroplast and mitochondrial DNA, experimental difficulties do not seem great, and one may hope to see this approach adopted widely, particularly in studies where electrophoresis has proven ambiguous.

SUMMARY

Investigations of polyploidy using electrophoresis are at present severely limited by several areas of difficulty which limit all applications of this technique. The technical problems inherent in electrophoresis of plants, namely extraction of active extracts and maximizing resolution of electrophoretic variants through investigation of gel and especially assay conditions, have never been addressed explicitly. No rationale for initiating work on a new species is available. Analytical approaches to defining the conditions which limit resolution are rare. Gel-to-gel variation is poorly controlled, seldom monitored. The individual nature of electrophoretic investigations limits the comparability of data among labs. In short, "hit-and-miss" approaches predominate, and these limit investigation. Techniques are now available which one can hope will greatly improve the experimental situation.

LITERATURE CITED

1. Powell, J., 1975, Protein variation in natural populations of animals. Evol. Biol. 8: 79-119.

2. Hamrick, J., 1979, Genetic variation and longevity, pp. 84-113, <u>in</u> Solbrig, O.T., et al. (eds.), "Topics in Plant Population Biology," Columbia University Press, New York.

3. Kelley, W.A., Adams, R.P., 1977, Preparation of extracts from juniper leaves for electrophoresis. Phytochem. 16: 513-516.

4. Anderson, J.W., 1968, Extraction of enzymes and subcellular organelles from plant tissues. Phytochem. 7: 1973-1988.

5.   Enama, M., 1977, Molecular weight variation of phosphoenolpyruvate carboxylases from C4 plants. Carnegie Inst. Wash. Yearb. 75: 409–410.

6.   Johnson, G., 1976, Hidden alleles at the α-glycerophosphate dehydrogenase locus in Colias butterflies. Genetics 83: 149–167.

7.   Singh, R., Lewontin, R., Felton, A., 1976, Genetic heterogeneity within electrophoretic "alleles" of xanthine dehydrogenase in Drosophila pseudoobscura. Genetics 84: 609–629.

8.   Coyne, J., 1976, Lack of genic similarity between two sibling species of Drosophila as revealed by varied techniques. Genetics 84: 593–607.

9.   Johnson, G., Simonsen, V., Pohlman, C., 1979, The influence of temperature on the electrophoretic behavior of polymorphic enzymes alleles. (Submitted to Biochem. Genetics)

10. Johnson, G., 1979, Genetically controlled variation in conformation of enzymes. Prog. Nucleic Acid Res./Molec. Biol. 22: 293–326.

11. Allard, R.W., Kahler, A.L., Clegg, M.T., 1977, Estimation of mating cycle components of selection in plants. Lecture Notes in Biomath. 19: 1–21.

12. Nei, M., 1972, Genetic distance between population. Amer. Nat. 106: 283–292.

13. Johnson, G., 1977, Assessing electrophoretic similarity: the problem of hidden heterogeneity. Ann. Rev. Ecol. Syst. 8: 309–328.

MOLECULAR TECHNIQUES APPLIED TO POLYPLOIDS

Virginia Walbot, Roger N. Beachy, and Meng-Chao Yao

Department of Biology
Washington University
St. Louis, MO 63130

We have learned a great deal about the patterns of evolution
through examination of species differences at the phenotypic
level: isozyme patterns, secondary metabolic products, morphological changes, karyotype, or other criteria. Such studies are
inherently limited to studying those changes visible to us; many
changes in the genome of a particular species may not result in
visible phenotypic change. In the last 10 years many innovations
in examining the average composition of genomes by reassociation
analysis, thermal denaturation of interspecific hybrid DNA
molecules, and other procedures have provided a means for examining
the total divergence between related genomes. Such procedures
can be used to chart the general trends of species-specific
changes in genome composition over time, including both individual
base changes and phenomena such as loss or amplification of
sequences. DNA reassociation procedures necessarily give information on typical patterns, but new methods developed over the
last five years can yield information on the evolution of specific gene sequences. These new methods include restriction
enzyme digestion patterns and DNA sequencing; in order to accomplish these analyses it is usually necessary to clone a specific
sequence of eukaryotic DNA in a phage or plasmid vector. The
fine scale resolution provided by DNA sequencing of particular
sequences can be combined with knowledge gained from DNA reassociation experiments on the average divergence of all sequences to
understand the trends in genome evolution.

DNA HYBRIDIZATION METHODS

DNA hybridization experiments are designed to test the
extent of homology and proportion of sequences sharing some

homology. Such measurements can be used to calculate the extent
of divergence among species and to follow the overall organization
of individual genomes. For example, one percent mismatching of
duplexes can be readily detected and used to date the divergence
of taxa at the species and genus level, 5-10 MY (1).

Hybridization experiments require pure nucleic acid samples
and a careful experimental design. Protocols for DNA preparation
and a thorough review of the rationale of various hybridization
experiments is provided in Britten et al., (2). The results
obtained in hybridization experiments depend on the criterion
conditions chosen; the combination of salt concentration, and
temperature used in an experiment determines how closely matched
sequences must be to be counted as a duplex. Stringent criterion
conditions can be chosen so that only very closely matched sequences
will be found in duplex; low stringency conditions can be used to
define sequences of limited homology. Stringency parameters are
empirically determined to optimize the analysis of sequences of
varying degrees of homology.

Reassociated DNA molecules can be analyzed to determine the
proportion of nucleotides in duplex by thermal denaturation or by
S_1 nuclease digestion and to determine the proportion of molecules
containing some duplex region by hydroxyapatite chromatography.
The extent of mismatching of reassociated duplexes is typically
determined by thermal denaturation in which the depression of Tm
(the melting temperature at which 50% of hyperchromicity has
occurred) can be measured and compared to the Tm of native DNA of
similar length. Electron microscopy of reassociated duplexes can
be used to determine the average length and spacing between DNA
sequences of specific reiteration values. Data analysis of DNA
reassociation experiments is based on assumptions of ideal second
order reaction kinetics by DNA molecules in solution with provision
for correction for variables such as DNA length, reaction rate
influences, and other factors (2).

For an introduction to the major experimental designs utilized
in analyzing complex genomes of high DNA content, the following
references are suggested: Walbot and Dure (3), Flavell and Smith
(4), Zimmerman and Goldberg (5), Goldberg (6), and Walbot and
Goldberg (7). The role of genome organization in gene regulation
and evolution is discussed in the following references: Davidson
and Britten (8), Lewin (9), Thompson (10) and Wilson et al.
(1).

ISOLATION OF SPECIFIC DNA SEQUENCES

In order to make interspecific or interfamily comparisons of
particular gene sequences it is first necessary to isolate, in
pure form, the desired DNA; only then can nucleotide sequence and
restriction endonuclease digestion maps be constructed. The
following section will outline these procedures.

If the gene under study codes for a protein found in large
amounts in a particular tissue, such as a seed storage protein,
it may be possible to isolate the respective messenger RNA (mRNA)
from polyribosomes (11,12), identifying the function of the mRNA
by in vitro protein synthesis (13,14). The mRNA under study can
be partially purified by sucrose density gradient centrifugation
and/or by electrophoresis in, and extraction from an agarose gel
(15). If the mRNA is expected to be present in low amounts (< 1%
of the mRNA in the cell) it may be necessary to immune precipitate
polyribosomes containing peptides antigenically related to the
protein in question (16,17). There are many pitfalls in the
isolation, characterization and in vitro translation of mRNA, the
greatest being ribonuclease contamination, primarily from the
starting material. This problem can, however, usually be minimized
by procedural precautions.

After isolating a specific or enriched fraction of mRNA(s),
DNA complementary in sequence to the mRNA can be produced using
the enzyme reverse transcriptase (18,19), followed by the synthesis
of second strand DNA with DNA polymerase I (18). The ends of the
now double-stranded DNA can be modified to permit in vitro recombination with any one of a number of bacterial plasmids (20).
After transfection of an appropriate bacterial host (according to
NIH Guidelines on Recombinant DNA Research) colonies bearing
recombinant molecules can be identified on the basis of colony
phenotype. Further identification of the cloned DNA can be done
by any of several methods (20,21), including the isolation of a
specific mRNA by hybridization-purification (22) and its identification by in vitro protein synthesis.

Once the proper cDNA clones are identified they can be used
to select a particular mRNA from several plant species (assuming
that the genes for the proteins in question are closely related).
Direct base sequence analysis of the mRNA can be carried out
(23).

Comparing the relatedness of genomic DNA may be more informative than studies with cDNA. Fragments of genomic DNA can,
after in vitro recombination with plasmid or viral DNA followed
by amplification in an appropriate host, be identified by molecular
hybridization with characterized cDNA clones. If the procedure
outlined above were carried through authentic genes coding for
the synthesis of seed storage proteins, for example, could be
isolated. Likewise recombinant DNA clones containing the genes
for the ribosomal or transfer RNAs can be identified using in
vivo- or in vitro-labeled RNAs as hybridization probes. Isolated
DNA would then be ready for further characterizations.

RESTRICTION MAPPING AND DNA SEQUENCING

Through cloning or direct fractionation one normally obtains
a segment of DNA whose length varies from a few hundred base
pairs to thousands of base pair long. Analysis of this long

segment of DNA has been greatly simplified by the recent discovery
of restriction endonucleases (24). This group of enzymes recognizes
specific nucleotide sequences and cleave the DNA at or near those
sites. As a result the DNA is broken down to smaller fragments
of defined sizes and can be further separated by electrophoresis
in an agarose gel (25). Thus, a unique "restriction pattern" is
obtained for a given DNA when digested by a given enzyme. Using
this method one can compare in good detail very closely related
DNAs. Since agarose gel electrophoresis separates DNA according
to size, this method is most powerful in detecting insersion or
deletion of more than a few base pairs. It could also detect
translocations, inversions, and substitutions involving restriction
sites. This method is simple and rapid. It is most useful in
analysing divergence of genes in different populations or in
closely related species. Currently more than 100 restriction
enzymes have been identified (26) and many of them are commercially
available.

When more than a few sequences are to be compared by restriction mapping, a simple modification is available which eliminates
the need for purifying all but one of the sequences involved. In
this modification unfractionated genomic DNA instead of cloned
sequence is digested with restriction enzymes and analysed by
electorphoresis. The DNA is then blotted directly onto a nitro-
cellulose filter after denaturation (27). The sequence of interest
can be detected among other genomic DNA by hybridization using
the cloned sequence as a probe. Thus, once a sequence is purified,
it is possible to detect and compare as many related sequences as
desired without the need for further purification. This technique
is extremely sensitive and has been used to detect single copy
genes in mammalian genomes (28). It has also been used widely to
compare similar genes in different genomes, such as ribosomal RNA
genes in mammals (29) and human β-globin genes in different
individuals (30).

The sensitivity of the restriction mapping method is limited
in detecting simple base substitutions. Most enzymes recognize
sequences four to six nucleotides long, which occur on the average
once every several hundred nucleotides in most DNA. Only on rare
occasions will the base change occur right on one of the restriction sites and be detected. For ultimate comparison, DNA
sequencing is probably the only method available. Lately the
method has been greatly improved and it is now possible to sequence
up to a few thousand nucleotides with only a moderate effort.
The method essentially involves radioactively labelling the
purified DNA fragment at or from one end and interrupting the
polymer at a specific nucleotide in varying distances from the
labelled end, either by chemical means or by using chain termi-
nators (31,32). The interrupted fragments are then separated by
gel electrophoresis and detected by autoradiography. By comparing
fragments terminated at all four nucleotides, it is possible to
read out up to a few hundred nucleotide sequence in a single gel.

The accuracy of this method is extremely high and would normally exceed 99%. It allows one to determine the entire information content of a gene without ambiguity. For detecting slight difference between closely related alleles or slight homology between distantly related genes, DNA sequencing is probably the best method available.

LITERATURE CITED

1. Wilson, A.C., Carlson, S.S., White, T.J., 1977, Biochemical evolution. Ann. Rev. Biochem. 46: 573-639.
2. Britten, R.J., Graham, D.E., Neufeld, B.R., 1974, An analysis of repeating DNA sequences by reassociation, pp. 363-418, Grossman, L.,Moldave, K. (eds.), in "Methods In Enzymology," Vol. 29E, Academic Press, New York.
3. Walbot, V., Dure, L.S., III, 1976, Developmental Biochemistry of cotton seed embryogenesis and germination. VII. Characterization of the cotton genome. J. Mol. Biol. 101: 503-536.
4. Flavell, R.B., Smith, D.B., 1976, Nucleotide sequence organization in the wheat genome. Heredity 37: 231-252.
5. Zimmerman, J.L., Goldberg, R.B., 1977, DNA sequence organization in the genome of Nicotiana tabacum. Chromosoma 59: 227-252.
6. Goldberg, R.B., 1978, DNA sequence organization in the soybean plant. Biochem. Genet. 16: 45-68.
7. Walbot, V., Goldberg, R., Plant genome organization and its relationship to classical plant genetics, in Hall, T., Davies J. (eds.), "Nucleic Acids in Plants," CRC Press, West Palm Beach, Florida (in press).
8. Davidson, E.H., Britten, R.J., 1973, Organization, transcription, and regulation in the animal genome. Quart. Rev. Biol. 48: 555-613.
9. Lewin, B.L., 1975, "Gene Expression - 2," Wiley, New York.
10. Thompson, W.F., 1978, Prespectives on the evolution of plant DNA. Carnegie Inst. Ann. Rep. Plant Biology 1977-1978, pp. 310-316.
11. Jackson, A.O., Larkins, B., 1976, Influence of ionic strength, pH, and chelation of divalent metals on isolation of polyribosomes from tobacco leaves. Pl. Physiol. 57: 5-10.
12. Beachy, R.N., Thompson, J.E., Madison, J.T., 1978, Isolation of polyribosomes and messenger RNA active in in vitro synthesis of soybean seed proteins. Pl. Physiol. 61: 139-144.
13. Roberts, B.E., Paterson, B.M., 1973, Efficient translation of tobacco mosaic virus RNA and rabbit globin as RNA in a cell-free system from commercial wheat germ. Proc. Nat. Acad. Sci. USA 70: 2330-2334.
14. Marcu, K., Dudock, B., 1974, Characterization of a highly efficient protein synthesizing system derived from commercial wheat germ. Nucleic Acids Res. 1: 1385-1397.

15. Langridge, J., Langridge, P., Bergquist, P.L., 1979, Extrac-
     tion of nucleic acids from agarose gels. Analyt. Biochem.
     (in press).
16. Palacios, R., Palmiter, R., Schimke, R.T., 1972, Identifi-
     cation and isolation of ovalbiemin-synthesizing polysomes I.
     Specific binding of ^{125}I-anti-ovalbumin to polysomes. J.
     Biol. Chem. 247: 2316-2321.
17. Tunis, M.A., Miller, D.L., 1977, Quantitation of rat α-
     fetoprotein messenger RNA with a complementary DNA probe.
     J. Biol. Chem. 252: 8469-8475.
18. Efstratiadis, A., Kafatos, F.C., Maxam, A.M., Maniates, T.,
     1976, Enzymatic in vitro synthesis of globin genes. Cell 7:
     279-288.
19. Myers, J.C., Spiegelman, S., 1978, Sodium pyrophosphate
     inhibition of RNA·DNA hybrid degradation by reverse trans-
     criptase. Proc. Nat. Acad. Sci. USA 75: 5329-5333.
20. Scott, W.A., Werner, R., 1977, "Molecular Cloning of Recom-
     binant DNA," Academic Press, New York.
21. Paterson, B.M., Roberts, B.E., Kuff, E.L., 1977, Structural
     gene idenfitication and mapping by DNA·mRNA hybrid-arrested
     cell-free translation. Proc. Nat. Acad. Sci. USA 74:
     4370-4374.
22. Smith, D.F., Searle, P.E., Williams, J.G., 1979, Characteri-
     zation of bacterial clones containing DNA sequences derived
     from Xenopus laevis vitellogenin mRNA. Nucleic Acids Res.
     6: 487-506.
23. Zain, B.S., Roberts, R.J., 1979, Sequences from the beginning
     of the fiber messenger RNA of adenovirus-2. J. Mol. Biol.
     131: 341-352.
24. Smith, H., 1979, Nucleotide sequence specificity of restric-
     tion endonucleases. Life Science 205: 455-462.
25. Helling, R.B., Goodman, H.M., Boyer, H.W., 1974, Analysis of
     endonuclease R-EcoR1 fragments of DNA from lambdoid bacteri-
     ophages and other viruses by agarose-gel electrophoresis.
     J. Virol. 14: 1235-1244.
26. Roberts, R.J., 1978, Restriction and modification enzymes
     and their recognition sequences. Gene 4: 183-193.
27. Southern, E.M., 1975, Detection of specific sequences among
     DNA fragments separated by gel electrophoresis. J. Mol.
     Biol. 98: 503-517.
28. Botchan, M., Topp, W., Sambrook, J., 1976, The arrangement
     of simian virus 40 sequences in the DNA of transformed
     cells. Cell 9: 269-287.
29. Arnheim, N., Southern, E.M., 1977, Heterogeneity of the
     ribosomal genes in mice and man. Cell 11: 363-370.
30. Jeffreys, A.J., 1979, DNA sequence variants in the $^{G}\gamma$-, $^{A}\gamma$-,
     δ- and β-globin genes of man. Cell 18: 1-10.
31. Maxam, A.M., Gilbert, W., 1977, A new method for sequencing
     DNA. Proc. Nat. Acad. Sci. USA 74: 560-564.

32. Sanger, F., Nicklen, S., Coulson, A.R., 1977, DNA sequencing
     with chain terminating inhibitors. Proc. Nat. Acad. Sci.
     USA 74: 5463-5467.

PRINCIPLES OF DEMOGRAPHIC ANALYSIS APPLIED TO NATURAL

POLYPLOID POPULATIONS

Otto T. Solbrig

Department of Biology and Gray Herbarium
Harvard University
Cambridge, MA   02138

The general principles of demographic analysis apply equally well to diploid or polyploid populations. The question is whether the morphological, physiological, or behavioral characteristic of polyploid populations will affect their demographic development.

Evidence was presented by Solbrig from his work with the genus Viola and from the literature showing that in many if not most herbaceous plants survivorship and fecundity are size and not age dependent. It was also shown that seedlings have different survivorship probabilities from adults and furthermore it was indicated that seedling mortality is several times greater than adult mortality.

Polyploid plants are known to be larger than their diploid ancestors at least in certain cases, and particularly in the case of allopolyploids. All other things being equal polyploids exhibiting gigas characteristics should have higher survivorships and fecundities than their diploid counterparts in a population where survivorship and fecundity are size and not age dependent. This demographic act alone could explain the prevalence of polyploidy among herbaceous perennials.

Another question that has been raised is the problem of establishment of a polyploid individual in a population of diploids, since the probability of such an occurrence is very low. However, if fecundity is size dependent and a few individuals account for over 90% of the seed contribution in the population as was shown with the populations of Viola, the problem of establishment of polyploids is considerably reduced. In effect, effective population size may be less than 10 rather than over 100 increasing considerably the probability of establishment of a fecund polyploid.

Finally the question of seedling establishment was raised. If polyploidy increases the rate of growth of seedlings and the size they can attain in a year, their probability of establishment should increase. However, instances are known where polyploids have a slower growth rate. Unless compensated by increase size, decreased growth rate will decrease the probability of establishment.

The workshop concluded that more research on these questions should be undertaken, especially to establish the relationship between size, survivorship, and fecundity in polyploids.

NEWLY ATTAINED POLYPLOIDY AND/OR CLONAL REPRODUCTION IN ANIMALS:

THE BRINK OF EXTINCTION, OR THRESHOLD TO NEW FRONTIERS?

Charles J. Cole

Department of Herpetology
American Museum of Natural History
New York, N.Y. 10024

Polyploid and parthenogenetic or apomictic species of verte-brates were unknown less than 20 years ago, although such species were recognized among invertebrates (1-3) and a few unisexual populations of fishes were being investigated (4,5). In the last 15 years, however, many examples of polyploidy and several kinds of reproduction in unisexual species have been carefully docu-mented among numerous animals, including amniote vertebrates, as illustrated by speakers at this symposium (Lokki and Saura, Schultz, Bogart). Today, examples of autopolyploidy and allo-ploidy are known, a relationship between polyploidy and parthe-nogenesis is recognized (but note Bogart's examples of polyploid and bisexually reproducing frogs), and it is well established that the origin of many unisexual and/or polyploid vertebrates (and some invertebrates) involved interspecific hybridization between previously existing diploid bisexual species. Thus, much of the theory concerning evolution of polyploidy and apomixis in plants, which botanists, geneticists, and cytogeneticists have developed over several decades (6) is being applied successfully to animals.

With some basic problems solved, documenting the existence of polyploid and unisexual species of animals, several zoologists now are emphasizing analyses of intraspecific variation in these animals, their potential as ecological competitors, and their evolutionary adaptability. Theory suggests that polyploid and especially clonal-reproducing organisms should be at a selective disadvantage compared to diploid bisexual organisms, due to extremely limited means of incorporating new gene combinations and mutations into their genomes; particularly considering the greatly reduced probability that favorable recessive mutations will become expressed in polyploids. Consequently, polyploid and unisexual organisms have been referred to as "evolutionary dead ends," highly susceptible to extinction.

Putting semantic problems aside (i.e., an "evolutionary dead end" might not be capable of rapid adaptation, but it may survive and reproduce for millions of years, evolving slowly, as long as it occupies a niche), some investigations in morphology (e.g., 7,8), ecology (e.g., 9), karyotypes (e.g., 10-12), genetics (e.g., 13), electrophoretic mobilities of proteins (e.g., 14-18), and tissue histocompatibilities (e.g., 19,20) have revealed more variability among polyploid and/or unisexual animals than many biologists expected. Now, in addition to expanding our knowledge of the extent of polyploidy and clonal reproduction, more comparative studies of variation are required to determine its significance. Questions that seem pertinent are:

1) How can we determine date of origin for various polyploid and/or unisexual species?

2) What mechanisms of gene regulation and dosage compensation occur within polyploids, and how do these effect their adaptability or individual plasticity in interactions between organism and environment?

3) What really is a "recessive" gene, how important is fixation of such genes in evolution in general (not only in polyploids), and how does this compare with the evolutionary significance of codominant alleles and epistatic interactions? If recessive mutations do not have the importance in evolution that often is ascribed to them, theoretical difficulties of their gaining expression in polyploids would not constitute a significant obstacle to the adaptability of polyploid species.

4) Is the mutation rate higher in some polyploid and unisexual species than in their diploid bisexual relatives?

5) Does somatic crossing over occur more frequently than has been generally recognized, and if this is an important source of variation in polyploid and unisexual organisms, might it not also be more significant than we realize among diploid bisexual species?

6) How can one distinguish with reasonable certainty among possible alternative sources of variation, such as: that stemming from recombination or mutation following the establishment of polyploidy or unisexuality in a lineage; or that stemming from the moment of origin of polyploidy or unisexuality, which may occur several times through separate events of hybridization involving gametes bearing different genes (i.e., separate founder events)? If, indeed, most of the variation observed in polyploid and/or unisexual animals stems merely from separate founder events, it might be reasonably correct to refer to these species as "evolutionary dead ends," afterall.

7) But what are the relative degrees of variability among animals of different levels of ploidy and among unisexual species that reproduce by different means (hybridogenesis, gynogenesis, parthenogenesis or apomixis)?

Nearly all of the work on polyploid and/or unisexual animals in the last few years has been in basic research. The results indicate that the main advantages of clonal reproduction include the perpetuation of highly successful gene combinations together generation after generation, and highly efficient reproduction, as all normal individuals produce additional individuals similar to themselves. Perhaps it is not too daring to consider that research in the near future might be directed toward understanding the processes involved in switching from bisexual to unisexual reproduction, and learning to take advantage of genes controlling this phenomenon to develop new breeds of plants and animals of agricultural importance.

LITERATURE CITED

1. Suomalainen, E., 1950, Parthenogenesis in animals. Adv. Genet. 3: 193–253.
2. Suomalainen, E., 1959, On polyploidy in animals. Sitzungsber. Finnischen Akad. Wiss. 1958, 105–119.
3. White, M.J.D., 1954, "Animal Cytology and Evolution," ed. 2, Cambridge Univ. Press, Cambridge. xiv + 454 pp.
4. Hubbs, C.L., 1955, Hybridization between fish species in nature. Syst. Zool. 4: 1–20.
5. Miller, R.R., Schultz, R.J., 1959, All-female strains of the teleost fishes of the genus Poeciliopsis. Science 130: 1656–1657.
6. Stebbins, G.L., 1971, "Chromosomal Evolution in Higher Plants," Addison-Wesley, Reading, MA, viii + 216 pp.
7. Zweifel, R.G., 1965, Variation in and distribution of the unisexual lizard, Cnemidophorus tesselatus. Amer. Mus. Novitates, no. 2235, 1–49.
8. Atchley, W.R., 1977, Biological variability in the parthenogenetic grasshopper Warramaba virgo (Key) and its sexual relatives. I. The eastern Australian populations. Evolution 31: 782–799.
9. Vrijenhoek, R.C., 1978, Coexistence of clones in a heterogeneous environment. Science 199: 549–552.
10. Wright, J.W., Lowe, C.H., 1967, Evolution of the alloploid parthenospecies Cnemidophorus tesselatus (Say). Mammal. Chromos. Newsletter 8 (2): 95–96.
11. Lowe, C.H., Wright, J.W., Cole, C.J., Bezy, R.L., 1970, Natural hybridization between the teiid lizards Cnemidophorus sonorae (parthenogenetic) and Cnemidophorus tigris (bisexual). Syst. Zool. 19: 114–127.
12. Cole, C.J., 1979, Chromosome inheritance in parthenogenetic lizards and evolution of allopolyploidy in reptiles. J. Heredity 70: 95–102.

13. Leslie, J.F., Vrijenhoek, R.C., 1978, Genetic dissection of
     clonally inherited genomes of Poeciliopsis. I. Linkage
     analysis and preliminary assessment of deleterious gene
     loads. Genetics 90: 801-811.
14. Lokki, J., Suomalainen, E., Saura, A., Lankinen, P., 1975,
     Genetic polymorphism and evolution in parthenogenetic animals.
     II. Diploid and polyploid Solenobia triquetrella (Lepi-
     doptera: Psychidae). Genetics 79: 513-525.
15. Uzzell, T., Berger, L., 1975, Electrophoretic phenotypes of
     Rana ridibunda, Rana lessonae and their hybridogenetic
     associate, Rana esculenta. Proc. Acad. Nat. Sci. (Phila-
     delphia) 127: 13-24.
16. Parker, E.D., Selander, R.K., 1976, The organization of
     genetic diversity in the parthenogenetic lizard Cnemidophorus
     tesselatus. Genetics 84: 791-805.
17. Selander, R.K., Parker, E.D., Jr., Browne, R.A., 1978,
     Clonal variation in the parthenogenetic snail Campeloma
     decisa (Viviparidae). Veliger 20: 349-351.
18. Vrijenhoek, R.C., Angus, R.A., Schultz, R.J., 1978, Variation
     and clonal structure in a unisexual fish. Amer. Nat. 112:
     41-55.
19. Kallman, K.D., 1962, Population genetics of the gynogenetic
     teleost, Mollienesia formosa (Girard). Evolution 16: 497-504.
20. Cuellar, O., 1977, Genetic homogeneity and speciation in the
     parthenogenetic lizards Cnemidophorus velox and C. neo-
     mexicanus: Evidence from intraspecific histocompatibility.
     Evolution 31: 24-31.

CYTOGENETICS AND CROP IMPROVEMENT

G. Kimber and E. R. Sears

Department of Agronomy, University of Missouri, and
Science and Education Administration of USDA
Columbia, MO 65201

Most consideration was given to the question of the potential usefulness in plant breeding of the new technologies, such as tissue culture, microspore culture, and protoplast culture. Are improvements in crop plants more likely to come from these techniques than from conventional breeding procedures? Particular attention was paid to the transfer of desirable characters to crop plants from related species.

There appeared to be a consensus that with such polyploids as wheat, oats, and various forage grasses, where aneuploids are either available or presumably obtainable, conventional cytogenetic techniques are capable of a degree of precision in the transfer of alien genes not likely soon to be realized by the new techniques. In other crop plants barriers to hybridization may not be so easily overcome, and attempts to apply the protoplast-fusion technique may therefore be more easily justified.

There are special situations where protoplast fusion is a particularly attractive possibility. For example, a sterile plant may have a potentially valuable character that cannot be used in a conventional breeding program, but can be introduced through cell culture and protoplast fusion. Desirable characters of plants with long life cycles can be used in protoplast-fusion breeding without the long wait for flowering. Hybrids produced by protoplast fusion are not subject to the restriction that they must immediately produce viable plants; thus modifications of the chromosome constitution can occur in culture that may ultimately result in potentially valuable, but otherwise unobtainable, materials such as addition and substitution lines at the diploid level.

A question as to which polyploid crop plants besides <u>Triticum</u> have a genetic system for the suppression of homoeologous pairing brought out that some certainly, and most others probably, have such a system. <u>Avena</u> is known to have a major suppressor, like <u>Triticum</u>; and <u>Gossypium</u> and <u>Fragaria</u> clearly have genetic suppression, not yet analyzed in detail. Where hybrids of the parental species have a significant amount of chromosome pairing but haploids produced by the amphiploid do not, genetic suppression must be suspected.

PARTICIPANTS IN THE CONFERENCE ON
POLYPLOIDY: BIOLOGICAL RELEVANCE HELD
AT WASHINGTON UNIVERSITY, ST. LOUIS, MAY 24-27, 1979

Anderson, J. M.
  N.E. Oklahoma State University
  Tahlequah, Oklahoma   74464

Alonso-Arnedo L. C.
  University of Missouri
  Columbia, Missouri   65201

Al-Falluji, Raof Ali
  University of Missouri
  Columbia, Missouri   65201

Amos, J.
  University of Northern Iowa
  Cedar Falls, Iowa   50613

Argus, G. W.
  Museum of Natural Sciences
  Ottawa, Ontario

Averett, J. E.
  University of Missouri
  St. Louis, Missouri 63131

Badr, E. A.
  Alexandria University
  Shatby, Alexandria, Egypt

Baker, R. K.
  Washington University
  St. Louis, Missouri   63130

Banek, H.
  University of British Columbia
  Vancouver, British Columbia,

Banks, D. J.
  USDA, Oklahoma State University
  Stillwater, Oklahoma   74074

Banks, J.
  Ohio State University
  Columbus, Ohio   43201

Bauchan, G. R.
  Michigan State University
  East Lansing, Michigan   48824

Beachy, R. N.
  Washington University
  St. Louis, Missouri   63130

Bedigian, D.
  University of Illinois
  Urbana, Illinois   61801

Beitel, J.
  University of Michigan
  Ann Arbor, Michigan   48105

Bingham, E. T.
  University of Wisconsin
  Madison, Wisconsin   53705

Bodkin, N. L
  James Madison University
  Harrisonburg, Virginia   22801

Bogart, J. P.
  University of Guelph
  Guelph, Ontario

Boom, B.
  University of Tennessee
  Knoxville, Tennessee   37916

Bowers, M. C.
  Northern Michigan University
  Marquette, Michigan   49855

Bowman, V.
  Washington University
  St. Louis, Missouri   63130

Bretting, P.
  Indiana University
  Bloomington, Indiana   47401

Bringhurst, R. S.
  University of California
  Davis, California   95616

Brouillet, L.
  University of Waterloo
  Waterloo, Ontario

Carr, B.
  Washington University
  St. Louis, Missouri   63130

Casey, J.
  Texas Tech University
  Lubbock, Texas   79414

Chinnappa, C. C.
  University of Waterloo
  Waterloo, Ontario

Christy, A. L.
  Monsanto Agricultural
    Products Company
  St. Louis, Missouri   63166

Clausen, K. E.
  Southern Illinois University
  Carbondale, Illinois   62958

Coffey, J. C.
  University of South Carolina
  Columbia, South Carolina   29208

Cole, C. J.
  American Museum
  of Natural History
  New York, New York   10024

Coulthart, M. B.
  University of Alberta
  Edmonton, Alberta

Crosby, M. R.
  Missouri Botanical Garden
  St. Louis, Missouri   63110

Davidse, G.
  Missouri Botanical Garden
  St. Louis, Missouri   63110

Dawe, J.
  University of Alaska
  Fairbanks, Alaska   99701

Decker, J. M.
  Ohio Wesleyan University
  Ostrander, Ohio   43061

Delevoryas, T.
  University of Texas
  Austin, Texas   78758

Denford, K.
  University of Alberta
  Edmonton, Alberta

Dewey, D. R.
  USDA, Utah State University
  Logan, Utah   84322

Douglass, K. L.
  University of Oklahoma
  Norman, Oklahoma   73069

Doyle, J. J.
  Indiana University
  Bloomington, Indiana 47401

Ehrendorfer, F.
  University of Vienna
  Vienna, Austria

Eisendrath, E. R.
  Washington University
  St. Louis, Missouri 63130

Eizenga, G.
  University of Missouri
  Columbia, Missouri 65201

Erickson, H. T.
  Purdue University
  W. Lafayette, Indiana 47906

Erickson, Mrs. H. T.
  Purdue University
  W. Lafayette, Indiana 47906

Essig, F. B.
  University of South Florida
  Tampa, Florida 33620

Estes, J. R.
  University of Oklahoma
  Norman, Oklahoma 73071

Fadan, R. B.
  Field Museum
  of Natural History
  Chicago, Illinois 60637

Fairchild, R. S., Sr.
  University of Arkansas
  Fayetteville, Arkansas 72701

Feldmann, K. A.
  University of Northern Iowa
  Cedar Falls, Iowa 50613

Funk, V. A.
  Ohio State University
  Columbus, Ohio 43210

Gentry, A.
  Missouri Botanical Garden
  St. Louis, Missouri 63110

Gereau, R. E.
  Michigan State University
  East Lansing, Michigan 48823

Gereau, Mrs. R. E.
  Michigan State University
  East Lansing, Michigan 48823

Goldman, M.
  Purdue University
  W. Lafayette, Indiana 47907

Goldblatt, P.
  Missouri Botanical Garden
  St. Louis, Missouri 63110

Gomez, L. D.
  National Museum of Costa Rica
  San Jose, Costa Rica

Griesbach, R. J.
  Michigan State University
  East Lansing, Michigan 48824

Griffin, J. D.
  Michigan State University
  East Lansing, Michigan 48824

Hancock, J. F., Jr.
  University of South Carolina
  Columbia, South Carolina 29208

Hansen, D. J.
  Monsanto Agricultural
    Products Company
  St. Louis, Missouri 63166

Hart, G. E.
  Texas A & M University
  Bryan, Texas 77801

Haufler, C.
  Missouri Botanical Garden
  St. Louis, Missouri 63110

Heithauf, J. J.
  Monsanto Agricultural
    Products Company
  St. Louis, Missouri   63166

Herman, P. L.
  Univeristy of Pittsburgh
  Pittsburgh, Pennsylvania   15218

Hickok, L. G.
  University of Tennessee
  Knoxville, Tennessee   37920

Hoch, P.
  Missouri Botanical Garden
  St. Louis, Missouri   63110

Honegger, J.
  Monsanto Agricultural
    Products Company
  St. Louis, Missouri   63166

Hoshaw, R. W.
  University of Arizona
  Tucson, Arizona   85721

Hunsperger, J.
  Michigan State University
  East Lansing, Michigan   48824

Jackson, R. C.
  Texas Tech University
  Lubbock, Texas   79413

Jaworski, E. G.
  Monsanto Agricultural
    Products Company
  St. Louis, Missouri   63166

Johnson, G. B.
  Washington University
  St. Louis, Missouri   63130

Joseph, C.
  University of Missouri
  Columbia, Missouri   65211

Kerr, K.
  University of Texas
  Austin, Texas   78722

Kimber, G.
  University of Missouri
  Columbia, Missouri   62511

King, N.
  Washington University
  St. Louis, Missouri   63130

Kupfer, P.
  Institut de Botanique
  Neuchatel, Switzerland

Lake, S.
  Washington University
  St. Louis, Missouri   63130

Leto, K. J
  University of Illinois
  Champaign, Illinois   61820

Levetin, E.
  University of Tulsa
  Tulsa, Oklahoma   74105

Levin, D. A.
  University of Texas
  Austin, Texas   78721

Levy, M.
  Purdue University
  W. Lafayette, Indiana   47907

Lewis, W. H.
  Washington University
  St. Louis, Missouri   63130

Lewis, Mrs. W. H.
  Washington University
  St. Louis, Missouri   63130

Liang, G. H.
  Kansas State University
  Manhattan, Kansas   66506

Lissant, E.
  Washington University
  St. Louis, Missouri   63130

Lissant, K.
  Petrolite Corporation
  St. Louis, Missouri   63102

Liu, C. W.
  Michigan State University
  East Lansing, Michigan   48824

Lokki, J.
  University of Helsinki
  Helsinki, Finland

Loshman, C. A.
  University of Northern Iowa
  Cedar Falls, Iowa   50613

McArthur, E. D.
  USDA Forest Service, Utah
  Provo, Utah   84601

McGirk, B. F.
  Washington University
  St. Louis, Missouri   63130

Maha, G. C.
  University of Illinois
  Urbana, Illinois   61801

Maniotis, J.
  Washington University
  St. Louis, Missouri   63130

Martin, G.
  Michigan State University
  East Lansing, Michigan   48824

Marvel, J. T.
  Monsanto Agricultural
    Products Company
  St. Louis, Missouri   63166

Mears, J. A.
  Academy of Natural Sciences
  Philadelphia, Pennsylvania 19088

Mitten, D. H.
  Monsanto Agricultural
    Products Company
  St. Louis, Missouri   63166

Moffler, M. D.
  Marine Research Laboratory
  Tampa, Florida   33604

Mujeeb, K. A.
  Kansas State University
  Manhattan, Kansas   66506

Murphy, R. P.
  Cornell University
  Ithaca, New York   14850

Nesom, G. L.
  Ohio State University
  Columbus, Ohio   53210

Newell, C. A.
  University of Illinois
  Champaign, Illinois   61820

Newhouse, K.
  Iowa State University
  Ames, Iowa   50010

Nichols, H. W.
  Washington University
  St. Louis, Missouri   63130

Ninan, C. A.
  University of Kerala
  Trivandrum, India

Olson, K. C.
  School of the Ozarks
  Branson, Missouri   65616

Oresky, D.
  University of Maryland
  Adelphi, Maryland   20783

Pate, D.
  University of Missouri
  St. Louis, Missouri   63121

Payne, W. W.
  Cary Arboretum, New York
    Botanical Garden
  Millbrook, New York   12545

Peng, C. I.
  Washington University
  St. Louis, Missouri   63130

Polley, D.
  Wabash College
  Crawfordsville, Indiana   47933

Poston, M.
  Missouri Botanical Garden
  St. Louis, Missouri   63110

Pringle, J. S.
  Royal Botanical Garden
  Hamilton, Ontario

Pullen, T. M.
  University of Mississippi
  University, Mississippi   38677

Pusateri, W.
  Miami University
  Oxford, Ohio   45056

Ouinlivan, E.
  University of Northern Iowa
  Waterloo, Iowa   50702

Rivin, C.
  Washington University
  St. Louis, Missouri   63130

Robinson, W. A.
  University of Pittsburgh
  Pittsburgh, Pennsylvania   15218

Roose, M.
  SUNY at Stony Brook
  Stony Brook, New York   11794

Sadanaga, K.
  Iowa State University
  Ames, Iowa   50010

St. Amand, W.
  University of Mississippi
  Oxford, Mississippi   38655

St. Amand, G. S.
  University of Mississippi
  Oxford, Mississippi   38655

Sarkar, P.
  University of Toronto
  Toronto, Ontario

Sarkar, Mrs. P.
  University of Toronto
  Toronto, Ontario

Saura, A.
  University of Helsinki
  Helsinki, Finland

Schilling, E.
  University of Texas
  Austin, Texas   78705

Schultz, R. J.
  University of Connecticut
  Storrs, Connecticut   06268

Sears, E. R.
  University of Missouri
  Columbia, Missouri   65211

Semple, J. C.
  University of Waterloo
  Waterloo, Ontario

Sexton, O. J.
  Washington University
  St. Louis, Missouri   63130

Sleper, D. A.
  University of Missouri
  Columbia, Missouri   65201

Solbrig, O. T.
  Harvard University
  Cambridge, Massachusetts   02138

Solomon, J.
  Washington University
  St. Louis, Missouri 63130

Sorrells, M. E.
  Cornell University
  Ithaca, New York 14850

Speisiale, A. J.
  Monsanto Agricultural
    Products Company
  St. Louis, Missouri 63166

Stalker, H. D.
  Washington University
  St. Louis, Missouri 63130

Steadman, J.
  Purdue University
  W. Lafayette, Indiana 47906

Stebbins, G. L.
  University of California
  Davis, California 85616

Storbeck, T.
  Indiana University
  Bloomington, Indiana 47401

Tal, M.
  Ben Gurion University
  Beer Sheva, Israel

Tempelton, A. R.
  Washington University
  St. Louis, Missouri 63130

Thach, R. E.
  Washington Universtiy
  St. Louis, Missouri 63130

Thomas, D. B., Jr.
  University of Missouri
  Columbia, Missouri 65201

Thorgaard, G. H.
  University of California
  Davis, California 85616

Torne, S. G.
  S.P.C. College
  Margao, Goa, India

Tseng, C. C.
  Purdue University
  W. Lafayette, Indiana 47906

Tseng, Mrs. C. C.
  Purdue University
  W. Lafayette, Indiana 47906

Tyrl, R. J.
  Oklahoma State University
  Stillwater, Oklahoma 74074

Varner, J. E.
  Washington University
  St. Louis, Missouri 63130

Victor, R.
  University of Waterloo
  Waterloo, Ontario

Vinay, P.
  Washington University
  St. Louis, Missouri 63130

Wagner, W. H., Jr.
  University of Michigan
  Ann Arbor, Michigan 48104

Wagner, F.S.
  University of Michigan
  Ann Arbor, Michigan 48104

Walbot, V.
  Washington University
  St. Louis, Missouri 63130

Walker, K. A.
  Monsanto Agricultural
    Products Company
  St. Louis, Missouri 63166

Ward, G. H.
  Knox College
  Galesburg, Illinois 61401

Wasserman, A. O.
  The City College
  New York, New York   10031

Wasserman, A. L.
  Washington University
  St. Louis, Missouri   63130

Watrud, L. S.
  Monsanto Agricultural
    Products Company
  St. Louis, Missouri   63166

Weimarck, A.
  University of Lund
  Lund, Sweden

Werth, C. R.
  Miami University
  Oxford, Ohio   45056

deWet, J. M. J.
  University of Illinois
  Urbana, Illinois   61801

Wideman, M.
  Monsanto Agricultural
    Products Company
  St. Louis, Missouri   63166

Woodland, D. W.
  McGill University
  Montreal, Quebec

Worstell, J.
  University of Missouri
  Columbia, Missouri   65201

Yao, M. C.
  Washington University
  St. Louis, Missouri   63130

Yates, W. J., Jr.
  Butler University
  Indianapolis, Indiana   46208

Yen, S. T.
  Cornell University
  Ithaca, New York   14850

York, D. W.
  Monsanto Agricultural
    Products Company
  St. Louis, Missouri   63166

Yungbluth, A.
  Western Kentucky University
  Bowling Green, Kentucky   42101

Zeven, A. C.
  Agricultural University
  Wageningen, The Netherlands

Zinger, V.
  Washington University
  St. Louis, Missouri   63130

LIST OF CONTRIBUTORS

Dr. John E. Averett
  Department of Biology
  University of Missouri-St. Louis
  St. Louis, Missouri 63121

Dr. Roger N. Beachy
  Department of Biology
  Washington University
  St. Louis, Missouri 63130

Dr. Edwin T. Bingham
  Department of Agronomy
  University of Wisconsin
  Madison, Wisconsin 53706

Dr. James P. Bogart
  Department of Zoology
  University of Guelph
  Guelph, Ontario N1G 2W1
  Canada

Mr. Bruce Carr
  Department of Biology
  Washington University
  St. Louis, Missouri 63130

Ms. Jane Casey
  Department of Biological
    Sciences
  Texas Tech University
  Lubbock, Texas 79409

Dr. Charles J. Cole
  Department of Herpetology
  American Museum
    of Natural History
  Central Park West at 79th St.
  New York, New York 10024

Dr. Marshall C. Crosby
  P.O. Box 299
  Missouri Botanical Garden
  St. Louis, Missouri 63166

Dr. Theordore Delevoryas
  Department of Botany
  University of Texas
  Austin, Texas 78712

Dr. Douglas R. Dewey
  Crops Research Laboratory, USDA
  Utah State University
  Logan, Utah 84322

Prof. Dr. Friedrich Ehrendorfer
   Botanisches Institut
   Universitat Wien
   A-1030, Wein
   Austria

Dr. Peter Goldblatt
   P.O. Box 299
   Missouri Botanical Garden
   St. Louis, Missouri 63166

Dr. Ray C. Jackson
   Department of Biological
      Sciences
   Texas Tech University
   Lubbock, Texas   79409

Dr. George B. Johnson
   Department of Biology
   Washington University
   St. Louis, Missouri   63130

Dr. Gorden Kimber
   Department of Agronomy
   University of Missouri
   Columbia, Missouri 65201

Dr. Walter H. Lewis
   Department of Biology
   Washington University
   St. Louis, Missouri 63130

Dr. Juhani Lokki
   Department of Genetics
   University of Helsinki
   SF-00100 Helsinki 10
   Finland

Dr. James Maniotis
   Department of Biology
   Washington University
   St. Louis, Missouri 63130

Dr. James A. Mears
   Department of Botany
   Academy of Natural Sciences
   19th and the Parkway
   Philadelphia,Pennsylvania 19103

Dr. H. Wayne Nichols
   Department of Biology
   Washington University
   St. Louis, Missouri 63130

Dr. Anssi Saura
   Department of Genetics
   University of Helsinki
   SF-00100 Helsinki 10
   Finland

Dr. R. Jack Schultz
   Biological Sciences Group
   University of Connecticut
   Storrs, Connecticut   06268

Dr. Ernest R. Sears
   Department of Agronomy
   University of Missouri
   Columbia, Missouri 65201

Dr. Owen J. Sexton
   Department of Biology
   Washington University
   St. Louis, Missouri   63130

Dr. Otto T. Solbrig
   Gray Herbarium
   22 Divinity Avenue
   Harvard University
   Cambridge, Massachusetts   02138

Dr. G. Ledyard Stebbins
   Department of Genetics
   University of California
   Davis, California   95616

Dr. Moshe Tal
   Department of Biology
   Ben Gurion University
      of the Negev
   Beer Sheva, Isreal

Dr. Florence S. Wagner
   Department of Botany
   University of Michigan
   Ann Arbor, Michigan   48109

Dr. W. H. Wagner, Jr.
  Department of Botany
  University of Michigan
  Ann Arbor, Michigan   48109

Dr. Virginia Walbot
  Department of Biology
  Washington University
  St. Louis, Missouri   63130

Dr. Keith A. Walker
  Monsanto Agricultural
    Products Company
  800 N. Lindbergh Blvd.
  St. Louis, Missouri   63166

Dr. J. M. J. deWet
  Department of Agronomy
  University of Illinois
  Urbana, Illinois   61801

Dr. Meng-Chao Yao
  Department of Biology
  Washington University
  St. Louis, Missouri   63130

Dr. A. C. Zeven
  Institute of Plant Breeding
  Center of Agricultural Sciences
  166 Lawickse Allee
  Wageningen
  The Netherlands

INDEX TO NAMES OF ORGANISMS[1]

Abatia 246
Abelmoschus 265
Abutilon 247,265
Acacia 265
Aclypha 265
Acanthaceae 253,262,267
Acanthus 267
Acer 266
Aceraceae 251,266
Achillea 107,135,267,509
Achlya 169,181,182,184
Achlys 109,118,263
Achyranthes 264
Acipenser 321
Acipenseridae 321
Acomastylis 265
Aconitum 243,263
Acrotrema 53
Actaea 243,263
Actinidia 264
Actinidiaceae 245,264
Actinostrobeae 218
Adansonia 265

Adesmia 265
Adenia 246,264
Adenocaulon 508,510
Adenophora 267
Adhotoda 267
Adiantum 205
Adonis 243,263
Adoxa 266
Adoxaceae 252,266
Aechmea 299
Aegilops 87,89,95,96,395,414,415, 464
Aegle 266
Aegopodium 266
Aeonium 265
Aerua 264
Aeschynanthus 267
Aesculus 251,266,390
Aethionema 264
Aframomum 230
Agamidae 343,511
Agapanthus 233
Agastachys 249

---

[1]Latin names of plants and animals excluding subgeneric, specific, and subspecific taxa, and including vernacular names of genera as appropriate. Vernacular names of broad application are found in the Subject Index.

SUBJECT INDEX

579